MW01028077

Workbook to Accompany

Thomson Delmar Learning's

COMPREHENSIVE MEDICAL ASSISTING

Administrative and Clinical Competencies

Third Edition

THOMSON
DELMAR LEARNING

Workbook to Accompany

Thomson Delmar Learning's

COMPREHENSIVE MEDICAL ASSISTING

Administrative and Clinical Competencies

3rd Edition

Prepared by
Barbara M. Dahl,
CMA, CPC

THOMSON
DELMAR LEARNING

Workbook to Accompany Thomson Delmar Learning's Comprehensive Medical Assisting: Administrative and Clinical Competencies, Third Edition
Prepared by Barbara M. Dahl

Vice President, Health Care Business Unit:
William Brottmiller

Editorial Director:
Matthew Kane

Acquisitions Editor:
Rhonda Dearborn

Developmental Editor:
Sarah Duncan

Editorial Assistant:
Debra Gorgos

Marketing Director:
Jennifer McAvey

Marketing Coordinator:
Kimberly Duffy

Technology Director:
Laurie K. Davis

Technology Project Manager:
Mary Colleen Liburdi

Technology Project Coordinator:
Carolyn Fox

Production Director:
Carolyn Miller

Production Manager:
Barbara A. Bullock

Production Editor:
Jack Pendleton

Project Editor:
Natalie Pashoukos

Printed in the United States of America
2 3 4 5 6 7 8 XXX 09 08 07 06

For more information, contact Thomson Delmar Learning, 5 Maxwell Drive, Clifton Park, NY 12065
Or find us on the World Wide Web at http://www.delmarlearning.com

ISBN 13: 978-1-4018-8125-2
ISBN 10: 1-4018-8125-4

Contents

Unit 5: Managing Facility Finances

SECTION III: CLINICAL PROCEDURES

Unit 6: Integrated Clinical Procedures

Unit 7: Assisting with Specialty Examinations and Procedures

Unit 8: Advanced Techniques and Procedures

Unit 9: Laboratory Procedures

SECTION IV: PROFESSIONAL PROCEDURES

Unit 10: Office and Human Resources Management

Unit 11: Entry into the Profession

To the Learner

This workbook is part of a dynamic learning system that will help reinforce the essential competencies you need to enter the field of medical assisting and become a successful, multiskilled medical assistant. It has been completely revised to challenge you to apply the chapter knowledge from *Thomson Delmar Learning's Comprehensive Medical Assisting: Administrative and Clinical Competencies*, *Third Edition*, to develop basic competencies, use critical thinking skills, and integrate your knowledge effectively.

WORKBOOK ORGANIZATION

The workbook chapters are divided into the following sections: Chapter Pre-Test, Performance Objectives, Vocabulary Builder, Learning Review, Certification Review, Case Study, Self-Assessment, and Chapter Post-Test. Each chapter also contains checklists for evaluation of chapter knowledge, certification criteria, and competency assessments.

The content of the workbook has been conceived to give you a creative and interpretive forum to apply the knowledge you have learned, not simply to repeat information to answer questions. Realistic simulations appear throughout the workbook referencing characters referred to in the textbook. This gives the material a real-world feel that comes as close as possible to your future experiences in an ambulatory setting. Clinical principles, such as infection control or sterilization, are repeatedly reinforced through simulation exercises that require the ability to use your knowledge effectively and readily.

CHECKLISTS

Evaluation of Chapter Knowledge sheets are incorporated at the end of each chapter to review theoretical understanding and define competency while at the same time incorporating essential interpersonal communication and professional skills. The assessment and grading of these sheets is done by self-evaluation.

Certification Criteria Checklists are provided at the end of each chapter to help you track your progress in learning the content covered on the certification examinations from AAMA and AMT. As you complete each chapter of the text and workbook, use the Certification Criteria Checklists and checklists at the end of the workbook to highlight the examination criteria covered in that chapter. The checklists correlate to each of the three examinations: CMA, RMA, CMAS.

Competency Assessment Checklists are designed to set criteria or standards that should be observed while a specific procedure is being performed. They follow the same procedural steps as listed in the textbook. As you perform each procedure, the evaluation section of this checklist can be used to judge your performance. The instructor will use this checklist to evaluate your competency in performing this skill. A master Competency Assessment Tracking Sheet is also provided for you in the front of the workbook to use as an overview of all competency assessment checklists in the workbook. This tracking sheet can serve as a table of contents for all checklists, as well as a guide to easily view your performance on the assessment checklists.

The format of the Competency Assessment Checklists is designed to provide specific conditions, standards, skill steps, and evaluation and documentation sections for essential skills necessary for an entry-level medical assistant.

MEDICAL OFFICE SIMULATION SOFTWARE

Six case studies are found in Appendix A of this workbook. They are designed to give you experience using practice management software in performing some of the tasks that medical assistants complete on a daily basis.

Medical Office Simulation Software (MOSS) is a highly interactive medical practice management software CD-ROM included with the workbook. MOSS includes eight basic components, common to most practice management software, including Patient Registration, Appointment Scheduling, Procedure Posting, Insurance Billing, Posting Payments, Patient Billing, Report Generation, and File Maintenance.

Refer to Appendix A in the workbook for setup and usage instructions to install MOSS on your computer.

FINAL THOUGHTS

- Feel certain that each procedure and concept you master is an important step toward preparing your skills and knowledge for the workplace. The textbook, student software CD, workbook, and online companion have all been coordinated to meet the core objectives. Review the performance objectives at the beginning of each chapter in the workbook before you begin to study; they are a road map that will take you to your goals.
- Remember that you are the learner, so you can take credit for your success. The instructor is an important guide on this journey, and the text, workbook, student software CD, and externships are tools, but whether or not you use the tools wisely is ultimately up to you.
- Evaluate yourself and your study habits. Take positive steps toward improving yourself, and avoid habits that could limit your success. For example, do you let family responsibilities or social opportunities interfere with your study? If so, sit down with your family and plan a schedule for study that they will support and to which you will adhere. Find a special place to study that is free from distraction.
- Because regulations vary from state to state regarding which procedures can be performed by a medical assistant, it will be important to check specific regulations in your state. A medical assistant should never perform any procedure without being aware of legal responsibilities, correct procedure, and proper authorization.

Enjoy your career in medical assisting!

Competency Assessment Tracking Sheet

Student Name: ______________________________

Procedure Number and Title	Date Assessment Completed and Competency Achieved			
	School Date/Initials	Externship Date/Initials	Externship Date/Initials	Externship Date/Initials
EXAMPLE: 22-1 Medical Asepsis Hand Washing	2/23/XX MP	3/15/XX BG	4/20/XX SD	5/1/XX JP
9-1 Control of Bleeding				
9-2 Applying an Arm Splint				
9-3 Abdominal Thrusts for a Conscious Adult				
9-4 Abdominal Thrusts for an Unconscious Adult or Child				
9-5 Abdominal Thrusts for a Conscious Child				
9-6 Back Blows and Chest Thrusts for a Conscious Infant Who Is Choking				
9-7 Back Blows and Chest Thrusts for an Unconscious Infant				
9-8 Rescue Breathing for Adults				
9-9 Rescue Breathing for Children				
9-10 Rescue Breathing for Infants				
9-11 CPR for Adults				
9-12 CPR for Children				
9-13 CPR for Infants				
11-1 Software Installation				
11-2 Hardware Installation				
12-1 Answering and Screening Incoming Calls				
12-2 Transferring a Call				
12-3 Taking a Telephone Message				
12-4 Handling Problem Calls				
12-5 Placing Outgoing Calls				
12-6 Recording a Telephone Message on an Answering Device or Voice Mail System				
13-1 Checking In Patients and Sharing Office Policies				
13-2 Cancellation Procedures				
13-3 Establishing the Appointment Matrix				
13-4 Scheduling of Inpatient and Outpatient Admissions and Procedures				
13-5 Making an Appointment on the Telephone				
14-1 Steps for Manual Filing with a Numeric System				
14-2 Steps for Manual Filing with a Subject Filing System				
14-3 Correcting a Paper Medical Record				
14-4 Correcting an Electronic Medical Record				
14-5 Establishing a Paper Medical Chart for a New Patient				

Procedure Number and Title	Date Assessment Completed and Competency Achieved			
	School Date/Initials	Externship Date/Initials	Externship Date/Initials	Externship Date/Initials
15-1 Preparing and Composing Business Correspondence Using All Components (Computerized Approach)				
15-2 Addressing Envelopes According to United States Postal Regulations				
15-3 Folding Letters for Standard Envelopes				
15-4 Creating a Mass Mailing Using Mail Merge				
15-5 Preparing Outgoing Mail According to United States Postal Regulations				
15-6 Preparing, Sending, and Receiving a Fax				
17-1 Recording/Posting Patient Charges, Payments, and Adjustments				
17-2 Balancing Day Sheets in a Manual System				
17-3 Preparing a Deposit				
17-4 Reconciling a Bank Statement				
17-5 Balancing Petty Cash				
17-6 Recording a Nonsufficient Funds Check				
18-1 Screening for Insurance				
18-2 Obtaining Referrals and Authorizations				
19-1 Current Procedural Terminology Coding				
19-2 International Classification of Diseases, 9th Revision, Clinical Modificaiton Coding				
19-3 Applying Third-Party Guidelines				
19-4 Completing a Medicare CMS-1500 Claim Form				
20-1 Explaining Fees in the First Telephone Interview				
20-2 Prepare Itemized Patient Accounts for Billing				
20-3 Post/Record Adjustments and Refunds, Including Collection Agency Payments				
21-1 Preparing Accounts Receivable Trial Balance				
22-1 Medical Asepsis Hand Wash				
22-2 Removing Contaminated Gloves				
22-3 Transmission-Based Precautions: Donning a Gown, Mask, Gloves, and Cap (Isolation Technique)				
22-4 Sanitization of Instruments				
22-5 Chemical "Cold" Sterilization of Endoscopes				
22-6 Wrapping Instruments for Sterilization in Autoclave				
22-7 Sterilization of Instruments (Autoclave)				
23-1 Taking a Medical History				
24-1 Measuring an Oral Temperature Using an Electronic Thermometer				
24-2 Measuring an Aural Temperature Using a Tympanic Thermometer				
24-3 Measuring a Rectal Temperature Using a Digital Thermometer				
24-4 Measuring an Axillary Temperature				
24-5 Measuring an Oral Temperature Using a Disposable Oral Strip Thermometer				
24-6 Measuring a Radial Pulse				
24-7 Taking an Apical Pulse				
24-8 Measuring the Respiration Rate				

Procedure Number and Title	Date Assessment Completed and Competency Achieved			
	School Date/Initials	Externship Date/Initials	Externship Date/Initials	Externship Date/Initials
24-9 Measuring Blood Pressure				
24-10 Measuring Height				
24-11 Measuring Adult Weight				
25-1 Positioning Patient in the Supine Position				
25-2 Positioning Patient in the Dorsal Recumbent Position				
25-3 Positioning Patient in the Lithotomy Position				
25-4 Positioning Patient in the Fowler's Position				
25-5 Positioning Patient in the Knee-Chest Position				
25-6 Positioning Patient in the Prone Position				
25-7 Positioning Patient in the Sims' Position				
25-8 Assisting with a Complete Physical Examination				
26-1 Assisting with Routine Prenatal Vists				
26-2 Instructing Patient in Breast Self-Examination				
26-3 Assisting with Pelvic Examination and Pap Test (Conventional and ThinPrep® Methods)				
26-4 Wet Prep/Wet Mount and Potassium Hydroxide (KOH) Prep				
26-5 Amplified DNA ProbeTec Test for Chlamydia and Gonorrhea				
27-1 Maintaining Immunization Records				
27-2 Measuring the Infant: Weight, Length, Head, and Chest Circumference				
27-3 Taking an Infant's Rectal Temperature with a Digital Thermometer				
27-4 Taking an Apical Pulse on an Infant				
27-5 Measuring Infant's Respiration Rate				
27-6 Obtaining a Urine Specimen from an Infant or Young Child				
28-1 Instructing Patient in Testicular Self-Examination				
30-1 Obtain Urine Sample for Drug Screening				
30-2 Performing a Urinary Catheterization on a Female Patient				
30-3 Performing a Urinary Catheterization on a Male Patient				
30-4 Fecal Occult Blood Test				
30-5 Performing Visual Acuity Testing Using a Snellen Chart				
30-6 Measuring Near Visual Acuity				
30-7 Performing Color Vision Test Using the Ishihara Plates				
30-8 Performing Eye Instillation				
30-9 Performing Eye Patch Dressing Application				
30-10 Performing Eye Irrigation				
30-11 Performing Audiometry				
30-12 Performing Ear Irrigation				
30-13 Performing Ear Instillation				
30-14 Assisting with Nasal Examination				
30-15 Cautery Treatment of Epistaxis				
30-16 Performing Nasal Instillation				
30-17 Administer Oxygen by Nasal Cannula for Minor Respiratory Distress				
30-18 Instructing Patient in Use of Metered Dose Nebulizer				
30-19 Spirometry Testing				

Procedure Number and Title	Date Assessment Completed and Competency Achieved			
	School Date/Initials	Externship Date/Initials	Externship Date/Initials	Externship Date/Initials
30-20 Pulse Oximetry				
30-21 Assisting with Plaster Cast Application				
30-22 Cast Removal				
30-23 Assisting the Physician during a Lumbar Puncture or Cerebrospinal Fluid Aspiration				
30-24 Assisting the Physician with a Neurologic Screening Examination				
31-1 Applying Sterile Gloves				
31-2 Setting Up and Covering a Sterile Field				
31-3 Opening Sterile Packages of Instruments and Supplies and Applying Them to a Sterile Field				
31-4 Pouring a Sterile Solution into a Cup on a Sterile Field				
31-5 Assisting with Office/Ambulatory Surgery				
31-6 Dressing Change				
31-7 Wound Irrigation				
31-8 Preparation of Patient Skin before Surgery				
31-9 Suturing of Laceration or Incision Repair				
31-10 Sebaceous Cyst Excision				
31-11 Incision and Drainage of Localized Infection				
31-12 Aspiration of Joint Fluid				
31-13 Hemorrhoid Thrombectomy				
31-14 Suture/Staple Removal				
31-15 Application of Sterile Adhesive Skin Closure Strips				
33-1 Transferring Patient from Wheelchair to Examination Table				
33-2 Transferring Patient from Examination Table to Wheelchair				
33-3 Assisting the Patient to Stand and Walk				
33-4 Care of the Falling Patient				
33-5 Assisting a Patient to Ambulate with a Walker				
33-6 Teaching the Patient to Ambulate with Crutches				
33-7 Assisting a Patient to Ambulate with a Cane				
36-1 Administration of Oral Medications				
36-2 Withdrawing Medication from a Vial				
36-3 Withdrawing Medication from an Ampule				
36-4 Administration of Subcutaneous, Intramuscular, and Intradermal Injections				
36-5 Administering a Subcutaneous Injection				
36-6 Administering an Intramuscular Injection				
36-7 Administering an Intradermal Injection of Purified Protein Derivative (PPD)				
36-8 Reconstituting a Powder Medication for Administration				
36-9 Z-Track Intramuscular Injection Technique				
37-1 Perform Single-Channel or Multichannel Electrocardiogram				
37-2 Perform Holter Monitor Application				
39-1 Using the Microscope				
40-1 Palpating a Vein for Venipuncture				
40-2 Venipuncture by Syringe				

Procedure Number and Title	Date Assessment Completed and Competency Achieved			
	School Date/Initials	Externship Date/Initials	Externship Date/Initials	Externship Date/Initials
40-3 Venipuncture by Vacuum Tube System				
40-4 Venipuncture by Butterfly Needle System				
40-5 Capillary Puncture				
40-6 Obtaining a Capillary Specimen for Transport Using a Microtainer Transport Unit				
41-1 Hemoglobin Determination (HemoCue®)				
41-2 Microhematocrit				
41-3 Erythrocyte Sedimentation Rate				
41-4 Obtaining Blood for Blood Culture				
42-1 Assessing Urine Volume, Color, and Clarity				
42-2 Using the Refractometer to Measure Specific Gravity				
42-3 Performing a Urinalysis Chemical Examination				
42-4 Preparing Slide for Microscopic Examination of Urine Sediment				
42-5 Performing a Complete Urinalysis				
42-6 Utilizing a Urine Transport System for C&S				
42-7 Instructing a Patient in the Collection of a Clean-Catch, Midstream Urine Specimen				
43-1 Procedure for Obtaining a Throat Specimen for Culture				
43-2 Wet Mount and Hanging Drop Slide Preparations				
43-3 Performing Strep Throat Testing				
44-1 Pregnancy Test				
44-2 Performing Infectious Mononucleosis Test				
44-3 Obtaining Blood Specimen for Phenylketonuria (PKU) Test				
44-4 Screening Test for PKU				
44-5 Measurement of Blood Glucose Using an Automated Analyzer				
44-6 Cholesterol Testing				
45-1 Preparing a Meeting Agenda				
45-2 Supervising a Student Practicum				
45-3 Making Travel Arrangements				
45-4 Making Travel Arrangements via the Internet				
45-5 Developing and Maintaining a Procedure Manual				
46-1 Develop and Maintain a Policy Manual				
46-2 Prepare a Job Description				
46-3 Conduct Interviews				
46-4 Orient Personnel				

Workbook to Accompany

Thomson Delmar Learning's

COMPREHENSIVE MEDICAL ASSISTING

Administrative and Clinical Competencies

Third Edition

CHAPTER 1

Complete Evaluation of Chapter Knowledge on Pg 13 - turn in.

Medical Assisting as a Profession

DW

CHAPTER PRE-TEST

Perform this test without looking at the book. This is just to see how well you have understood and can recall the information in this chapter after you have read it, but before you have completed the workbook exercises. You will not be graded on this portion (other than the grade you give yourself). Justify any "false" answers.

1. Are medical assistants licensed, registered, or certified? (circle all that apply)
2. Anyone can take the national (AAMA) medical assisting examination without going to a special program. (T or F)
3. Medical assistants are only allowed to work in the back office. (T or F)
4. Medical assistants can become office managers. (T or F)
5. Medical assistants work as medical receptionists, medical bookkeepers, medical insurance coders and billers, transcriptionists, office managers, laboratory assistants, surgery assistants, and clinical assistants. (circle all that apply)
6. Choosing to attend an accredited medical assisting program is not as important as getting trained as quickly as possible so you can get a job. (T or F)
7. Medical assistants do not have to be credentialed to work in the field. (T or F)

INTRODUCTION

Medical assisting is a fairly conservative career that requires many professional traits. Professionalism includes things such as mature work ethics, attitude, and behaviors.

Your appearance is also an important part of professionalism. When you come to work, make sure you are dressed appropriately in clean, pressed scrubs (do not forget about clean shoes!), with clean, well-kept hair, and clean, clipped, unpolished nails. Use good personal hygiene and keep your teeth in good health. Your clothes and personal appearance should look clean, fresh, and healthy. Your appearance sets the tone for the office. If you want to wear jewelry and makeup, make sure the jewelry is small and do not wear rings other than your engagement and wedding rings. Makeup should be conservative and natural looking. Wear deodorant, but not perfume.

Your work ethics should include coming to work on time and showing responsibility for performing your job well. Sometimes we forget that we are being paid for every minute of our time spent at work and our physician–employers deserve value for their money. We should stay busy at work and work hard for our employers. Your professional ethics include using proper language, treating all your patients and coworkers with respect, and being helpful and cheerful.

Other parts of professionalism include obtaining and maintaining your credentials and certificates, continuing your education, being actively involved in your professional organizations, and networking with other medical assistants. Chapter 47 of your textbook more completely covers these attributes.

Personal attributes of a medical assistant include traits such as empathy, dependability, initiative, flexibility, desire to learn, ability to communicate (written and orally), and, of course, professionalism. These attributes are covered individually in your textbook.

How we treat people—our patients, coworkers, employers, other members of the health care team, and the general public—helps us form our professional behaviors and demeanor. We need to learn to treat all people with respect, empathy, impartial behavior, tact, and diplomacy, without judgment. Remember, as a medical assistant, you are a professional.

PERFORMANCE OBJECTIVES

After successful completion of this chapter, you should be able to list and justify professional attributes and personal traits required of medical assistants. You should be able to explain the difference between accreditation, certification, receiving a certificate or diploma, and licensure, and to compare the Certified Medical Assistant (CMA) with the Registered Medical Assistant (RMA) credentials as far as educational and training requirements. You also should be familiar with the two main medical assisting program accrediting organizations, Accrediting Bureau of Health Education Schools (ABHES) and Commission on Accreditation of Allied Health Education Programs (CAAHEP). In addition, you should know how to treat people and how to act and look like a professional. Try not to look back at the introductory section of this workbook as you complete the following exercise. If necessary, reread the Introduction. *The following statements are related to your learning objectives for this chapter. Fill in the blanks with the appropriate term(s):*

To be a good medical assistant you will need to acquire many (1) ______________ traits. These traits include mature (2) __________ ____________, (3) ____________ and (4) _____________. (5) __________________ also is important. Your scrubs should be (6) ______________ and (7) ________________. Your personal appearance should be (8) _____________, (9) _______, and (10) ________________. If you wear jewelry or makeup, the jewelry should be (11) __________ and the makeup should be (12) ____________ and (13) ______________ _____________. Wear (14) ________________ but not (15) _________________________. Work ethics should include (16) ____ and showing (17) ________________________ ________________ your job well. Our physician–employers deserve (18) _____________ for their money, and we provide that by (19) ____________________ and (20) ____________________. Professional ethical behaviors include (21) ____, (22) ________________________________, and being (23) ____________________________ and (24) ________________________. As a professional medical assistant, you should obtain and maintain your (25) ____________________ and (26) ____________________ and continue your

(27) ____________. You should become actively involved in your (28) ________________ ________________ and (29) ______________________________ with other medical assistants. You should strive to obtain personal attributes such as (30) ____________________, (31) ____________________, (32) ______________________, (33) __________________, (34) __________________________, (35) __________________________, and of course, (36) ______________________. Treat all people with (37) ________, (38) ____________, (39) ________________, (40) _______________, and (41) _______________.

VOCABULARY BUILDER

Find the words below that are misspelled; circle them, and then correctly spell them in the spaces provided. Then replace the highlighted words in the following paragraph with the correct vocabulary terms from the list. (Be sure to spell them all correctly!)

acredits	complience	integrate
ambulatory care setting	credential	liscensed
attributes	disposition	licensure
associate's	empathy	litiguous
certify	facilitates	practicums
competancy	improvising	versatile

__________________ __________________ __________________

__________________ __________________

The medical assistant is a **multiskilled** (1) ________________________ health care professional who performs many clinical and administrative duties in physicians' offices and **outpatient facilities** (2) ___________________________. In today's **lawsuit-prone** (3) ________________________ society, health care consumers are demanding educated, skilled health care professionals. The American Association of Medical Assistants is a national organization that **recognizes qualifying standards for** (4) _____________________________ medical assisting education programs and **practical applications of theory** (5) ______________________; provides national **proficiency** (6) _______________________ examinations that **guarantee** (7) _________________________ the skills of medical assistants at entry-level job, earning them the **official credit** (8) _______ __________________ of CMA; and encourages continuing education. Medical assistants are educated at community, junior, and technical colleges and proprietary schools in programs that are in **agreement** (9) _______________________________ with essential guidelines and standards, and they sometimes earn **2-year** (10) ___________________________ college degrees. The medical assistant must **combine** (11) ____________________________ several **characteristics** (12) _______________________ that will enhance a professional appearance and attitude. Several of these include a warm and friendly **temperament** (13) ______________________ that **allows for easy** (14) _______________________ communication, **an insight into another's feelings or emotions** (15) ____________________________, and a talent for **performing without previous**

preparation (16) ______________________________ good solutions to unexpected situations. Medical assistants work with **legally authorized to practice** (17) ______________________________ medical and nursing professionals, who have gone through a process of **granting of licenses to practice** (18) ______________________________.

From the vocabulary list below, select the term that best fits the sentences.

accreditation	certification examination	competency
CMA	credentialed	diploma
license	RMA	

Medical Assisting Programs undergo (1) ______________ processes that prove they are covering the right curriculum and properly serving the education/training needs of their students. Included in this process is proof that each required (2) ___________ has been assessed.

When you graduate from your medical assisting program, you will be given a (3) ______________ (sometimes called a certificate), which proves that you have taken all the courses necessary to graduate from the program.

After taking and passing a national (4) __________________ examination offered by either AAMA or AMT, you will be (5) _____________ as either an (6) _______ or a (7) __________.

None of the above documents or processes should be confused with having a (8) ___________, which requires a state-mandated scope of practice.

Word Game

Find the words in the grid below. They may go in any direction. The first four lines of unused letters contain a hidden message.

B	L	E	C	O	M	E	C	E	R	T	I	F	I	E	D	Z	B	E	C	G	O
M	I	P	I	H	S	N	R	E	T	X	E	E	I	N	L	I	C	E	N	S	E
V	T	O	L	V	E	D	Q	Y	C	N	E	T	E	P	M	O	C	I	C	O	S
N	I	T	C	I	N	I	U	E	E	L	E	A	R	N	I	N	T	G	S	Z	I
B	G	C	L	E	E	T	N	Z	M	Z	W	Q	M	Z	K	T	K	H	C	P	V
M	I	D	H	J	R	C	L	T	R	P	Y	V	M	T	E	K	D	L	O	R	O
N	O	L	T	X	X	T	N	G	E	R	A	F	Q	S	A	R	M	R	P	O	R
O	U	D	V	N	K	L	I	A	G	G	A	T	E	B	R	M	D	N	E	F	P
I	S	W	Z	G	N	C	L	F	I	C	R	R	H	J	R	E	O	Q	O	E	M
T	P	J	R	W	M	F	X	J	I	L	A	A	G	Y	L	R	D	L	F	S	I
A	R	J	K	A	M	K	B	L	P	C	P	X	T	A	F	W	D	D	P	S	L
T	R	L	Y	X	R	J	I	I	Y	P	A	M	I	E	B	P	I	E	R	I	N
I	D	B	R	R	X	T	H	R	R	M	Z	T	O	K	R	T	S	T	A	O	D
D	T	J	V	R	A	S	O	A	Y	T	N	P	I	C	Q	M	P	A	C	N	Y
E	R	T	Q	T	N	T	C	K	P	E	W	N	C	O	C	C	O	V	T	A	V
R	F	K	E	R	A	T	T	P	D	Z	K	P	R	W	N	Z	S	I	I	L	Y
C	Z	W	E	L	I	R	V	E	F	N	D	G	F	K	L	M	I	T	C	I	F
C	Y	T	U	C	M	W	R	X	K	Q	P	N	A	D	N	Z	T	L	E	S	N
A	N	B	U	L	T	C	T	N	H	L	K	N	R	M	R	T	I	U	D	M	V
I	M	M	T	T	R	W	R	N	D	H	K	V	M	R	R	Z	O	C	J	M	R
A	M	B	Y	H	A	T	T	R	I	B	U	T	E	V	Y	D	N	Z	Q	K	Z
G	D	E	X	T	E	R	I	T	Y	Y	R	A	T	E	I	R	P	O	R	P	K

accreditation
ambulatory care setting
attribute
certified
CMA
competency
compliance
credentialed
cultivate
dexterity
diploma
disposition
empathy
externship
facilitate
improvise
integrate
internship
license
litigious
practicum
professionalism
proprietary
RMA
scope of practice

LEARNING REVIEW

True or False

Mark true statements with a T and false statements with an F. Then rewrite each false statement to make it true.

____ 1. Medical assistants are licensed by each state. ____________________

____ 2. All medical assisting programs are accredited by either CAAHEP or ABHES. ____________________

____ 3. Anyone can call themselves a medical assistant, but professional medical assistants have graduated from an accredited program and obtained a credential to prove their competency. ____________________

____ 4. If you graduate from a medical assisting program and get a diploma or certificate, then you are automatically credentialed. ____________________

____ 5. Medical assistants continue their education by attending seminars, workshops, and professional meetings. ____________________

____ 6. Both RMAs and CMAs are required to obtain continuing education units (CEUs) to recertify. ____________________

____ 7. Medical assistants must be either a CMA or an RMA to join the AAMA or the AMT. ____________________

____ 8. The AAMA "owns" the CMA credential, and no person may call themselves a CMA unless they have passed the national AAMA Certification Examination. ____________________

Matching

A. externship
B. scope of practice
C. mandatory
D. voluntary
E. continuing education units

1. Recertification as a CMA may be obtained by either retaking the examination or obtaining ____.
2. Going into a medical setting to practice skills while still a student is called ____.
3. A description of a health care professional's job and legal boundaries is called a ____.
4. Certification and registration as a CMA/RMA is still ____.
5. Licensure is ____ for many professions.

Fill in the Blanks

Medical assistants learn a variety of clinical, administrative, and general skills in their courses. Write a C next to each clinical course, an A next to each administrative course, and a G next to each general course.

1. Medical Records ____
2. Therapeutic Relations ____
3. Medical Law & Ethics ____
4. Medical Computers ____

5. Pathology C
6. Transcription A
7. Coding and Insurance A
8. Receptioning A
9. Ambulatory Surgery C
10. Anatomy and Physiology G
11. Pharmacology A
12. Laboratory Procedures C
13. Terminology A
14. Taking Vital Signs C

15. Write the name, address, phone number, and Web site address for the AAMA. 20 N. Wacker Dr., Suite 1575, Chicago, IL 60606-2963, 1800-228-2262 www.AAMA-ntl.org

16. Write the name, address, phone number, and Web site address for the AMT. 1800-275-1268 AMT, 710 Higgins Rd Park Ridge, IL 60068, www.amt1.com

17. Name the nine personal attributes of a professional medical assistant. Then, for each attribute, write a sentence that describes how possessing it contributes to better patient care and good relationships with coworkers and employers.

(1) ______________________________

(2) ______________________________

(3) ______________________________

(4) ______________________________

(5) ______________________________

(6) ______________________________

(7) ______________________________

(8) ____

____

____

(9) ____

____

____

18. Name four reasons why the medical assisting profession has grown to require more formal, skilled education and credentialing for medical assistants.

    (1) ____

    ____

    (2) ____

    ____

    (3) ____

    ____

    (4) ____

    ____

19. The U. S. Department of Labor, Bureau of Statistics, lists medical assisting as the fastest growing allied health profession. Name eight settings where medical assistants are usually employed.

    (1) hospitals (5) insurance companies
    (2) doc's offices (6) clinics
    (3) medical labs (7) pharmaceutical companies
    (4) optometrists (8) podiatrists

Choose the Correct Answer

1. *Circle the two correct responses.* Medical assistants must recertify their credential every five years. The two ways to recertify for the CMA credential are:

   a. Accumulate approved continuing education hours.

   b. Obtain a good recommendation from a physician–employer.

   c. Become licensed.

   d. Retake the certification examination.

2. *Circle the two correct responses.* The Role Delineation Components is a list of competencies compiled by practicing medical assistants. These competencies are used by medical assisting program directors to develop curricula that ensure:

   a. certification

   b. employment preparedness

   c. continuing education

   d. high-quality medical assisting education

3. A system of values that each individual has that determines perceptions of right and wrong is called:
   a. laws
   b. ethics
   c. attributes
   d. attitudes

4. Stepping into a patient's place, discovering what the patient is experiencing, then recognizing and identifying with those feelings is:
   a. sympathy
   b. association
   c. flexibility
   d. empathy

5. Recertification of the CMA credential must be undertaken every:
   a. year
   b. six months
   c. seven years
   d. five years

6. Courses in a professional medical assisting program include a complement of general knowledge classes such as anatomy and physiology and:
   a. assisting with minor surgery
   b. CPR
   c. medical terminology
   d. computer applications

7. The type of regulation for health care providers that is legislated by each state and is mandatory to practice is:
   a. licensure
   b. registration
   c. certification
   d. a and c

CERTIFICATION REVIEW

The following questions are designed to mimic the certification examinations. You can use these questions like a small "Certification Examination Study Guide," but this is not meant to take the place of the more extensive study guides. Use this section to determine where to concentrate your efforts when studying for the certification examination.

1. Medical assistants may take the AAMA examination to obtain which credential?
   a. CMAS
   b. RMA
   c. CMA
   d. CPC
   e. AMT

2. Select the following statement that best describes the professional medical assistant.
   a. has good written and oral communication skills
   b. looks and acts professional at all times
   c. is aware of her or his scope of practice and stays within her or his legal boundaries
   d. assists the physician in all areas of the ambulatory care setting
   e. all of the above

3. Good medical assistants portray their professional attitude by:
   a. discussing their personal lives at work because it is therapeutic for them
   b. gossiping with their coworkers to help them with their problems
   c. reminding their physicians that they only work 7.5 hours per day
   d. helping patients in a friendly and empathetic manner
   e. being too busy to do more than the basic workload

4. To become involved with their professional organization, medical assistants could:
   a. attend local chapter or state meetings
   b. attend a national conference or state convention
   c. join their national organization
   d. offer to serve on a local, state, or national committee
   e. all of the above

CASE STUDIES

Case 1

During your course of studies to become a medical assistant, you volunteer to help out at a multi-doctor urgent care center in the center of a large city to gain some firsthand experience in a professional setting.

Discuss the following issues:

1. What about this opportunity is interesting to you to the extent that you want to volunteer in a professional setting?
2. Even though you are a volunteer, why is it important to look and behave like a professional? What does this entail?
3. You ask the CMA if you can be allowed to watch the performance of some basic clinical procedures. The CMA must get permission from the center's office manager and physician and obtain the consent of the patient. Why are these permissions necessary? How are patients' rights affected by your request?
4. After volunteering at the urgent care center for a period of time, you decide to try volunteering in another setting to get a new experience. How are your personal interests and goals important in choosing the right setting? Why are different personal qualities and ambitions needed in each setting; for example, how does a hospital setting differ from a medical laboratory?

Case 2

You are scheduled to go for your yearly complete physical examination. You decide to use this as an opportunity to study an ambulatory care setting.

Consider the following:

1. How is a patient's first impression of the physician's office and staff important in establishing a good relationship between the patient and the health care professionals who work there?
2. What, if anything, would you change about the experience to make it more successful from the patient's point of view?
3. Describe how the CMA at the physician's office interacted with patients. How did the CMA interact with the other health care professionals there? What kind of duties did the CMA perform?

Case 3

Michelle Lucas is preparing for externship. Michelle is an excellent student, detail oriented, responsible, and professional in her dress and attitude. Michelle is eager to do her externship with a large general practice or clinic with open hours built into the schedule for emergency patients, such as Inner City Health Care. Michelle is intrigued by the idea of working with a group of physicians and a diverse patient population where she can really work on improving her triage skills. Michelle, however, is shy and quiet; she has difficulty meeting new people and relies on a core group of friends.

Discuss the following:

1. Is Michelle really suited to externship at Inner City Health Care? What are the potential advantages or disadvantages of this externship placement?
2. Consider your own short- and long-range goals. How important is it to challenge yourself, personally and professionally, with experiences that contribute to your growth and knowledge? How can you use your externship placement to work toward fulfilling your goals?

SELF-ASSESSMENT

1. As you begin your education as a medical assistant, you may not be sure whether you want to work in the administrative and clerical area or in the clinical and laboratory areas. What are some ways for you to explore the various options?

2. For each of the personal attributes used in your textbook to describe a professional, identify individuals from your family, friends, work, or community who possess one or more of those traits. Explain why you chose them.

3. Imagine your first day in your externship. What will you wear? How will you prepare the night before? Would you change anything about your hairstyle? Makeup? Jewelry?

CHAPTER POST-TEST

This test is similar to the Pre-Test. Perform this test without looking at the book. This is just to see how well you have understood and can recall the information presented in this chapter after you have studied it and completed the workbook exercises. You will not be graded on this portion (other than the grade you give yourself), but this is an excellent preparation for your instructor's test. You may use this Post-Test to determine what areas you need to study more. Justify any "false" answers.

1. Medical assistants may be either licensed, registered, or certified. (T or F)
2. The AAMA medical assisting certification examination is available to anyone, even people who have not been formally trained. (T or F)
3. Medical assistants only work in the clerical parts of the office. (T or F)
4. The position of Office Manager is a career option for a medical assistant. (T or F)
5. Medical assistants work as medical receptionists, medical bookkeepers, medical insurance coders and billers, transcriptionists, office managers, laboratory assistants, surgery assistants, and clinical assistants. (circle all that apply)
6. Getting trained as quickly as possible is more important than attending an accredited medical assisting program. (T or F)
7. Medical assistants may work in their field even without being credentialed. (T or F)

CHAPTER 2

Complete Evaluation of Chap knowledge on pg 23 - turn in.

Health Care Settings and the Health Care Team

CHAPTER PRE-TEST

Perform this test without looking at the book. This is just to see how well you have understood and can recall the information in this chapter after you have read it, but before you have completed the workbook exercises. You will not be graded on this portion (other than the grade you give yourself). Justify any "false" answers.

1. Doctors who work in sole proprietorships work alone and employ no other doctors. (T or F)
2. Two doctors make up a partnership, and three doctors make up a corporation. (T or F)
3. Urgent care centers are like emergency rooms and do not offer routine well-patient services. (T or F)
4. Medical assistants do not generally work in urgent care centers. (T or F)
5. Managed care may set limits on the services your doctor can provide to a patient. (T or F)
6. Physicians are licensed to practice nationally so they can move freely from state to state. (T or F)
7. Doctors of chiropractic medicine work only on the musculoskeletal systems. (T or F)
8. Acupuncturists treat pain and a variety of disorders in the gastrointestinal urogenital, gynecologic, circulatory, respiratory, neuromusculoskeletal, and many other systems. (T or F)

INTRODUCTION

The medical assistant is one member of a dynamic, growing health care industry. As medical settings evolve to meet the challenges of technology and societal needs, the medical assistant represents a vital link in the health care team and is responsible for many duties, both clinical and administrative. Students beginning a course of study to become a medical assistant can use this workbook chapter to understand the medical settings where medical assistants are employed, learn about the shift of the health care industry toward managed care, and discover the wide range of health care professionals the medical assistant comes into contact with in various medical settings.

PERFORMANCE OBJECTIVES

After successful completion of this chapter, you should be able to list four or more physician specialists, at least three alternative health care specialists, and five allied health professionals. You should understand the differences in education and training between medical assistants and nurses and the different levels of nursing. You also should be able to define health maintenance organizations (HMOs), preferred provider organizations (PPOs), independent physician associations (IPAs), and managed care plans, including their purposes, limitations, and benefits. Try not to look back at the textbook as you fill in the blanks in the following paragraphs. *The following statements are related to your learning objectives for this chapter. Fill in the blanks with the appropriate term(s):*

Originally, (1) ______________ were designed to serve patients more efficiently and effectively while cutting costs. Critics charge that patients under HMO plans are often denied many services because they are not considered (2) ______________________. Physicians have joined together to form large (3) __________________________ to control costs within their practices. Controlling costs also has caused many insurers to direct dollars away from hospitals and toward (4) ___________________ care.

The medical assistant works directly under the supervision of the physician and serves as an important link between the physician and the (5) ________________. Although nurses are educated and trained to work in (6) ______________________, extended care facilities, and inpatient settings, many do work side by side with medical assistants in the clinic setting.

Alternative therapies, which include biofeedback, hypnotherapy, aromatherapy, massage therapy, and (7) ___________________________, are widely accepted.

VOCABULARY BUILDER

Find the words below that are misspelled; circle them, and then correctly spell them in the spaces provided. Then insert the correct vocabulary terms from the list that best fit the descriptions below.

A. accupuncture
B. frindge benefits
C. health maintainance organizations (HMOs)
D. intagrative medicine
E. independent physician association (IPA)
F. managed care operations
G. prefered provider organization (PPO)
H. ambulatory care settings
I. triage
J. homeopathy

_________________ _________________ _________________

_________________ _________________

1.____ Organizations designed to provide a full range of health care services under one roof, or, more recently, through a network of participating physicians within a defined geographic area

2.____ Advantages added to the terms of employment, such as health insurance and vacation time

3.____ An independent organization of physicians, whose members agree to treat patients for an agreed-on fee

4._____ The theory that large doses of drugs that produce symptoms of a disease in healthy people will cure the symptoms when given in small amounts

5._____ This kind of medical setting includes environments such as a medical office, an urgent or primary care center, and a managed care organization

6._____ A nontraditional medical approach proving to be effective in treating drug dependency and managing pain that requires insertion of needles at specified sites of the body

7._____ Organizations in which physicians network to offer discounts to employers and other purchasers of health care

8._____ Alternative forms of health care increasingly perceived as complements to traditional health care

9._____ Determine priorities for medical action and assess patient needs

10._____ A standard of patient care that seeks to provide quality care while containing costs

LEARNING REVIEW

1. How has managed care changed medical settings as the health care profession works to offer high-quality, cost-effective care to patients? What is the medical assistant's role in contributing to the efforts of the health care team in an era of managed care?

____

____

____

____

____

____

2. For each of the three forms of medical practice management, list appropriate medical settings. Then describe the patient's experience with care under each form of medical practice management. Note how patient experiences may differ and why this is possible.

Sole Proprietorships:

A. Medical settings ____

____

B. Patient experience ____

____

____

Partnerships:

A. Medical settings ____

____

B. Patient experience ____

____

____

Corporations:

A. Medical settings ______________________________

____

B. Patient experience ______________________________

____

____

3. Name three ways in which insurers, providers, and patients are working creatively to meet the challenge of managed care to keep costs down.

(1) ______________________________

____

____

(2) ______________________________

____

____

(3) ______________________________

____

____

4. A. Name six administrative duties of the medical assistant as a member of the health care team.

(1) ______________ (4) ______________

(2) ______________ (5) ______________

(3) ______________ (6) ______________

B. Name five clinical duties of the medical assistant as a member of the health care team.

(1) ______________________________

(2) ______________________________

(3) ______________________________

(4) ______________________________

(5) ______________________________

5. A. In the medical field, the abbreviation *Dr.* is used and the title *doctor* is addressed to the person qualified by education, training, and licensure to practice medicine. List the medical degree associated with each of the following credentials, and define each specialty.

MD ______________________________

____

____

DPM ____

____

____

DC____

____

____

ND____

____

____

DO____

____

____

OD____

____

____

DDS____

____

____

B. Using a medical dictionary or encyclopedia to help you, define the following six medical and surgical specialists. Refer to your textbook for a complete listing of medical and surgical specialties.

(1) Radiation oncologist ______________________________

____

____

(2) Obstetrician/gynecologist ______________________________

____

____

(3) Neurologist______________________________

____

____

(4) Gerontologist______________________________

____

____

(5) Ophthalmologist ______________________________

____

____

(6) Pediatrician ______________________________

____

____

6. Medical assistants are only one of many allied health and other health care professionals who form the health care team. Although medical assistants may not work directly with each professional, they are likely to come into contact with many of them through telephone, written, or electronic communication. List six of those types of professionals.

(1) ______________________________
(2) ______________________________
(3) ______________________________
(4) ______________________________
(5) ______________________________
(6) ______________________________

7. In an effort to receive alternative therapies, many health care providers and patients are pursuing integrative medicine as a complement to traditional health care. Name seven alternative forms of health care that may be currently perceived to supplement traditional health care.

(1) ______________________________
(2) ______________________________
(3) ______________________________
(4) ______________________________
(5) ______________________________
(6) ______________________________
(7) ______________________________

CERTIFICATION REVIEW

These questions are designed to mimic the certification examinations. You can use these questions like a small "Certification Examination Study Guide," but this is not meant to take the place of the more extensive study guides. Use this portion to determine where to concentrate your efforts when studying for the certification examination.

1. The form of medical practice management that states that personal property cannot be attached in litigation is a:

   a. partnership
   b. sole proprietorship
   c. corporation
   d. group practice

2. The minimum amount of time it takes to become an MD without specialization is:
   a. 6 years
   b. 9 years
   c. 12 years
   d. 4 years

3. Critical care medicine and pain management may require subspecialty certificates to practice:
   a. anesthesiology
   b. family practice
   c. pathology
   d. radiology

4. The American Society of Clinical Pathology is the professional organization that oversees credentialing and education in what allied health area?
   a. nurses
   b. medical laboratory
   c. registered dietitian
   d. physical therapy

5. The specialty that treats patients using the relationship between mind, body, spirit, and nature is called:
   a. chiropractic
   b. osteopathy
   c. podiatry
   d. naturopathy

CASE STUDIES

In each of the following scenarios, consider the following: (1) How can the patients be encouraged to consider themselves as a part of the health care team? and (2) What is the role of the medical assistant?

Abigail Johnson is an older woman in her 70s with mature-onset diabetes. She is having trouble managing her diet; she lives alone but craves social contact and seems to enjoy her visits to the family physician's office.

Herb Fowler is an African-American man in his early 50s. Herb is a heavy smoker, is significantly overweight, and has a chronic cough. He believes the cough is caused by bronchitis and stubbornly insists on being prescribed antibiotics.

Juanita Hansen is a single mother in her mid-20s with one son, Henry. Juanita arrives at the urgent care clinic for the fourth time in a month. Henry has fallen twice, suffered a burn on the hand, and is now refusing to eat.

Lenore McDonell is a disabled woman in her early 30s who lives independently, with the aid of a motorized wheelchair. Lenore functions well in her home environment but has grown fearful of venturing out, even to the physician's office for her routine follow-up examinations. She has canceled three appointments in a row.

SELF-ASSESSMENT

As you were deciding to become a medical assistant, what other careers were you considering? List the three reasons you were considering that other career, and then list three reasons you chose medical assisting instead. Keep in mind not just the time, money, and education involved, but also the profession itself, the day-to-day duties, the type of work, the people involved, and so forth.

Other career:

(1) ____________________

(2) ____________________

(3) ____________________

Medical assisting:

(1) ____________________

(2) ____________________

(3) ____________________

Think about the similarities between the two careers. Are there more similarities than differences? Are you going to be using some of the same skills? Is there a way that these two different careers will come together at any point in the future?

CHAPTER POST-TEST

This test is similar to the Pre-Test. Perform this test without looking at the book. This is just to see how well you have understood and can recall the information presented in this chapter after you have studied it and completed the workbook exercises. You will not be graded on this portion (other than the grade you give yourself), but this is an excellent preparation for your instructor's test. You may use this Post-Test to determine what areas you need to study more. Justify any "false" answers.

1. Sole proprietors work alone and do not employ other doctors. (T or F)
2. Partnerships are made up of two physicians, and corporations are made up of three or more physicians. (T or F)
3. Urgent care centers are for emergencies only. (T or F)
4. Urgent care centers require skills that medical assistants do not generally have. (T or F)
5. Managed care cannot set limits on the services your doctor provides to a patient. (T or F)
6. Physicians are licensed to practice state by state. (T or F)
7. Chiropractors only work on musculoskeletal conditions. (T or F)
8. Acupuncture can be helpful when dealing with pain and a variety of disorders in the gastrointestinal, urogenital, gynecologic, circulatory, respiratory, neuromusculoskeletal, and many other systems. (T or F)

CHAPTER 3

History of Medicine

CHAPTER PRE-TEST

Perform this test without looking back at the textbook or the workbook. This is just to see how well you have understood and can recall the information in this chapter after you have read it, but before you have completed the workbook exercises. You will not be graded on this portion (other than the grade you give yourself). Justify any "false" answers.

1. The practice of medicine began when we started keeping medical records. (T or F)
2. Plants used to be the basis of all medications, but are not anymore. (T or F)
3. Cultural differences do not and should not influence the way we treat our patients. (T or F)
4. Magic has played a vital role in medicine. (T or F)
5. Ancient Eastern treatments included curing the spirit and nourishing the body. (T or F)
6. Acupuncture uses the placement of needles in thousands of points on the body. (T or F)
7. Women were not accepted as medical doctors in Western culture until the 1800s. (T or F)
8. The Father of Preventive Medicine was Louis Pasteur. (T or F)
9. Edward Jenner developed the smallpox vaccine in the late 1700s. (T or F)
10. The Oath of Hippocrates mentions mischief, sexual misconduct, and slaves. (T or F)
11. Medical assisting has only been around for a few years. (T or F)

INTRODUCTION

The medical assistant is a part of the constantly evolving history of medicine. Medicine developed from the contributions of individuals from various cultures throughout history who held many different theories and attitudes about medicine and the treatment of patients. Today, the advances made in medicine continue to be shaped by more than one discipline or philosophy of care and treatment. Students of medical assisting can use this workbook chapter to discover the rich history of medicine and to think about the medical assistant's role in the future of medicine and health care.

PERFORMANCE OBJECTIVES

After successful completion of this chapter you will be able to discuss the effects that culture, religion, magic, and science have had on modern medicine. You will be able to discuss common treatments used in the past and three theories or practices of ancient medicine that still are prevalent today. You will know the historical roles of specialists and women and be able to trace the progression of medical education. You will become familiar with several significant contributions to medicine, including three recent developments. *The following statements are related to your learning objectives for this chapter. Fill in the blanks with the appropriate term(s).*

Ancient Chinese beliefs states that there were several methods of treatment; they were to cure the (1) ______________, nourish the (2) ______________, give (3) ______________, treat the whole (4) ______________, and use (5) ______________ and (6) ______________. Many of these ancient beliefs are still excellent (7) ______________ for today's health care. Religion is still an important part of health and healing. In ancient times and in some present-day cultures, certain gods were/are called on for (8) ______________ through (9) ______________, (10) ______________, and (11) ______________. Magic was used to chase away (12) ______________. Common treatments used in the past were (13) ______________, to cause vomiting, and (14) ______________, to purge from the rectum. Women were accepted as (15) ______________ in primitive societies, and later were allowed to care for (16) ______________ and to assist in (17) ______________. They were considered unqualified to become doctors in Western cultures until the (18) ______________ century. Medical education in established universities began in the (19) ______________ century. (20) ______________ made anatomical preparations from which he produced drawings of the skeletal, muscular, nervous, and vascular systems. Sadly, his accurate sketch of the spinal vertebrae went undiscovered for more the (21) ______________ years! We are all familiar with the Father of Bacteria, (22) ______________, but have you heard of (23) ______________, who discovered x-rays? We certainly have come a long way since then. More recently, we are finding noninvasive methods of "looking" into the body and seeing great detail. The (24) ______________, (25) ______________, and (26) ______________ assist in diagnosis now. Organ and tissue transplants, easy and quick laboratory tests, vaccines, and medicines are only a few of the wonderful new (27) ______________ in medicine.

VOCABULARY BUILDER

Find the words below that are misspelled; circle them, and then correctly spell them in the spaces provided. Then insert the correct vocabulary terms from the list that best fit the descriptions below.

acupuncture	malaria	septacemia
alopathic	moxibustion	typhis
asepsis	pharmacopoeias	yellow fever
bubonic plague	pluralistic	

__________________ __________________ __________________

__________________ __________________

1. In our ________________________ society, we rely on several philosophies of medicine that serve an individual's needs by respecting ethnic, cultural, and religious traditions while providing the best standard of care to patients and their families.
2. ________________________ is an ancient Chinese technique that requires the use of a powdered plant substance that is made into a small mound on the patient's skin and then burned, usually leaving a blister.
3. The piercing of the skin by long needles into any of 365 points along 12 meridians that transverse the body and transmit an active life force called *chi* is the practice of ________________________, an ancient Chinese technique thought by many today to be effective in the treatment of chronic pain.
4. That bacteria can enter the bloodstream to cause infection, __________________, was observed in the nineteenth century by Hungarian physician and obstetrician Ignaz Philipp Semmelweis. He proved that physicians who came from an autopsy directly to the care of postpartum women, without scrubbing their hands and washing instruments, carried infection with them that often caused puerperal fever and death in new mothers.
5. In the twentieth century, the discovery of antibiotics, the development of vaccines, and the institution of proper health and sanitation measures have largely contributed to the containment of many infectious diseases, including ________________________, ____________________, and ____________________. However, new drug-resistant strains of tuberculosis, __________________, and other diseases are not responding to known treatments, presenting medical researchers with new challenges for the twenty-first century.
6. Homeopathic physicians treat illness and disease by nonsurgical methods using small doses of medicine, based on the theory that "like cures like." __________________ physicians treat illness and disease with medical and surgical interventions intended to alleviate the condition or effect a cure.
7. World cultures throughout history have compiled unique________________________: books describing drugs and their preparation that detail plant, animal, and mineral substances as essential ingredients in effecting cures.

8. In the nineteenth century, ____________________, the process of sterilizing surgical environments to discourage the growth of bacteria, and anesthesia, the process of alleviating pain during surgery, revolutionized surgical practices throughout the world.

LEARNING REVIEW

1. A. Religion, magic, and science all play a vital part in the history of medicine. Why?

Religion ____

____

____

Magic ____

____

____

Science ____

____

____

B. *For each of the following, write an* R *if belief in religion, an* M *if belief in magic, or an* S *if belief in science underlies the treatment or practice.*

____ 1. A recent research study involved two groups of patients with AIDS: one group received daily prayers from an anonymous prayer group hundreds of miles away, and the other received no prayers. The group receiving the prayers responded better to treatment.

____ 2. Trephination was used by prehistoric cultures to release evil spirits responsible for illness.

____ 3. Chinese acupuncture techniques are used to control pain or treat drug dependency.

____ 4. Botanicals are effective in treating certain conditions. The Chinese pharmacopoeia is rich in the use of herbs.

____ 5. Some Native Americans believe that someone recovering from a serious illness might hold extraordinary powers.

____ 6. Some physicians throughout history have held to the belief that healing involves not just medical treatment, but attention to the purity of the patient's soul and an attention to the faith of the individual as well.

2. Name the five methods of treatment important to the practice of medicine according to ancient Chinese tradition. How are these methods relevant for allopathic physicians today?

(1) ____

____

(2) ____

____

(3) ____

____

(4) ____

____

(5) ____

____

3. Individual cultures and people throughout history have conferred different, and often changing, status to women in medicine. For each of the five cultures below, describe the status of women in medicine.

Primitive societies ____

____

____

____

____

Chinese ____

____

____

____

____

Muslim ____

____

____

____

____

Italian ____

____

____

____

____

American ____

____

____

____

____

4. Trace the progression of medical education by listing the important advances, discoveries, or medical philosophies for each period or century listed. What do you expect for the twenty-first century?

Prehistoric times ______________________________

Ancient times ______________________________

Seventh century ______________________________

Ninth century ______________________________

Renaissance ______________________________

Nineteenth century ______________________________

Twentieth century ______________________________

Twenty-first century

5. Attitudes toward illness have changed throughout the history of medicine and also often differ between cultures. For each situation listed, give both historical and current attitudes toward the sick person. Discuss how attitudes toward illness may, or may not, have changed through history.

   A. Elderly and infirm people are encouraged to end their own lives or are outcast from society.

   B. Individuals with a frightening illness, for which there is no cure, are shunned or quarantined.

   C. Sickness is seen as a moral or spiritual failing of an individual.

   D. Survivors of illness are viewed as heroic individuals.

   E. People with disabilities are valued as individuals and receive care that allows them to function in mainstream society.

6. Name 12 infectious or epidemic diseases that have been controlled in the twentieth century through medical advances and discoveries such as antibiotics, vaccines, asepsis, and insulin.

(1) __________	(6) __________	(11) __________
(2) __________	(7) __________	(12) __________
(3) __________	(8) __________	
(4) __________	(9) __________	
(5) __________	(10) __________	

7. The Hippocratic Oath, which originated in ancient Greece, embodied within it many ethical standards of treatment and care that physicians espouse even today. List, in contemporary layperson's language, the five basic standards contained in the oath.

(1) ______________________________

(2) ______________________________

(3) ______________________________

(4) ______________________________

(5) ______________________________

8. *Match each individual with their contribution to the history of medicine. In the space following each name, fill in the century in which the individual lived.*

____ 1. Andreas Vesalius _______
____ 2. Sir Alexander Fleming _______
____ 3. W. T. G. Morton _______
____ 4. Moses _______
____ 5. Edward Jenner _______
____ 6. Clara Barton _______
____ 7. Louis Pasteur _______
____ 8. Elizabeth Blackwell _______
____ 9. Hippocrates _______
____ 10. René Laënnec _______
____ 11. Robert Koch _______
____ 12. Florence Nightingale _______
____ 13. Anton van Leeuwenhoek _______
____ 14. Wilhelm Roetgen _______
____ 15. John Hunter _______
____ 16. Elizabeth G. Anderson _______
____ 17. Leonardo da Vinci _______
____ 18. Joseph Lister _______
____ 19. Jonas Salk _______
____ 20. Frederick G. Banting _______

A. developed a vaccine for poliomyelitis
B. Father of Medicine
C. developed smallpox vaccine
D. discovered penicillin
E. Father of Bacteriology
F. advocate of health rules in Hebrew religion
G. invented the stethoscope
H. first female physician in the United States
I. rendered accurate anatomical drawings of body systems
J. wrote first anatomical studies
K. laid the groundwork on asepsis
L. started the American Red Cross
M. founder of modern nursing
N. introduced ether as anesthetic
O. discovered lens magnification
P. discovered x rays
Q. founder of scientific surgery
R. developed culture-plate method
S. discovered insulin
T. first female physician in Britain

9. The ancient culture that believed that illness was a punishment by the gods for violations of moral codes was the:
   a. Chinese
   b. Egyptian
   c. Mesopotamian
   d. Indian

10. Ancient healing priests performed many functions that involved the welfare of the entire community or village and were referred to as:
    a. shaman
    b. chi
    c. lipuria
    d. polypenia

11. Medical education in established universities began in what century?
    a. second
    b. fifteenth
    c. eighteenth
    d. ninth

12. What country today quarantines everyone who tests positive for HIV, even if they show no signs of the disease?
    a. Africa
    b. Cuba
    c. Korea
    d. Canada

13. In 1922, insulin was founded as a treatment for diabetes by:
    a. Lister
    b. Pasteur
    c. Salk and Sabin
    d. Banting and Best

CERTIFICATION REVIEW

These questions are designed to mimic the certification examinations. You can use these questions like a small "Certification Examination Study Guide," but this is not meant to take the place of the more extensive study guides. Use this portion to determine in what areas to concentrate your efforts when studying for the certification examination.

1. Who of the following was not a scientist who contributed to the study of bacteriology?
   a. Louis Pasteur
   b. Robert Koch
   c. Joseph Lister
   d. John Hunter

2. The first female physician in the United States was:
   a. Clara Barton
   b. Elizabeth Blackwell
   c. Florence Nightingale
   d. Joan of Arc

3. The Oath of Hippocrates:
   a. establishes guidelines for all health care providers
   b. establishes guidelines for the practice of medicine
   c. is a well-known document about the ethics of ancient medicine
   d. was the first scientific journal of significance

CASE STUDY

When 52-year-old Margaret Thomas, Martin Gordon's younger sister, begins to experience mild hand tremors and balance problems, Martin suggests that Margaret go see Dr. Winston Lewis, Martin's primary care physician assisting in the treatment of his prostate cancer. Feeling more comfortable with a female physician, Margaret chooses to make an appointment with Dr. Lewis's associate in the group practice, Dr. Elizabeth King. On the day of the examination, she brings her 25-year-old daughter with her to the physician's office.

After taking a detailed patient history and undertaking a thorough physical examination of Margaret Thomas, Dr. King makes note of signs and symptoms, including a resting tremor, shuffling gait, muscle rigidity, and difficulty in swallowing and speaking. Margaret also complains of a "hot feeling" and odd, uncharacteristic moments of defective judgment when "she just can't keep things straight." Dr. King suspects Parkinson's disease and tells Margaret and her daughter that she'd like to refer Margaret to a neurologist for more specific examination and medical tests. Dr. King explains that there are effective drug therapies for controlling the disease, although it has no known cure, and that the neurologist will outline Margaret's treatment options if a diagnosis of Parkinson's is made. Margaret seems to be shaken but takes Dr. King's words in stride.

Dr. King leaves Margaret and her daughter in the examination room with Audrey Jones, C.M.A., who has assisted Dr. King throughout the examination and asks Audrey to be sure to give Mrs. Thomas the referral to the neurologist. Margaret's daughter asks Audrey if Parkinson's is the disease that has shown promise in fetal tissue research, and if her mother might be a candidate. Before Audrey can answer, Margaret becomes visibly distressed. "We're a good Catholic family, I could never consider that. Me, a grandmother." Looking to Audrey, she adds, "Please tell me I won't be involved with such a thing."

Discuss the following:

1. What part does the role of women in medicine and in society play in this situation?
2. How should medical assistant Audrey Jones reply to Mrs. Thomas and her daughter? What course of action, if any, should she take?
3. How do religious beliefs make an impact on the attitude toward illness held by the patient? How might these beliefs affect a treatment plan?
4. Discuss the issues that arise when a potential medical breakthrough involves controversial or radical ideas that challenge long-held cultural viewpoints and beliefs.

SELF-ASSESSMENT

A. Make a list of the various ethnic, religious, and cultural groups you and your family members participate in or are descended from.

B. Interview family members to determine how their ethnic, religious, or cultural beliefs make an impact on the kind of medical care and treatment they expect to receive and how attitudes may have changed or evolved from generation to generation. Write a brief summary of your family's beliefs.

C. Write down any folk or home remedies used by your parents or grandparents that may or may not still be used by your family today. Why might these remedies have been more widely relied on by previous generations? Is there a scientific basis for each remedy?

CHAPTER POST-TEST

This is similar to your Pre-Test. Perform this test without looking at the book. This is just to see how well you have understood and can recall the information presented in this chapter after you have studied it and completed the workbook exercises. You will not be graded on this portion (other than the grade you give yourself), but this is an excellent preparation for your instructor's test. You may use this Post-Test to determine what areas you need to study more. Justify any "false" answers.

1. The practice of medicine began long before we started keeping medical records. (T or F)
2. Plants remain the basis of many medications. (T or F)
3. Cultural differences do and should influence the way we treat our patients. (T or F)
4. Magic has never played a vital role in medicine. (T or F)
5. Ancient Eastern treatments did not include working with the human spirit. (T or F)
6. Acupuncture uses the placement of needles in 365 points on the body. (T or F)
7. Women were accepted as medical doctors in Chinese culture long before Western cultures. (T or F)
8. The Father of Preventive Medicine was Joseph Lister. (T or F)
9. Edward Jenner developed the smallpox vaccine in the late 1800s. (T or F)

EVALUATION OF CHAPTER KNOWLEDGE

	Student Self-Evaluation		
Skills	Good	Average	Poor
I am sensitive to cultural, ethnic, and religious beliefs of others.	_____	_____	_____
I understand the importance of mutual respect in the physician–patient relationship.	_____	_____	_____
I have the ability to identify attitudes toward illness.	_____	_____	_____
I have the ability to trace major discoveries and contributions to history of medicine.	_____	_____	_____
I recognize major figures of medical history.	_____	_____	_____
I show patience and open-mindedness toward others.	_____	_____	_____
I have the ability to describe the role of the medical assistant in the future of medicine.	_____	_____	_____

CHAPTER 4

Therapeutic Communication Skills

CHAPTER PRE-TEST

Perform this test without looking at the book. This is just to see how well you have understood and can recall the information in this chapter after you have read it, but before you have completed the workbook exercises. You will not be graded on this portion (other than the grade you give yourself). Justify any "false" answers.

1. Gestures and expressions have nothing to do with what a person is thinking or feeling. (T or F)
2. You can make sick patients "feel better" just by the way you communicate with them. (T or F)
3. Everyone enjoys a hug. (T or F)
4. While speaking on the phone a patient can tell how you are feeling. (T or F)

INTRODUCTION

The word *therapeutic* basically means "to aid in health" or to "make better." Therapeutic communication implies that the interaction (verbal or nonverbal) between you, as the medical assistant, and your patients should help them heal or at least should make them feel better. And, studies show, when we feel better, we are healthier. If we extend the therapeutic communication to our coworkers, our physician–employers, and into our personal lives, we all benefit.

Now all we have to agree on is: What makes up therapeutic communication? Some people enjoy a more intimate interaction, perhaps a touch on the arm, whereas others prefer a more distant, formal interaction. Some of these preferences come from our families and how we were raised, some are cultural, and some are developed through our personal experiences. However we obtain our personal preferences on how we like to be treated, we can all probably agree that a caring, professional manner is always appreciated. The traditional Golden Rule says: "Do unto others as you would have them do unto you"; in essence, treat people how you would like to be treated. The new Golden Rule says: "Treat others as they want to be treated." To abide by the new Golden Rule, we must understand other people; that is, where they come from, their culture, their heritage, and their attitudes toward health care.

Use this workbook chapter to explore the many components of effective therapeutic communication, cultivate the ability to learn and observe, recognize and respond to messages communicated both verbally and nonverbally, consider patients' needs with empathy and impartiality, and adapt your communication to meet the receivers' abilities to understand. In personal, face-to-face communication, as well as in telephone conversations, the medical assistant's goal is to achieve a level of therapeutic communication that enhances the patient's comfort level and eases the pathway of communication between the patient and the health care team.

PERFORMANCE OBJECTIVES

After successful completion of this chapter, you should be able to explain what therapeutic means, to differentiate between verbal and nonverbal communication, and be aware of your own communication style. You should have learned how to communicate with your patients, family, coworkers, and supervisors using effective and professional communication skills. Try not to look back at the introductory section of this workbook chapter as you fill in the blanks in the following paragraph. If necessary, reread the Introduction. *The following statements are related to your learning objectives for this chapter. Fill in the blanks with the appropriate term(s):*

The word *therapeutic* basically means (1) ______________________ or to (2) ______________________. Therapeutic (3) ______________________ can be either (4) ______________ or (5) ______________________, but it should always help your patient (6) ______________________. Therapeutic communication should also encompass your (7) ______________________, (8) ______________________, and (9) ______________________. Our communication preferences come from (10) ______________________, (11) ______________________, our (12) ______________________ and even (13) ______________________. Most people prefer a (14) ______________________ and (15) ______________________ manner, though. The new Golden Rule says: (16) ______________________. To honor this method of treating people, we must understand (17)______________________, (18) ______________________, (19) ______________________, and (20) ______________________. This chapter will help you explore therapeutic communication and (21) ______________________, (22) ______________________, (23) ______________________ and (24) ______________________.

VOCABULARY BUILDER

Find the words below that are misspelled; circle them, and then correctly spell them in the spaces provided. Then insert the correct vocabulary terms from the list that best fit the descriptions below.

active listening	decode	open-ended questions
biases	encode	perseption
body language	hierarcky of needs	prejudices
buffer words	indirect statements	roadblocks to communication
closed questions	interview technigues	therapuetic communication
cluster	kinesics	
congruancy	masking	

________________ ________________ ________________

________________ ________________

1. ________________________ Communication that allows patients to feel comfortable, even when receiving difficult or unpleasant information, achieved through use of specific and well-defined professional communication skills.
2. The italicized words in the following statement are examples of: ____________________.
   "*Good afternoon, this is* Inner City Health Care. *This is* Walter Seals. How may I help you?"
3. ________________________ Adept use of these methods encourages the best communication between health care professionals and patients, equalizing the relationship as much as possible.
4. ________________________ The specific order or rank within which a person's needs are met, moving from the most basic needs to self-actualization.
5. ________________________ These types of questions require only a yes or no answer: "Mrs. Leonard, are you feeling dizzy now?"
6. ________________________ These potential verbal or nonverbal messages that prevent a successful cycle of communication can be overcome by the medical assistant's sensitivity to patients' personalities and needs.
7. ________________________ The study of body language explores methods of nonverbal communication that accompany speech.
8. ________________________ These statements turn a question into a topic of interest that allows the patient to speak without feeling directly questioned: "Mr. Taylor, tell me about any difficulties your father's dementia presents with daily living activities at home."
9. ________________________ As Marilyn Johnson takes his family history for the patient record, Jim Marshall says repeatedly, "I am worried because my father died from a heart attack at a young age." Marilyn uses this kind of therapeutic communication to rephrase the message by responding, "You are concerned about your cardiovascular health and your genetic risk?"

10. ______________________ These personal preferences denote a predisposition for one particular belief or viewpoint over another.
11. ______________________ These beliefs or viewpoints represent preconceived notions an individual may have formed before all the facts are known.
12. ______________________ John O'Keefe sat with a sullen expression, eyes downcast, his arms folded across his chest, as he spoke to medical assistant Joe Guerrero about the financial hardships his family would face if his wife, Mary, were pregnant again. Joe relies on Mr. O'Keefe's nonverbal communication to convey his repressed feelings of anger.
13. ______________________ These types of questions require more than a yes or no answer: "Ms. Johnson, how are you doing with the special diet Dr. Lewis suggested?"
14. ______________________ This attempt to hide from or repress obscures one's true feelings or real message.
15. ______________________ Nonverbal messages grouped together to form, in aggregate, a statement or conclusion.
16. ______________________ Medical assistant Karen Ritter nods her head yes as she explains to Annette Samuels that insurance will cover any medical tests related to her stomach cramps. Karen's nonverbal message agrees with her verbal message.
17. ______________________ The receiver must interpret the meaning of the message to understand it.
18. ______________________ The sender creates a message carefully crafted to match the receiver's ability to receive and interpret it properly.
19. ______________________ This kind of intuitive realization involves an active understanding of one's own feelings *and* the feelings of others.

Crossword Puzzle

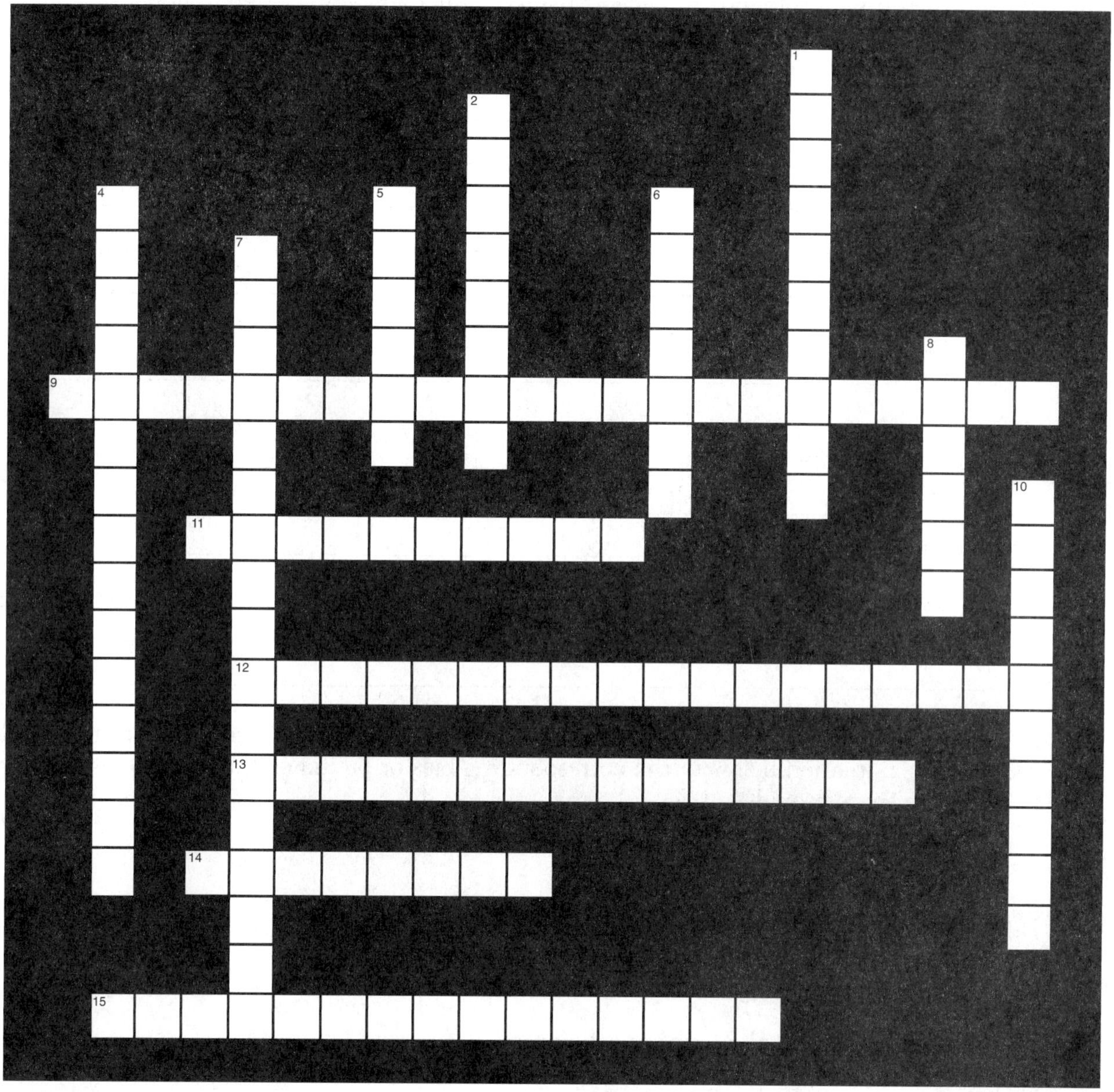

Across

9. Gestures and expressions together with body poses
11. Moving back to a former stage to escape conflict
12. Involves sending and receiving messages, verbal and nonverbal
13. The art of really hearing another person's message and sometimes verifying with them what you are hearing
14. The study of body movements
15. Questions that can be answered with a simple yes or no

Down

1. An opinion or judgement that is formed before all the facts are known
2. Giving the speaker information about what you are hearing
4. The act of justification, usually illogically, that people use to keep from facing the truth
5. The rejection or refusal to acknowledge information
6. The position of the body and parts of the body
7. Behavior that protects people from feelings of guilt, anxiety, and shame
8. A slant toward a particular belief
10. Sometimes referred to as temporary amnesia

LEARNING REVIEW

1. Culture presents a profound influence on successful therapeutic communication. For the seven cultural influences that follow, list one way in which each of them makes an impact on therapeutic communication.

   Ethnic heritage ______________________________

   ____

   Geographic location and background ______________________________

   ____

   Genetics ______________________________

   ____

   Economics ______________________________

   ____

   Educational experiences ______________________________

   ____

   Life experiences ______________________________

   ____

   Personal value systems ______________________________

   ____

2. Biases and prejudices common in today's society have the potential to create hostility. Match each difficult situation below to the corresponding bias or prejudice that motivates it. Put a letter in the space provided.

   A. A preference for Western-style medicine.

   B. The tendency to choose female rather than male physicians.

   C. Prejudice related to a person's sexual preference.

   D. Discrimination based on race or religion.

   E. Hostile attitudes toward persons with a value system opposite your own.

   F. A belief that persons who cannot afford health care should receive less care than someone who can pay for full services.

   ____ 1. Mr. Gordon refuses to accept a referral to an acupuncturist to help alleviate the chronic pain of advancing prostate cancer.

   ____ 2. Medical assistant Bruce Goldman mistakenly assumes that patient Bill Schwartz has AIDS when he arrives at the clinic with a gentleman friend, seeking attention for a recurring black mole on this calf.

   ____ 3. Rhoda and Lee Au fear they will not receive adequate medical care because they use Chinese as their first language and speak only broken English.

____ 4. Corey Boyer resists his gym teacher's efforts to get him to the clinic to check out a recurring rash on his arm because his family has no health insurance.

____ 5. Mary O'Keefe is relieved to find that the practice's OB/GYN is a female physician, Dr. Elizabeth King.

____ 6. Edith Leonard, a widow in her 70s, counsels medical assistant Liz Corbin that she should settle down and get married instead of pursuing a dream to attend medical school and become a pediatrician.

3. The four modes of communication most pertinent in our everyday exchange are:

(1) ______________________ (3) ______________________

(2) ______________________ (4) ______________________

4. Active listening is an important element of therapeutic communication. To practice active listening skills, rephrase each of the messages listed for verification from the sender; also include a therapeutic response.

A. "I don't know what to do. My father takes so many pills he can't remember which is the right one, so he ends up refusing to take any of them."

____

____

____

B. "I can't give you my insurance card; I lost it, and I don't remember the name of the company either. But you've always taken care of it before."

____

____

____

C. "I can't help being worried. The doctor just suggested a referral for treatment at that hospital where somebody had their wrong foot operated on. What do you think?"

____

____

____

D. "I feel dizzy just thinking about having my blood taken. Do you really need to do it?"

____

____

5. *Circle the five correct responses.*

The five Cs of communication are:

clear	complete	courteous
coherent	concise	credible
cohesive	constant	curious
comment	cooperative	curt

6. Abraham Maslow, the founder of humanistic psychology, postulated that a person's needs move from the most basic of survival to the state of self-actualization. Self-actualization occurs when the person realizes the maximum of human potential. Each level of need must be met before an individual can proceed successfully to the next level. Understanding Maslow's hierarchy will help medical assistants assess patients' needs and facilitate therapeutic communication. For each level, list a minimum of three needs that meet it.

   Survival or physiological needs ______________________________

   ____

   ____

   Safety needs ______________________________

   ____

   Belongingness and love needs ______________________________

   ____

   ____

   Prestige and esteem needs ______________________________

   ____

   ____

7. Identify eight significant roadblocks to communication.

   (1) ____________________ (5) ____________________
   (2) ____________________ (6) ____________________
   (3) ____________________ (7) ____________________
   (4) ____________________ (8) ____________________

8. Edith Leonard arrives at the clinic for a routine 6-month follow-up examination. At her last visit, she had been referred to an ophthalmologist for removal of a cataract in her right eye. Compose a closed question, open-ended question, and indirect statement regarding Ms. Leonard's condition.

   Closed question ______________________________

   ____

   Open-ended question ______________________________

   ____

   Indirect statement ______________________________

   ____

9. Telephone communication between medical assistants and patients is an important kind of therapeutic communication. Tone and pace of voice, together with word choice, carry the message when there is no visual feedback. List four tools of communication essential to conducting successful telephone conversations.

   (1) ______________________________
   ____

   (2) ______________________________
   ____

   (3) ______________________________
   ____

   (4) ______________________________
   ____

10. The conscious awareness of one's own feelings and the feelings of others is:
    a. congruency
    b. perception
    c. bias
    d. masking

11. The founder of humanistic psychology is:
    a. Jacobi
    b. Freud
    c. Erikson
    d. Maslow

12. The lifeline of the physician's office is:
    a. the facsimile machine
    b. telecommunication conferencing
    c. the telephone
    d. e-mail

13. The grouping of nonverbal messages into statements or conclusions is known as:
    a. assimilating
    b. feedback
    c. clustering
    d. introjection

CERTIFICATION REVIEW

These questions are designed to mimic the certification examinations. You can use these questions like a small "Certification Examination Study Guide," but this is not meant to take the place of the more extensive study guides. Use this portion to determine where to concentrate your efforts when studying for the certification examination.

1. Which of the following is not part of communication?
   a. speech
   b. facial expression
   c. gestures
   d. attitude
   e. body positioning

2. Which is the most basic of Maslow's hierarchy of needs?
   a. food
   b. safety
   c. status and self-esteem
   d. need for knowledge
   e. self-actualization

3. Your patient refuses to accept a diagnosis, claiming the doctor "must be mistaken." Assuming the doctor is correct, which self-defense mechanism is the patient using?
   a. repression
   b. denial
   c. projection
   d. compensation
   e. rationalization

4. Congruency in communication can be described as:
   a. when the verbal message matches the facial expression
   b. when the verbal message does not match the gestures
   c. when the verbal message can be interpreted in two or more different ways
   d. when two different messages are interpreted as the same

CASE STUDY

Wayne Elder arrives at the clinic for an examination to check on a recurrent ear infection that has been treated with antibiotics. Wayne, who is slightly retarded and lives in a group home, is still reporting dizziness and pain in his ear. He has come to the clinic by himself, taking a bus from his job as a part-time dishwasher. Wayne's boss asked him to return to the clinic because Wayne could not concentrate at work.

Clinical medical assistant Wanda Slawson discovers from Wayne that he has not been taking his medication properly; he stopped taking pills once his ear began to feel better. She must politely ask Wayne to repeat himself several times before she can clearly understand his slurred speech, and she has difficulty holding his attention or maintaining eye contact.

Wanda conveys Wayne's situation to Dr. Ray Reynolds, who examines Wayne and gives him a new prescription for antibiotics, gently explaining the need to finish the entire prescription to get well. After Dr. Reynolds leaves the examination room, however, it is clear to Wanda that Wayne is still confused about why he must take the medication even after he begins to feel better. Wanda carefully explains to Wayne that the infection will continue to heal even though he no longer feels sick. To be sure he understands, Wanda asks Wayne to repeat to her what he must do and why; she then asks Dr. Reynolds to step in briefly to remind Wayne once more to complete the prescription.

Discuss the following issues:

1. How does the unequal relationship that exists between patients and health care professionals have an impact on the therapeutic communication between physician, medical assistant, and patient?
2. How must medical assistant Wanda Slawson tailor her verbal and nonverbal messages to meet the abilities of her receivers: the physician (Dr. Ray Reynolds) and the patient (Wayne Elder)?
3. How does Wanda use active listening? Which interview techniques are the most effective in facilitating therapeutic communication? Does nonverbal communication play a role?
4. Using Maslow's hierarchy of needs, discuss how the health care team meets Wayne's special needs resulting from his disability.
5. Do you think the medical assistant acted appropriately? What else could she have done? What should she not do in this situation?

SELF-ASSESSMENT

Think about your own facial expressions and body language. Are you always portraying the message you want to send? List two situations in which you have been misinterpreted through your nonverbal communication, or situations in which you have misinterpreted someone else's message. Then think of what would have been a verbal message to help make the situation more accurate. That is, explain what you could have said to the person to determine if he or she was really hearing the message you meant to send.

(1) ____

____

____

(2) ____

____

____

CHAPTER POST-TEST

This is similar to the Pre-Test. Perform this test without looking at the book. This is just to see how well you have understood and can recall the information presented in this chapter after you have studied it and completed the workbook exercises. You will not be graded on this portion (other than the grade you give yourself), but this is an excellent preparation for your instructor's test. You may use this Post-Test to determine what areas you need to study more. Justify any "false" answers.

1. Gestures and expressions can always tell you what a person is thinking or feeling. (T or F)
2. You can make a sick patient "feel worse" just by the way you communicate with them. (T or F)
3. Hugs are universally acceptable as a means of communicating. (T or F)
4. While speaking on the phone you can tell how a patient is feeling. (T or F)

CERTIFICATION CRITERIA CHECKLIST

As you go through your education and training, keep in mind the national certification examination that you will take when you graduate. Each chapter of the textbook and workbook covers a different section of the examination criteria. To keep track of your preparation for the certification examination, turn to the back of this workbook and highlight the following CMA, RMA, or CMAS certification examination criteria (if you have already highlighted them from a previous chapter, put a check mark by the criteria):

CMA

C. Psychology
   1. Basic principles
   3. Hereditary, cultural and environmental influences on behavior
   4. Defense mechanisms

E. Communication
   2. Recognizing and responding to verbal and nonverbal communication
   4. Professional communication and behavior
      a. Professional situations
      b. Therapeutic relationships
   5. Evaluating and understanding communication

RMA

I. General Medical Assisting Knowledge
   E. Human Relations
      1. Patient relations
      2. Interpersonal relations

CMAS

1. Medical Assisting Foundation
   - Professionalism
3. Medical Office Clerical Assisting
   - Communication

COMPETENCY ASSESSMENT

Procedure 4-1 Identifying Community Resources

Performance Objectives: To have a list of community resources available for patient use. Perform this objective within 30 minutes with a minimum score of 20 points.

Supplies/Equipment: Computer and printer, multiple resources from a variety of community services.

Charting/Documentation: Enter appropriate documentation/charting in the box.

____

____

____

____

Instructor's/Evaluator's Comments and Suggestions:

____

____

____

____

____

____

SKILLS CHECKLIST Procedure 4-1: Identifying Community Resources

Name ______________________

Date ______________________

No.	Skill	Check #1 20 pts ea	Check #2 10 pts ea	Check #3 5 pts ea	Notes
1	Determine the type of information to be in your data base.				
2	Contact the sources and request any listings they may have.				
3	Search the Internet to obtain the desired resources.				
4	Develop a database on your computer so you can search easily for the resource when needed. Maintain a notebook with the resource information printed and indexed.				
Student's Total Points					
Points Possible					
Final Score (Student's Total Points / Possible Points)					

	Notes
Start time:	
End time:	
Total time:	

EVALUATION OF CHAPTER KNOWLEDGE

	Student Self-Evaluation		
Skills	Good	Average	Poor
I can identify my personal communication strengths.	_____	_____	_____
I can indentify areas for improvement in my personal communication style.	_____	_____	_____
I listen well.	_____	_____	_____
I cultivate sharp observation skills.	_____	_____	_____
I recognize and respond to verbal and nonverbal communication.	_____	_____	_____
I understand the communication cycle.	_____	_____	_____
I can adapt my communication to individuals' abilities to understand.	_____	_____	_____
I consider patients' needs with empathy and impartiality.	_____	_____	_____
I have the ability to identify roadblocks to communication and defense mechanisms.	_____	_____	_____
I know how to use proper telephone technique.	_____	_____	_____
I practice successful therapeutic communication.	_____	_____	_____

CHAPTER 5

Coping Skills for the Medical Assistant

Complete Self Assesment on pg 59-60 to be handed in.

CHAPTER PRE-TEST

Perform this test without looking at the book. This is just to see how well you have understood and can recall the information in this chapter after you have read it, but before you have completed the workbook exercises. You will not be graded on this portion (other than the grade you give yourself). Justify any "false" answers.

1. Stress is always something bad. (T or F)
2. Stress is something we cannot prevent. (T or F)
3. If you have a lot of responsibility in your job, you cannot avoid burnout. (T or F)
4. Setting goals helps relieve stress (T or F)

INTRODUCTION

Medical assistants and other health care professionals occasionally feel the stress of working in the demanding and challenging field of medicine and health care. Health care professionals must maintain a high level of skill and proficiency and possess knowledge about new technologies and medical advances. Whether juggling a full patient schedule, facing difficult—and sometimes life-or-death—situations with patients, or balancing administrative duties with a constant flow of paperwork, medical assistants take part in every phase of patient care. Students learning about medical assisting can use this workbook chapter to learn about handling stress in the workplace environment of the ambulatory care setting; discover how the body adapts to stress and how to use techniques for coping with stress and avoiding burnout; and consider possible short- and long-range career goals that can act as a centering and motivating influence, further reducing stress and increasing confidence.

PERFORMANCE OBJECTIVES

After successful completion of this chapter you will understand what stress is and how you can control your personal reactions to stressors. You will recognize the stages leading up to burnout and how to avoid burnout. You will also be able to set goals, both short and long range, at work and in your personal life. Try not to look back at the textbook as you fill in the blanks in the following paragraph. If necessary, reread the textbook chapter. *The following statements are related to your learning objectives for this chapter. Fill in the blanks with the appropriate term(s):*

Medical assistants are likely to feel the (1) ______________ of stress from time to time, even in the most (2) __________ ______________ ambulatory care settings. We need to learn how to (3) ____________ stress and handle (4) ________________ in both our everyday personal lives and in our (5) ____________. One of the ways to decrease stress is to recognize our personal (6) __________ so that we can gain control over our reactions to them. Another way to gain control is to set (7) ___________, both (8) ___________ range and (9) _________ range. The research shows that if we don't have control over our lives, (10) ____________________ _________ ________________. Stress and frustration can lead to (11) _____________. The four stages leading to this damaging state are: (12) _______________, (13) _______________, (14) ______________, and (15) ________________. If we learn to (16) ______________ these stages, we can regain (17) _______________ over our situations and take steps to make (18) ____________________.

VOCABULARY BUILDER

Find the words below that are misspelled; circle them, and then correctly spell them in the spaces provided. Then insert the correct letter of the vocabulary terms from the list that best fits the descriptions below.

A. burnout	D. long-range goals	G. short-range goals
B. goal	E. outer-directed people	H. stress
C. inter-directed people	F. self-actuazation	I. stressers

_________________ _________________ _________________

1. ____ James Whitney is a physician at Inner City Health Care. He hopes to go into private practice after gaining a few more years' experience at the urgent care center where he now works. James eventually would like to practice family medicine.

2. ____ Mark Woo, another physician at Inner City Health Care, prefers emergency medicine and often pulls double shifts working with emergency patients. Although he loves the work, Mark is experiencing chronic fatigue, frequently becomes angry at coworkers, and is prone to sudden and explosive displays of emotion.

3. ____ Ellen Armstrong, CMA, is usually a calming influence in the offices of Drs. Lewis and King. Lately, however, it seems to Ellen that circumstances beyond her control are threatening to pull her down. An influx of new patients into the group practice has Ellen continually backed up with filing and paperwork, her steady baby-sitter announced she'll be unavailable for the summer months, and today her car broke down on the way to work.

4.____ When Dr. Mark Woo tells emergency patient Annette Samuels that her severe stomach cramps may be caused by problems with her ovaries or appendix, she begins to feel panicky. Annette's blood pressure goes up, her breathing becomes rapid as her pulse quickens, and her eyes grow wide.

5.____ Audrey Jones, CMA, enrolls at a local college for a night-school biology class as a first step toward her goal of obtaining a bachelor's degree.

6.____ Dr. Elizabeth King, now in her mid-30s, always knew what she wanted to do with her life. After graduating from Kansas University and Stanford University Medical School, Beth searched for a physician with whom to begin a group practice and found the perfect partner in Winston Lewis.

7.____ Marilyn Johnson, CMA, office manager at the offices of Lewis and King, MD, enjoys her work and her life. Her children are grown and successful. With a master's degree in education, Marilyn teaches part-time at a local community college and is active in her town's music and art circles. She is a past president of the local chapter of the AAMA. Marilyn has worked hard to achieve the full potential of her abilities and talents and is now reaping the benefits of effort well spent.

8.____ Maria Jover takes what life gives her, deeply believing that she has no power to change her circumstances or take charge of her life. Now, Dr. King says her chronic fatigue and gynecology problems may be symptoms of AIDS, contracted from a blood transfusion she received after a severe car accident that happened several years ago. "This horrible disease will take over my life," Maria tells Dr. King.

9.____ Leo McKay is an elderly Irish Catholic man who has been laid off from his manufacturing job of 20 years. Leo asks easygoing Bruce Goldman, CMA, as he prepares Leo for a routine physical examination, "Do you have something you're working toward, some ambition for yourself—big or small?"

Word Search

Find the words in the grid below. They may go in any direction. When you are finished, the first few unused letters will form a hidden message.

T	A	K	E	C	A	R	E	O	F	Y	O	U	R	N	S	E	L	E	F
S	R	O	S	S	E	R	T	S	X	K	L	E	G	O	J	D	M	L	Y
L	L	J	C	K	L	K	K	C	Y	F	L	G	M	I	E	X	R	P	T
T	R	T	F	O	L	F	J	R	G	O	P	W	J	T	X	D	R	O	B
K	H	T	P	H	P	S	G	M	R	T	X	E	Z	A	H	R	S	E	H
L	W	G	R	R	T	I	X	X	Y	N	M	J	M	T	A	F	H	P	H
T	T	F	I	R	I	F	N	T	R	I	G	L	J	P	U	H	O	D	S
H	G	C	E	L	C	O	U	G	T	F	M	L	T	A	S	L	R	E	L
R	R	S	I	R	F	O	R	G	S	F	F	Z	X	D	T	B	T	T	A
M	S	R	R	L	N	R	N	I	R	K	J	K	D	A	I	M	R	C	O
N	C	B	M	R	F	I	O	U	T	L	I	Q	R	T	O	K	A	E	G
N	G	T	U	X	G	N	S	T	Q	I	X	L	L	Y	N	P	N	R	E
Y	Q	B	V	A	C	T	O	R	H	R	Z	H	L	K	Q	Z	G	I	G
T	W	J	N	D	R	Z	C	C	P	G	L	I	Z	S	M	Z	E	D	N
C	R	A	J	A	H	F	F	Z	E	R	I	Z	N	T	H	K	G	R	A
W	M	T	T	J	G	D	V	T	V	L	Q	F	T	G	B	Y	O	E	R
H	Y	I	C	O	N	T	R	O	L	T	O	T	H	N	M	R	A	N	G
Z	O	R	R	S	L	A	O	G	Q	N	T	R	C	M	P	T	L	N	N
N	Z	R	T	J	Z	K	H	N	L	C	V	K	Y	N	M	V	S	I	O
O	U	T	E	R	D	I	R	E	C	T	E	D	P	E	O	P	L	E	L

adaptation
burnout
control
coping skills
exhaustion
fight or flight
frustration
goals
inner-directed people
long-range goals
managing time
outer-directed people
prioritizing
role
role conflict
short-range goals
stress
stressors

LEARNING REVIEW

1. Han Selye's general adaptation syndrome (GAS) theory proposes that adaptation to stress occurs in four stages. Identify each stage in the order in which it is manifested and describe the physiologic changes that occur during each stage.

   (1) ____

   ____

   ____

   (2) ____

   ____

   ____

   (3) ____

   ____

   ____

   (4) ____

   ____

   ____

2. Match each of the following activities to its correct approach for coping with stress in the workplace.

   A. Plan ahead
   B. Arrive early
   C. Managing your lifestyle
   D. Laugh
   E. Music/Color/Light
   F. Breaks
   G. Work smarter, not harder

   ____ 1. Soothe and promote relaxation by softly playing a calming classical CD in the reception area.

   ____ 2. Go to the gym for an energizing yoga class twice a week after work.

   ____ 3. Keep up an ability to see the humor in life's events.

   ____ 4. Join your local chapter of the AAMA and participate in continuing education activities so you will have the CEUs you need to recertify.

   ____ 5. Keep a list of any special patient problems or needs by reviewing patient charts before formal office hours begin.

   ____ 6. Take a walk in a local park during a scheduled morning break.

   ____ 7. Learn how to practice self-motivation on tasks performed independently; feel free to contribute ideas and comments on group projects.

3. List and define the five considerations important in determining a goal.

   (1) ____

   ____

   (2) ____

   ____

(3) ____

____

(4) ____

____

(5) ____

____

4. For each consideration important in determining a goal, list a personal goal of your own that meets its particular requirements. Choose different goals for each answer; do not use the same goal twice.

(1) ____

____

(2) ____

____

(3) ____

____

(4) ____

____

(5) ____

____

5. Burnout is stress-related energy depletion that takes place in the working world. In the military world, burnout is called *battle fatigue*. Burnout occurs gradually over a period of continued stress.

Place a P *next to those items that promote burnout and an* R *next to those that reduce the risk for burnout.*

____ 1. Keep work separate from your home life.

____ 2. Have regular physical examinations.

____ 3. Work harder than anyone else in the office.

____ 4. Feel a greater need than others to do a job well for its own sake.

____ 5. Prioritize tasks and perform the most difficult ones first.

____ 6. Prefer to tackle projects yourself rather than consult a supervisor.

____ 7. Never stop until you achieve your goals, regardless of the personal cost to yourself or loved ones.

____ 8. Postpone vacation time.

____ 9. Give up unrealistic goals and expectations.

____ 10. Maintain a positive self-image and your self-esteem.

____ 11. Develop interests outside your profession.

____ 12. Procrastinate.

____ 13. Wear loose-fitting, comfortable clothes and shoes.

____ 14. Stretch or change positions. Walk around and deliver charts or laboratory specimens.

____ 15. Know your limits and be aware of your body's needs.

6. The "wear and tear" our bodies experience as we continually adjust to a changing environment is called:

   a. adaptation

   b. stress

   c. prioritizing

   d. conditioning

7. The fight-or-flight response includes all but which one of the following reactions?

   a. respirations and heart rate increases

   b. digestion is activated

   c. hormones are released into the bloodstream

   d. blood supply is increased to the muscles

8. One of the characteristics associated with burnout is when the employee does not know what is expected and how to accomplish it. This is often called:

   a. role conflict

   b. role overload

   c. role ambiguity

   d. role reversal

9. When individuals with a high need to achieve do not reach their goals, they are apt to feel:

   a. angry and frustrated

   b. tired and lonely

   c. distrustful and leery

   d. motivated and enthusiastic

10. The best way to treat burnout is to:

    a. cover it up

    b. get a prescription to help you cope

    c. prevent it

    d. encourage it

CERTIFICATION REVIEW

These questions are designed to mimic the certification examinations. You can use these questions like a small "Certification Examination Study Guide," but this is not meant to take the place of the more extensive study guides. Use this portion to determine where to concentrate your efforts when studying for the certification examination.

1. The body's response to mental or physical change is called:
   a. stress
   b. adaptation
   c. denial
   d. burnout

2. Which of the following is not part of Hans Selye's general adaptation syndrome?
   a. exhaustion
   b. alarm
   c. fear
   d. fight or flight
   e. return to normal

3. The four parts of the process leading to burnout are the Honeymoon stage, the Reality stage, the Dissatisfaction stage, and the:
   a. Sad stage
   b. Angry stage
   c. Retaliation stage
   d. Giving Up stage

CASE STUDY

Angie Esposito is a physician at Inner City Health Care. It was her dream, even as a child, to become a physician and work in an environment where she could help people and benefit the community as well. Proud of her accomplishments, she is the first woman in her family to attend college, and she got herself through medical school with scholarships and student loans. Angie works hard, often pulling double shifts. Liz Corbin, CMA, has a similar dream and is working to save money to attend medical school to become a pediatrician. Dr. Esposito does her best to encourage Liz's ambitions and has taken Liz under her wing.

Late one night, Liz assists Dr. Esposito in treating three difficult emergency patients in a row. "That's it," Angie Esposito says. "We're taking a 15-minute break. Ask Dr. Woo if he can cover for a short time." When Liz catches up with Dr. Esposito in the employee lounge, she finds Angie in frustrated tears. "These double shifts," Angie says. "I'm so tired. And the patients just keep coming. I want to help them all," she sighs and her voice trails off, "I just can't help them all..."

Discuss the following:

1. Dr. Angie Esposito is experiencing burnout. What personality traits are promoting her burnout? Identify the stressors in Angie's life.
2. Liz Corbin, CMA, sees her mentor breaking down under stress. Should Liz reevaluate her own long-range goals?
3. Discuss the importance of keeping goals in perspective.
4. What is Liz's best therapeutic response to Dr. Esposito?

SELF-ASSESSMENT

Determining how well you now handle stress will help you to identify personal strengths and weaknesses and point you toward the skills you will need to develop to be successful on the job as a medical assistant. Complete the following stress self-test.

For each question, circle the response that best describes you.

1. I exercise:
   a. three times a week
   b. less than three times a week
   c. only if I am forced to
2. When something stressful happens in my life, I:
   a. eat too much
   b. make sure I eat regular meals
   c. stop eating for days
3. If I am struggling with a problem or project, I am most likely to:
   a. consult someone who may be able to help
   b. become determined to solve the problem or finish the project on my own
   c. abandon the project or just hope the problem goes away
4. When I encounter difficult personalities, I:
   a. leave the scene and avoid the person in the future
   b. lose my temper and get into arguments
   c. practice the art of the diplomatic response
5. When offered a new challenge or responsibility that requires obtaining new skills or training, I:
   a. get tension headaches
   b. respond with enthusiasm and an open mind
   c. express concern about taking on a new duty
6. In emergency situations, I:
   a. react calmly and efficiently
   b. feel paralyzed
   c. wait for someone else to take charge
7. I feel confident and competent in group situations:
   a. only when I know everyone present
   b. most of the time
   c. hardly ever; conversations with others make me uncomfortable
8. I think meditating or taking time to be quiet and calm during a busy day is:
   a. a terrific waste of time: I always have to be doing something
   b. good for other people: I've tried it more than once, but I can't seem to get into meditation
   c. a great way to relax and refocus my mind
9. The key to handling stressful situations lies in:
   a. staying out of stressful situations
   b. examining my view of the situation from a new direction
   c. insisting that everyone agree with my point of view
10. To accomplish my personal goals, I:
    a. am willing to get up an hour earlier each day
    b. will give up sleep altogether
    c. find myself losing sleep because I am worrying about how I am going to get everything done
11. I usually complete projects:
    a. on time
    b. at the last minute
    c. late—but only by a day
12. As I prepare for a day's activities, I:
    a. prioritize and use time management skills to budget time carefully
    b. do not prepare; I like to be spontaneous
    c. find myself overwhelmed and unable to complete anything
13. When I focus on setting a long-range goal, I:
    a. think through the short-range goals necessary to achieve it
    b. become impatient
    c. talk constantly about the goal without making plans to achieve it
14. I volunteer to take on:
    a. more tasks than any one person can easily accomplish—then amaze everyone by pulling them off
    b. only what I know I can reasonably accomplish
    c. only what is required to get the job done
15. After a stressful day, the best way to unwind is to:
    a. talk all night with family or friends about what happened
    b. rent a funny movie
    c. work late to prepare for tomorrow
16. People think of me as:
    a. a person who is unpredictable. No one knows what I will do next
    b. someone fixed in life roles
    c. someone who is confident about who I am, but who also is willing to grow and change as worthy opportunities arise

Scoring: In the "My Score" column, record the number of points earned for each of your answers. The higher your score, the less you are prone to stress. The highest possible score is 160 points. If your score is low, consider the areas you need to focus on to reduce stress in your life.

	My Score
1. a. 10 points b. 5 points c. 0 point Regular exercise reduces stress.	______
2. a. 0 point b. 10 points c. 0 point Eating regular meals reduces stress.	______
3. a. 10 points b. 5 points c. 0 point Problems rarely just go away; ask for help before struggling on your own.	______
4. a. 5 points b. 0 point c. 10 points You won't always be able to avoid a difficult person, and argument leads to stress. Tact and grace are needed.	______
5. a. 0 point b. 10 points c. 5 points Worrying to the point of causing physical symptoms is not productive. Close-mindedness could keep you from enjoying something new and cause stressful reactions.	______
6. a. 10 points b. 0 point c. 5 points Feelings of helplessness increase stress.	______
7. a. 5 points b. 10 points c. 0 point The ability to interact comfortably with others in group situations reduces stress.	______
8. a. 0 point b. 5 points c. 10 points The more you can separate your sense of well-being from daily events by taking time to relax and refocus, the less stress you will experience.	______
9. a. 0 point b. 10 points c. 0 points Stressful situations cannot always be avoided; keeping a flexible instead of a rigid viewpoint will reduce stress.	______
10. a. 10 points b. 0 point c. 0 point Sleep is important in reducing stress. However, making time by getting up earlier is a good time-management technique.	______
11. a. 10 points b. 5 points c. 0 point Lateness causes stress for everyone.	______
12. a. 10 points b. 0 points c. 0 point Unexpected things can always happen, but prioritizing and budgeting time can help keep a handle on the day's events and reduce stress.	______
13. a. 10 points b. 5 points c. 0 point Achieving long-range goals takes perseverance and determination. Being realistic about goals reduces stress.	______
14. a. 0 point b. 10 points c. 5 points Taking on too much responsibility leads to stress.	______
15. a. 0 point b. 10 points c. 0 point Humor is an effective stress reducer—so is separating work from your home life.	______
16. a. 0 point b. 0 point c. 10 points Being grounded but open to new experiences reduces stress.	______
Total	______

CHAPTER POST-TEST

This is similar to your Pre-Test. Perform this test without looking at the book. This is just to see how well you have understood and can recall the information presented in this chapter after you have studied it and completed the workbook exercises. You will not be graded on this portion (other than the grade you give yourself), but this is an excellent preparation for your instructor's test. You may use this Post-Test to determine what areas you need to study more. Justify any "false" answers.

1. Stress is never a good thing. (T or F)
2. Stress is something we can always prevent. (T or F)
3. Even if you have a lot of responsibility at work, you can still avoid burnout. (T or F)
4. Setting goals eliminates stress (T or F)

CHAPTER 6

The Therapeutic Approach to the Patient with a Life-Threatening Illness

CHAPTER PRE-TEST

Perform this test without looking at the book. This is just to see how well you have understood and can recall the information in this chapter after you have read it, but before you have completed the workbook exercises. You will not be graded on this portion (other than the grade you give yourself). Justify any "false" answers.

1. Patients from different cultures will view death and life-threatening illnesses in different ways. (T or F)
2. The strongest influences in managing life-threatening illnesses in the life of the patient comes from the medical team. (T or F)
3. Health care professionals are responsible for making sure that patients have all their legal documents in order when diagnosed with a life-threatening illness. (T or F)
4. Alternative methods of treatment should be discussed with the patient, as well as no treatment at all. (T or F)
5. When facing a life-threatening illness, setting goals is no longer important. (T or F)

INTRODUCTION

As a member of the health care team, the medical assistant will be involved in the care of patients with life-threatening illnesses. In addition to providing medical, surgical, and psychological care, the health care team relies on its skills of empathy and compassion in building a strong therapeutic approach to the treatment and care of patients with life-threatening illness. As a source of information for these patients and their families and significant others, medical assistants need to be sensitive, supportive, and respectful of people who have a life-threatening disease. It is important for medical assistants to remain impartial and professional, making patients as comfortable and confident as possible in the ambulatory care setting.

PERFORMANCE OBJECTIVES

After successful completion of this chapter you will be able to discuss the needs, both legal and emotional, of patients facing life-threatening illnesses. You will be familiar with the feelings the patients might be experiencing and be able to sympathize and empathize with them and their families. You will recognize the influences of various cultures regarding death and dying. You will have an understanding and an ability to assist patients who are experiencing life-threatening situations. Try not to look back at the textbook as you fill in the blanks in the following paragraph. If necessary, reread the textbook chapter. *The following statements are related to your learning objectives for this chapter. Fill in the blanks with the appropriate term(s):*

Everything learned in the previous chapter about therapeutic communication is heightened and considerably more difficult when the patient has a (1) __________ ______________ ____________. It is essential for the medical assistant to recognize that the (2) _______________ of the patients will change when handling a life-threatening illness. No two individuals will respond to a life-threatening illness in the same way. Some patients will respond with (3) ________________. Some patients will prepare for death by altering their lives drastically. Some patients will quietly continue their lives with little obvious (4) ______________. Although the health care professionals are not (5) ____________________ for providing legal advice and documents for the patient, it is in the best interest of the patient and the health care team to raise topics for discussion during the course of the patient's life-threatening illness.

VOCABULARY BUILDER

Find the word below that is misspelled; circle it, and then correctly spell it in the space provided. Then insert the correct vocabulary terms from the list that best fit the descriptions below.

durible power of attorney for health care	physician's directive
living will	psychomotor retardation

____

1. ______________________________ allows the surrogate to make decisions related to health care when the patient is no longer able to do so.
2. _________________________________ and ______________________ allow the patients to make decisions (before becoming incapacitated) of whether life-prolonging medical or surgical procedures are to continue or be withheld.
3. ___________________________ is the slowing of mental responses, decreased alertness, and apathy.

Crossword Puzzle

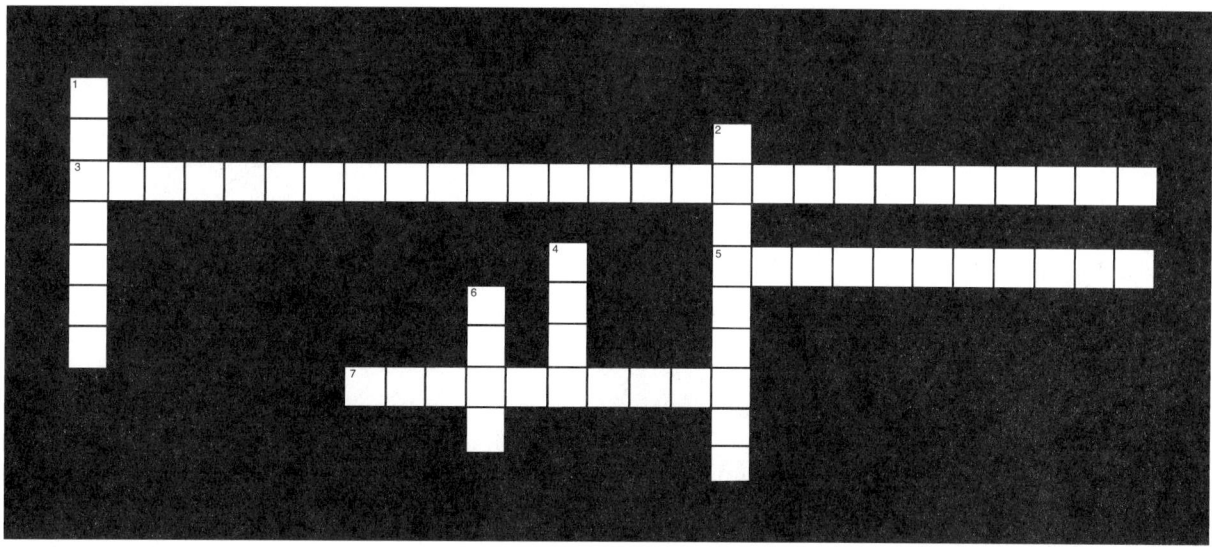

Across

3. This 1990 Act gave all patients in institutions that were Medicare or Medicaid funded certain rights
5. Aiding health, healthful
7. This emotion is common in patients dealing with life-threatening illnesses

Down

1. Recognition of another person's feelings by entering into those feelings
2. This type of support is vital when dealing with a life-threatening illness
4. Late stages of HIV infection
6. End-stage renal disease

LEARNING REVIEW

1. List five issues that are appropriate to discuss with a patient facing a life-threatening illness.
   (a) ______________________________
   (b) ______________________________
   (c) ______________________________
   (d) ______________________________
   (e) ______________________________

2. Discuss the pros and cons of using the words terminal illness or life-threatening illness. Which term seems more comfortable to you? Defend your rationale.

3. The federal government passed the Patient Self-Determination Act in ____________, giving all patients receiving care in institutions that receive payments from Medicare and Medicaid written information about their right to accept or refuse medical or surgical treatment.
   a. 1962
   b. 1990
   c. 1998
   d. 1973

4. What patients fear, more than anything else, when facing a life-threatening illness is:
   a. pain and loss of independence
   b. dementia
   c. financial issues
   d. becoming addicted to some medications

5. In caring for individuals with life-threatening illnesses, it can be helpful to remember:
   a. family members have the strongest influences on patients
   b. pain must be considered within a cultural perspective
   c. choices and decisions regarding treatment belong to the patient
   d. all of the above

6. One of the most common problems that a patient with life-threatening illness may exhibit is:
   a. displacement
   b. denial
   c. depression
   d. assimilation

7. Referrals to community-based agencies or service groups may include:
   a. health departments
   b. social workers
   c. hospice
   d. all of the above

CERTIFICATION REVIEW

These questions are designed to mimic the certification examinations. You can use these questions like a small "Certification Examination Study Guide," but this is not meant to take the place of the more extensive study guides. Use this portion to determine where to concentrate your efforts when studying for the certification examination.

1. Your patient's culture influences:
   a. his or her views on illness
   b. his or her views about treatment
   c. his or her views about death
   d. all of the above

2. When a person is faced with a life-threatening illness, he or she will go through certain stages of grieving. (T or F)

3. Your patient has just been diagnosed with a life-threatening illness. She tells you that she would much rather die quickly than to suffer through this disease. She asks you not to say anything about her comment to the doctor. What is your best response?
   a. You have had quite a shock. Dr. King would like to talk to you about those feelings. I'll go get him for you.
   b. You, above anyone else, know what is best for your life.
   c. I know what you mean, I would feel the same way
   d. Don't worry about that right now. Dr. King will give you medication to help with the pain.

CASE STUDIES

In working with patients with life-threatening illnesses, medical assistants hone their personal coping skills, capitalizing on strengths, maintaining hope, and showing continued human care and concern. For each case scenario presented, answer the following questions:

1. What is the best therapeutic response of the medical assistant?
2. On what criteria do you base this response as the best therapeutic approach?

Case 1

Jaime Carrera, a Hispanic man in his late 20s, is brought to Inner City Health Care, an urgent care center, by coworkers when he injures his head in an accident at a construction site where he is working. His head is bleeding profusely. As Jaime's coworkers watch the health care team implement Standard Precautions for infection control, one of them, his own shirt and hands covered with Jaime's blood, pulls the medical assistant aside and whispers frantically, "What are you doing? Does he have AIDS?"

Case 2

John Dukane, a longtime and much loved patient of the clinic, has end-stage renal disease. A kidney transplant is not appropriate, and his age of 83 years has led John to determine that he will not choose renal dialysis as a treatment. That decision has been made clear in his physician's directive and durable power of attorney for health care. He is healthy otherwise, and his family members think he should try the dialysis, which could extend his life a few weeks or months. Discuss the arguments on both sides of the decision.

SELF-ASSESSMENT

1. If you were faced with a life-threatening illness, would you choose to sustain your life regardless of the probable outcome? How far would you go with treatments? What four factors would enter into your decision? Have you discussed these issues with your family and physician?

CHAPTER POST-TEST

This is similar to the Pre-Test. Perform this test without looking at the book. This is just to see how well you have understood and can recall the information presented in this chapter after you have studied it and completed the workbook exercises. You will not be graded on this portion (other than the grade you give yourself), but this is an excellent preparation for your instructor's test. You may use this Post-Test to determine what areas you need to study more. Justify any "false" answers.

1. Patients view death and life-threatening illnesses in different ways depending on their culture. (T or F)
2. The strongest influences in managing life-threatening illnesses in the life of the patient comes from his or her family members. (T or F)
3. Health care professionals are not responsible for making sure that patients have all their legal documents in order when diagnosed with a life-threatening illness. (T or F)
4. Alternative methods of treatment, as well as the option of no treatment at all, should be discussed with the patient. (T or F)
5. When facing a life-threatening illness, setting goals is still important. (T or F)

CERTIFICATION CRITERIA CHECKLIST

As you go through your education and training, keep in mind the national certification examination that you will take when you graduate. Each chapter of the textbook and workbook covers a different section of the examination criteria. To keep track of your preparation for the certification examination, turn to the back of this workbook and highlight the following CMA, RMA, or CMAS certification examination criteria (if you have already highlighted them from a previous chapter, put a check mark by the criteria):

CMA
C. Psychology
    1. Basic principles
    3. Hereditary, cultural and environmental influences on behavior
E. Communication
    1. Adapting communication to an individual's ability to understand
    4. Professional communication and behavior
    5. Evaluating and understanding communication
M. Resource Information and Community Services
    4. Patient advocate

RMA
I. General Medical Assisting Knowledge
    E. Human Relations
        1. Patient relations
        2. Interpersonal relations
    F. Patient Resource Materials

CMAS
1. Medical Assisting Foundation
    • Professionalism

EVALUATION OF CHAPTER KNOWLEDGE

Evaluate your own strengths and weaknesses in administering a therapeutic approach to the patient with a life-threatening illness.

	Student Self-Evaluation		
Skills	Good	Average	Poor
I can recognize psychological problems that accompany life-threatening illnesses.	___	___	___
I can identify my personal fears or concerns about assisting in the care and treatment of patients with life-threatening illnesses.	___	___	___
I have the ability to treat patients and families with empathy, impartiality, and respect.	___	___	___
I recognize the demands of providing therapeutic care for patients with life-threatening illnesses in the ambulatory care setting.	___	___	___
I have the skills to avoid emotional burnout when caring for patients with life-threatening illnesses.	___	___	___
I understand the use of Standard Precautions for infection control in protecting myself.	___	___	___

CHAPTER 7

Legal Considerations

CHAPTER PRE-TEST

Perform this test without looking at the book. This is just to see how well you have understood and can recall the information in this chapter after you have read it, but before you have completed the workbook exercises. You will not be graded on this portion (other than the grade you give yourself). Justify any "false" answers.

1. You may discuss a person's confidential medical information as long as you do not say the patient's name. (T or F)
2. Your physician does not have a contract with the patient until he or she treats the patient. (T or F)
3. A physician practicing medicine without a license would come under *(circle one)*: criminal law or civil law?
4. A physician may stop treating a patient immediately if the patient refuses to pay his or her bill. (T or F)
5. Medical assistants do not have to worry about a "standard of care" because their physician–employers are ultimately responsible for everything the medical assistant does under their direction. (T or F)

INTRODUCTION

Medical assistants and other health care professionals are employed in the medical profession, where laws regulate medical and business practices at both the state and the federal levels. Regulatory agencies act to investigate the quality of health care and control health care costs while providing equitable access to care. Medical assistants need to be aware of the laws and regulations that govern the practices and procedures followed by health care professionals in the ambulatory care setting. In a society that strongly advocates the individual's right to seek redress in a court of law, the potential for litigation in medical settings must be considered. As responsible health care professionals, medical assistants need to understand the regulations and laws that affect their daily experiences on the job and to behave appropriately within the scope of their training and knowledge.

PERFORMANCE OBJECTIVES

After successful completion of this chapter you will be able to discuss the four sources of law, compare civil law with criminal law, and identify the three major areas of civil law that affect the medical profession. You will be able to recall at least seven of the nine administrative laws important to the medical profession. You will be able to define administering, prescribing, and dispensing medications and cite how these actions are applied to controlled substances. You will know three main goals of the Health Insurance Portability and Accountability Act (HIPAA), the differences between implied and expressed contracts; the three main reasons for the physician–patient contract to be terminated and how to go about instituting a termination. You will be able to discuss torts, the four Ds of negligence, and what constitutes battery in the ambulatory care setting; describe two forms of defamation of character; and cite at least 10 practices to help in risk management. You will be able to discuss informed consent, the types of minors, the necessary steps in a civil litigation, and how a medical assistant might be involved. You will understand subpoenas and be able to recall special issues of confidentiality, statute of limitations, public duties, and AIDS. *The following statements are related to your learning objectives for this chapter. Fill in the blanks in the following paragraphs with the appropriate term(s).*

Law may come from five different sources: (1) ________________, (2) ________________, (3) ________________, (4) ________________, and (5) ________________. The main difference between civil and criminal law is that civil law addresses crimes (6) ________________, and criminal law addresses crimes (7) ________________. The three major areas of civil law that affect the medical profession are (8) ________________, (9) ________________, and (10) ________________.

Three main goals of HIPAA are (11) ________________, (12) ________________, and (13) ________________.

Medical assistants are considered (14) ________________ of the physicians they serve and as such should be cautious in their actions and (15) ________________. A physician is obligated to continue care on a patient unless one of three things happens: The (16) ________________ may discharge the physician, the (17) ________________ formally withdraws, or the (18) ________________ no longer (19) ________________ ________________. A (20) ________________ law is a wrongful act, other than a breach of contract, resulting in injury to one person by another. The four Ds of negligence are: (21) ________________, (22) ________________, (23) ________________, and (24) ________________. The touching of another person without their consent is considered (25) ________________. Defamation of character consists of the injury of another person's (26) ________________, (27) ________________, or (28) ________________, either through (29) ________________ or (30) ________________ words. Consent may be either (31) ________________ or implied. Implied consent may occur when the patient is in a life-threatening situation or when the patient is (32) ________________ or unable to respond. Implied consent may also occur in more

(33) ____________________ ways. Persons who are under the age of 18 years, but are free from parental care are called (34) ______________________ ______________________. You may be protected from being sued if you give first aid at the scene of an accident provided you stay within your (35) ____.

VOCABULARY BUILDER

Find the words below that are misspelled; circle them, and then correctly spell them in the spaces provided. Then insert the correct vocabulary terms from the list that best fit the descriptions below.

A. agents
B. civil law
C. malfeasance
D. defendents
E. doctrins
F. durable power of attorney for health care
G. emanciated minor
H. expert witness
I. expressed contract
J. implied consent
K. constitutional law
L. incompetant
M. lible
N. litigation
O. malpractice
P. administrative law
Q. miner
R. negligance
S. noncompliant
T. plaintiffs
U. risk management
V. slander
W. statutes
X. supoena
Y. tort

____
____
____
____
____
____
____
____

1.____ Establishes agencies given power to enact regulations having the force of law

2.____ Designation of health care surrogate

3.____ Law that includes 27 amendments, 10 of which are the Bill of Rights

4.____ A 17-year-old person serving in the U.S. armed forces

5.____ Medical practice acts, or laws, that regulate the practice of medicine, such as licensure and standards of care

6.____ A patient who refuses needed care, such as a cancer patient who will not complete a series of chemotherapy treatments

7.____ A physician or health care professional who testifies in court to establish a reasonable and expected standard of care with respect to a specific medical situation so that jurors can understand the nature of medical information

8.____ The failure to exercise the standard of care that a reasonable person would exercise in similar circumstances

9.____ A patient sues a laboratory for money damages for delivering an incorrect analysis of a specimen that results in misdiagnosis by a physician

10.____ In a state where medical assistants must be licensed to perform venipuncture, charges are brought against a person who is performing this invasive procedure without the proper licensure

11.____ Persons who bring charges in a civil case

12.____ Medical assistants are _____________ of their physician–employers

13.____ A written lease for office space

14.____ A patient tilts her head back and opens her eyes wide for instillation of medicated eyedrops from a medical assistant without any verbal instructions to do so

15.____ Professional negligence

16.____ *Respondeat superior* and *res ipsa loquitur*

17.____ Although the patient, a competent adult, forcibly draws back, the medical assistant proceeds to administer an injection, breaking off the needle in the skin

18.____ Court order

19.____ Persons against whom charges are brought

20.____ A medical assistant writes in the patient's record, "Jim Marshall is a ruthless, rude man who is very full of himself. Be careful around him."

21.____ A patient says loudly in the reception area of Inner City Health Care, filled to capacity with waiting patients, "Dr. Reynolds should retire. I know he's not up on the latest medical techniques."

22.____ Lawsuit

23.____ A 17-year-old student who lives with his or her parents

24.____ A person found by the court to be insane, inadequate, or not an adult

25.____ Actions that make the medical assistant and the physician–employer less vulnerable to litigations

Crossword Puzzle

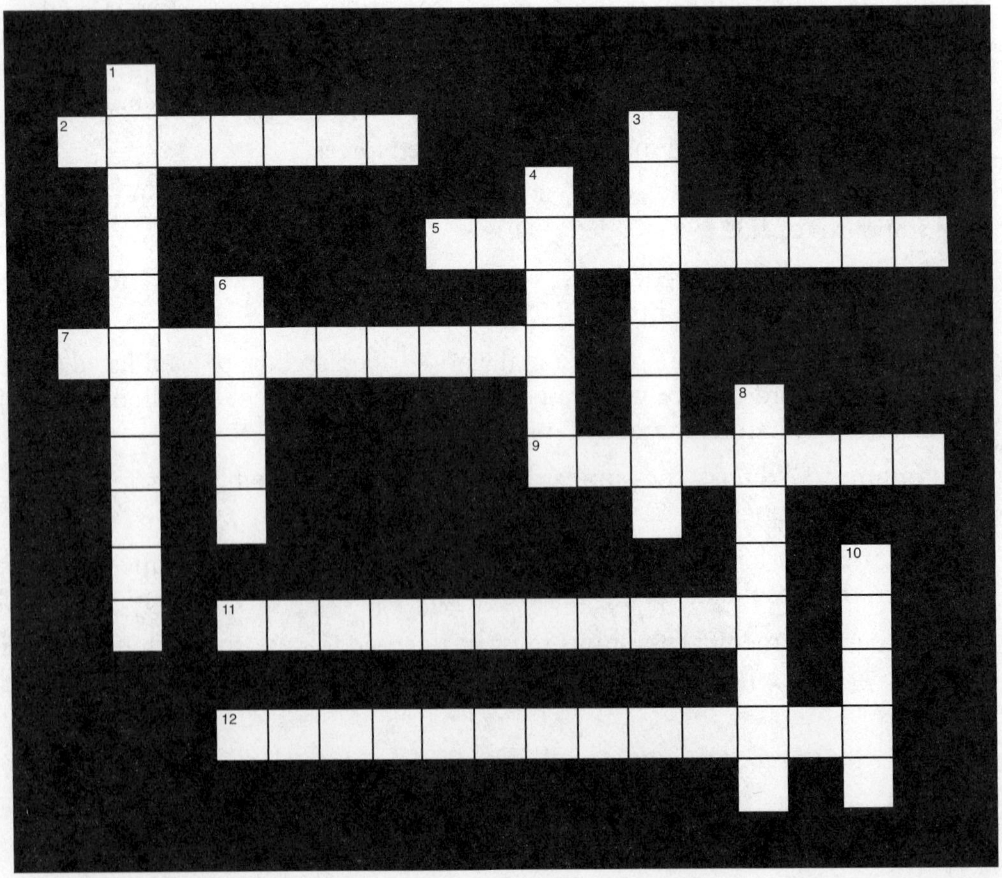

Clues

Across

2. The type of consent that is given when a patient is unconscious
5. When a doctor should have treated a patient, but did not, it can sometimes be called this
7. Another word for lawsuit
9. Another word for laws
11. A type of lawsuit in which the doctor is accused of harming a patient
12. When a patient does not follow the doctor's orders, such as not taking medication that is prescribed

Down

1. Minors (under 18 years old) who are no longer under parental authority
3. Law that governs criminal acts
4. Medical assistants are ___ of our physician–employers
6. Law that governs issues between persons
8. This document is a legal force that you must comply with
10. When someone harms another person's reputation by saying something untrue

LEARNING REVIEW

1. Civil law is a branch of the law in which restitution is awarded to individuals, usually in monetary form, when a civil wrong has been committed. Crimes against the safety and welfare of society as a whole, however, are addressed by criminal law, in which the punishment is usually incarceration and/or a fine.

   Identify whether the following actions fall under the domain of civil law (CV) or criminal law (CM).

   ____ A. A physician is siphoning off narcotics from an urgent care center's locked drug cabinet and continuing to treat patients while under the influence of the drugs.

   ____ B. A woman, in the advanced stages of breast cancer, sues her insurer when it refuses to provide benefits for a bone marrow transplant.

   ____ C. An office manager steals, or embezzles, funds from the medical practice.

2. Contracts are expressed or implied. Expressed contracts are written or verbal agreements that specify the exact duties of each party. Implied contracts depend on the power of action and circumstance; the actions performed would have been intended had an expressed contract existed.

   Identify each of the following as an expressed (E), implied (I), or invalid (X) contract.

   ____ A. professional negligence contract

   ____ B. living will

   ____ C. rescue breathing

   ____ D. patient appointment scheduled over the telephone

   ____ E. a purchase order for office supplies

   ____ F. completing a consent form for major abdominal surgery

   ____ G. a physician's directive signed by a patient with progressive Alzheimer's disease

   ____ H. a medical decision made by a health care surrogate for a patient suffering a debilitating cerebral vascular accident (CVA)

   ____ I. setting the fractured arm of a 6-year-old child rushed to the emergency department after a playground fall, and the parent has not consented

   ____ J. confirming verbal acceptance of a job offer as a clinical medical assistant by a handshake with the office manager of the medical practice

3. List and define the four Ds of negligence.

   (1) ______________________________

   ____

   (2) ______________________________

   ____

   (3) ______________________________

   ____

   (4) ______________________________

   ____

4. List at least 11 strategies for risk management in an ambulatory care setting that will lessen the potential for litigation.

   (1) ______________________________

   ____

   (2) ______________________________

   ____

   (3) ______________________________

   ____

   (4) ______________________________

   ____

   (5) ______________________________

   ____

   (6) ______________________________

   ____

   (7) ______________________________

   ____

   (8) ______________________________

   ____

   (9) ______________________________

   ____

   (10) ______________________________

   ____

   (11) ______________________________

   ____

5. Before any invasive or surgical procedure is performed, patients are asked to sign consent forms, which become a permanent part of the medical record. What four things must the patient know to give informed consent?

   (1) ____________________

   (2) ____________________

   (3) ____________________

   (4) ____________________

6. The unauthorized touching of one person by another is:
   a. invasion of privacy
   b. defamation
   c. libel
   d. battery

7. The federal government established laws in 1968 to allow people to make a gift of all or part of their body. It is known as:
   a. Occupational Safety and Health Act (OSHA)
   b. Uniform Anatomical Gift Act
   c. Family Gift Act
   d. Death Act of 1968
   e. Body Right Act of 1968

8. Protection of health care professionals who may provide medical care in an emergency without fear of being sued is called the:
   a. Good Samaritan laws
   b. physician's directives
   c. durable power of attorney for health care
   d. litigation

9. The law mandates that certain diseases and injuries are reported to the proper authorities; these include:
   a. rape
   b. gunshot and knife wounds
   c. child abuse
   d. elder abuse
   e. all of the above
   f. c and d only

10. An order for a physician to appear in court with a medicine record is:
    a. *res ipsa loquitur*
    b. *subpoena duces tecum*
    c. *respondeat superior*
    d. an interrogatory

CERTIFICATION REVIEW

These questions are designed to mimic the certification examinations. You can use these questions like a small "Certification Examination Study Guide," but this is not meant to take the place of the more extensive study guides. Use this portion to determine which areas to concentrate your efforts when studying for the certification examination.

1. The Patient's Self-Determination Act, which includes advanced directives, is to ensure that patients are able to:
   a. choose their own physician
   b. control their own health care decisions
   c. have guaranteed confidentiality
   d. have health care benefits
2. Which of the following covers the relationship between physicians and their patients?
   a. informed consent
   b. locum tenens
   c. medical ethics
   d. contract law
3. *Res ipsa loquitur* means:
   a. the thing speaks for itself
   b. the physician is ultimately responsible
   c. the record must be opened in court
   d. patients have a right to their records
4. The 4 Ds of negligence are:
   a. duty, dereliction, danger, damage
   b. danger, duty, direct cause, disaster
   c. duty, dereliction, direct cause, damage
   d. disaster, damage, direct cause, disaster
5. A 17-year-old individual who is in the navy is considered to be:
   a. *respondeat superior*
   b. an emancipated minor
   c. privileged
   d. a naval dependent

CASE STUDIES

For each of the following cases, what errors are made that could leave the medical assistants and physician-employers vulnerable to litigation? How might the errors leave the health care professionals open to potential lawsuits? How could the errors have been avoided through effective risk management techniques?

Case 1

On a busy afternoon at Inner City Health Care, the reception area is filled with walk-in patients and the staff struggles to keep up with the patient load. Administrative medical assistant Liz Corbin, CMA, gives the patient file for Edith Leonard to clinical medical assistant Bruce Goldman, CMA. "Dr. Reynolds wants a CBC done stat on the older adult woman in exam room 1," she tells Bruce, handing him the file.

Bruce proceeds to examination room 1; without identifying the patient, he performs a venipuncture on Cele Little, who has come to the clinic for a hearing problem. Cele asks Bruce why the procedure needs to be performed and doesn't want to have it. Bruce insists that the physician has ordered the procedure and performs the venipuncture anyway. The procedure frightens Cele, and she begins to fear her hearing loss is indicative of a more serious illness.

Case 2

Dr. Elizabeth King has just completed a routine physical examination of Abigail Johnson. Elizabeth asks Anna Preciado, RMA, to administer a flu shot to Abigail before she leaves the office. Abigail, an older African-American woman, is accompanied by her daughter. When Anna attempts to administer the flu vaccine, Abigail says, "Is that a flu shot? They make me sick; I don't want it."

Abigail's daughter says, "Yes, she does want it. Go ahead and give it to her."

Abigail begins to laugh. "Okay," Anna says, "may I give you the vaccination?"

Abigail says nothing, but she rolls up her sleeve. As Anne administers the parenteral injection, the older woman looks up at her seriously and says, "I didn't want any flu shot. My daughter makes me get it every year." However, Abigail does not withdraw physically.

Case 3

Dr. Elizabeth King is going over the daily list of scheduled patients with Ellen Armstrong, CMA. They are standing at the front desk close to the reception area; several patients are waiting for the first appointments of the day. Elizabeth's eye moves down the list and stops over the name Mary O'Keefe. "Mary O'Keefe," she mutters, "she's so neurotic and pestering. It's a small wonder her husband hasn't left her yet; just wait till they have that third child. . . . I don't think I have the patience for Mary today."

Case 4

Lydia Renzi, a deaf woman with some residual hearing, comes to Inner City Health Care with a recurrent vaginal discharge. Lydia is diagnosed by Dr. Angie Esposito with candidiasis, a yeast infection caused by the fungus *Candida albicans;* Angie prescribes a vaginal suppository and asks Wanda Slawson, CMA, to give Lydia instructions for using the prescription. Lydia wears a hearing aid and has chosen not to be accompanied to the clinic by a sign language interpreter. Lydia has trouble understanding Wanda, who is soft spoken; Wanda is also standing against a brightly lit window, and Lydia has trouble seeing her face. Lydia writes on a pad she has brought with her, "Is this a sexually transmitted illness?"

In frustration, Wanda begins shouting, "You just have a yeast infection; it's not like you have herpes or anything." At that moment, Bruce Goldman, CMA, is escorting a male patient past the open door of the examination room. Both men turn their heads away, though it is clear they have overheard.

Case 5

Construction workers Jaime Carrera and Ralph Samson are required to take a preemployment drug-screening test before they can be hired to work on a new site to which they have applied. Jaime and Ralph come to Inner City Health Care, where urine specimens are collected for examination. The test comes back positive for Jaime, and his potential employer does not give him the job. Ralph tests negative. Two weeks later, Ralph returns to Inner City Health Care for a routine physical examination.

"Whatever happened to Jaime Carrera?" Ralph asks Bruce Goldman, CMA. "I haven't seen him around the site."

"Oh," Bruce replies, "he tested positive for chemical substance abuse, and now he's in a rehab program Dr. Whitney suggested."

SELF ASSESSMENT

1. Have you ever been in a situation in which you were asked to disclose information about another person that might have been considered confidential? Or have you ever been told confidential information? If this has happened (or if it happens in the future), what should you have done or said? What will you do/say in the future?

CHAPTER POST-TEST

This is similar to your Pre-Test. Perform this test without looking at the book. This is just to see how well you have understood and can recall the information presented in this chapter after you have studied it and completed the workbook exercises. You will not be graded on this portion (other than the grade you give yourself), but this is an excellent preparation for your instructor's test. You may use this Post-Test to determine where you need to study more. Justify any "false" answers.

1. As long as you do not say the patient's name you may discuss the patient's illnesses and treatments with anyone. (T or F)
2. The patient–physician contract begins when the patient makes the appointment. (T or F)
3. A physician practicing medicine without a license is breaking a *(circle one)*: criminal law or civil law.
4. If patients refuse to pay their bills, a physician may stop treating them immediately. (T or F)
5. Because our physician–employers are ultimately responsible for everything the medical assistant does under their direction, medical assistants do not have to worry about a "standard of care." (T or F)

CHAPTER 8

Ethical Considerations

CHAPTER PRE-TEST

Perform this test without looking at the book. This is just to see how well you have understood and can recall the information in this chapter after you have read it, but before you have completed the workbook exercises. You will not be graded on this portion (other than the grade you give yourself). Justify any "false" answers.

1. Ethics has to do with what is right and wrong. (T or F)
2. Bioethics has to do with ethical issues dealing with human life. (T or F)
3. When abuse is suspected, the physician and medical assistant have ethical responsibilities to report it. (T or F)
4. When a patient has HIV, the physician may refuse to treat the patient. (T or F)
5. A physician and medical assistant can refuse to perform abortions. (T or F)

INTRODUCTION

Laws and regulations that govern the practice of medicine ensure that basic requirements and guidelines for protecting both patients and health care providers are observed. Medical assistants and all health care professionals are charged with the ethical responsibility to follow the law and to perform their duties within the scope of their training and practice. Laws and regulations find their origins in a system of ethics, or what is considered to be right and wrong behavior. As medical technology continues to advance, ethical dilemmas are created that challenge traditional codes of behavior. Medical ethics often confront ethical issues of great social controversy, such as in the field of bioethics. Medical assistants need to examine carefully their own deeply held values and beliefs, opinions, and their system of personal ethics, to build a strong foundation with which to face the ethical dilemmas encountered in the ambulatory care setting. We must strive to remain impartial and nonjudgmental in providing care.

PERFORMANCE OBJECTIVES

After successful completion of this chapter you will be able to discuss the reasons for a medical Code of Ethics, the eight characteristics of principle-centered leadership, the five Ps of ethical power, and the ethical guidelines for doctors, and you will be able to cite a few examples. You will be able to relate the five principles of the AAMA code to patient care and restate the dilemmas encountered in certain current bioethical issues. *The following statements are related to your learning objectives for this chapter. Fill in the blanks in the following paragraphs with the appropriate term(s).*

Another word for ethics might be (1) ________________. Ethics are often identified in a set of principles and guidelines called (2) ________________. The physician's code of ethics is called (3) ________________________________. There are more than (4) __________ different codes of ethics; seven of them are worldwide. (5) ________________ refers to those ethics that have to do with life issues such as abortion, fetal tissue research, right to die, among others.

VOCABULARY BUILDER

Find the words below that are misspelled; circle them, and then correctly spell them in the spaces provided. Then insert correct vocabulary terms from the list that best fit into the descriptive sentence below.

bioethics	genetic enginering	macroallocation
criopreservation	microallocation	serrogate
ethics		
________________	________________	________________

1. ______________________________ Someone who substitutes for another
2. ______________________________ Branch of ethics resulting from sophisticated medical research
3. ______________________________ Medical decisions made by Congress
4. ______________________________ Defined as a code of what is right or wrong
5. ______________________________ Medical decisions made by individuals and physicians
6. ______________________________ Biotechnology used to diagnose diseases, produce medicines, and so forth
7. ______________________________ The use of freezing to preserve tissue for later use

Word Game

Find the words in the grid below. They may go in any direction. When you are finished, the first few unused letters in the grid will spell out a hidden message.

S	T	R	R	E	S	O	U	R	C	E	S	I	S	V	E	T
O	Y	M	D	C	E	O	W	H	A	T	I	C	S	M	M	E
O	G	I	R	O	S	R	E	W	O	P	I	A	A	L	L	N
L	O	C	Y	D	U	A	L	W	S	T	N	C	D	G	E	G
A	L	R	T	E	B	A	R	E	E	C	R	H	N	I	C	I
C	O	O	S	S	A	O	L	N	A	O	I	I	A	L	L	N
I	N	A	P	N	N	Y	E	L	A	D	S	H	R	I	M	E
H	H	L	R	G	O	G	G	L	O	I	E	S	T	O	H	E
T	C	L	O	T	L	I	L	G	T	C	A	R	R	E	Y	R
E	E	O	T	N	N	O	S	R	R	M	A	A	S	G	Q	I
O	T	C	E	K	C	T	E	I	M	I	L	T	P	H	W	N
I	O	A	C	A	L	V	P	E	C	L	G	L	I	Y	I	G
B	I	T	T	V	D	P	L	R	Y	E	N	H	P	O	R	P
T	B	I	I	A	Z	I	Y	M	V	V	D	G	T	N	N	W
M	O	O	N	N	D	L	Y	R	E	S	E	A	R	C	H	R
N	X	N	G	E	T	A	G	O	R	R	U	S	N	K	D	D
P	C	O	N	F	I	D	E	N	T	I	A	L	I	T	Y	G

abuse
advertising
allocation
bioethical
biotechnology
codes
confidentiality
decisions
dilemmas
engineering
ethics
genetics
leadership
macroallocation
microallocation
morally
power
protecting
research
resources
right
surrogate
wrong

LEARNING REVIEW

1. The AAMA Code of Ethics presents five basic principles that medical assistants must pledge to honor as members of the medical assisting profession.

   For each situation presented, identify the AAMA ethical principle that applies.

   A. Render service with full respect for the dignity of humanity.

   B. Respect confidential information.

   C. Uphold the honor and integrity of the profession.

D. Pursue continuing education activities and improve knowledge and skills.

E. Participate in community service and education.

____ 1. Marilyn Johnson, CMA, in conversation with co-office manager Shirley Brooks, CMA, refuses to speculate about whether a diagnosis of AIDS will be confirmed for patient Maria Jover.

____ 2. Administrative medical assistant Karen Ritter joins a study group to prepare for the CMA certification examination as a method of securing her recertification of credentials, which is required every 5 years.

____ 3. Clinical medical assistant Anna Preciado agrees to speak to a group of high school students who are interested in pursuing a career in the medical assisting profession.

____ 4. Liz Corbin, CMA, politely reminds older adult patient Edith Leonard that she is a medical assistant, not a nurse, but assures Edith that she is qualified to perform the instillation of medicated eyedrops ordered by Dr. Susan Rice.

____ 5. When patient Dottie Tate makes an appointment at Inner City Health Care for follow-up treatment of chronic back pain and a recent history of frequent falls, Bruce Goldman, CMA, prearranges for a wheelchair to accommodate Dottie's office visit.

____ 6. Karen Ritter, CMA, volunteers at the local community office of Planned Parenthood on weekends.

____ 7. Jane O'Hara, CMA, gently and kindly guides patient Wayne Elder, whose mild retardation often causes him to become confused in unfamiliar settings, back to the proper examination room when she finds him wandering down the hallway in search of Dr. Ray Reynolds.

____ 8. When filing a group of recent laboratory reports into the correct patient files, Ellen Armstrong, CMA, takes care to complete the task quickly and efficiently. She performs the task at a private office station away from the general reception area and does not leave the charts open or unattended as she works.

____ 9. Audrey Jones, CMA, approaches office manager Shirley Brooks, CMA, about opportunities for obtaining advanced training to become qualified to perform a wider array of clinical procedures in the ambulatory care setting.

____ 10. Clinical medical assistant Wanda Slawson, who assisted Dr. Mark Woo in the treatment of patient Rhoda Au, diagnosed with lupus erythematosus, believes the patient is foolhardy when she rejects Mark's treatment plan of Western drug therapy in favor of an approach that integrates Chinese medicine. However, she respects the patient's heritage and right to choose her own health care.

2. According to the *Current Opinions of the Council on Ethical and Judicial Affairs of the* AMA, advertising by physicians is considered ethical if the ad follows certain requirements. Which of the following are appropriate types of physician advertisements? *Circle each correct response*.

   A. Testimonials from patients cured of serious illnesses or whose conditions were reversed or controlled under the care and treatment of the physician.

   B. Physicians' credentials, together with physicians' hospital or community affiliations.

C. A description of the practice, facility hours of operation, and the types of services available to health care consumers.

D. Photographs of health care professionals performing their duties at a medical facility. For example, a physical therapist applying ultrasound, a deep-tissue modality, to a patient experiencing chronic lower back pain.

E. Guarantees of cure promised within a specific time frame.

F. Word-of-mouth advertisement from patients.

3. Patient medical records are confidential legal documents. Name three instances, however, in which health professionals are allowed or required to reveal confidential patient information by law.

   (1) ______________________________

   (2) ______________________________

   (3) ______________________________

4. Which state recently passed a physician-assisted suicide law?
   a. Florida
   b. California
   c. Oregon
   d. Texas

5. Revealing information about patients without consent unless otherwise required to do so by law is:
   a. a breach of confidentiality
   b. bioethics
   c. a conflict of interest
   d. genetic manipulation

6. Allocation of scarce resources may refer to:
   a. rationing of health care
   b. denied services
   c. advertising by health care professionals
   d. a and b only

7. *Roe v. Wade* refers to guidelines for:
   a. artificial insemination
   b. surrogacy
   c. abortion
   d. fetal tissue transplant

8. Codes of ethics:
   a. remain constant over time
   b. constantly change and evolve
   c. enhance professionalism
   d. are challenged and examined
   e. all but a
   f. none of the above

CERTIFICATION REVIEW

These questions are designed to mimic the certification examinations. You can use these questions like a small "Certification Examination Study Guide," but this is not meant to take the place of the more extensive study guides. Use this portion to determine in what areas to concentrate your efforts when studying for the certification examination.

1. The AAMA Code of Ethics includes all but which one of the following?
   a. We should render service with respect for the dignity of our patients.
   b. We should be paid an equitable salary/wage.
   c. We should respect confidential information.
   d. We should accept the disciplines of the profession.
   e. We should seek to improve our knowledge and skills.

2. Physicians may choose who to treat but may not refuse treatment based on certain criteria. Which of the following is untrue?
   a. Physicians may not refuse to treat patients based on race, color, religion, or national origin.
   b. It is unethical for a physician to refuse to treat a patient who is HIV-positive.
   c. Physicians must inform a patient's family of a patient's death and not delegate that responsibility to others.
   d. Physicians who know they are HIV-positive should tell their patients.
   e. Physicians should report unethical behaviors committed by other physicians.

CASE STUDY

Lourdes Austen arrives at the offices of Drs. Winston Lewis and Elizabeth King for her annual physical examination. It has been one year since Lourdes had surgery to remove a tumor in her breast by lumpectomy with axillary lymph node dissection, followed by a course of radiation. Lourdes's one-year mammogram and follow-up examinations with her surgeon and radiologist find no evidence of a recurrence of the cancer. Lourdes is a single woman in her late 30s. As Elizabeth begins the routine physical examination, assisted by Anna Preciado, RMA, Lourdes begins to cry. "I'm so happy to be alive," Lourdes says. "And so afraid of the cancer coming back. But I want to celebrate life. I've talked to my boyfriend about it and we want to get pregnant. What should I do?"

Elizabeth takes Lourdes's hand. "I know that living with cancer is hard. You are doing well. There are many things to consider . . . "

Discuss the following:

1. What bioethical dilemma exists in Lourdes's situation? In your opinion, is Lourdes's choice to become pregnant an ethical one?
2. How do deeply held beliefs and attitudes about parenthood and the role of women in our society have an impact on the patient's decision? How could these beliefs have an impact on the health care team's response to Lourdes?
3. What is Elizabeth's best therapeutic response to Lourdes? What medical issues should the health care team consider if Lourdes becomes pregnant?
4. What is the role of the medical assistant in this situation?

SELF-ASSESSMENT

A. List and describe the five Ps of ethical power and identify how you are able to demonstrate the five Ps in your own life.

(1) ____

____

____

____

(2) ____

____

____

____

(3) ____

____

____

____

(4) ____

____

____

____

(5) ____

____

____

____

B. List the eight questions adapted from Stephen Covey's book that can be used as guidelines for making ethical decisions. Identify how your life fits into these guidelines and where/if you are striving to do better.

(1) ____________________

____

(2) ____________________

____

(3) ____________________

____

(4) ____________________

____

(5) ____________________

____

(6) ____________________

____

(7) ____________________

____

(8) ____________________

____

CHAPTER POST-TEST

This is similar to the Pre-Test. Perform this test without looking at the book. This is just to see how well you have understood and can recall the information presented in this chapter after you have studied it and completed the workbook exercises. You will not be graded on this portion (other than the grade you give yourself), but this is an excellent preparation for your instructor's test. You may use this Post-Test to determine what areas you need to study more. Justify any "false" answers.

1. Doing what is right is called ethical behavior. (T or F)
2. Ethical issues dealing with human life is called bioethics. (T or F)
3. The physician and medical assistant have ethical responsibilities to report suspected abuse. (T or F)
4. A physician may refuse to treat an HIV-positive patient. (T or F)
5. Whether to perform abortions is a choice each physician and medical assistant can make for themselves. (T or F)

CHAPTER 9

Emergency Procedures and First Aid

Visit the American Red Cross Web site for information on cardiopulmonary resuscitation (CPR) guidelines at: http://www.redcross.org.

CHAPTER PRE-TEST

Perform this test without looking at the book. This is just to see how well you have understood and can recall the information in this chapter after you have read it, but before you have completed the workbook exercises. You will not be graded on this portion (other than the grade you give yourself). Justify any "false" answers.

1. Of the following, which is the most important in an emergency?
   a. if the patient has medical insurance
   b. if the patient is HIV-positive
   c. if the patient is taking any medication
   d. if the patient is breathing
2. The ABCs of CPR are:
   a. attitude, breathing, circulation
   b. airway, bleeding, circulation
   c. airway, breathing, circulation
   d. airway, bleeding, cardiac
3. As a medical assistant, you are required to perform CPR and first aid in an emergency. (T or F)
4. A first-degree burn is the worst because it has damaged deeper tissues. (T or F)
5. Whenever a person has a penetrating object imbedded in his or her body, it is important that you remove it as soon as possible so you can treat the wound. (T or F)

INTRODUCTION

Medical assistants may encounter emergency situations and should be familiar with the many types of potential emergencies that may occur both within the ambulatory care setting and outside of the office environment. In the ambulatory care setting, primarily designed to see patients in nonemergency situations, a physician is usually available to provide emergency care. The ambulatory care setting also contains medical equipment and supplies to address various emergency situations. The medical assistant, however, is often the first health care professional to interact with an emergency patient. The physician–employer will establish policies and procedures for emergency situations in an emergency policies and procedures manual for the ambulatory care setting that all employees, including medical assistants, will follow in emergency situations. The manual should be reviewed at regularly scheduled staff meetings. Emergency care is provided under the physician's instruction and according to the guidelines established in the emergency policies and procedures manual. Medical assistants must develop the essential skills of triaging emergency situations, that is, of recognizing emergency situations and correctly identifying the measures that must be taken to provide immediate care. As with any health care professional, medical assistants should provide emergency care only within the scope of their knowledge and training. Certified medical assistants (CMAs) must be provider care level CPR and First Aid certified from either American Red Cross, American Heart, American Safety and Health Institute, or National Safety Council.

PERFORMANCE OBJECTIVES

After successful completion of this chapter you will be able to recognize, prepare for, and respond to emergencies. You will understand the precautions you should take when rendering first aid or CPR. You will be able to identify different types of open or closed wounds, burns, and injuries to muscles, bones, and joints, and will be able to describe heat- and cold-related illnesses, the different kinds of shock, and the symptoms of a heart attack or stroke. You also will be able to perform the abdominal thrust maneuver, rescue breathing, and CPR. You should be able to obtain provider level competency to become certified in CPR and First Aid. *The following statements are related to your learning objectives for this chapter. Fill in the blanks in the following paragraphs with the appropriate term(s).*

It is important that medical assistants are able to (1) ____________________, (2) ____________________, and (3) ____________________ to emergencies. Certain (4) ____________________ should be taken when rendering CPR and first aid, including assessing that the scene of the emergency is (5) ____________________. Wounds may be categorized as either (6) ____________ or (7) ____________________. Burns are categorized according to their severity. A (8) ____________________ -degree burn is usually superficial, a (9) ________________ -degree burn has burned through partial thickness of the skin, and a (10) ________________ -degree burn has damaged the full thickness of the skin. Bone fractures are categorized according to the style of break, whether the bone has broken through the skin, as in a (11) ____________________ fracture, whether the bone has been twisted, as seen in a (12) __________________ fracture, and if the bone has fragmented into several pieces, as in a

(13) ________________________ fracture. The main difference between a strain and a sprain is that a (14) _____________________ involves a joint, whereas a (15) ________________ is a muscle injury. Heat stroke differs from heat exhaustion in that the person experiencing heat (16) ________________ will be sweating. Although both heat stroke and heat exhaustion are serious, heat (17) ____________ is critical. (18) ________________ ________________________ is a method of giving the victim your oxygen until they can breathe on their own. (19) ___________________________________ is a method of helping a person who is choking, and (20) _____________ is the treatment of choice when a person's heart has stopped beating.

VOCABULARY BUILDER

Find the key vocabulary below that are misspelled; circle them, and then correctly spell them in the spaces provided.

anaphalaxis
automated external defibillator
cardiapulmonary resusitation
cardioversion
crepidation
explicit
fracture
Heimlich manuever
hypothermia
occlusion
syncopy

_________________ _______________________ ____________________
_________________ _______________________ ____________________

Word Game

Find the words in the grid. Pick them out from left to right, top line to bottom line. Words can go horizontally, vertically, and diagonally in all eight directions. When you are finished, the first few unused letters in the grid will spell out a hidden message.

B	E	A	W	A	R	E	E	O	F	Y	O	U	R	O	W	N	S	A	F
E	T	T	R	I	A	G	E	U	Y	A	S	S	Y	O	U	C	A	G	Y
R	E	F	O	R	O	T	S	H	C	P	E	R	S	I	N	A	S	R	C
N	E	M	E	R	G	P	E	N	R	S	C	Y	X	X	M	D	T	E	N
S	Y	T	M	L	I	P	R	A	Z	Z	E	C	Q	L	E	Y	R	E	E
Q	P	H	V	R	Q	P	I	B	K	K	C	R	H	T	L	S	A	N	G
D	C	L	A	R	C	N	W	S	G	Y	V	O	U	D	M	H	I	S	R
N	F	L	I	T	C	O	R	K	Y	N	G	N	M	Q	K	O	N	T	E
E	D	V	G	N	U	R	V	K	R	N	I	M	X	P	Q	C	K	I	M
G	K	V	N	N	T	V	R	W	I	M	C	H	Q	X	O	K	T	C	E
A	K	L	D	H	M	N	L	S	M	R	D	O	T	W	L	U	D	K	M
D	L	S	F	L	M	Z	S	O	R	J	I	J	P	A	B	T	N	L	Z
N	H	T	T	Z	C	E	C	P	T	J	A	D	R	E	E	R	D	D	L
A	V	G	D	P	R	C	B	R	N	T	T	Y	Q	P	R	R	L	K	D
B	W	L	R	D	N	D	F	M	Y	R	S	Z	T	Q	K	R	B	D	Z
C	A	R	D	I	A	C	G	W	C	P	R	G	N	I	D	E	E	L	B
V	G	E	R	U	T	C	A	R	F	H	I	J	L	N	V	T	Q	N	N
N	O	I	S	S	E	R	P	E	D	L	F	N	K	Z	J	M	F	M	W
F	A	N	A	P	H	Y	L	A	X	I	S	W	L	N	H	B	N	T	N
Z	D	T	H	Y	P	O	T	H	E	R	M	I	A	K	T	H	B	K	P

anaphylaxis
bandage
bleeding
breathing
cardiac
comminuted
compound
CPR
depression
dressing
emergency
first aid
fracture
greenstick
hypothermia
rescue
shock
spiral
splint
sprain
strain
syncope
triage
wounds

Identify each of the following correct vocabulary terms as an emergency condition (EC), an emergency or first aid procedure performed by health care professionals (EP), emergency equipment (EQ), or an emergency service provided to assist in emergency situations (ES).

A. _____ A. first aid

_____ B. triage

_____ C. syncope

_____ D. shock

_____ E. wounds

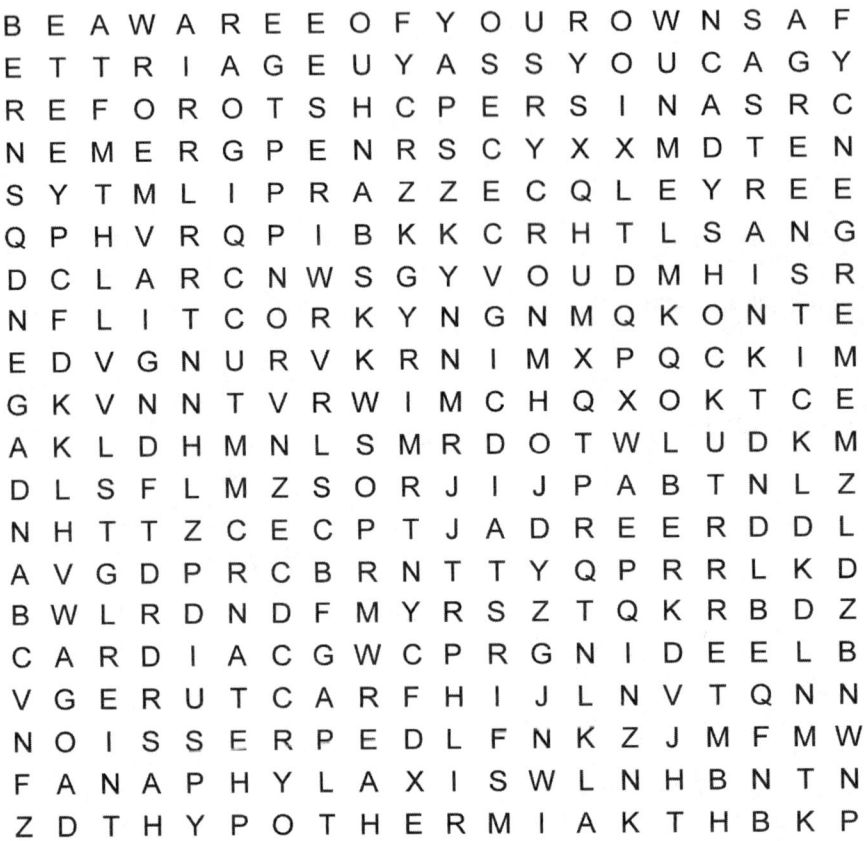

_____ F. crash tray or cart
_____ G. Heimlich maneuver
_____ H. occlusion
_____ I. universal emergency medical identification symbol and card
_____ J. hypothermia
_____ K. Standard Precautions
_____ L. CPR
_____ M. sprain
_____ N. emergency medical services (EMS)
_____ O. fractures
_____ P. splints
_____ Q. strain
_____ R. rescue breathing

B. *Match each key vocabulary term given in part A with its definition listed below.*

_____ 1. A break in a bone. There are several types, but all are classified as open or closed.
_____ 2. A tray or portable cart that contains medications and supplies needed for emergency and first aid procedures.
_____ 3. An injury to the soft tissue between joints that involves the tearing of muscles or tendons and occurs often in the neck, back, or thigh muscles.
_____ 4. A break in the skin or underlying tissues, categorized as open or closed.
_____ 5. Closure of a passage.
_____ 6. An injury to a joint, often an ankle, knee, or wrist, that involves a tearing of the ligaments. Most are minor and heal quickly; others are more severe, include swelling, and may not heal properly if the patient continues to put stress on the affected joint.
_____ 7. A local network of police, fire, and medical personnel trained to respond to emergency situations. In most communities, the system is activated by calling 911.
_____ 8. Abdominal thrusts designed to overcome breathing difficulties in patients who are choking.
_____ 9. Identification sometimes carried by individuals to identify any health problems they might have.
_____ 10. Any device used to immobilize a body part. Often used by EMS personnel.
_____ 11. An extremely dangerous cold-related condition that can result in death if the individual does not receive care and if the progression of the condition is not reversed. Symptoms include shivering, cold skin, and confusion.
_____ 12. Fainting.
_____ 13. The immediate care provided to persons who are suddenly ill or injured, typically followed by more comprehensive care and treatment.
_____ 14. A condition in which the circulatory system is not providing enough blood to all parts of the body, causing the body's organs to fail to function properly.

_____15. The combination of rescue breathing and chest compressions performed by a trained individual on a patient experiencing cardiac arrest.

_____16. To assess patients' conditions and prioritize the need for care.

_____17. Performed in individuals in respiratory arrest, this is a mouth-to-mouth (using appropriate protective equipment) or mouth-to-nose procedure that provides oxygen to the patient until emergency personnel arrive.

_____18. Guidelines issued by the Centers for Disease Control and Prevention (CDC) in 1996 that combine many of the basic principles of Universal Precautions and body substance isolation techniques. These augmented 1996 guidelines represent the new requirements for infection control measures and are intended to protect health care professionals, patients, and visitors.

LEARNING REVIEW

1. Keen observation skills are necessary to recognize potential emergency situations; medical assistants rely on sight, hearing, and even smell, and they must be acutely sensitive to unusual behaviors. To identify the nature of the emergency and respond effectively, what five things must the medical assistant do to triage, or assess, the patient's situation?

   (1) ____

   (2) ____

   (3) ____

   (4) ____

   (5) ____

2. In an urgent care setting, two or more patients may present with emergency symptoms. The order in which emergency patients will receive care depends on the health care professionals' abilities to triage patients' symptoms to determine who needs care most urgently.

   The following five patients present simultaneously on New Year's Eve at Inner City Health Care, an urgent care center. Office manager Walter Seals, CMA, is working the evening shift with Dr. Mark Woo. In what order will Walter and Mark triage the priority of treatment?

   Number the patients 1 through 5 to correspond to the urgency of their conditions, one being most critical. For each patient, list the emergency conditions he or she is suffering from, in order of severity, and name the emergency procedures the health care team will initiate to treat the patient.

   A. A patient presents with a gunshot wound to the leg that is bleeding severely. The patient is conscious but his pupils are dilated and he is unable to answer simple questions put to him by Walter and Dr. Woo. He cradles his right arm and will not let anyone touch it, although there is no immediate evidence of an open wound to the arm.

   Urgency of Condition: ______________________________

   ____

   ____

   ____

B. An elderly man, brought in by his grandson, describes debilitating chest pains and nausea after eating a large family dinner. The man is a regular patient of Dr. Ray Reynolds, another physician at Inner City Health Care. The patient's medical record indicates that he has a hiatal hernia, slipped disks, high blood pressure, and mild angina. His vital signs are within a normal range for his general physical condition. The man is walking and speaking with moderate distress and is extremely anxious.

Urgency of Condition: ______________________________

____

____

C. A young woman presents with her boyfriend. She appears to have multiple abrasions on her right palm and knee, with damage to the right knee and ankle joints sustained after a fall on in-line skates. Both joints are swollen and painful. She received the skates as a Christmas gift from her boyfriend.

Urgency of Condition: ______________________________

____

____

D. A man in his mid-30s presents with the cotton tip of a cotton swab stuck in his ear canal. The tip became lodged in his ear while he was showering and dressing for a New Year's Eve party. Although the man feels a dull consistent pain in the ear, he says he has no trouble hearing. The outside of the ear appears normal, and the man appears annoyed but not distressed.

Urgency of Condition: ______________________________

____

____

E. A young woman presents with a group of friends, all college students, with an eye injury sustained by a champagne cork. The cork, which had a metal covering over its tip, hit the patient's eye; the students bring the cork with them. The young woman's eye is red and tearing, and she is experiencing severe pain in the eye.

Urgency of Condition: ______________________________

____

____

3. In administering emergency care in the ambulatory care setting, medical assistants and all health care professionals must follow Standard Precautions to protect themselves, their patients, and visitors. What five infection control measures can health care professionals follow to greatly reduce the risk for transmitting infectious disease when providing emergency care?

(1) ______________________________

(2) ______________________________

(3) ______________________________

(4) ______________________________

(5) ______________________________

4. The medical crash cart or tray contains emergency or first aid supplies and medications health care professionals commonly use in treating emergencies. Using a medical encyclopedia or reference such as the *Physician's Desk Reference* (PDR), describe the following emergency medications and identify potential uses for each. Remember that only a physician can order medications or treatment.

   A. Lidocaine ______________________________

   ____

   ____

   B. Verapamil ______________________________

   ____

   ____

   C. Atropine ______________________________

   ____

   ____

   D. Insulin ______________________________

   ____

   ____

   E. Nitroglycerin ______________________________

   ____

   ____

   F. Marcaine ______________________________

   ____

   ____

   G. Diphenhydramine ______________________________

   ____

   ____

   H. Diazepam ______________________________

   ____

   ____

5. Shock requires immediate medical attention. Progressive shock can reach an irreversible point and is life threatening. Shock occurs when the circulatory system is not providing enough blood to all parts of the body, causing the body's organs to function improperly.

   For each of the patient symptoms or conditions below, identify the type of shock that is most likely.

   ____________ A. Patient suffers heart attack

   ____________ B. Patient experiences severe infection after colon surgery

   ____________ C. Patient experiences syncope after witnessing a traumatic event

   ____________ D. Patient experiences reaction to food allergy

_______________ E. Choking patient has extreme difficulty breathing

_______________ F. Diabetic patient lapses into a coma

_______________ G. Patient has serious head trauma

_______________ H. Accident victim experiences extreme loss of blood

6. A common procedure for treating closed wounds is to RICE them. What do the letters of this acronym stand for?

   R_______________ I_______________ C_______________ E_______________

7. Match each type of open wound to its defining characteristics.

   A. incision
   B. puncture
   C. laceration
   D. avulsion
   E. abrasion

   _____ 1. A wound that pierces and penetrates the skin. This wound may appear insignificant, but actually can go quite deep.

   _____ 2. These wounds commonly occur at exposed body parts such as the fingers, toes, and nose. Tissue is torn off and wounds may bleed profusely.

   _____ 3. A wound that results from a sharp object such as a scalpel blade.

   _____ 4. A painful wound that involves nerve endings. The epidermal layer of the skin is scraped away.

   _____ 5. A wound that results in a jagged tear of body tissues and may contain debris.

8. For each type of wound, describe proper emergency concerns, care, and treatment.

   Incision ____

   ____

   ____

   Puncture ____

   ____

   ____

   Laceration ____

   ____

   ____

   Avulsion ____

   ____

   ____

   Abrasion ____

   ____

   ____

9. Name three sources other than heat that can cause burns. For each, describe the proper emergency concerns, care, and treatment.

   (1) ______________________________

   ____

   ____

   ____

   (2) ______________________________

   ____

   ____

   ____

   (3) ______________________________

   ____

   ____

   ____

10. Musculoskeletal injuries, or injuries to muscles, bones, and joints, can be difficult to triage, especially for closed fractures. List five assessment techniques health care professionals can use to determine the seriousness of musculoskeletal injuries.

    (1) ______________________________

    (2) ______________________________

    (3) ______________________________

    (4) ______________________________

    (5) ______________________________

11. For each set of symptoms that follows, identify the most likely emergency condition and describe emergency concerns, care, and treatment.

    ____________ A. Off-color, cold skin with a waxy appearance

    ____

    ____

    ____________ B. Hives, itching, lightheadedness

    ____

    ____

    ____________ C. Cold, clammy skin; profuse sweating; abdominal cramps; headache; general weakness

    ____

    ____

    ____________ D. Lightheadedness, weakness, nausea, unsteadiness

    ____

    ____

_______________ E. Moist, pale skin; drooling; lack of appetite; diplopia; full pulse

_______________ F. Numbness in face, arm, and leg on one side of body; slurred speech; nausea and vomiting

_______________ G. Fever, convulsions, clenched teeth

_______________ H. Cold, clammy skin; anxiety; dilated pupils; weak pulse; rigid boardlike abdomen postsurgery for hysterectomy

12. Identify the method of entry into the body for each of the following poisons:

_______________ A. carbon monoxide

_______________ B. insect stingers

_______________ C. chemical pesticides used in the garden

_______________ D. spoiled food

_______________ E. poison oak

_______________ F. cleaning fluid fumes

Emergency Procedure 1

13. Lenore McDonell, a wheelchair-bound woman in her early 30s, experiences a serious laceration to the right arm sustained from a fall while performing an independent transfer from the examination table to her wheelchair. Joe Guerrero, CMA, assists Dr. Winston Lewis in administering emergency care.

    A. What Standard Precautions must the health care professionals follow before administering emergency treatment?

    B. Joe and Dr. Lewis attempt to control Lenore's bleeding by applying a dressing and pressing firmly.

        (1) When the bleeding does not stop, what two actions should the health care professionals perform?

            (a) _______________

            (b) _______________

(2) In the unlikely event that bleeding continues, what piece of medical equipment will the health care team use in substitution of a tourniquet? Why is this alternative equipment effective and widely used today?

C. The bleeding stops, and Joe applies a pressure bandage over the dressing.

(1) This patient is prone to fractures, and a radiograph will need to be taken. What is the next emergency procedure Dr. Lewis will perform? Why is this procedure necessary, and what equipment will the physician and medical assistant require?

(2) Before applying a sling, what do the health care professionals check to be sure that the medical equipment used has not been too tightly applied?

D. What Standard Precautions will the health care team follow after the emergency treatment of the patient is successfully completed?

E. What information will the health care team include in documenting the procedure for the patient's medical record?

Emergency Procedure 2

14. New patient Grace Fisher comes to the offices of Drs. Lewis and King for a well-baby visit for infant Joseph Michael. In the reception area, the baby is fussy; Grace picks him up and holds him at her chest, rocking and gently patting the baby's back. Suddenly, the baby's face becomes red; he begins to cough and wheeze. When the baby does not quickly resume normal breathing, Ellen Armstrong, CMA, alerts Dr. King over the office intercom. As Ellen takes the baby from a bewildered and frightened Grace to begin rescue breathing in a nearby

empty examination room, she motions to coworker Joe Guerrero, CMA, to accompany them to attend to the mother's needs.

A. What four steps will Ellen perform to initiate rescue breathing?

(1) ____________________

(2) ____________________

(3) ____________________

(4) ____________________

B. Ellen checks [illegible] of the brachial artery. The pulse is present but the baby seems to have increased difficulty breathing. What sequence [illegible] Ellen follow next? How long should Ellen continue this sequence?

____

____

____

C. After 3 minutes, the baby is still conscious and has a pulse but is no longer able to cough, cry, or breathe. Dr. King has joined Grace and Ellen in the examination room.

(1) What procedure does Dr. King initiate at this time?

____

(2) What four steps does Dr. King follow to perform this procedure?

(a) ____________________

____

(b) ____________________

____

(c) ____________________

____

(d) ____________________

____

(3) How long will Dr. King continue this procedure?

____

D. The infant, Joseph Michael, loses consciousness. Grace becomes hysterical.

(1) As she shakes the infant to check for consciousness, Dr. King gives what two instructions to Joe?

(a) ____________________

(b) ____________________

(2) Dr. King begins to administer what procedure? How long will Dr. King administer this procedure? What happens if the baby loses a pulse?

____

____

E. On the second set of back blows and thrusts after the baby loses consciousness, Dr. King sweeps a bead out of the baby's mouth. Joseph Michael begins to cough and cry. A bead from Grace's sweater had come loose and lodged in the baby's trachea. "We've caught this just in time," Dr. King announces to a grateful and relieved mother.

What follow-up procedures will the health care team initiate?

____

____

____

F. What information will the health care team include in documenting the procedure in the infant's medical record? In Grace's medical record?

(1) *Joseph Michael Fisher:*

____

____

____

____

(2) *Grace Fisher:*

____

____

____

____

Emergency Procedure 3

15. Edith Leonard, a frail widow in her early 70s, participates in the knitting club at the local senior center. As she knits, Edith becomes restless and begins to rub her chest and massage her jaw. Her breathing becomes shallow. Bruce Goldman, CMA, who volunteers at the senior center, remembers Edith as a patient at Inner City Health Care, where he works. When Edith slumps in her chair, Bruce rushes over.

A. When Bruce calls Edith's name, she nods her head. However, Edith seems to have extreme difficulty breathing, and her face is contorted with pain. What is Bruce's first action?

____

B. Edith is no longer breathing. What procedure should Bruce initiate? What steps does Bruce follow in performing the procedure?

____

____

____

____

____

C. Edith is still not breathing and no pulse is present.

(1) What procedure does Bruce initiate?

____

____

(2) What is the correct method to administer chest compressions?

____

____

(3) How many slow breaths will Bruce administer after completing the chest compressions?

____

____

(4) How many times will Bruce repeat the sequence of chest compressions and rescue breathing before again checking Edith's pulse?

____

____

D. Under what four conditions is it acceptable for Bruce to stop administering this technique of chest compressions and rescue breathing?

(1) ____

(2) ____

(3) ____

(4) ____

E. After 10 minutes, EMS personnel arrive and transport Edith to a local hospital.

(1) What Standard pPrecautions will Bruce practice at the senior center after EMS personnel have transported the patient from the scene of the emergency?

____

____

____

(2) What supplies and equipment would the medical assistant have used if this emergency had taken place in an ambulatory care setting?

____

____

16. Shock that occurs as a result of overwhelming emotional factors such as fear, anger, or grief is called:

a. neurogenic

b. psychogenic

c. anaphylactic

d. septic

17. The type of burn that may occur resulting in an entrance and exit burn wound area is:
    a. chemical
    b. electrical
    c. solar radiation

18. In burn depth classifications, third-degree burns are also called:
    a. superficial
    b. full thickness
    c. partial thickness

19. The type of fracture often caused by falling on an outstretched hand that involves the distal end of the radius is called:
    a. greenstick
    b. spiral
    c. colles
    d. implicated

20. Jaw and left shoulder pain; a rapid, weak pulse; excessive perspiration; and cold, clammy skin may be symptomatic of:
    a. seizure
    b. heart attack
    c. stroke
    d. sepsis

CERTIFICATION REVIEW

These questions are designed to mimic the certification examinations. You can use these questions like a small "Certification Examination Study Guide," but this is not meant to take the place of the more extensive study guides. Use this portion to determine in what areas to concentrate your efforts when studying for the certification examination. Justify any "false" answers.

1. Which of the following is not an appropriate treatment for hypothermia?
    a. Give the victim warm liquids to drink.
    b. Remove any wet clothing.
    c. Rub the victim's skin vigorously to increase circulation.
    d. Use warm water to warm the person if possible.

2. A diabetic emergency should be treated with sugar. (T or F)

3. In anaphylactic shock, the patient will:
    a. feel a constriction in his or her throat and chest
    b. have difficulty breathing
    c. have swelling and tingling of the lips and tongue
    d. all of the above

4. When performing CPR, the breaths and chest compressions should be at a rate of
   a. 12 to 5
   b. 5 to 12
   c. 15 to 5
   d. 2 to 15

CASE STUDY

Mary O'Keefe calls Dr. King's office in a panic. Ellen Armstrong, CMA, answers the telephone. "Oh my God, help me. I need Dr. King."

"This is Ellen Armstrong, CMA. Who is this calling and what is the situation?"

"It's my baby, oh God, get Dr. King."

"Dr. King is unavailable, but we can help you. Now, tell me your name."

"It's Mary O'Keefe. Help me, I think my baby is dead."

"Are you at home?"

"Yes."

"Good. Tell me what's happened."

"My son Chris pried the plug off an outlet and he's electrocuted himself!" Mary cries. "He's just lying there. I'm so scared; if I touch him will I electrocute myself? Oh my God, my baby, my baby. What should I do?"

Ellen, who has been writing the details on a piece of paper motions to Joe Guerrero, another CMA in the office, and hands him her notes. Joe immediately accesses the O'Keefe's address from the patient database and uses another telephone line to call EMS with the nature of the emergency situation and directions to the O'Keefe's residence. Meanwhile, Ellen remains on the line with Mary. Dr. King is on rounds at the hospital this morning and will not be in the office for at least another hour.

"Mary, we're calling EMS, and they will be there as soon as possible. In the meantime, I'm going to need you to focus and answer my questions. Okay?"

Discuss the following:

1. What steps does the medical assistant take to triage the emergency situation?
2. What questions should Ellen ask Mary regarding the emergency situation? Based on Mary's answers, what instructions should Ellen give Mary to begin emergency treatment?
3. What should the medical assistant do after EMS arrives and takes over emergency care? What follow-up procedures are necessary?

SELF-ASSESSMENT

1. A. *On a scale of 1 to 5, rate your personal comfort in regard to the following emergency situations medical assistants may find themselves involved with in an ambulatory or urgent care setting.*

   1. Extremely uncomfortable
   2. Uncomfortable
   3. Somewhat comfortable
   4. Comfortable
   5. Very comfortable

   _____ Assisting in treatment of patients with injuries clearly sustained by an act of violence or abuse

   _____ Performing the Heimlich maneuver on an unconscious person

   _____ Administering CPR to a child

_____ Administering back blows and thrusts to a conscious infant

_____ Performing rescue breathing on someone who has poor personal hygiene

_____ Bandaging the open wound of an HIV-infected person

_____ Caring for a person experiencing a seizure

_____ Administering care to a patient who faints after venipuncture

_____ Administering care to a patient in extreme pain

_____ Administering care to a patient who is verbally abusive or uncooperative

B. *On a scale of 1 to 5, rate your level of agreement with the statements that follow.*

1. Never
2. Occasionally
3. Sometimes
4. Most of the time
5. All of the time

_____ Life-threatening emergencies frighten me.

_____ I respond well under pressure.

_____ I am bothered by the sight of blood.

_____ I lose my temper easily, becoming openly frustrated and angry.

_____ I become frustrated and overwhelmed by feelings of helplessness in emergency situations.

_____ I remain calm and clearheaded in emergency situations.

_____ I forget about myself completely and focus on the emergency victim.

_____ I am concerned about administering care in emergency situations in which danger to myself may exist when giving such care.

_____ I am comfortable speaking to the family or friends of emergency victims.

CHAPTER POST-TEST

This test is similar to the Pre-Test. Perform this test without looking at the book. This is just to see how well you have understood and can recall the information presented in this chapter after you have studied it and completed the workbook exercises. You will not be graded on this portion (other than the grade you give yourself), but this is an excellent preparation for your instructor's test. You may use this Post-Test to determine what areas you need to study more. Justify any "false" answers.

1. Of the following, which is the most important in an emergency?
   a. if the patient has medical insurance
   b. if the patient is HIV-positive
   c. if the patient is taking any medication
   d. if the patient is breathing

2. In ABCs of CPR are:
   a. attitude, breathing, circulation

b. airway, bleeding, circulation
c. airway, breathing, circulation
d. airway, bleeding, cardiac

3. As a medical assistant, you are required to perform CPR and first aid in an emergency. (T or F)

4. A first-degree burn is the worst because it has damaged deeper tissues. (T or F)

5. Whenever a penetrating object has been imbedded in a person's body, it is important that you remove it as soon as possible so you can treat the wound. (T or F)

CERTIFICATION CRITERIA CHECKLIST

As you go through your education and training, keep in mind the national certification examination that you will take when you graduate. Each chapter of the textbook and workbook covers a different section of the examination criteria. To keep track of your preparation for the certification examination, turn to the back of this workbook and highlight the following CMA, RMA, or CMAS certification examination criteria (if you have already highlighted them from a previous chapter, put a check mark by the criteria).

CMA

T. Patient Preparation and Assisting the Physician
    1. Performing telephone and in-person screening

X. Emergencies
    1. Preplanned action
    2. Assessment and triage

Y. First Aid
    1. Establishing and maintaining an airway
    2. Identifying and responding to (first aid)
    3. Signs and symptoms
    4. Management (first aid)

RMA

I. General Medical Assisting Knowledge
    A. Anatomy and Physiology
        1. Body systems: Identify the structure and function of
        2. Disorders and diseases: Identify and define various

CMAS

2. Basic Clinical Medical Office Assisting
    - Medical office emergencies

COMPETENCY ASSESSMENT

Procedure 9-1 Control of Bleeding

Performance Objectives: To control bleeding caused by an open wound. Perform this objective within 15 minutes with a minimum score of 30 points.

Supplies/Equipment: Sterile dressings, sterile gloves, mask, eye protection, a gown, biohazard waste container

Charting/Documentation: Enter appropriate documentation/charting in the box.

Instructor's/Evaluator's Comments and Suggestions:

SKILLS CHECKLIST Procedure 9-1: Control of Bleeding

Name ____________________

Date ____________________

No.	Skill	Check #1 20 pts ea	Check #2 10 pts ea	Check #3 5 pts ea	Notes
1	Wash hands and gather equipment quickly.				
2	Apply gloves and other PPE; eye mask, gown if splashing likely.				
3	Apply pressure bandages and apply pressure for 10 minutes. If bleeding continues, elevate arm above heart. If continues, press adjacent artery against bone.				
4	Dispose of waste in biohazard container.				
5	Wash hands.				
6	Document procedure.				
Student's Total Points					
Points Possible		120	60	30	
Final Score (Student's Total Points / Possible Points)					
		Notes			
Start time:					
End time:					
Total time: (15 min goal)					

COMPETENCY ASSESSMENT

Procedure 9-2 Applying an Arm Splint

Performance Objectives: To immobilize the area above and below the injured part of the arm to reduce pain and prevent further injury. Perform this objective within 15 minutes with a minimum score of 30 points.

Supplies/Equipment: Thin piece of rigid board and gauze roller bandage

Charting/Documentation: Enter appropriate documentation/charting in the box.

Instructor's/Evaluator's Comments and Suggestions:

SKILLS CHECKLIST Procedure 9-2: Applying an Arm Splint

Name ______________________________

Date ______________________________

No.	Skill	Check #1 20 pts ea	Check #2 10 pts ea	Check #3 5 pts ea	Notes
1	Place a padded splint under the injured area.				
2	Hold the splint in place with roller gauze.				
3	Check circulation (note color and temperature of skin and nails, and check pulse).				
4	Apply sling to keep arm elevated.				
5	Wash hands.				
6	Document procedure.				
Student's Total Points					
Points Possible		120	60	30	
Final Score (Student's Total Points / Possible Points)					

	Notes
Start time:	
End time:	
Total time: (15 min goal)	

COMPETENCY ASSESSMENT

Procedure 9-3 Abdominal Thrusts for a Conscious Adult

Performance Objectives: To open a blocked airway. Perform this objective within 15 minutes with a minimum score of 25 points.

Supplies/Equipment: None.

Charting/Documentation: Enter appropriate documentation/charting in the box.

Instructor's/Evaluator's Comments and Suggestions:

SKILLS CHECKLIST Procedure 9-3: Abdominal Thrusts for a Conscious Adult

Name ______________________

Date ______________________

No.	Skill	Check #1 20 pts ea	Check #2 10 pts ea	Check #3 5 pts ea	Notes
1	Place thumb side of fist against the middle of the abdomen above the umbilicus and below the xiphoid process.				
2	Grasp the fist with the free hand and give quick upward thrusts.				
3	Repeat until the patient coughs up the object. If the patient loses consciousness, perform abdominal thrusts for unconscious adult.				
4	Wash hands.				
5	Document procedure.				
Student's Total Points					
Points Possible		100	50	25	
Final Score (Student's Total Points / Possible Points)					

	Notes
Start time:	
End time:	
Total time: (15 min goal)	

COMPETENCY ASSESSMENT

Procedure 9-4 Abdominal Thrusts for an Unconscious Adult or Child

Performance Objectives: To open a blocked airway on an unconscious victim. Perform this objective within 15 minutes with a minimum score of 60 points.

Supplies/Equipment: Gloves, a resuscitation mouthpiece, biohazard waste receptacle

Charting/Documentation: Enter appropriate documentation/charting in the box.

Instructor's/Evaluator's Comments and Suggestions:

SKILLS CHECKLIST Procedure 9-4: Abdominal Thrusts for an Unconscious Adult or Child

Name ______________________

Date ______________________

No.	Skill	Check #1 20 pts ea	Check #2 10 pts ea	Check #3 5 pts ea	Notes
1	Appoint someone to call emergency services.				
2	Apply gloves.				
3	Lie patient on back and tilt patient's head back.				
4	Open victim's mouth and look for foreign object, then position resuscitation.				
5	Give breaths.				
6	If air will not go in, retilt head and try again. If air will not go in, place heel of the hand against the abdomen and the umbilicus and below the xiphoid process of the sternum.				
7	Kneel astride the patient's thighs and give five abdominal thrusts.				
8	Lift the jaw and sweep out the mouth.				
9	Tilt the head back, lift the chin, and give breaths again. Continue giving breaths and thrusts, sweeping the mouth until breaths go in.				
10	Dispose of waste in biohazard waste receptacle.				
11	Wash hands.				
12	Document procedure.				
Student's Total Points					
Points Possible		240	120	60	
Final Score (Student's Total Points / Possible Points)					

	Notes
Start time:	
End time:	
Total time: (15 min goal)	

COMPETENCY ASSESSMENT

Procedure 9-5 Abdominal Thrusts for a Conscious Child

Performance Objectives: To open a blocked airway. Perform this objective within 15 minutes with a minimum score of 20 points.

Supplies/Equipment: None.

Charting/Documentation: Enter appropriate documentation/charting in the box.

____

____

____

____

Instructor's/Evaluator's Comments and Suggestions:

____

____

____

____

____

____

SKILLS CHECKLIST Procedure 9-5: Abdominal Thrusts for a Conscious Child

Name ______________________________

Date ______________________________

No.	Skill	Check #1 20 pts ea	Check #2 10 pts ea	Check #3 5 pts ea	Notes
1	Place thumb side of fist against the middle of the umbilicus and below the xiphoid process.				
2	Grasp the fist with the free hand and give quick upward thrusts. Repeat until the object is expelled or until the victim loses consciousness.				
3	Wash hands.				
4	Document procedure.				
Student's Total Points					
Points Possible		80	40	20	
Final Score (Student's Total Points / Possible Points)					
		Notes			
Start time:					
End time:					
Total time: (15 min goal)					

COMPETENCY ASSESSMENT

Procedure 9-6 Back Blows and Chest Thrusts for a Conscious Infant Who Is Choking

Performance Objectives: To open a blocked airway and assist a conscious infant who is choking. Perform this objective within 15 minutes with a minimum score of 30 points.

Supplies/Equipment: None.

Charting/Documentation: Enter appropriate documentation/charting in the box.

____

____

____

____

Instructor's/Evaluator's Comments and Suggestions:

____

____

____

____

____

____

SKILLS CHECKLIST Procedure 9-6: Back Blows and Chest Thrusts for a Conscious Infant Who Is Choking

Name ______________________

Date ______________________

No.	Skill	Check #1 20 pts ea	Check #2 10 pts ea	Check #3 5 pts ea	Notes
1	With infant facedown on the forearms, give five back blows between the infant's shoulder blade with the heel of the hand.				
2	Position infant faceup on the forearm.				
3	Give five chest thrusts on about the center of the breastbone.				
4	Look in infant's mouth for the object and repeat back blows and chest thrusts, looking for the object until the infant can breathe on his or her own. If the infant loses consciousness, activate EMS, then use back blows and chest thrust techniques for unconscious infant.				
5	Wash hands.				
6	Document procedure.				
Student's Total Points					
Points Possible		120	60	30	
Final Score (Student's Total Points / Possible Points)					

	Notes
Start time:	
End time:	
Total time: (15 min goal)	

COMPETENCY ASSESSMENT

Procedure 9-7 Back Blows and Chest Thrusts for an Unconscious Infant

Performance Objectives: To open a blocked airway by delivering back blows and chest thrusts for an unconscious infant. Perform this objective within 15 minutes with a minimum score of 85 points.

Supplies/Equipment: Gloves, resuscitation mouthpiece

Charting/Documentation: Enter appropriate documentation/charting in the box.

Instructor's/Evaluator's Comments and Suggestions:

SKILLS CHECKLIST Procedure 9-7: Back Blows and Chest Thrusts for an Unconscious Infant

Name ____________________

Date ____________________

No.	Skill	Check #1 20 pts ea	Check #2 10 pts ea	Check #3 5 pts ea	Notes
1	Appoint someone to call emergency services.				
2	Don gloves.				
3	Tap the infant gently to check for consciousness.				
4	Gently tilt back the infant's head.				
5	Apply resuscitation mouthpiece.				
6	Listen and watch for breathing.				
7	Give two breaths, covering the infant's nose and mouth.				
8	If air does not go in, retilt head and make another attempt.				
9	If breaths still do not go in, position the infant facedown on the forearms.				
10	Give back blows with the heel of the hand between the shoulder blades.				
11	Position the infant faceup on the forearms.				
12	Give five chest thrusts on about the center of the breastbone.				
13	Lift the jaw and tongue to check for objects, sweeping it out.				
14	Tilt the head back and give breaths again.				
15	Repeat breaths, back blows, and chest thrusts, and check for objects until the infant is breathing on his or her own.				
16	Wash hands.				
17	Document procedure.				
Student's Total Points					
Points Possible		340	170	85	
Final Score (Student's Total Points / Possible Points)					

	Notes
Start time:	
End time:	
Total time: (15 min goal)	

COMPETENCY ASSESSMENT

Procedure 9-8 Rescue Breathing for Adults

Performance Objectives: To respond to a breathing emergency. Perform this objective within 15 minutes with a minimum score of 60 points.

Supplies/Equipment: Gloves, resuscitation mouthpiece, biohazard waste receptacle

Charting/Documentation: Enter appropriate documentation/charting in the box.

Instructor's/Evaluator's Comments and Suggestions:

SKILLS CHECKLIST Procedure 9-8: Rescue Breathing for Adults

Name ______________________

Date ______________________

No.	Skill	Check #1 20 pts ea	Check #2 10 pts ea	Check #3 5 pts ea	Notes
1	Appoint someone to call emergency services.				
2	Don gloves.				
3	Shout "Are you all right?"				
4	Tilt head back and lift chin; position resuscitation mouthpiece and pinch the nose closed.				
5	Give two slow breaths into the patient, turn face to the side, listen, and watch for air return.				
6	Check for pulse on carotid attery.				
7	If pulse is present but the victim is not breathing, give 1 slow breath every 5 seconds for 1 minute.				
8	Recheck pulse and breathing status every minute.				
9	Continue rescue breathing as long as pulse is present and the victim is not breathing. Continue breathing until breathing is restored or someone else takes over.				
10	Disposes of waste in the biohazard container.				
11	Wash hands.				
12	Document procedure.				
Student's Total Points					
Points Possible		240	120	60	
Final Score (Student's Total Points / Possible Points)					

	Notes
Start time:	
End time:	
Total time: (15 min goal)	

COMPETENCY ASSESSMENT

Procedure 9-9 Rescue Breathing for Children

Performance Objectives: To respond to a breathing emergency involving a child. Perform this objective within 15 minutes with a minimum score of 65 points.

Supplies/Equipment: Gloves, resuscitation mouthpiece, biohazard waste receptacle

Charting/Documentation: Enter appropriate documentation/charting in the box.

Instructor's/Evaluator's Comments and Suggestions:

SKILLS CHECKLIST Procedure 9-9: Rescue Breathing for Children

Name ______________________________

Date ______________________________

No.	Skill	Check #1 20 pts ea	Check #2 10 pts ea	Check #3 5 pts ea	Notes
1	Appoints someone to call emergency services				
2	Don gloves.				
3	Position resuscitation mouthpiece.				
4	Tilt head back and lift chin, pinch nose closed, and give two short breaths.				
5	If air does not go in, retilt head and breathe again.				
6	Check for pulse on carotid attery.				
7	If pulse is present but the victim is not breathing, give 1 slow breath every 3 seconds for 1 minute.				
8	Recheck pulse and breathing status every minute.				
9	Continue rescue breathing as long as pulse is present and the victim is not breathing. Continue breathing until breathing is restored or someone else takes over.				
10	Wash hands.				
11	Document procedure.				
Student's Total Points					
Points Possible		260	130	65	
Final Score (Student's Total Points / Possible Points)					

	Notes
Start time:	
End time:	
Total time: (15 min goal)	

COMPETENCY ASSESSMENT

Procedure 9-10 Rescue Breathing for Infants

Performance Objectives: To restore breathing to an infant. Perform this objective within 15 minutes with a minimum score of 55 points.

Supplies/Equipment: Gloves, resuscitation mouthpiece, biohazard waste receptacle

Charting/Documentation: Enter appropriate documentation/charting in the box.

Instructor's/Evaluator's Comments and Suggestions:

SKILLS CHECKLIST Procedure 9-10: Rescue Breathing for Infants

Name ______________________

Date ______________________

No.	Skill	Check #1 20 pts ea	Check #2 10 pts ea	Check #3 5 pts ea	Notes
1	Appoint someone to call emergency services.				
2	Don gloves and resuscitation mouthpiece.				
3	Tilt head back.				
4	Seal lips tightly around infant's nose and mouth.				
5	Give two slow breaths into the infant until the chest rises.				
6	Check for pulse on brachial artery.				
7	If pulse is present but the victim is not breathing, give 1 slow breath every 3 seconds for 1 minute.				
8	Recheck pulse and breathing status every minute.				
9	Continue rescue breathing as long as pulse is present and the victim is not breathing. Continue breathing until breathing is restored or someone else takes over.				
10	Wash hands.				
11	Document procedure.				
Student's Total Points					
Points Possible		220	110	55	
Final Score (Student's Total Points / Possible Points)					

	Notes
Start time:	
End time:	
Total time: (15 min goal)	

COMPETENCY ASSESSMENT

Procedure 9-11 CPR for Adults

Performance Objectives: To restore breathing and cardiac activity in an emergency. Perform this objective within 15 minutes with a minimum score of 55 points.

Supplies/Equipment: Gloves, resuscitation mouthpiece, biohazard waste receptacle

Charting/Documentation: Enter appropriate documentation/charting in the box.

Instructor's/Evaluator's Comments and Suggestions:

SKILLS CHECKLIST Procedure 9-11: CPR for Adults

Name ______________________

Date ______________________

No.	Skill	Check #1 20 pts ea	Check #2 10 pts ea	Check #3 5 pts ea	Notes
1	Ask "Are you okay, are you okay?" If no response, appoint someone to call emergency services.				
2	Don gloves and resuscitation mouthpiece.				
3	Tilt head back and lift chin.				
4	Look, listen, and feel for breathing for 10–15 seconds. If the patient is not breathing, keep the airway open, pinch the nose, insert mouthpiece, and give two breaths.				
5	Check pulse at the carotid artery for 10–15 seconds; if the patient does not have a pulse, start chest compressions.				
6	After locating the area on the abdomen, 2 inches above the xiphoid, position the shoulders over the hands and compress the chest 15 times.				
7	Give two slow breaths, pinching the nose closed.				
8	Do 3 more sets of 15 compressions and two breaths.				
9	Check the pulse and breathing for 10–15 seconds.				
10	If there is no pulse, continue sets of 15 compressions to 2 breaths.				
11	Disposes of waste in biohazard container.				
Student's Total Points					
Points Possible		220	110	55	
Final Score (Student's Total Points / Possible Points)					

	Notes
Start time:	
End time:	
Total time: (15 min goal)	

COMPETENCY ASSESSMENT

Procedure 9-12 CPR for Children

Performance Objectives: To respond to a cardiac arrest emergency involving a child. Perform this objective within 15 minutes with a minimum score of 60 points.

Supplies/Equipment: Gloves, resuscitation mouthpiece

Charting/Documentation: Enter appropriate documentation/charting in the box.

Instructor's/Evaluator's Comments and Suggestions:

SKILLS CHECKLIST Procedure 9-12: CPR for Children

Name ______________________

Date ______________________

No.	Skill	Check #1 20 pts ea	Check #2 10 pts ea	Check #3 5 pts ea	Notes
1	Tap child to check for consciousness level; if no response, appoint someone to call emergency services.				
2	Don gloves and resuscitation mouthpiece.				
3	Tilt head back, look, listen, and feel for breathing. If there is no breathing, give two slow breaths.				
4	Check carotid artery.				
5	Locate one hand on the breastbone and the other hand on the forehead to maintain an open airway. Using the heel of one hand only, position shoulders over the patient's chest and compress the chest five times.				
6	Give one slow breath while pinching the nose closed.				
7	Repeat cycles of 5 compressions and 1 breath for 1 minute.				
8	Check pulse and breathing for about 5–10 seconds.				
9	If there is no pulse, continue sets of five compressions and one breath.				
10	Recheck the pulse and breathing every few minutes.				
11	Wash hands.				
12	Document procedure.				
Student's Total Points					
Points Possible		240	120	60	
Final Score (Student's Total Points / Possible Points)					

	Notes
Start time:	
End time:	
Total time: (15 min goal)	

COMPETENCY ASSESSMENT

Procedure 9-13 CPR for Infants

Performance Objectives: To restore the heartbeat in a cardiac arrest emergency involving an infant. Perform this objective within 15 minutes with a minimum score of 65 points.

Supplies/Equipment: Gloves, resuscitation mouthpiece

Charting/Documentation: Enter appropriate documentation/charting in the box.

Instructor's/Evaluator's Comments and Suggestions:

SKILLS CHECKLIST Procedure 9-13: CPR for Infants

Name ______________________

Date ______________________

No.	Skill	Check #1 20 pts ea	Check #2 10 pts ea	Check #3 5 pts ea	Notes
1	Tap child to check for consciousness level; if no response, appoint someone to call emergency services.				
2	Don gloves and resuscitation mouthpiece.				
3	Tilt head back, look, listen, and feel for breathing. If there is no breathing, give two slow breaths.				
4	Check brachial artery for pulse for 5–10 seconds.				
5	Find finger position on the center of sternum.				
6	Compress the infant's chest five times about 0.5–0.75 inch.				
7	Give one slow breath.				
8	Repeats cycle of 5 compressions and 1 breath for 1 minute.				
9	Recheck brachial pulse and breathing for 5–10 seconds.				
10	If there is no pulse, continue cycles for five compressions and one breath.				
11	Rechecks pulse and breathing every few minutes.				
12	Wash hands.				
13	Document procedure.				
Student's Total Points					
Points Possible		260	130	65	
Final Score (Student's Total Points / Possible Points)					

	Notes
Start time:	
End time:	
Total time: (15 min goal)	

EVALUATION OF CHAPTER KNOWLEDGE

Skills	Student Self-Evaluation Good	Average	Poor
I recognize emergency situations.	_____	_____	_____
I understand the need for emergency preparation and the function of emergency medical services (EMS).	_____	_____	_____
I possess the ability to triage emergency cases in person and over the telephone.	_____	_____	_____
I understand legal and health considerations of emergency caregiving.	_____	_____	_____
I understand the necessity of providing emergency care only within the scope of training and knowledge.	_____	_____	_____
I can assemble a medical crash tray or cart.	_____	_____	_____
I understand the use of Standard Precautions in emergency situations.	_____	_____	_____
I can identify signs and symptoms of shock, types of shock, and treatment of shock.	_____	_____	_____
I can identify classification and care of wounds.	_____	_____	_____
I can identify dressings, bandages, and their applications.	_____	_____	_____
I can identify first-, second-, and third-degree burns and burn care.	_____	_____	_____
I can identify musculoskeletal injuries, including types of fractures and strategies for care.	_____	_____	_____
I can identify heat- and cold-related illnesses and priorities for care.	_____	_____	_____
I understand how poisons enter the body.	_____	_____	_____
I can identify sudden illnesses such as syncope, seizures, diabetes, and hemorrhage.	_____	_____	_____
I recognize cerebral vascular accident (CVA) and priorities for immediate emergency care.	_____	_____	_____
I recognize heart attack and priorities for immediate emergency care.	_____	_____	_____
I can identify and name steps for performing these emergency procedures:			
Control of bleeding	_____	_____	_____
Applying a splint	_____	_____	_____
Abdominal thrusts	_____	_____	_____
Rescue breathing	_____	_____	_____
Cardiopulmonary resuscitation (CPR)	_____	_____	_____

CHAPTER 10

Creating the Facility Environment

CHAPTER PRE-TEST

Perform this test without looking at the book. This is just to see how well you have understood and can recall the information in this chapter after you have read it, but before you have completed the workbook exercises. You will not be graded on this portion (other than the grade you give yourself). Justify any "false" answers.

1. A reception area should:
   a. be comfortable
   b. be clean and uncluttered
   c. contain current reading materials for all ages
   d. all of the above
2. It is considerate, but not required, to provide at least one handicapped patient parking space. (T or F)
3. Keeping the reception area clean is a responsibility of:
   a. the receptionist
   b. the bookkeeper
   c. the medical assistant
   d. the office manger
   e. all of the above

INTRODUCTION

Medical assistants are generally employed in ambulatory care settings, such as the medical office or clinic. The physical environment of the health care facility is an important contributing factor to patient comfort. Effective facility design and layout can also increase efficiency and boost the medical facility's functional utility. Medical assistants recognize that maintaining a professional, welcoming environment for patient care promotes health and increases patient confidence in the physician and in the entire health care team. Complying with the Americans with Disabilities Act (ADA) also ensures that the physically challenged have equal access to care.

PERFORMANCE OBJECTIVES

After successful completion of this chapter you will be able to describe a comfortable and efficient reception area, list and describe the specific items that should be present, and describe the arrangement of the furnishings, the role of Health Insurance Portability and Accountability Act (HIPAA) on the reception area, and the effect your reception area has on your patients. You will be able to discuss the requirement of the ADA for your office entrance and space. You will be able to describe the characteristics of a good medical receptionist and cite the procedures to follow when the patient's appointment is delayed. You will also know how to open and close the office. *The following statements are related to your learning objectives for this chapter. Fill in the blanks in the following paragraph with the appropriate term(s).*

The reception area should make the patient feel (1) ________________________, secure, and comfortable. Proper seating should be available with adequate (2) ____________________ for reading. The furnishings should be able to accommodate at least (3) ______________ hour's patients per physician, assuming that one friend or relative will accompany each patient. If the clinic sees children or expects that patients will bring children, a special (4) ________________ area should be set aside with appropriate (5) _______________ and books. The receptionist should have the (6) ________________________ and (7) _____________________ to handle many situations without getting upset. He or she must be willing to assist patients whenever necessary and keep the schedule flowing smoothly. Although keeping the reception area neat and clean is probably the responsibility of the (8) __________________, all employees should contribute by noticing and correcting any untidy or unclean situation. When opening the facility in the morning, the reception area should be checked, the patient (9) _____________ should be prepared if not done so the day before, and the answering (10) ________________________ should be checked for messages. When closing the facility, all equipment should be checked to make sure it is (11) ___________________________, doors and (12) _______________________ should be secured, all (13) _______________ material should be locked away or covered, and the (14) ____________________ cash should be locked away.

VOCABULARY BUILDER

Find the words below that are misspelled; circle them, and then correctly spell them in the spaces provided. Then insert vocabulary terms from the list that best fit into the descriptive sentences below.

accessibility	characteristic	infomatics
accountibility	enviroment	receptionist
____________________	____________________	____________________

1. ____ Information available through the Internet or other electronic format
2. ____ The physical space of the reception area

3. ______________________________ A typical or distinguishing quality
4. ______________________________ The medical assistant who greets the patient and begins the patient visit process: this person may also answer the phones
5. ______________________________ Being ultimately responsible
6. ______________________________ Being readily reachable

Word Game

Find the words in the grid. Pick them out from left to right, top line to bottom line. Words can go horizontally, vertically, and diagonally in all eight directions. When you are finished, the first few unused letters in the grid will spell out a hidden message.

L	S	C	I	T	A	M	R	O	F	N	I	O	O	P	E
K	E	A	T	Y	F	A	C	I	L	I	T	Y	L	S	N
O	U	L	R	R	E	C	E	P	G	T	I	A	O	C	V
N	A	R	B	E	A	A	S	N	A	A	Y	P	G	I	I
A	D	E	L	A	Y	S	I	T	C	I	T	E	N	T	R
N	T	W	O	U	T	D	L	C	D	S	V	I	I	S	O
D	E	L	W	A	A	R	E	I	I	T	.	F	T	I	N
T	E	F	I	E	A	S	O	N	K	T	K	V	I	R	M
J	J	S	R	G	S	P	O	F	G	P	B	T	V	E	E
F	N	N	I	I	H	I	I	N	M	T	Y	T	N	T	N
R	N	Z	B	G	T	T	I	H	K	O	M	O	I	C	T
L	D	L	H	P	N	M	I	Z	Z	R	C	Y	A	A	V
K	E	V	E	L	L	H	B	N	Z	N	Q	S	D	R	K
N	T	C	W	A	G	P	L	Q	G	M	Z	M	A	A	L
R	E	L	C	B	G	N	I	M	O	C	L	E	W	H	V
R	K	M	N	R	F	U	R	N	I	T	U	R	E	C	G

accessible
ADA
calming
characteristics
comfortable
delays
design
environment
facility
furniture
HIPAA
informatics
inviting
lighting
play
reading
receptionist
toys
welcoming

LEARNING REVIEW

1. A. What is the purpose of the ADA?

____

____

____

____

   B. When creating the facility environment, why is accessibility a major consideration?

____

____

____

____

   C. Name four ways an ambulatory care setting can accommodate the physically challenged.

   (1) ____

   (2) ____

   (3) ____

   (4) ____

2. The physical office environment can contribute to the patient's sense of confidence and comfort, or it can be viewed by the patient as intimidating or anxiety producing. For each office area below, describe why the area could be perceived by patients as a frightening place. What can be done to make each area a more comforting environment for patients?

   Reception area ____

____

____

____

____

   Corridors ____

____

____

____

   Examination rooms ____

____

____

____

3. Health care professionals should strive to empower the patient with as much control and dignity as possible. For each of the following situations listed, identify strategies that health care professionals can use to respect the patient's dignity and lessen the sense of disproportion between health care providers and the patient.

A. Bill Schwartz is referred to a dermatologist by Dr. Ray Reynolds for examination of a suspicious mole on his calf. The dermatologist tells Bill that a full-body inspection will need to be done to ensure that no other areas of the skin are affected. Bill must appear disrobed in front of the dermatologist and medical assistant, who are both female.

B. Martin Gordon, diagnosed with prostate cancer, begins a series of radiation treatments. At the radiation clinic, he is required to disrobe from the waist down and put on a hospital gown. While waiting for access to the treatment room, Martin must sit in a common area with other patients, male and female, who are also waiting for radiation treatments.

C. Ellen Armstrong, CMA, places a Holter monitor on patient Charles Williams. After the Holter monitor is in place, Charles has several questions about the patient activity diary that he would prefer to discuss with Dr. Winston Lewis.

4. The medical receptionist, often a medical assistant with other duties to perform as well, is the person who sets the social climate for the interchange between the patient and the health care team. A friendly, reassuring demeanor and an ability to triage situations are essential skills. For each situation listed, what is the best action or response of the medical receptionist?

A. A patient with intense stomach pain doubles over, and then bolts up to the reception desk, saying, "I'm going to throw up."

B. When presented with a bill, the patient exclaims, "I can't pay for all of this now! Every time I come here it seems like the doctor bill goes up a hundred dollars."

C. A patient is looking for the correct exit from the examination area to the waiting area and makes a wrong turn into the receptionist's area. He asks, "Where do I go?"

____

____

D. A patient new to an HMO plan does not realize that a separate referral form is needed for a follow-up visit with the gastroenterologist one week after a colonoscopy test has been performed. She says, "I drove an hour to get to this appointment. No one told me I needed another form."

____

____

____

____

5. Identify at least four things to be done in the reception area to accommodate children.
   (1) ____
   (2) ____
   (3) ____
   (4) ____

6. A. Create a checklist of five activities to perform on opening a medical facility.
   (1) ____
   (2) ____
   (3) ____
   (4) ____
   (5) ____

   B. Create a checklist of five activities to perform on closing a medical facility.
   (1) ____
   (2) ____
   (3) ____
   (4) ____
   (5) ____

7. Making facilities and equipment available to all users is called:
   a. maintenance
   b. accessibility
   c. promotion
   d. standardization

8. HIPAA requires that clinic facilities:
   a. have adequate corridors and bathrooms to accommodate wheelchair patients
   b. place a receptionist in an area seen and heard by all patients

c. protect the confidentiality of patients checking in at the reception desk

d. provide space for children in the clinic

9. The primary goal of maintaining a comfortable environment in which patient care is given is to:

 a. feed anxiety

 b. aggravate illness

 c. promote health

 d. stimulate the senses

10. Space planners suggest:

 a. that the reception area accommodate at least 2 hours' patients per physician

 b. that the reception area can accommodate a friend or relative who might accompany each patient

 c. that there be 2.5 seats in the reception area for each examination room

 d. only b and c

11. Any drugs kept in the office that are identified as controlled substances must always be kept:

 a. in the refrigerator

 b. in a locked, secure cabinet

 c. in the physician's desk drawer

 d. in the receptionist's desk drawer

CERTIFICATION REVIEW

These questions are designed to mimic the certification examinations. You can use these questions like a small "Certification Examination Study Guide," but this is not meant to take the place of the more extensive study guides. Use this portion to determine where to concentrate your efforts when studying for the certification examination.

1. HIPAA has changed the way we organize our entrance and reception areas in the following way:

 a. Patients must be able to see the receptionist at all times.

 b. Patients must have adequate parking.

 c. Patients must not be able to see or hear confidential information about other patients.

 d. The magazines must be current.

2. ADA states that:

 a. Patients must not know the names and diagnoses of other patients.

 b. Handicapped patients must have access to all patient areas with reasonable accommodations.

 c. Visually impaired patients must have adequate lighting and contrast for better viewing.

 d. An interpreter must be present with any non–English-speaking patient.

3. Patient safety within the reception area is accomplished by:
   a. providing chairs that are sturdy and in good repair
   b. containing wires and cords and keeping them out of reach
   c. attaching rugs to the flooring without loose edges
   d. containing toys within a designated play area
   e. all of the above

CASE STUDY

Lydia Renzi, a deaf woman with some residual hearing, is a patient of Dr. Angie Esposito's at Inner City Health Care. Lydia is fluent in American Sign Language (ASL) and usually wears a hearing aid when she is away from home.

Lydia calls to make her appointment at Inner City Health Care using a telecommunications device for the deaf (TDD) and the services of a government-funded relay operator. Although Lydia often chooses not to be accompanied by an interpreter, Inner City Health Care always provides the option to supply the services of a qualified professional sign language interpreter in compliance with the ADA. When Lydia arrives at Inner City Health Care with a high fever and a suspected case of the flu, the staff accommodates Lydia's special needs in several simple ways. Remembering that deaf people rely on visual images to receive and to convey messages, Liz Corbin, CMA, always faces Lydia directly so that the patient can see her facial expressions and lip movements. Liz holds eye contact with Lydia and does not break it until she is sure that Lydia understands her message and has time to think and respond. Special care is taken to provide Lydia with written instructions for prescriptions and for following through on home care.

Discuss the following:

1. What are the special communication needs of the hearing-impaired patient in the ambulatory care setting?
2. How can the medical assistant's actions make a direct impact on the quality of care given to hearing-impaired patients?
3. Suppose that Lydia is an elderly woman who is embarrassed and sensitive about her hearing loss and will not admit that she has trouble hearing others. How might the medical assistant accommodate the special needs of this patient?

SELF-ASSESSMENT

1. Visualize your last visit to a medical facility. Was the reception area clean, tidy, welcoming, and comfortable? What would you do to improve it?

   ____

   ____

   ____

   ____

2. List at least three things you would add to any reception area to make it even more accommodating. Think of items not mentioned in the textbook.

   ____

   ____

   ____

   ____

CHAPTER POST-TEST

This is similar to the Pre-Test. Perform this test without looking at the book. This is just to see how well you have understood and can recall the information presented in this chapter after you have studied it and completed the workbook exercises. You will not be graded on this portion (other than the grade you give yourself), but this is an excellent preparation for your instructor's test. You may use this Post-Test to determine what areas you need to study more. Justify any "false" answers.

1. A receptioning area should:
   a. be comfortable, clean, and uncluttered
   b. contain current reading materials for all ages
   c. have adequate lighting for reading
   d. contain accommodations for patients with disabilities
   e. all of the above
2. It is required to provide at least one handicapped patient parking space. (T or F)
3. Keeping the reception area clean is a responsibility of:
   a. the receptionist
   b. the bookkeeper
   c. the medical assistant
   d. the office manger
   e. all employees

CERTIFICATION CRITERIA CHECKLIST

As you go through your education and training, keep in mind the national certification examination that you will take when you graduate. Each chapter of the textbook and workbook covers a different section of the examination criteria. To keep track of your preparation for the certification examination, turn to the back of this workbook and highlight the following CMA, RMA, or CMAS certification examination criteria (if you have already highlighted them from a previous chapter, put a check mark by the criteria):

CMA

F. Medicolegal Guidelines & Requirements
   2. Legislation
   3. Documentation/reporting

O. Managing the Office
   1. Maintaining the physical plant

RMA

II. Administrative Medical Assisting
   C. Medical Receptionist/Secretarial/Clerical
      2. Reception
      5. Records and chart management
      9. Office safety

CMAS

3. Medical Office Clerical Assisting
   - Reception
4. Medical Records Management
   - Systems
   - Confidentiality

EVALUATION OF CHAPTER KNOWLEDGE

	Student Self-Evaluation		
Skills	Good	Average	Poor
I can identify tasks in opening and closing the facility.	_____	_____	_____
I recognize the importance of the medical receptionist.	_____	_____	_____
I can relate the physical environment of the facility to the patient's care and comfort.	_____	_____	_____
I can relate the physical environment of the facility to optimal functionality and efficiency.	_____	_____	_____
I know how to safeguard patient privacy.	_____	_____	_____
I understand the purpose of the ADA and can describe methods of compliance.	_____	_____	_____
I am able to empathize with the patient experience of the health care facility.	_____	_____	_____

CHAPTER 11

Computers in the Ambulatory Care Setting

CHAPTER PRE-TEST

Perform this test without looking at the book. This is just to see how well you have understood and can recall the information in this chapter after you have read it, but before you have completed the workbook exercises. You will not be graded on this portion (other than the grade you give yourself). Justify any "false" answers.

1. One main advantage of e-mail is:
   a. you have an immediate response
   b. messages are secure
   c. everybody has access
   d. you do not have to play "telephone tag"

2. To ensure that your work in the computer is safe, you should:
   a. use only formatted discs
   b. defragment frequently
   c. use firewalls
   d. backup frequently

3. Circle each of the following that is a computer function:
   a. keeping track of appointments
   b. keeping track of accounts receivable
   c. keeping track of accounts payable
   d. processing insurance claims

4. The "brain" of the computer is called the:
   a. motherboard
   b. math coprocessor

c. video card
d. central processing unit (CPU)

5. To prevent unauthorized use of your clinic computers, you should:
   a. keep the computer in a locked cabinet at all times
   b. keep the computer in a locked cabinet at night
   c. assign every employee a password
   d. have only one person on the computer at a time

6. The difference between a spreadsheet and a database is:
   a. Databases keep track of numbers.
   b. Spreadsheets calculate numbers.
   c. Databases organize information.
   d. Spreadsheets organize information.
   e. They are both the same and function the same.

INTRODUCTION

Ambulatory care settings have made the transition from manual to computerized systems. Medical assistants with a knowledge of computer equipment, or hardware, and computer programs, or software, are a strong asset to the medical office. Today, computers are used in complex clinical applications such as assisting in performing sensitive surgeries, diagnosing illnesses, and developing patient treatment strategies. In the ambulatory care setting, physicians purchase computer systems to perform administrative tasks, such as patient data collection, correspondence, reports, billing, and insurance claim filing. Confidentiality of computerized patient records must be strictly maintained. Medical assistants are expected to be able to learn and use office computer applications. Often, medical assistants are involved in researching and implementing computer applications for specific administrative office functions. Medical assisting students are encouraged to explore the potential of computers. Perhaps intimidating at first, with a little experience computers can become user-friendly tools that offer valuable methods for streamlining tasks and increasing efficiency in the ambulatory care setting.

PERFORMANCE OBJECTIVES

After successful completion of this chapter you will be able to define the correct vocabulary terms in this chapter, describe the basic elements of a computer system, identify main types of computers, list examples of input and output devices, explain how computer information can be stored, describe networks, explain the various uses for computers in the medical clinic, explain ergonomics, cite ways to prevent computer viruses, use various computer software applications, and explain how Health Insurance Portability and Accountability Act (HIPAA) regulations can be maintained within a computerized office. You will be able to follow professional behavior while using clinic computers. *The following statements are related to your learning objectives for this chapter. Fill in the blanks in the following paragraph with the appropriate term(s).*

The four fundamental elements of a computer are (1) ______________________________, (2) ______________________________, (3) ______________________________, and (4) ______________________________. Four main types of computers are

(5)______________________________, (6) ______________________________,
(7) ______________________________, and (8) ______________________________.
Two examples of commonly used input devices are (9) ______________________________ and (10) ______________________________. Two examples of output devices are (11) ______________________________ and (12) ______________________________.
Three common ways to store computer information are (13) ______________________________, (14) ______________________________, and (15) ______________________________.
Networks might best be described as an (16) ______________________________connection of two or more computers for the purpose of sharing information. Hardwired networks are referred to as (17) ________________. Wireless systems are capable of a much (18) (more or less) rapid rate of data transmission than the hard-wired systems. Hard-wired systems are (19) (more or less) secure from hacking or other unauthorized access. One way of protecting the clinic computer from damage from an outside source is to install (20) ______________________________ software and keep it updated. HIPAA privacy rules require that no (21) ____________________ persons be allowed access to private medical and personal information. One way to accomplish this when patient information is stored on computers is to use (22) ______________________.

VOCABULARY BUILDER

A. *Find the words below that are misspelled; circle them, and then correctly spell them in the spaces provided. Then insert the correct vocabulary terms from the list that best fit the descriptions below.*

A. erganomics	G. modom
B. hardware	H. personal computer
C. Internet	I. RAM
D. maneframe computer	J. supercomputer
E. microcomputer	K. system
F. minicomputer	

____________________ ____________________ ____________________

______ 1. A device used by a computer to communicate to a remote computer through phone lines

______ 2. The scientific study of work and space, including factors that influence workers' productivity and that affect workers' health

______ 3. A large computer system capable of processing massive volumes of data

______ 4. A personal, or desktop, computer

______ 5. Acronym for random access memory, a type of computer memory that can be written to and read from

______ 6. The physical equipment used by the computer system to process data

______ 7. Larger than a microcomputer and smaller than a mainframe

______ 8. A worldwide computer network available via modem

______ 9. The fastest, largest, and most expensive computers currently being manufactured

______ 10. Also known as microcomputer

______ 11. A unit composed of a number of parts that function together to perform a particular task

B. *Find the words below that are misspelled; circle them, and then correctly spell them in the spaces provided. Then insert the correct vocabulary terms from the list that best fit the descriptions below.*

A. applications software
B. bit
C. byte
D. communications software
E. data
F. database managment software
G. documentation
H. electronic mail
I. feilds
J. footers
K. graphics software
L. headers
M. information retieval systems
N. macros
O. merge mail
P. operating system
Q. orphen
R. record
S. software
T. sort
U. spreadsheat software
V. widow
W. word processing software

____________________ ____________________ ____________________

____________________ ____________________

______ 1. A page formatting feature that allows the bottom of all pages to be marked consistently with keyed-in data

______ 2. The raw material; the collection of characters and numbers entered into a computer

______ 3. A word processing operation designed to produce form letters

______ 4. Software that provides instructions to the computer hardware and also runs computer programs

______ 5. Systems that allow electronic access to large databases for the retrieval of information

______ 6. Related fields, grouped together and organized in the same order

______ 7. Smallest unit of data a computer can process

______ 8. Applications software used to create pictorial representations

______ 9. A frequently used data processing operation that arranges data in a particular sequence or order

______ 10. In typesetting, a term describing the situation in which a new paragraph begins on the last line of a printed page

______ 11. Communications that take place online from computer to computer by means of a modem

______ 12. Equivalent of a computer program or programs

______ 13. Amount of memory needed to store one character

______ 14. A page formatting feature that allows the top of a page to be printed with identifying information

______ 15. A series of keystrokes that have been saved under a separate file name that can be used and inserted repeatedly into a document or documents

______ 16. Software that performs a specific data processing function

______ 17. A computer application that allows the user to format and edit documents before printing

______ 18. A basic data category within the database

______ 19. Computer applications packages that act as "number crunchers" because of their mathematical processing capabilities

______ 20. Written material that accompanies purchased software, containing the information necessary for using the software appropriately

______ 21. Applications software used for the transfer of data from one computer system to another

______ 22. In typesetting, a term describing the situation in which a line of text that is the end of a paragraph ends on a new page of printed text

______ 23. Applications software designed for the manipulation of data within a database

LEARNING REVIEW

1. Medical assistants may encounter many types of software in the ambulatory care setting, including scheduling (S); word processing (WP); clinical (C); accounting (A); billing, collecting, and insurance (BCI); and practice management (PM).

   Identify the tasks listed below according to the type of software used to perform them by placing the proper letters in the spaces provided.

   _____ A. inventories and drug supplies
   _____ B. medical records
   _____ C. aging accounts receivable
   _____ D. patient reminders
   _____ E. employee vacation records
   _____ F. charge slips
   _____ G. insurance claim processing
   _____ H. check writing
   _____ I. labels and addressing
   _____ J. prescription writing
   _____ K. payroll
   _____ L. thank you letters
   _____ M. consultation reports
   _____ N. treatment plans

2. Computer systems are great assets to any ambulatory care setting in streamlining tasks and increasing productivity. Special steps need to be taken to keep the systems operating at peak efficiency. Name three steps medical assistants should take in the care and handling of computer components.

   (1) ______________________________

   (2) ______________________________

   (3) ______________________________

3. There are six operations that are fundamental to the operation of any computer software. Identify the proper operation in the examples below.

_______________ A. Administrative medical assistant Ellen Armstrong, CMA, working in the offices of Drs. Lewis and King, makes adjustments in format and corrects spelling and punctuation errors in a thank you letter the practice sends to new patients.

_______________ B. Ellen prepares a hard copy of Martin Gordon's treatment plan for Dr. Winston Lewis.

_______________ C. Office manager Marilyn Johnson, CMA, asks Ellen to add columns to the existing drug inventory spreadsheet.

_______________ D. Ellen enters data on employee vacation and sick time into the new spreadsheet software.

_______________ E. After entering all of the patient addresses into a single file, Ellen makes sure that the file will be retained permanently.

_______________ F. On request from Dr. Elizabeth King, Ellen produces the most recent correspondence sent to patient Maria Jover.

4. Word processing is largely concerned with the production of textual material and is an integral part of the ambulatory care setting. Match the following common word processing features with the correct descriptions.

A. multicolumn output
B. macros
C. page formatting
D. sorting
E. import and export
F. block operations

_____ 1. These allow the user to highlight and move text to another position within the document

_____ 2. This refers to the rearrangement of information

_____ 3. Allows users to carry a text file into another applications program

_____ 4. Keystrokes that have been saved separately so the saved keystrokes may be inserted into any document

_____ 5. The arrangement of text on a page in two or more columns

_____ 6. This is used to create a variety of looks for the printed page

5. Spreadsheet software "crunches," or calculates, numbers. Define the following elements of spreadsheet programs.

A. Cell location _______________

B. Worksheet _______________

C. Values _______________

D. Labels _______________

Name three tasks for which spreadsheet software is particularly useful.

(1) ____________________

(2) ____________________

(3) ____________________

6. A. Databases or database management systems (DBMS) are built from the concept of data organization. Name four elements that comprise the organization of data.

(1) ____________________ (3) ____________________

(2) ____________________ (4) ____________________

B. Ellen Armstrong, CMA, is creating a patient database for the offices of Drs. Lewis and King. The office currently maintains information on 1,000 patients. List 10 fields of information the database should contain to track the patients.

(1) ____________________

(2) ____________________

(3) ____________________

(4) ____________________

(5) ____________________

(6) ____________________

(7) ____________________

(8) ____________________

(9) ____________________

(10) ____________________

7. The use of computerized databases in the delivery of health care services is becoming an established methodology for patient care. However, the trend toward computerizing medical records and the electronic processing of insurance claims presents challenges in preserving patient confidentiality.

A. Name the federal legislation that protects against unauthorized access or interception of data communication.

____

B. The ____________________ has put forth guidelines to follow for the enactment of laws that protect individual privacy and confidentiality.

8. The American Medical Association (AMA) has published computer confidentiality guidelines to assist physicians and computer service organizations in maintaining the confidentiality of information in medical records when that information is stored in computerized databases.

A. Confidential medical information should be entered into the computer-based patient record only by ____________________.

B. The person making any additions to the record should be ______________________.

C. The computerized medical database should be online to the computer terminal only when ____________________________ are being used.

D. Name three security measures that can be used to control access to the computerized database.

(1) ____

(2) ____

(3) ____

9. The monitor or screen that provides a real-time feedback of what is taking place with input data is:
   a. data storage
   b. data output
   c. formatting
   d. retrieval

10. Accounting, scheduling, and insurance coding are examples of:
    a. application software
    b. system software
    c. word processing software
    d. database management

11. Arrangement of information so that it is concise, easy to read, and in word processing files includes setting margins, line spacing, and tab settings is:
    a. editing
    b. file creation
    c. retrieval
    d. formatting

12. One of the health hazards associated with repetitive computer use is:
    a. Ménière's disease
    b. Bell's palsy
    c. carpal tunnel syndrome
    d. rheumatoid arthiritis

13. A term used for the precautions taken to prevent persons from hacking into computer systems through the Internet is:
    a. dam
    b. firewall
    c. stonewall
    d. retention wall

CERTIFICATION REVIEW

These questions are designed to mimic the certification examinations. You can use these questions like a small "Certification Examination Study Guide," but this is not meant to take the place of the more extensive study guides. Use this portion to determine what areas to concentrate your efforts when studying for the certification examination.

1. A flashing bar that indicates where you are on the computer screen is called the:
   a. scroll bar
   b. cursor
   c. flash bar
   d. input bar
2. A flash drive is a:
   a. memory device
   b. type of software device
   c. a DVD drive
   d. a safety warning
3. Hacker is a term given to:
   a. a computer operator with inconsistent word processing
   b. a computer operator with a very bad cough
   c. a computer that goes off and on for no reason
   d. a person who gets into a computer system without permission
4. RAM stands for:
   a. reality actuated memory
   b. random access memory
   c. right access mouse
   d. retrieval access motherboard
5. Firewalls will prevent:
   a. fires from damaging your information
   b. fires from damaging your computer
   c. damage from spreading from one area of your computer to another
   d. damage from unauthorized access
6. Defragmenting gets rid of:
   a. fragments of information that you do not need anymore
   b. old information no longer needed
   c. empty spaces within your database
   d. fragments of software that you do not use

CASE STUDY

The offices of Drs. Lewis and King recently experienced a pronounced surge in patient load when the physician–employers agreed to accept patients from several HMOs operating in the area. The group practice added two new staff members, co-office manager Shirley Brooks, CMA, and clinical medical assistant Anna Preciado, CMA. To handle the increased load of paperwork, Dr. Winston Lewis asks Shirley to devise a database to identify patient insurance variables. The practice already has a functional database of patient information.

Discuss the following:

1. What strategies will Shirley use to research the proper database software and to determine the desired organization of information within the new patient insurance database?
2. What information will the patient insurance database need to contain to allow for the streamlining of paperwork and claims processing?
3. What will the office manager do when she has completed her research and has devised a plan for assembling the patient insurance database?

SELF-ASSESSMENT

1. How comfortable are you with moving a computer from one area to another and hooking up all the cords, connections, and wires? What do you think you could do to become more comfortable with computer hardware connections. Look at the connections of your computer and its accessory hardware. Is it color coded or marked in some way?

2. How comfortable are you with installing a software program onto a computer? Would you be able to do it by yourself? How about defragmenting? Formatting a disc? Updating virus protection? Next time it is appropriate to perform these actions, ask your technical support person/department to let you watch, or ask a technically experienced person to show you how.

3. Have you explored all the options in your e-mail software system? Set up groups? Set up signatures? Asked for a return reply? Explore the options and set up these actions.

CHAPTER POST-TEST

This is similar to the Pre-Test. Perform this test without looking at the book. This is just to see how well you have understood and can recall the information presented in this chapter after you have studied it and completed the workbook exercises. You will not be graded on this portion (other than the grade you give yourself), but this is an excellent preparation for your instructor's test. You may use this Post-Test to determine what areas you need to study more. Justify any "false" answers.

1. A disadvantage of e-mail is:
   a. you do not have an immediate response
   b. messages are not secure
   c. not everyone has access
   d. all of the above

2. To ensure that your computer information is safe from unauthorized viewing:
   a. use only formatted discs
   b. defragment frequently
   c. use firewalls
   d. backup frequently

3. Which of the following is a not a computer function:
   a. keeping track of appointments
   b. keeping track of accounts receivable
   c. keeping track of accounts payable
   d. processing insurance claims
   e. fixing dinner

4. A circuit board that houses the chips for the CPU, RAM, and ROM is called the:
   a. motherboard
   b. math coprocessor
   c. video card
   d. CPU board

5. To prevent unauthorized use of your clinic's computers, you should:
   a. establish only one person who has access to the computer
   b. keep the computer in a locked cabinet at night
   c. assign every employee a password
   d. have only one person on the computer at a time

6. A database:
   a. keeps track of numbers and other information
   b. calculates numbers
   c. organizes information
   d. functions like a spreadsheet

CERTIFICATION CRITERIA CHECKLIST

As you go through your education and training, keep in mind the national certification examination that you will take when you graduate. Each chapter of the textbook and workbook covers a different section of the examination criteria. To keep track of your preparation for the certification examination, turn to the back of this workbook and highlight the following CMA, RMA, or CMAS certification examination criteria (if you have already highlighted them from a previous chapter, put a check mark by the criteria):

CMA

D. Professionalism
   4. Maintaining confidentiality

F. Medicolegal Guidelines & Requirements
   2. Legislation

G. Data Entry
   1. Keyboard fundamentals and functions

H. Equipment

I. Computer Concepts

RMA

II. Administrative Medical Assisting
   - C. Medical Receptionist/Secretarial/Clerical
      - 8. Computer applications

CMAS

7. Medical Office Information Processing
   - Fundamentals of computing
   - Medical office computer applications

COMPETENCY ASSESSMENT

Procedure 11-1 Software Installation

Performance Objectives: To add software to the computer system for later call up and use. Perform this objective within 15 minutes with a minimum score of 15 points for automatic installation and 25 points for manual installation.

Supplies/Equipment: Manual, computer, software program

Charting/Documentation: Enter appropriate documentation/charting in the box.

Instructor's/Evaluator's Comments and Suggestions:

SKILLS CHECKLIST Procedure 11-1: Software Installation

Name ______________________

Date ______________________

No.	Skill	Check #1 20 pts ea	Check #2 10 pts ea	Check #3 5 pts ea	Notes
Automatic Installation					
1	Close all open programs.				
2	Insert the CD provided with the program into the CD drive.				
3	Follow the instructions given by the software documentation and the Installation Wizard screens that appear.				
4	At the completion of the program, you will respond to questions appropriately. Example is the registration of the software package.				
Manual Installation					
1	Close all open programs.				
2	Insert CD. Click START, then select RUN from the menu.				
3	Respond to the questions appropriately, such as the name and address of the program you want to run for installation.				
4	Include the letter destination for the drive where the program is located (usually D drive). Common name is: Setup. Example: D:\setup.				
5	Follow onscreen instructions.				
Student's Total Points					
Points Possible (depending on type of installation)		60 or 100	30 or 50	15 or 25	
Final Score (Student's Total Points / Possible Points)					

	Notes
Start time:	
End time:	
Total time: (15 min goal)	

COMPETENCY ASSESSMENT

Procedure 11-2 Hardware Installation

Performance Objectives: To add hardware to the computer system for later use. Perform this objective within 15 minutes with a minimum score of 25 points for automatic installation and 15 points for manual installation.

Supplies/Equipment: Manual, computer, hardware to be installed

Charting/Documentation: Enter appropriate documentation/charting in the box.

Instructor's/Evaluator's Comments and Suggestions:

SKILLS CHECKLIST Procedure 11-2: Hardware Installation

Name ______________________

Date ______________________

No.	Skill	Check #1 20 pts ea	Check #2 10 pts ea	Check #3 5 pts ea	Notes
Using Automatic Initiation from Microsoft Windows® Installation Wizard					
1	Close all open programs.				
2	Answer questions appropriately such as: Manufacturer and Model Number of the hardware				
3	How the hardware is connected to the computer (Via USB, Parallel, or IEEE 1394 cable).				
4	Whether the driver was supplied with the hardware or already registered with Microsoft.				
5	Follow further directions.				
Using Manual Initiation of Microsoft Windows® Installation Wizard					
1	Close all open programs.				
2	Go to START, SETTINGS, CONTROL PANEL, and double click ADD HARDWARE.				
3	Follow onscreen instructions.				
Student's Total Points					
Points Possible (depending on type of installation)		100 or 60	50 or 30	25 or 15	
Final Score (Student's Total Points / Possible Points)					

	Notes
Start time:	
End time:	
Total time: (15 min goal)	

EVALUATION OF CHAPTER KNOWLEDGE

Skills	Student Self-Evaluation Good	Average	Poor
I understand how computers enhance office efficiency and can give examples of specific methods.	_____	_____	_____
I can identify types of computer hardware.	_____	_____	_____
I can distinguish between systems and applications software.	_____	_____	_____
I can identify categories of applications software and can describe the purpose of each.	_____	_____	_____
I can apply database management concepts to ambulatory care setting.	_____	_____	_____
I understand issues of preserving patient confidentiality and can identify guidelines for maintaining confidentiality.	_____	_____	_____
I recognize the potential of computer for locating resources and information.	_____	_____	_____
I can relate relevant ergonomic theories and give guidelines for setting up ergonomic workstations.	_____	_____	_____
I recognize the growing role of medical assistants as information managers.	_____	_____	_____
I can discuss the increasing role of computers in medicine for both clinical and administrative tasks.	_____	_____	_____

CHAPTER 12

Telecommunications

CHAPTER PRE-TEST

Perform this test without looking at the book. This is just to see how well you have understood and can recall the information in this chapter after you have read it, but before you have completed the workbook exercises. You will not be graded on this portion (other than the grade you give yourself). Justify any "false" answers.

1. When transferring a call, it is not necessary to obtain the patient's name and phone number. (T or F)
2. Some patients need to be handled with a firm voice on the phone. (T or F)
3. We do not always have time to ask patients if they can be put on hold. (T or F)
4. When taking a message, be as brief as possible. The patient's name and phone number is enough information. (T or F)
5. Patients cannot expect confidentiality on their home answering machines. (T or F)
6. All angry calls should be forwarded to the physician. (T or F)

INTRODUCTION

Telephone communication, including facsimile (fax) and electronic mail (e-mail) transmission, is crucial to the effective management of the ambulatory care setting. Medical assistants use the telephone to speak with patients; schedule appointments; respond to emergencies; and communicate with physicians, health care professionals, and others. To become efficient, successful communicators, medical assistants must be familiar with proper telephone etiquette, understand the extent of their authority when answering questions and releasing information, and develop proficiency in the use of various telephone systems and technologies. Upholding patient confidentiality and maintaining a professional telephone manner are essential skills of the medical assistant.

PERFORMANCE OBJECTIVES

After successful completion of this chapter you will be able to explain the proper techniques for answering the telephone, list at least five courtesies you could use while on the telephone, discuss proper screening and routing techniques, correctly take a phone message including all the right information, and differentiate calls that you or other office staff can handle from calls that should be referred to your physician–employer. *The following statements are related to your learning objectives for this chapter. Fill in the blanks in the following paragraph with the appropriate term(s).*

There are four things that will define your "tone of voice" while on the phone. One is the volume of your voice, the other three are (1) ______________________, (2) ______________________, and (3) ______________________. If you are occasionally asked to repeat yourself while on the phone, you should assess those four factors. Ask a colleague to help you determine which quality you could improve. When answering a multiline phone, you often need to place a caller on hold. You should always politely ask the first caller to hold, go to the second line, and (4) ____.
If at all possible, answer all calls by the (5) ________________ ring. When taking a message, you should (6) ______________ the information to ensure that you have not misunderstood the caller.

When ending a call, (7) ________________ for a moment to see if the caller has any additional questions. Some calls can be handled by the office staff, and others should be referred to the physician. All complaints about medical care and treatments should be (8) ____________________. Telephone triage is one of the most important functions of the person answering the phone. Triage takes (9) __________________ and (10) ____________________ to do well.

VOCABULARY BUILDER

A. *Find the words below that are misspelled; circle them, and then correctly spell them in the spaces provided. Then insert the correct vocabulary terms from the list that best fit the descriptions below.*

answering services	ethical	jargon
articulate	etiguette	modulated
buffer words	faximile	obfucation
cellular phones	fluant	pagers
communication	Good Samaritan laws	pronounciation
enunciate	handheld devices	triage
________________	________________	________________
________________	________________	

When speaking on the telephone, medical assistants must use proper telephone (1) ______________________, which means being courteous and professional to others. To ensure that listeners understand what is said, it is important to (2) ______________________, or say the words clearly. Simple terms rather than medical (3) ______________________ promote mutual understanding rather than confusion or (4) ______________________. The use of slang words and expressions is considered unprofessional and disrespectful. When speaking with a caller who is not (5) ______________________ in English, it is helpful to speak slowly and use short sentences. Proper (6) ______________________ of all words in a carefully (7) ______________________ voice will also help people understand what you are saying, especially non–English-speaking people. Good (8) ______________________ skills are of real benefit to a medical assistant when using the telephone and when speaking directly to patients. The use of (9) __________ ______________________ can help the sentences make sense to the patient. Responding with empathy conveys an appreciation for the caller's concerns and needs. Medical assistants will screen and route calls that come into the medical facility to ensure that callers speak to the appropriate staff member who can (10) ______________________ their medical problems. Because complete patient confidentiality is considered a legal and (11) ______________________ obligation, medical assistants must not discuss patients outside of the professional environment or share any patient information with nonmedical professionals without written patient permission. And, of course, always remember that the (12) ______ ______________________ __________ will only protect those medical assistants who stay within their scope of practice when interacting with patients or the public.

B. *Match the following devices or services listed in Column A with corresponding descriptions in Column B.*

Column A

1. _______ pager
2. _______ answering service
3. _______ cellular phone
4. _______ automated routing unit
5. _______ fax
6. _______ e-mail

Column B

A. Takes calls when the office is closed

B. Sends a message via phone lines to an electronic mailbox located in another person's computer

C. A one-way communication device used to contact staff when away from the office

D. A portable telephone

E. A document sent over telephone lines from one facsimile machine or modem to another

F. A system that allows callers to reach specific people or departments by pressing a specified number on a touch-tone telephone

LEARNING REVIEW

1. Effective telephone communication requires prompt and professional responses from medical assistants. For each of the scenarios listed below, what should the medical assistant say to give the best telephone response?

   A. Karen Ritter, CMA, answers the first call of the morning at Inner City Health Care.

   Medical assistant: ____

   ____

   ____

   B. Patient Nora Fowler calls with a question about medication prescribed for her rheumatoid arthritis and insists on a call back from Dr. Elizabeth King. Dr. King is presently on rounds at the hospital and will not be available until 4:30 PM. Nora's tone of voice indicates that she is distrustful of the medication and of the physician's reliability, and it is clear from the conversation that Nora has discontinued taking her medication.

   Medical assistant: ____

   ____

   ____

   C. While speaking on telephone line 1 with patient Bill Schwartz, who is calling to schedule a physical examination, medical assistant Wanda Slawson receives another call on line 2 from a laboratory with a summary of emergency test results for another patient. Wanda knows Dr. Susan Rice is waiting for the test results.

   Medical assistant: ____

   ____

   ____

   D. Bruce Goldman, CMA, takes a call from patient Juanita Hansen. Juanita is inquiring about a bill and indicating that her insurance carrier, Blue Cross, did not pay the entire fee for her son's last examination, which left her with a balance owed to Inner City Health Care. Office manager Walter Seals is responsible for managing insurance claims and inquiries.

   Medical assistant: ____

   ____

   ____

2. Showing compassion and concern for the well-being of the caller allows both potential and established patients to feel confident about the high quality of care they receive.

   A. Name four reasons why a potential patient will contact an ambulatory care facility by telephone.

   (1) ____

   (2) ____

   (3) ____

   (4) ____

B. What seven pieces of information should a medical assistant record in the appointment book when scheduling an initial appointment with the physician?

(1) ______________________ (5) ______________________

(2) ______________________ (6) ______________________

(3) ______________________ (7) ______________________

(4) ______________________

3. Indicate the calls described below that fall within the scope of practice for a medical assistant (MA) to respond to and the calls that should be directed to the physician (P). For each call handled by a medical assistant, describe the information needed to address the needs of the caller. For each call referred to the physician, give reasons why a physician must handle the call.

_____ A. Insurance questions

____

____

_____ B. Scheduling patient testing and office appointments

____

____

_____ C. Medical emergencies

____

____

_____ D. Requests for prescription refills

____

____

_____ E. Complaints about medical care or treatment

____

____

_____ F. General information about the practice

____

____

_____ G. Poor progress reports from a patient

____

____

_____ H. Requests for medications other than prescription refills

____

____

______ I. Medical questions

____

____

______ J. Salespeople

____

____

4. Answering services and answering machines are two methods of taking calls after hours. Answering services are staffed by live operators who take messages for the physician and medical practice when the office is closed. Answering machines can also be used for taking the majority of after-hours calls, with a telephone number given in the outgoing message that will connect callers with a live operator in the event of an emergency.

   A. Compose an appropriate outgoing message for the offices of Drs. Lewis and King.

   ____

   ____

   ____

   ____

   ____

   B. Each morning, administrative medical assistant Ellen Armstrong is responsible for transcribing messages left on the medical practice's answering machine the evening before. Using the message pad slips in Figure 12-1, transcribe each message completely and appropriately. In the space for "Attachments," list any records, files, or documents that should be attached to the message slip for the recipient's review.

   Message 1. "Ellen, this is Anna Preciado. Can you tell [office manager,] Marilyn, that I won't be in tomorrow for the afternoon shift? I've got a 101 degree temperature and bad flu symptoms. Maybe Joe Guerrero can come in to sub for me as the clinical medical assistant; yesterday, he said he might be available if I wasn't feeling well enough to come in. I know Dr. Lewis has several patients scheduled for clinical testing in the afternoon. I'm at 555-6622. Thanks."

   Message 2. "This is Heidi from Dr. Kwiczola's office calling for Dr. Lewis. We have a new patient, Marsha Beckman, in our psychiatric practice who is experiencing symptoms of fatigue, anxiety, palpitations, and weight loss. Dr. Kwiczola suspects this patient may be suffering from hyperthyroidism. Dr. Kwiczola will be in the office tomorrow from 2 PM to 7 PM and can be reached at 555-7181."

   Message 3. "This is Martin Gordon, a patient of Dr. Lewis's. I need to talk to Shirley Brooks, the office manager who handles insurance. I've got a question about my out-of-pocket maximum."

   Message 4. "This is Charles Williams. Dr. Lewis put me on a Holter monitor today. It's about 11 PM. and one of the leads came off. I put it back on, but I'm worried about whether I'll have to do this test again. Can you call me at home before eight at 555-6124 or at the office after nine at 555-8125?"

Person	Yes, without signed release	No	Yes, with signed release
H. Members of the office staff, as necessary for patient care	☐	☐	☐
I. Patient's insurance carrier	☐	☐	☐
J. Other patients	☐	☐	☐
K. People outside the office (friends, family, acquaintances of the medical assistant)	☐	☐	☐
L. Patient's parent or legal guardian, except concerning issues of birth control, abortion, or sexually transmitted diseases	☐	☐	☐

6. Many physicians and health care professionals use paging systems. Paging systems allow the medical assistant to alert a physician or other health care professional who is not on-site to call in for an important message. Name and describe four paging system options.

(1) ______________________________

(2) ______________________________

(3) ____

____

____

(4) ____

____

____

7. The term that best describes speaking clearly and articulating carefully is:
   a. pronunciation
   b. modulation
   c. enunciation
   d. fluency

8. The act of evaluating the urgency of a medical situation and prioritizing treatment is:
   a. screening
   b. referral
   c. triage
   d. etiquette

9. To ensure sensible risk management when making calls, you should protect the patient's privacy at all times; this is referred to as:
   a. confidentiality
   b. jargon
   c. elaboration
   d. screening

10. Many hospitals and ambulatory care settings have telephone systems to manage heavy telephone traffic; these are called:
    a. ARU
    b. CPU
    c. ATT
    d. BLS

11. No call should be left unattended for more than:
    a. 1 minute
    b. 2 minutes
    c. 20–30 seconds
    d. 5 minutes

CERTIFICATION REVIEW

These questions are designed to mimic the certification examinations. You can use these questions like a small "Certification Examination Study Guide," but this is not meant to take the place of the more extensive study guides. Use this portion to determine in what areas to concentrate your efforts when studying for the certification examination.

1. Telephone calls that may be handled by the medical assistant include all but which one of the following?
   a. billing questions
   b. appointment changes
   c. requests for prescription refills
   d. calls from other physicians

2. When a medical assistant is talking to a patient on the telephone and another line rings, what should the medical assistant do?
   a. Put the first call on hold, answer the second call, put that caller on hold, and go back to the first caller to finish up.
   b. Put the first call on hold, answer the second call and handle that issue, then go back to the first caller.
   c. Let the second line ring; it will be picked up by an answering system.
   d. Finish with the first caller, then answer the second line.

3. Which of the following is not a good idea in a medical office?
   a. using a speaker phone to listen to voice messages
   b. speaking quietly on the telephone so other patients cannot hear
   c. using a privacy screen to reduce the chance of being overheard on the telephone
   d. using only e-mail so you will not be overheard

4. After-hours telephone messages are usually directed to:
   a. the physician's home
   b. the medical manager's home
   c. a voice mail system or answering service/machine
   d. an e-mail system

5. When talking to older adult patients on the phone:
   a. If the patient is hearing impaired, speak slower, clearer, and a little louder.
   b. Assume they are senile or at least forgetful and repeat all the information several times.
   c. If the person has difficulty understanding, simplify the information, ask if there are any questions, and try to explain patiently in simple terms.
   d. all of the above
   e. a and c only

6. Health Insurance Portability and Accountability Act (HIPAA) guidelines for telephone communications include:
   a. Determine if the patient has specific instructions on who has been granted privilege to their private medical information.
   b. Determine if the patient has a particular number they want called for confidential communications.
   c. Ask if it is acceptable to leave a message if the patient is not at the number provided.
   d. All of the above.

CASE STUDY

As Inner City Health Care, an urgent care center, continues to grow, increasing both patient load and staff, the existing telephone system consisting of a simple intercom and four telephone lines is no longer sufficient to handle the call volume and allow for full, immediate accessibility for all staff members. Callers are frustrated by the length of time it takes to get through and by long amounts of time spent on hold. Messages are often late in getting properly routed. Administrative medical assistant Karen Ritter suggests to office manager Jane O'Hara that an automated routing unit (ARU) might be more efficient for the growing clinic's needs. At the next regularly scheduled staff meeting, the physician–employers give the go-ahead to research an ARU.

Discuss the following:

1. ARU systems provide several options for callers that identify specific departments or services that callers can be connected with directly. What kinds of caller options might be appropriate for Inner City Health Care?
2. What can be done so emergency patients or hearing-impaired patients can speak automatically to a "live" operator?
3. How can an ARU help staff members receive their calls more efficiently?
4. How can the office manager and medical assistant implement the ARU system with a minimum of disruption to physicians, staff, and patients?

SELF-ASSESSMENT

Discuss the following questions with another classmate or in a small group. During the discussion, consider how different people react in different ways, depending on their personalities, their patience, and their confidence levels. After the discussion, spend a moment in self-reflection to think of ways you can improve your telephone communication skills.

1. Have you ever conversed with someone on the telephone whom you could not understand?
2. Was it his or her language, accent, enunciation, or volume?
3. Would it have been easier to understand him or her if you were face to face with him or her?
4. How did you handle the situation? Did you ask the person to speak louder, slower, or more clearly?
5. How do you think most people would handle a situation in which they could not hear the speaker clearly? Older adults? Non–English speakers? People in pain or very ill?

Of the following telecommunication devices and methods, with which are you familiar and which will you need to learn more about? What do you think is the best way to become more familiar with the devices and methods?

1. e-mail
2. pagers
3. handheld devices
4. multiline phones
5. cellular phones
6. instant messaging
7. fax machines
8. answering services

CHAPTER POST-TEST

This is similar to the Pre-Test. Perform this test without looking at the book. This is just to see how well you have understood and can recall the information presented in this chapter after you have studied it and completed the workbook exercises. You will not be graded on this portion (other than the grade you give yourself), but this is an excellent preparation for your instructor's test. You may use this Post-Test to determine what areas you need to study more. Justify any "false" answers.

1. When transferring a call, it is important to obtain the patient's name and phone number. (T or F)
2. Some patients will become defensive when a firm voice is used on the phone. (T or F)
3. We always have time to ask patients if they can be put on hold. (T or F)
4. When taking a message, be brief but thorough. The patient's name, phone number, questions, best time for a call back, and any other pertinent information are useful. (T or F)
5. Patients should expect confidentiality at all times, even on their home answering machines. (T or F)
6. The physician should be alerted to any angry calls regarding patient care and treatment. (T or F)

CERTIFICATION CRITERIA CHECKLIST

As you go through your education and training, keep in mind the national certification examination that you will take when you graduate. Each chapter of the textbook and workbook covers a different section of the examination criteria. To keep track of your preparation for the certification examination, turn to the back of this workbook and highlight the following CMA, RMA, or CMAS certification examination criteria (if you have already highlighted them from a previous chapter, put a check mark by the criteria):

CMA

E. Communication
  1. Adapting communication to an individual's ability to understand
  4. Professional communication and behavior
  5. Evaluating and understanding communication
  7. Receiving, organizing, prioritizing and transmitting information
  8. Telephone techniques

F. Medicolegal Guidelines & Requirements
  2. Legislation

H. Equipment
  1. Equipment operation

M. Resource Information and Community Services
   2. Appropriate referrals

P. Office Policies and Procedures
   3. Instructions for patients with special needs

RMA

II. Administrative Medical Assisting
   C. Medical Receptionist/Secretarial/Clerical
      4. Oral (and written) communication

CMAS

8. Medical Office Management
   - Office communications

COMPETENCY ASSESSMENT

Procedure 12-3 Taking a Telephone Message

Performance Objectives: To record an accurate message and follow up as required. Perform this objective within 5 minutes with a minimum score of 55 points.

Supplies/Equipment: Telephone, message pad, black ink pen, notepad, clock or watch

Charting/Documentation: Enter appropriate documentation/charting in the box.

Instructor's/Evaluator's Comments and Suggestions:

SKILLS CHECKLIST Procedure 12-3: Taking a Telephone Message

Name ______________________

Date ______________________

No.	Skill	Check #1 20 pts ea	Check #2 10 pts ea	Check #3 5 pts ea	Notes
1	Answer the phone following the steps outlined in Procedure 12-1.				
2	Use a message pad to gather the required information.				
	a. Name of person calling and numbers				
	b. Date and time call was received				
	c. Who the call is for				
	d. Reason for the call				
	e. Action to be taken				
	f. Your name/initials				
3	Repeat the above information back to the caller.				
4	If the patient already has a medical record, attach the phone message to it.				
5	Maintain copies of all calls.				
Student's Total Points					
Points Possible		220	110	55	
Final Score (Student's Total Points / Possible Points)					

	Notes
Start time:	
End time:	
Total time: (5 min goal)	

COMPETENCY ASSESSMENT

Procedure 12-4 Handling Problem Calls

Performance Objectives: To handle calls in a positive and professional manner while providing necessary comfort, empathy, and information to the caller to resolve the problem. Perform this objective within 15 minutes with a minimum score of 65 points.

Supplies/Equipment: Telephone, message pad, pen or pencil

Charting/Documentation: Enter appropriate documentation/charting in the box.

Instructor's/Evaluator's Comments and Suggestions:

SKILLS CHECKLIST Procedure 12-4: Handling Problem Calls

Name ______________________________

Date ______________________________

No.	Skill	Check #1 20 pts ea	Check #2 10 pts ea	Check #3 5 pts ea	Notes
1	Answer the call as outlined in Procedure 12-1.				
2	Remain calm and avoid becoming upset.				
3	Lower your voice both in pitch and volume.				
4	Listen to what the caller is upset about, then paraphrase back to the caller for verification.				
5	Use the words "I understand."				
6	Do not take the call personally.				
7	Offer assistance.				
8	Document the call accurately.				
9	If caller is hysterical or frightened, speak in a soothing voice.				
10	If the call is an emergency, begin triage procedures as needed.				
11	Always have the caller repeat instructions.				
12	Finalize and follow through on action to be taken.				
13	Always report problem calls to the office manager.				
Student's Total Points					
Points Possible		260	130	65	
Final Score (Student's Total Points / Possible Points)					

	Notes
Start time:	
End time:	
Total time: (15 min goal)	

COMPETENCY ASSESSMENT

Procedure 12-5 Placing Outgoing Calls

Performance Objectives: To place calls efficiently and effectively. Perform this objective within 3 minutes with a minimum score of 25 points.

Supplies/Equipment: Telephone, notepad, pen or pencil, all materials specifically applicable to the call

Charting/Documentation: Enter appropriate documentation/charting in the box.

Instructor's/Evaluator's Comments and Suggestions:

SKILLS CHECKLIST Procedure 12-5: Placing Outgoing Calls

Name ______________________________

Date ______________________________

No.	Skill	Check #1 20 pts ea	Check #2 10 pts ea	Check #3 5 pts ea	Notes
1	Preplan the call by preparing all materials.				
2	Make calls from a location that will not be disrupted.				
3	Schedule specific times of the day for calls. Be aware of time zones.				
4	Use appropriate language and tone, and follow proper telephone techniques.				
5	Document appropriately.				
Student's Total Points					
Points Possible		100	50	25	
Final Score (Student's Total Points / Possible Points)					

	Notes
Start time:	
End time:	
Total time: (3 min goal)	

COMPETENCY ASSESSMENT

Procedure 12-6 Recording a Telephone Message on an Answering Device or Voice Mail System

Performance Objectives: To provide clear and precise instructions to the caller when medical staff is not available to answer the call immediately. The words should be spoken clearly in a pleasant and well-modulated tone. Perform this objective within 15 minutes with a minimum score of 25 points.

Supplies/Equipment: Telephone and recording device, prepared written message to record

Charting/Documentation: Enter appropriate documentation/charting in the box.

____

____

____

____

Instructor's/Evaluator's Comments and Suggestions:

____

____

____

____

____

____

SKILLS CHECKLIST Procedure 12-6: Recording a Telephone Message on an Answering Device or Voice Mail System

Name ______________________

Date ______________________

No.	Skill	Check #1 20 pts ea	Check #2 10 pts ea	Check #3 5 pts ea	Notes
1	Write out message to be recorded.				
2	Check for completeness and accuracy, and read message aloud to determine its length.				
3	Record the message when distractions and noise are at a minimum.				
4	Play the message back to verify that it is accurate and includes all necessary information.				
5	Set the message device to the recorded message when you are not available to answer.				
Student's Total Points					
Points Possible		100	50	25	
Final Score (Student's Total Points / Possible Points)					

	Notes
Start time:	
End time:	
Total time: (15 min goal)	

EVALUATION OF CHAPTER KNOWLEDGE

Evaluate your own strengths and weaknesses in communicating with others on the telephone, performing triage, directing calls, and understanding telephone systems and technology.

Skills	Student Self-Evaluation Good	Average	Poor
I can adhere to the principles of preserving patient confidentiality.	____	____	____
I project empathy and enthusiasm.	____	____	____
I understand telephone procedures for new and existing patient appointments.	____	____	____
I have the ability to triage and respond to medical emergencies.	____	____	____
I possess good listening skills.	____	____	____
I can receive, prioritize, organize, and transmit information.	____	____	____
I understand the principles of successful telephone communication.	____	____	____
I can perform effective telephone triage.	____	____	____
I understand the use of communication technology such as a fax machine, automated routing units, and e-mail.	____	____	____
I have the ability to communicate effectively with people at their levels of understanding.	____	____	____
I can demonstrate the ability to make outgoing calls.	____	____	____
I can serve as an effective liaison between the physician and others.	____	____	____
I can perform within ethical boundaries.	____	____	____
I practice within the scope of my training and expertise.	____	____	____

CHAPTER 13

Patient Scheduling

CHAPTER PRE-TEST

Perform this test without looking at the book. This is just to see how well you have understood and can recall the information in this chapter after you have read it, but before you have completed the workbook exercises. You will not be graded on this portion (other than the grade you give yourself). Justify any "false" answers.

1. Circle the letter that lists correct types of scheduling systems:
   a. wave, modified wave, double booking, a mile-a-minute
   b. open hours, wave, clustering, stream
   c. first-come first-served, open hours, clustering
2. Below are guidelines to scheduling. Which one is correct?
   a. Urgent calls should be sent to the hospital, where they are better equipped to handle them.
   b. Urgent calls should be triaged/assessed before determining the best course of action.
   c. Referrals by other physicians need to be seen immediately.
   d. Appointments for pharmaceutical and medical supply representatives should be referred to the physician.
3. Information that should be obtained from all new patients includes all but which one of the following?
   a. the patient's full legal name
   b. the patient's birth date
   c. the patient's address and telephone numbers
   d. the patient's symptoms
   e. the patient's insurance information
   f. the patient's family health history

4. All medical offices are changing to electronic appointment scheduling. (T or F)

5. When a patient misses an appointment, we:
   a. call them to reschedule
   b. let them contact us
   c. release them from our practice
   d. charge them for our time

INTRODUCTION

The effective scheduling of patient appointments is an essential skill of the medical assistant. Achieving efficient patient flow requires that the medical assistant coordinate the schedules of physicians, staff, and patients. Use of staff and physical facilities are also considered in selecting the proper scheduling system. When scheduling appointments, medical assistants draw on administrative and computer skills, as well as communication skills. By considering and respecting the needs, time, and comfort of the patient, the medical assistant creates a positive impression of the physician and the medical practice.

PERFORMANCE OBJECTIVES

After successful completion of this chapter you will be able to list and describe six major scheduling options, explaining the advantages and disadvantages of each; list some scheduling guidelines and state the rationales for them; explain the importance of triaging calls and how to handle certain situations you might encounter; be able to demonstrate the proper documentation processes for canceled and missed appointments; and be able to review the office protocols and procedures for patients checking in for appointments. You will be able to establish a schedule matrix given the parameters, and also be able to successfully schedule an outpatient procedure or surgery according to the needs of your patient and physician–employer. *The following statements are related to your learning objectives for this chapter. Fill in the blanks with the appropriate term(s).*

Six major options in scheduling include (1) ________________________________, (2) ________________________, (3) ________________________, (4) ________________________, (5) ________________________, and (6) ________________________. One of the advantages of wave scheduling is that it can accommodate (7) ________________________ appointments. One of the staffing requirements when using wave scheduling is that the personnel must be skilled in (8) ________________________. Guidelines for scheduling appointments depend on many variables. Six of those variables are (9) ________________________, (10) ________________________, (11) ________________________, (12) ________________________, (13) ________________________, and (14) ____. When a patient misses an appointment, the medical assistant should contact the patient and attempt to (15) ________________________ the appointment. Both the missed appointment and the rescheduled appointment should be (16) ________________________ in the patient's medical record. When scheduling inpatient admissions and surgeries and outpatient procedures, it is important to consider the (17) ______________________________ of the patient, the physician(s), and the facilities, as well as the equipment and personnel, depending on the services being scheduled.

VOCABULARY BUILDER

Find the words below that are misspelled; circle them, and then correctly spell them in the spaces provided. Then replace the highlighted words in the following paragraph with the correct vocabulary terms from the list. (Be sure to spell them all correctly!)

clustering	modified wave scheduling	slack time
double booking	new patient	stream scheduling
encription technology	no-show	triage
estableshed patient	open hours	wave scheduling
matrics	practice based	
________________	________________	________________

1. ______________________________ Inner City Health Care reserves 9 AM to 12 PM on Thursday mornings for walk-in patients who are seen on a first-come, first-served basis within that time frame.

2. ______________________________ At the offices of Drs. Lewis and King, Ellen Armstrong, CMA, schedules Mary O'Keefe for a 1:00 PM appointment and Martin Gordon for a 1:00 PM appointment with Dr. Winston Lewis.

3. ______________________________ Lenny Taylor, an older adult patient with mild dementia, forgets his third appointment with Dr. James Whitney.

4. ______________________________ At Inner City Health Care, vaccinations are scheduled every 10 minutes from 10 AM to 12:20 PM on Mondays; Tuesday office hours are reserved for new patients only.

5. ______________________________ Three patients are scheduled to receive treatments in the first half hour of every hour.

6. ______________________________ Ellen Armstrong, CMA, takes a complete current medical history from patient Lourdes Austen on her first visit to Dr. Elizabeth King.

7. ______________________________ Joe Guerrero, CMA, asks patient Martin Gordon if the personal information in his medical chart is complete and up to date before escorting him to the examination room to be seen by Dr. Winston Lewis.

8. ______________________ Dr. Elizabeth King prefers to see patients for regular gynecologic examinations in consecutive appointments from 8:30 AM to 11:30 AM and patients who are pregnant from 1:00 PM to 3:30 PM.

9. ______________________ When patient Herb Fowler calls to set up an appointment with Dr. Winston Lewis for his chronic cough, Ellen Armstrong, CMA, asks Herb a series of screening questions to ascertain the nature, extent, and urgency of his condition.

10. ______________________ Dr. Winston Lewis prefers that two or more patients be scheduled at 30 or 60 minute intervals on a continuous basis throughout the day.

11. ______________________ An ophthalmologist schedules three patients at the beginning of each hour for comprehensive examinations, followed by single appointments every 10 to 20 minutes during the rest of the hour for quick, follow-up procedures such as removing eye patches or instilling eyedrops.

12. ______________________ Ellen Armstrong, CMA, uses empty or unscheduled periods for dictation or processing paperwork.

13. ______________________ On the 15th day of each month, office manager Walter Seals, CMA, who is responsible for efficient patient flow at Inner City Health Care, asks each of the urgent care center's five physicians to confirm their scheduling commitments for the upcoming month to block off unavailable times in the appointment book.

14. ______________________ The medical assistant uses software to protect the patients' confidentiality in electronic format.

11. The type of scheduling that requires visits to be set up around patients with specific chronic aliments such as diabetes and hypertension is called:
    a. triaging
    b. referral appointments
    c. group appointments
    d. stream appointments

12. The general rule for no-shows and cancellations is that after ______________ consecutive missed appointments, the physician will review the patient's record and could terminate care.
    a. five
    b. three
    c. two
    d. ten

13. What, more than anything else, determines the success of a day in the ambulatory care setting?
    a. patient care
    b. efficient patient flow
    c. operational functions
    d. interpersonal skills

CERTIFICATION REVIEW

These questions are designed to mimic the certification examinations. You can use these questions like a small "Certification Examination Study Guide," but this is not meant to take the place of the more extensive study guides. Use this portion to determine in what areas to concentrate your efforts when studying for the certification examination.

1. In scheduling, double booking means to keep two appointment books going for the same doctor. (T or F)
2. One major purpose of triage when scheduling appointments is to determine if the patient has an emergency or urgent situation/illness. (T or F)
3. After a patient has missed three appointments, most clinics refuse to schedule that patient again. (T or F)
4. The appointment book/record may be subpoenaed, and therefore is considered a legal document. (T or F)
5. Providing patients with appointment cards is an effective way to prevent missed appointments. (T or F)

CASE STUDY

When patient Lenore McDonell falls from the examination table and lacerates her arm while attempting an independent transfer from the table to her wheelchair, clinical medical assistant Joe Guerrero alerts Dr. Winston Lewis, and the two begin to implement emergency procedures to control Lenore's bleeding and assess damage to the arm. Lenore's fall occurred at the end of her appointment, a routine checkup with Dr. Lewis.

Administrative medical assistant Ellen Armstrong must adjust Dr. Lewis's schedule to accommodate the emergency situation. Martin Gordon, a man in his mid-60s diagnosed with prostate cancer, waits in the reception area for Dr. Lewis's next appointment. Mr. Gordon's appointment, a 6-month follow-up, is expected to take 30 minutes. Mr. Gordon is also being treated for depression related to his cancer diagnosis. Hope Smith, a new patient in good general health, is scheduled for a complete examination; she is due to arrive at the offices of Drs. Lewis and King at the Northborough Family Medical Group within 20 minutes. Jim Marshall, an impatient and aggressive businessman, is scheduled for the first afternoon appointment after Dr. Lewis's lunch commitment. Mr. Marshall's appointment, for a physical examination and ECG to investigate chest pains he has experienced recently, is expected to take 45 minutes. Dr. Lewis's schedule is completely booked for the rest of the day.

Discuss the following:

1. What scheduling alternatives will Ellen offer Mr. Gordon, who is already waiting in the reception area? What special considerations regarding Mr. Gordon should Ellen take into account and why?
2. What is Ellen's first action regarding Ms. Smith, Dr. Lewis's next patient due to arrive? What scheduling alternatives should Ellen offer to her?
3. What scheduling alternatives, if any, should Ellen present to Mr. Marshall? Explain your logic.
4. How is patient triage important to Ellen's rescheduling of Dr. Lewis's patients? What important administrative and communication skills will Ellen use to handle this emergency situation efficiently and professionally?

SELF-ASSESSMENT

1. When you call a doctor's office, do any of the following aggravate you? Do you think other people are aggravated by these?

   a. Being put on hold right away or too often

   b. The receptionist asking too many questions

   c. Not enough appointment time choices; that is, you have to wait too long for an appointment

   d. Not getting a real person; that is, having to listen to electronic choices and make selections

   e. Other (add your own idea) ____

   ____

2. Now go to each of the situations in Question 1 and determine an action that could alleviate all or some of the aggravation. Keep in mind that the situation might still exist (e.g., the receptionist might still have to ask a lot of questions), but how might he or she make the experience more pleasant?

3. When you visit a doctor's office, do any of the following aggravate you?

   a. The receptionist does not acknowledge you right away

   b. The wait is too long

   c. The waiting room is noisy, messy, or uncomfortable

   d. There are no magazines of interest to you

   e. Other (add your own idea) ____

   ____

4. Similar to the instructions in Question 2, go to each of the situations in Question 3 and determine solutions that could alleviate all or some of the causes of aggravation. Keep in mind that the solutions in this case are obvious and doable.

5. Think of your most pleasant interaction with a doctor's office as a patient making an appointment, scheduling a procedure, changing an appointment, or even canceling an appointment. What made the experience more pleasant? Was it the receptionist's voice? Tone? Actual words? The overall options? Or something else?

As you enter your career as a medical assistant, try to remember how the patient feels. Try to recall situations that bother you when you are a patient. Try to keep these issues in mind and see if you can eliminate or alleviate them to make your patients as comfortable as possible. Maybe you are just the person who will help to make the experience of seeing a doctor more pleasant for your patients. Try to be like the person you thought of for Question 5. This is not an easy thing to do when you are busy and stressed. Can you think of ways you can remind yourself every day of these lessons?

CHAPTER POST-TEST

This is similar to the Pre-Test. Perform this test without looking at the book. This is just to see how well you have understood and can recall the information presented in this chapter after you have studied it and completed the workbook exercises. You will not be graded on this portion (other than the grade you give yourself), but this is an excellent preparation for your instructor's test. You may use this Post-Test to determine what areas you need to study more. Justify any "false" answers.

1. Circle the letter that lists correct types of scheduling systems:

   a. modified wave, wave, clustering, and mile-a-minute

   b. stream, open hours, wave, grouping, separating

   c. first-come first-served, open hours, clustering

   d. open hours, wave, clustering, stream

2. Below are guidelines to scheduling. Which one is correct?
   a. Urgent calls should be scheduled into the next available appointment time.
   b. Urgent calls should be sent to the hospital, where they are better equipped to handle them.
   c. Calls from other physicians should be put through to the physician immediately, if possible.
   d. Appointments for pharmaceutical and medical supply representatives should be referred to the physician.

3. Information that should be obtained from all new patients includes all but which one of the following?
   a. the patient's full legal name
   b. the patient's birth date
   c. the patient's address and telephone numbers
   d. the patient's place of employment
   e. the patient's symptoms
   f. the patient's insurance information

4. Many medical offices are changing to electronic appointment scheduling. (T or F)

5. When a patient misses an appointment, we document it, and then we:
   a. call them to reschedule
   b. let them contact us
   c. release them from our practice
   d. charge them for our time

CERTIFICATION CRITERIA CHECKLIST

As you go through your education and training, keep in mind the national certification examination that you will take when you graduate. Each chapter of the textbook and workbook covers a different section of the examination criteria. To keep track of your preparation for the certification examination, turn to the back of this workbook and highlight the following CMA, RMA, or CMAS certification examination criteria (if you have already highlighted them from a previous chapter, put a check mark by the criteria):

CMA

E. Communication
   8. Telephone techniques

H. Equipment
   1. Equipment operation

I. Computer Concepts
   3. Computer applications

L. Scheduling and Monitoring Appointments

N. Managing Physician's Professional Schedule and Travel
  3. Integrating meetings and travel with office schedule

RMA

II. Administrative Medical Assisting
  C. Medical Receptionist/Secretarial/Clerical
    2. Reception
    3. Scheduling

CMAS

3. Medical Office Clerical Assisting
  - Appointment management and scheduling

COMPETENCY ASSESSMENT

Procedure 13-1 Checking In Patients

Performance Objectives: To ensure the patient is given prompt and proper care; to meet legal safeguards for documentation. Perform this objective within 25 minutes with a minimum score of 35 points.

Supplies/Equipment: Patient chart, black ink pen, required forms, check-in list or appointment book

Charting/Documentation: Enter appropriate documentation/charting in the box.

Instructor's/Evaluator's Comments and Suggestions:

SKILLS CHECKLIST Procedure 13-1: Checking In Patients

Name ______________________________

Date ______________________________

No.	Skill	Check #1 20 pts ea	Check #2 10 pts ea	Check #3 5 pts ea	Notes
1	Prepare a list of patients to be seen and assemble the charts.				
2	Check charts to see that everything is up to date.				
3	Acknowledge patients when they arrive.				
4	Check patient in, review vital information, and protect patient's privacy.				
5	Indicate patients arrival on daily worksheet and computer system.				
6	Ask patient to be seated and indicate wait time.				
7	Following office policy, place the chart where it can be picked up to route the patient to the appropriate location for the visit.				
Student's Total Points					
Points Possible		140	70	35	
Final Score (Student's Total Points / Possible Points)					

	Notes
Start time:	
End time:	
Total time: (25 min goal)	

COMPETENCY ASSESSMENT

Procedure 13-2 Cancellation Procedures

Performance Objectives: To protect the physician from legal complications; to free up care time for other patients; and to assure quality patient care. Perform this objective within 15 minutes with a minimum score of 20 points.

Supplies/Equipment: Patient chart, red ink pen, check-in list or appointment book

Charting/Documentation: Enter appropriate documentation/charting in the box.

Instructor's/Evaluator's Comments and Suggestions:

SKILLS CHECKLIST Procedure 13-2: Cancellation Procedures

Name ______________________

Date ______________________

No.	Skill	Check #1 20 pts ea	Check #2 10 pts ea	Check #3 5 pts ea	Notes
1	Indicate on the appointment sheet all appointments that were changed, canceled, or did not show.				
2	Reschedule those appointments by calling the patients.				
3	If unable to reschedule, record a reminder in the tickler file.				
4	Document action taken in the patient's medical record/ chart.				
Student's Total Points					
Points Possible		80	40	20	
Final Score (Student's Total Points / Possible Points)					
		Notes			
Start time:					
End time:					
Total time: (15 min goal)					

COMPETENCY ASSESSMENT

Procedure 13-3 Establishing the Appointment Matrix

Performance Objectives: To have a current and accurate record of appointment times available for scheduling patient visits. Perform this objective within 25 minutes with a minimum score of 25 points.

Supplies/Equipment: Appointment scheduler, physician's schedule, staff schedule, office calendar

Charting/Documentation: Enter appointment documentation/charting in the box.

Instructor's/Evaluator's Comments and Suggestions:

SKILLS CHECKLIST Procedure 13-3: Establishing the Appointment Matrix

Name ______________________

Date ______________________

No.	Skill	Check #1 20 pts ea	Check #2 10 pts ea	Check #3 5 pts ea	Notes
1	Mark in appointment book times that are not to be scheduled.				
2	Indicate all vacations, holidays, and other office closures.				
3	Note all physician meetings, hospital rounds, appointments, conferences, vacations, and other prescheduled commitments.				
4	Highlight the time frame for specific procedures.				
5	Have clearly established guidelines for scheduling specific types of appointments and procedures.				
Student's Total Points					
Points Possible		100	50	25	
Final Score (Student's Total Points / Possible Points)					
		Notes			
Start time:					
End time:					
Total time: (25 min goal)					

COMPETENCY ASSESSMENT

Procedure 13-4 Scheduling of Inpatient and Outpatient Admissions and Procedures

Performance Objectives: To assist patients in scheduling inpatient and outpatient admissions and procedures ordered by the physician. Perform this objective within 20 minutes with a minimum score of 45 points.

Supplies/Equipment: Calendar, black ink pen, telephone, referral slip, patient's schedule/calendar, physician's requests/orders regarding procedure/admittance

Charting/Documentation: Enter appropriate documentation/charting in the box.

____

____

____

____

Instructor's/Evaluator's Comments and Suggestions:

____

____

____

____

____

____

SKILLS CHECKLIST Procedure 13-4: Scheduling of Inpatient and Outpatient Admissions and Procedures

Name ______________________

Date ______________________

No.	Skill	Check #1 20 pts ea	Check #2 10 pts ea	Check #3 5 pts ea	Notes
1	Ensure privacy. Clarify with the patients that they understand the inpatient admission or outpatient procedure ordered.				
2	If required, seek permission from the patient's insurance company for the procedure or admissions.				
3	Produce a large, easily read calendar and check to see if the patient has one.				
4	Place telephone call to the facility. Identify yourself, your physician, your clinic, and the reason for calling.				
5	Identify any urgency. Request next available appointment.				
6	Confer with the patient for an immediate response.				
7	Provide receiver pertinent information related to the patient.				
8	Request special instructions or advanced data.				
9	Complete the referral slip for the patient; send or fax a copy to referred facility.				
Student's Total Points					
Points Possible		180	90	45	
Final Score (Student's Total Points / Possible Points)					

	Notes
Start time:	
End time:	
Total time: (20 min goal)	

COMPETENCY ASSESSMENT

Procedure 13-5 Making an Appointment on the Telephone

Performance Objectives: To schedule an appointment entering information in the appointment schedule according to office policy. Perform this objective within 15 minutes with a minimum score of 40 points.

Supplies/Equipment: Telephone, black ink pen, calendar, appointment book/computer screen/appointment worksheet

Charting/Documentation: Enter appropriate documentation/charting in the box.

Instructor's/Evaluator's Comments and Suggestions:

SKILLS CHECKLIST Procedure 13-5: Making an Appointment on the Telephone

Name ______________________________

Date ______________________________

No.	Skill	Check #1 20 pts ea	Check #2 10 pts ea	Check #3 5 pts ea	Notes
1	Answer the call following the steps outlined in Procedure 12-1.				
2	Make notes on your personal log sheet of patient's name and reason for calling.				
3	Determine if patient is new or established, physician to be seen, and reason for appointment.				
4	Discuss with the patient any special scheduling needs and search for an available time.				
5	Enter patient's name into the schedule.				
6	Repeat the date and time, and provide necessary instructions.				
7	End the call politely.				
8	Make certain all necessary information was transferred from your telephone log to appointment schedule. Draw line through your notes.				
Student's Total Points					
Points Possible		160	80	40	
Final Score (Student's Total Points / Possible Points)					

	Notes
Start time:	
End time:	
Total time: (15 min goal)	

EVALUATION OF CHAPTER KNOWLEDGE

Skills	Student Self-Evaluation Good	Average	Poor
I can choose appropriate scheduling tools and can describe advantages of each.	_____	_____	_____
I am able to establish an appointment matrix.	_____	_____	_____
I can prepare the daily appointment sheet.	_____	_____	_____
I can prepare the daily worksheet.	_____	_____	_____
I understand the importance of triage in scheduling patient appointments.	_____	_____	_____
I understand basic considerations in scheduling appointments.	_____	_____	_____
I know how to review procedures for cancellations, no-shows, and appointment changes.	_____	_____	_____
I know how to review procedures for patients checking in.	_____	_____	_____
I can recall three types of reminder systems.	_____	_____	_____
I can review six major scheduling systems.	_____	_____	_____
I recognize the importance of communication skills in the scheduling process.	_____	_____	_____

CHAPTER 14

Medical Records Management

CHAPTER PRE-TEST

Perform this test without looking at the book. This is just to see how well you have understood and can recall the information in this chapter after you have read it, but before you have completed the workbook exercises. You will not be graded on this portion (other than the grade you give yourself). Justify any "false" answers.

1. Out guides indicate when patient charts are out of order. (T or F)
2. Which of the following is not an important skill to have when filing?
   a. You should know the alphabet.
   b. You should know the basic rules of filing.
   c. You should pay attention to details.
   d. You should be good at math.
3. Medical records are important for many reasons. They provide information for medical care, legal protection, and research purposes. (T or F)
4. It is acceptable to release medical information to family members as long as they can show proper picture identification. (T or F)
5. When charting, you should write every detail of your conversation with the patient. (T or F)
6. All medical filing systems are based on the alphabet. (T or F)

INTRODUCTION

Accurate filing of patient medical records is an essential administrative task in the ambulatory care setting. To provide the highest quality care, patient medical records and other important files must be easily and promptly accessed by the physician and other members of the health care team.

The contents of all medical charts and other files must be kept complete and up to date. Medical assisting students can use this workbook chapter to review the filing systems commonly used in the ambulatory care setting and the correct procedures for medical records management.

PERFORMANCE OBJECTIVES

After successful completion of this chapter you should be able to explain the importance of medical records; discuss several methods of filing medical records, the rules for filing, and the order and steps for filing medical documents into the patient's chart or medical record, and describe several variations of filing systems. You should be able to define words such as tickler files, release marks, checkout systems, and cross-referencing. You should have a basic understanding of computer applications for medical records. You should know how an electronic medical record differs from a paper system in regard to retrieval, storage, making changes/corrections, access/transfers, and confidentiality. *The following statements are related to your learning objectives. Fill in the blanks with the appropriate term(s).*

There are five main purposes for medical records in the ambulatory care setting. One is to provide a base for (1) ______________________ patient care. Another is to provide (2) ________________ and (3) ______________________ communications as necessary. A third purpose is to (4) ____________________ a pattern to signal the physician of patient needs. The fourth purpose is to serve as a (5) ______________ for legal information necessary to (6) ______________ physicians, (7) ____________, and patients. The fifth and final purpose is to provide clinical data for (8) ____________. When filing documents into a medical record/chart, there are certain procedural steps that should be followed for efficiency. The steps are (9) ____________, (10) ____________, (11) ____________, and finally, (12) ____________________. There are many different methods of filing; some are alphabetical, some are numeric, and some are filed according to (13) ________________. A (14) ____________ ________ is a card system that helps you remember when an action is necessary in the future. Having the doctor initial laboratory reports before they are filed is a good example of (15) ______________ ____________ and helps to ensure the reports are not filed until the doctor has seen them. (16) ___________________________ consist of "place holders" sometimes called "out sheets," or (17) ___________________________. Medical records that are kept on computer are called (18) ____________________________________ and have distinct advantages and disadvantages. Regardless of how records are kept, patient (19) ____________________ is always a major concern, and safeguards must be in place to prevent unauthorized persons from seeing private medical information.

VOCABULARY BUILDER

Fill in the blanks in the following sentences using the words listed below.

accession record	key unit	shingling
captions	nonconsecutive filing	SOAP
coding	out guide	source-oriented medical record (SOMR)
consecutive or serial filing	problem-oriented medical record (POMR)	tickler file
cross-reference	purging	units
indexing		

1. To remember to check with the reference laboratory on Friday to obtain patient Martin Gordon's test results, Ellen Armstrong, CMA places a note in her ____________________.
2. When using the ____________________ approach for all progress notes, Dr. Lewis enters information about a patient's problem in this order: S—subjective impressions; O—objective clinical evidence; A—assessment or diagnosis; P—plans for further studies, treatment, or management.
3. Every 6 months, Marilyn Johnson, CMA, follows office policy and procedures for ____________________ inactive files to remove and archive those not in active use.
4. The organized method of identifying and separating items to be filed into small subunits is accomplished with the use of ____________________ units.
5. When Liz Corbin, CMA, retrieves Annette Samuels's chart for Dr. Woo, she places an ____________________ in the filing cabinet to show that the file has been removed from storage.
6. When returning a patient's chart to the filing cabinet, Walter Seals, CMA, inspects the patient's name to identify the indexing ____________________.
7. The ____________________ is a journal (or computer listing) where numbers in a numeric filing system are preassigned. The log sequentially lists numbers to be used to assign to numeric records.
8. The ____________________ filing system uses groups of two, three, or four or more digits, such as the patient's social security number or telephone number, as the filing reference in a numeric filing system.
9. The file for Kent Memorial Hospital contains three indexing ____________________ to be considered when preparing the filing label.
10. If a ____________________ card is required in the alphabetic card file of a numeric filing system, such as when making note of an established patient's married name, a card is prepared that includes an *X* next to the file number to indicate that this card does not designate the primary location card for the file.

11. In the ______________________ system of recordkeeping, patient problems are identified by a number that corresponds to the charting relevant to that problem number; that is, asthma #1; dermatitis #2; and so on.
12. When a filing system other than alphabetic is being used, the proper ______________________ must be determined for the chart or file so it can be retrieved.
13. Ellen Armstrong, CMA, uses the ______________________ method for filing laboratory reports; the reports are stacked across the page with the most recent report placed on top of the previous one.
14. Ellen Armstrong, CMA, uses the ______________________ method for handling invoices, sales orders, and requisitions; each record is numbered and filed in ascending order.
15. ______________________ are used to identify major sections of file folders by more manageable subunits, such as GA-GE, or Miscellaneous. Captions are marked on the tabs of the guides.
16. Inner City Health Care uses the ______________________ method of recordkeeping, which groups information according to its origin; for example, laboratories, examinations, physician notes, consulting physicians, and other types of information.

LEARNING REVIEW

1. Assign the correct units to the following items to be filed using the rule for filing patient records that is listed for each.
   A. Names that are hyphenated are considered one unit.
      1. Jackson Hugh Levine-Dwyer
         unit 1________________ unit 2________________ unit 3________________
      2. Leslie Jane Poole-Petit
         unit 1________________ unit 2________________ unit 3________________
   B. Seniority units are indexed as the last indexing unit.
      1. Keith Wildasin Sr.
         unit 1________________ unit 2________________ unit 3________________
      2. Gerald Maggart III
         unit 1________________ unit 2________________ unit 3________________
   C. Titles are considered as separate indexing units. If the title appears with first and last names, the title is considered the last indexing unit.
      1. Dr. Louise Udolf
         unit 1________________ unit 2________________ unit 3________________
      2. Prof. Valerie Rajah
         unit 1________________ unit 2________________ unit 3________________

D. The names of individuals are assigned indexing units respectively: last name, first name, middle, and succeeding names.

1. Lindsay Adair Martin

   unit 1__________________ unit 2__________________ unit 3__________________

2. Abigail Sue Johnson

   unit 1__________________ unit 2__________________ unit 3__________________

E. When indexing names of married women, the name is indexed by the legal name.

1. Mary Jane O'Keefe (Mrs. John)

   unit 1____________ unit 2____________ unit 3____________ unit 4____________

2. Nora Patrice Fowler (Mrs. Herb)

   unit 1____________ unit 2____________ unit 3____________ unit 4____________

F. Foreign language units are indexed as one unit with the unit that follows. Spacing, punctuation, and capitalization are ignored.

1. Joseph Jack de la Hoya

   unit 1__________________ unit 2__________________ unit 3__________________

2. Maurice John van de Veer

   unit 1__________________ unit 2__________________ unit 3__________________

2. Using the numbers 1, 2, and 3, label the patient names in each group according to the correct filing order of names in an alphabetic filing system.

A. ________ Larry Peter Sanders
   ________ Larry Paul Samuels
   ________ Lawrence Paul Sanders

B. ________ James Edward Reed Sr.
   ________ James Edward Reed
   ________ James Edward Reed Jr.

C. ________ Lynn Elaine Brenner
   ________ Lynn Ellen Brenner
   ________ Lynn Eloise Brenner

D. ________ Patrick Sam Saint
   ________ Patrick Sam St. Bartz
   ________ Paul Sam Saint

3. Circle the right answer(s) from the choices below.

A. Jane O'Hara, CMA, is filing patient records using a nonconsecutive numeric filing system. For the patient file labeled 618 32 6445, what is unit 1?

1. 6445
2. 618
3. 32 6445

B. The most important reason for using numeric filing is that:
   1. it preserves patient confidentiality.
   2. a larger number of records can be easily filed.
   3. a computer can more readily read numeric filing labels.

C. Walter Seals, CMA, is filing using a consecutive numeric filing system. For the patient file labeled 67 843, what is unit 1?
   1. 3
   2. 6
   3. 843

D. Outgoing correspondence is:
   1. friendly correspondence
   2. correspondence sent out of the medical office
   3. correspondence to be thrown away

E. Karen Ritter, CMA, is filing patient files using a numeric filing system. She comes across a file for a patient who has not yet been assigned a number. Karen should:
   1. put the file in the miscellaneous numeric file section.
   2. put the file in a pending filing bin until the physician can assign a number.
   3. put the file directly behind the rest of the files.

F. An out guide should contain:
   1. a record of when the chart was removed and the name of the person who has the chart
   2. the signature of the patient's physician
   3. a record of when the file is expected to be returned

4. State statutes have ruled that medical records are the property of the:
   a. state medical society
   b. ones who create them
   c. patient only
   d. none of the above

5. Any information to be released from the medical record:
   a. goes to medical insurance
   b. requires a physician's signature
   c. requires patient notification and approval
   d. requires a subpoena

6. Filing equipment:
   a. should have a locking capability
   b. is available in vertical or lateral styles
   c. is to be stored in an area accessible only to authorized personnel
   d. all of the above

7. EMR stands for:
   a. emergency room
   b. a popular color-coding system's trade name
   c. electronic medical records
   d. emergency medical rules

8. Release marks include:
   a. date stamp and initials
   b. out guides
   c. tabs
   d. SOAP

CERTIFICATION REVIEW

These questions are designed to mimic the certification examinations. You can use these questions like a small "Certification Examination Study Guide," but this is not meant to take the place of the more extensive study guides. Use this portion to determine in what areas to concentrate your efforts when studying for the certification examination.

1. The POMR is also known as:
   a. source-oriented medical record
   b. SOAP system
   c. traditional method
   d. problem-oriented medical record
   e. none of the above

2. SOAP stands for:
   a. a way to sanitize instruments
   b. patient electronic records
   c. a type of filing system
   d. a charting system
   e. none of the above

3. If a patient needs to return for another examination in 6 months, you might use a reminder system. What is the name of that system?
   a. reminder system
   b. recall system
   c. phone log
   d. tickler system
   e. out guide

4. The most common method of filing in today's medical office is:
   a. alphabetically
   b. numerically
   c. by insurance
   d. by subject
   e. color coding

5. If a medical document is filed in multiple places, you might use a(n):
   a. index
   b. out guide
   c. cross-reference
   d. multiple reference
   e. cross-filed card

CASE STUDY

At the offices of Drs. Lewis and King, co-office managers Marilyn Johnson and Shirley Brooks stress the importance of maintaining accurate, up-to-date, and complete documentation in all patient medical records. The practice uses the POMR method of recordkeeping for patient files within an alphabetical color-coded filing system. Drs. Lewis and King use the SOAP approach in charting patient progress notes. Twice each year, the office managers hold a special staff meeting devoted solely to a discussion of the filing system. The meeting is used to answer staff questions and consider ideas for streamlining the filing system to increase efficiency and ease of use.

Discuss the following:

1. Why is accurate, up-to-date, and complete documentation in patient medical records essential in the ambulatory care setting?
2. Why is the POMR system commonly used by family practice offices?
3. Why is a color-coding system effective in the ambulatory care setting?
4. How important is an effective, easy-to-use, and easy-to-access filing system to the efficiency of the ambulatory care setting?

SELF-ASSESSMENT

To perform this self-assessment, you must first perform an exercise: Go to your spice drawer, a stack of magazines, a bunch of bills/statements, or even your clothes closet, drawers, or the shelves you keep your towels on. Maybe organize something in your medical assisting classroom or laboratory area. Think of the best way to organize them. Is it by size, color, or both? Alphabetically? By date? Frequency of use? Perform the organization. What was the most difficult part; planning how to best accomplish it, or actually doing it? Did you have to take everything out and place it back in order, or were you able to just move things around? Was this a time-consuming exercise? Is the order now a useful tool? Did you have any decisions to make, such as do you file red pepper under red or pepper? Should your pants be organized with their matching tops, or should all the pants be together and all the tops together? Should the medications be organized in alphabetical order, or by classification (type of action)? Now choose another item to organize in a different way. How did this second exercise differ? I suspect your towels were organized by size or by color, whereas your spices would be organized alphabetically. Do you think another person would have chosen a different method? Who do you think decides in an office how a particular area is to be organized? Do you think there might be different ways? Let us pretend that your doctor's office has its patients' charts filed alphabetically, but now they are moving to more computerized records and want to change their files to a numeric system. Make a list of the supplies the staff will need, calculate the time it might take, and make up a plan on how to accomplish this (remember the files are still being used everyday). Does this seem like a major undertaking? Could any files be purged (pulled out of circulation) during this reorganization?

CHAPTER POST-TEST

This is similar to the Pre-Test. Perform this test without looking at the book. This is just to see how well you have understood and can recall the information presented in this chapter after you have studied it and completed the workbook exercises. You will not be graded on this portion (other than the grade you give yourself), but this is an excellent preparation for your instructor's test. You may use this Post-Test to determine what areas you need to study more. Justify any "false" answers.

1. When patient charts are out of order, we use out guides to help us see the error better. (T or F)

2. When filing, you need to be skilled in all but which one of the following?
   a. knowing the alphabet
   b. knowing the basic rules of filing
   c. being able to pay attention to details
   d. being good at math

3. Medical records are important for many reasons. Their most important purpose is for legal protection. (T or F)

4. It is acceptable to release medical information to a family member as long as you have written authorization from the patient. (T or F)

5. When charting, you should determine the relevant information and leave out the opinions and incidentals, unless they relate to the patient's medical care. (T or F)

6. Medical filing systems may be based on the alphabet, a numeric system, or by subject. (T or F)

CERTIFICATION CRITERIA CHECKLIST

As you go through your education and training, keep in mind the national certification examination that you will take when you graduate. Each chapter of the textbook and workbook covers a different section of the examination criteria. To keep track of your preparation for the certification examination, turn to the back of this workbook and highlight the following CMA, RMA, or

CMAS certification examination criteria (if you have already highlighted them from a previous chapter, put a check mark by the criteria):

CMA

D. Professionalism
  4. Maintaining confidentiality

F. Medicolegal Guidelines & Requirements
  3. Documentation/reporting
  4. Releasing medical information

J. Records Management

RMA

II. Administrative Medical Assisting
  C. Medical Receptionist/Secretarial/Clerical
    5. Records and chart management

CMAS

4. Medical Records Management

COMPETENCY ASSESSMENT

Procedure 14-1 Steps for Manual Filing with a Numeric System

Performance Objectives: To demonstrate an understanding of the principles of the numeric filing system. Perform this objective within 15 minutes with a minimum score of 35 points.

Supplies/Equipment: Documents to be filed, dividers with guides, miscellaneous number file section, alphabetic card file and cards, accession journal if needed

Charting/Documentation: Enter appropriate documentation/charting in the box.

Instructor's/Evaluator's Comments and Suggestions:

SKILLS CHECKLIST Procedure 14-1: Steps for Manual Filing with a Numeric System

Name ______________________

Date ______________________

No.	Skill	Check #1 20 pts ea	Check #2 10 pts ea	Check #3 5 pts ea	Notes
1	Inspect and index.				
2	Code for filing units.				
3	Write the number in the upper-right corner.				
4	If no number is assigned, check the miscellaneous file. If item is ready to be assigned, make a card and note number, cross out M, and make a chart file.				
5	If there is no card, make up an alphabetic card.				
6	Cross-reference if necessary and file the card properly.				
7	File in ascending order.				
Student's Total Points					
Points Possible		140	70	35	
Final Score (Student's Total Points / Possible Points)					

	Notes
Start time:	
End time:	
Total time: (15 min goal)	

COMPETENCY ASSESSMENT

Procedure 14-2 Steps for Manual Filing with a Subject Filing System

Performance Objectives: To demonstrate an understanding of the principles of the numeric filing system. Perform this objective within 15 minutes with a minimum score of 35 points.

Supplies/Equipment: Documents to be filed by subject, subject index list or index card filing listing subjects, alphabetic card file and cards

Charting/Documentation: Enter appropriate documentation/charting in the box.

Instructor's/Evaluator's Comments and Suggestions:

SKILLS CHECKLIST Procedure 14-2: Steps for Manual Filing with a Subject Filing System

Name ______________________________

Date ______________________________

No.	Skill	Check #1 20 pts ea	Check #2 10 pts ea	Check #3 5 pts ea	Notes
1	Review the item to find the subject.				
2	Match the subject of the item with an appropriate category.				
3	If neccessary, decide on proper cross-reference.				
4	Underline any subject title on the material.				
5	Write subject title in upper right corner and underline.				
6	Use wavy underline for cross-referencing; use an X as with alphabetic and numeric filing.				
7	Underline the first indexing unit.				
Student's Total Points					
Points Possible		140	70	35	
Final Score (Student's Total Points / Possible Points)					

	Notes
Start time:	
End time:	
Total time: (15 min goal)	

COMPETENCY ASSESSMENT

Procedure 14-3 Correcting a Paper Medical Record

Performance Objectives: To demonstrate the appropriate method to correct an error in a medical chart. Perform this objective within 3 minutes with a minimum score of 25 points.

Supplies/Equipment: Document containing error, document containing correction, red ink pen

Charting/Documentation: Enter appropriate documentation/charting in the box.

Instructor's/Evaluator's Comments and Suggestions:

SKILLS CHECKLIST Procedure 14-3: Correcting a Paper Medical Record

Name ______________________

Date ______________________

No.	Skill	Check #1 20 pts ea	Check #2 10 pts ea	Check #3 5 pts ea	Notes
1	Review information on correction of medical records.				
2	Draw single red line through error.				
3	Write in the correct information.				
4	Follow standard clinic protocol (options: make "error" or "correction" notation above error or corrected information).				
5	Initial and date the correction.				
Student's Total Points					
Points Possible		100	50	25	
Final Score (Student's Total Points / Possible Points)					

	Notes
Start time:	
End time:	
Total time: (3 min goal)	

COMPETENCY ASSESSMENT

Procedure 14-4 Correcting an Electronic Medical Record

Performance Objectives: To demonstrate the appropriate method of correction errors in electronic medical records. Perform this objective within 3 minutes with a minimum score of 30 points.

Supplies/Equipment: Computer with screen open to document containing error, document containing correction

Charting/Documentation: Enter appropriate documentation/charting in the box.

Instructor's/Evaluator's Comments and Suggestions:

SKILLS CHECKLIST Procedure 14-4: Correcting an Electronic Medical Record

Name ______________________________

Date ______________________________

No.	Skill	Check #1 20 pts ea	Check #2 10 pts ea	Check #3 5 pts ea	Notes
1	Review information on correcting EMRs.				
2	Set the software to track the area to be corrected.				
3	Line out the error using the dash key.				
4	Key in the correction to be made beside the error.				
5	Follow clinic protocol (option: key in "correction" or "error" near the corrected information/error).				
6	Initial and date the correction.				
Student's Total Points					
Points Possible		120	60	30	
Final Score (Student's Total Points / Possible Points)					

	Notes
Start time:	
End time:	
Total time: (3 min goal)	

COMPETENCY ASSESSMENT

Procedure 14-5 Establishing a Paper Medical Chart for a New Patient

Performance Objectives: To demonstrate an understanding of the principles for establishing a paper medical chart. Perform this objective within 15 minutes with a minimum score of 50 points.

Supplies/Equipment: File folder used in the facility (flip-up or book-style), divider pages used in the facility (SOAP, laboratory reports, HIPAA Information Sheets, etc.), adhesive twin-prong fasteners for divider pages, two-hole punch for twin-prong fasteners, selected tabs to identify folder and divider pages, demographic patient information completed before or at the first appointment

Charting/Documentation: Enter appropriate documentation/charting in the box.

____

____

____

____

Instructor's/Evaluator's Comments and Suggestions:

____

____

____

____

____

____

SKILLS CHECKLIST Procedure 14-5: Establishing a Paper Medical Chart for a New Patient

Name ______________________

Date ______________________

No.	Skill	Check #1 20 pts ea	Check #2 10 pts ea	Check #3 5 pts ea	Notes
1	Assemble all supplies at a desk or table.				
2	Punch holes in the manila file folder and any necessary dividers.				
3	Affix the adhesive twin-prong fasteners.				
4	Assemble the divider pages dictated by the practice and the office policy.				
5	Securely fasten twin-prong fasteners over the divider pages.				
6	Index and code the patient's name according to the filing system to be used.				
7	Affix appropriately labeled tabs to the folder cut.				
8	Transfer demographic data in black ink pen or office demographic divider sheet.				
9	Affix HIPAA required information, read and signed by patient.				
10	Place prepared chart in proper location.				
Student's Total Points					
Points Possible		200	100	50	
Final Score (Student's Total Points / Possible Points)					

	Notes
Start time:	
End time:	
Total time: (15 min goal)	

CHAPTER 15

Written Communications

CHAPTER PRE-TEST

Perform this test without looking at the book. This is just to see how well you have understood and can recall the information in this chapter after you have read it, but before you have completed the workbook exercises. You will not be graded on this portion (other than the grade you give yourself). Justify any "false" answers.

1. The four major letter styles are (circle four):
   a. full block
   b. modified block, standard
   c. facilitated block
   d. simplified block
   e. simplified
   f. modified block, indented

2. The part of a letter that includes a specially designed logo with the address and phone numbers is called the:
   a. salutation
   b. inside address
   c. letterhead
   d. reference heading
   e. enclosure

3. Whenever documents are to be included in a mailed letter, the word *enclosure* should be written out completely and placed one or two lines below the reference initials. (T or F)

4. Envelopes should be addressed using block (uppercase) letters and no punctuation. (T or F)

5. A computerized feature that allows you to send the same letter, although personalized, to many different people using a database is called:
   a. word processing letters
   b. mail merge
   c. database letters
   d. merge correspondence

6. E-mail is a casual correspondence method; therefore, spelling and grammar are not important. (T or F)

INTRODUCTION

Written correspondence in the ambulatory care setting has three important functions: it conveys necessary information to patients, other physicians, and health care organizations; it reflects on the professional standards of the office; and it provides permanent legal documentation in the event of any litigation. It is essential that medical assisting students understand the importance of written communication skills. Valuable skills include being able to distinguish between and compose the four major letter styles used in the ambulatory care setting; being able to proofread for spelling, grammar, and content; and being able to describe the significance of accuracy in, and the basic rules of, medical transcription.

PERFORMANCE OBJECTIVES

After successful completion of this chapter you should be able to discuss the purposes and uses of written communication in the ambulatory care setting, identify your responsibilities toward written communication, list major letter styles, compose and create appropriate business letters, use official proofreader's marks when proofing a document/letter, address envelopes according to acceptable postal regulations, use computers for electronic communication and to create mass mailings, and be able to sort and classify incoming mail properly according to your office policies. *The following statements are related to your learning objectives for this chapter. Fill in the blanks in the following paragraph with the appropriate term(s).*

All written communication should be of excellent quality because it (1) ________________ on the professionalism of the office. Written documents are (2) ________________ legal documents in the event of any litigation. Medical assistants should remember that there is a difference between (3) ________________________ and business correspondence. It is best to keep business letters to one page, if possible. It is important the business correspondence contain no (4) ____________________ errors and no words that are used incorrectly. Keep a dictionary handy for reference as needed. Computerized (5) ________________ tools are not infallible and should be relied on with caution. Components of a business letter include the (6) ________________ line, (7) ______________________ address, (8) ________________, (9) ________________ line, (10) ____________ of the letter, (11) ______________ closing, keyed (12) ____________________, and (13) ________________________ initials. Business letters may also include a (14) ____________ notation, (15) ____________ notation, (16) ________________, and continuation (17) ________________ heading. (18) ________________ marks are a universally accepted method of marking documents to highlight suggested changes, errors, and inaccuracies. There are many different styles of letters. The most widely accepted styles in a business setting are the (19) ________________, (20) ________________, and (21) ________________. Postal preferences for envelopes have been established to create a quicker, more efficient, and more reliable mail delivery system, especially with the use of (22) ________________ character readers. Among the suggestions are the elimination of all (23) ________________, use of a uniform (24) ________________ margin, preference toward all (25) ________________ letters, and the absence of all marks in the (26) ________________ of the envelope. The zip code should contain all (27) ________________ numbers. Mail (28) ________________ is an excellent use of computers in the medical office that eliminates the need to rekey the same letter many times when sent to a variety of people, and yet allows the letter to be personalized for each recipient. When handling incoming mail, the first step is to (29) ________________ it into different categories. Then the mail should be (30) ________________ with the date received and checked for a return (31) ________________. Then attach the letter/document to the (32) ________________ and either route it appropriately, attach supporting documentation, or reply as promptly as possible.

VOCABULARY BUILDER

Fill in the blanks in the passage below with the correct vocabulary terms.

bond paper
full block letter
keyed
mail merge
medical transcription
modified block letter
optical character reader (OCR)
simplified letter
voice recognition technology (VRT)
watermark
Zip+4

There are four major types of letters that medical assistants commonly write. Of these, the (1) ________________ is the most time-efficient, because it does not use excessive tab indentations for the address, complimentary close, or keyed signature. In the (2) ________________, all lines begin at the left margin with the exception of the date line, complimentary closure, and keyed signature. Medical assistants may choose to use the (3) ________________, the style of letter recommended by the Administrative Management Society. In this style, all lines are (4) ________________, or input by keystroke, flush with the left margin. When selecting paper supplies, the medical assistant should choose (5) ________________ with a (6) ________________, or image imprinted during the papermaking process that is visible when a sheet is held up to the light. When preparing letters for outgoing shipments, it is important for the medical assistant to pay attention to several factors, including addresses. Medical assistants should machine print addresses (including the (7) ________________ code) with a uniform left-hand margin so that the addresses can be read by the U.S. Postal Service's (8) ________________.

One of the most utilized aspects of written communication in the clinic is the management of the patient records, which are processed in the arena of (9) ____________________. One of the latest technical advances in this area is (10) ________________________________, by which physicians speak into a microphone that translates spoken words into a typed report via the computer. This new method can cut down on errors and aid medical assistants in maintaining confidentiality and protecting the privacy of patients in the process of medical documentation.

LEARNING REVIEW

1. Identify the letter style in Figure 15-1. ______________________

2. Proofread the letter in Figure 15-1, correcting all errors by inserting the proper proofreader's marks. Make your marks directly onto the text. Consult your textbook for a list of common proofreader's marks. Refer to a medical dictionary, if necessary.

3. To practice your skills of medical transcription, record the content of the letter in Figure 15-1 by speaking into a tape recorder. Play back the tape and transcribe the letter accurately on a sheet of stationery using the standard modified block style.

JAMES CARTER, MD, NEUROLOGY

Metropolitan University Medical Center, 8280 Wright Avenue, Northborough, OH 12382

February 2, 20XX

Elizabeth Kind, M.D
Inner City Health Care
The Offices of Lewis & King, MD
2501 Center Street
Nrothborough, OH 12345

RE: MARGARET THOMAS

Dear Dr. King:

Thank you for refering Margaret Thomas to my neurological practice. Margaret come to you recently as a new patient for a comprehensive physical examination to evaluate troubling symptoms she had been experiencing for several months. Margaret notices symtoms of tremor, difficulty walking, defective judgement, and hot flushes; she is not able to poinpoint the exac ttime symptoms began. Your physical examination suggested the possible diagnoisis of parkingson's Disease. Margaret presented today for a complete nuerological evaluation.

Figure 15-1

MEDICAL/SURGICAL HISTORY. The patient is posiitive for the usual childhood diseases and the births of three children, following normal pregnancies. Her surgical history includes an Appendectomy performed 10 years ago. She has a food allergy to shellfish, but no known allergies to medications. She takes Pepto-Bismol and Metamusil for frequent stomach upset and constipation. She is a widow with two children, ages twenty three, twenty-five, and 29, and is a retired homemaker. She does not smoke and has an occassional glass of wine. Her family history is positive for colon cancer in her mother and parenteral grandfather and for lung cancer in her father.

PYHSICALEXAMINATION. VITAL SIGNS: The patient has normal vital signs for a 52-year old Caucasian female. HEENT: The patient had a normacephalic and atraumatic exam. There is mild bobing of the head and facial expressions appear fixed. Pupils equal, round, regular, react to light and acommodation. The fundi were benign. There was normal cup to disc ratio of 0.3. Tympanic Membranes were both clear and mobile. Her nose was clear, the oropharynz ws clear without any evidence of lezions. There was not cervical adenopathy, no thyromegely, or other masses. NECK: Musles of the neck are quite rigid and stiff. CHEST: Cear to percussion and auscultation. HEART: Regular rate and rhythm without murmurs or gallops. there was no jugular venous distention, no peripheral edema, no carotid buits. Pulses were 2+ and symetrical. Abdomen. Some what obese, but benigh. There was not organomegaly or masses. Bowel tones were normal. There was no rebound tenderness. BACK: Examination reveals loss of posturalreflexe and patient stands with head bent forward and wals as if in danger of falling forward. There is difficulty in pivoting and loss of balance. GENITOURINARY: Normal. EXTREMITIES: Thre is moderate bradykinesia. Chracteristic slow, turning motion (pronation-supination) of, the forearm and the hand and a motion of the thumb against the fingers as if rolling a pill between the fingers is noted. This condition seems to worsen when the patient is concentrating or feeling anxious.

NEUROLOGICAL. The patient was cooperative and answered all questions. There is no history past of mental disorders or cardiovascular disease. There is muscle weakness and rigidity in all four extremities. Intellect remains intact;

LABORATORY DATA: Urinanalysis reveals low levels of dopamin. Cat scan reveals degeneration of nerve cells occuring in the basel ganglia.

ASSESSMENT. Based on the patient history and neurologic examination, it appears most likely that the patient has mild to moderate Parkinsons Disease.

PLAN. 1. Recommend physical therapy focussed on learning how to manage diffi-cult movements such as descneding stairs safely.
2. Exercises to maintain flexibility, motility, and mental well-being.
3. Levadopa to increase dopamine levels in the brain to control symptoms. Please advise the patient that alchohol consumption shoudl be limited because it acts antegonistically to levodopa.
4. Relaxation and stress management counseling.

PROGNOSIS. Parkinson's disease progresses slowly. Patient should be follow on a regular basis and observed for any signs of damentia which may result in about 1-third of cases.

Sincerely,

James Carter, MD

DD: February 2, 20XX
DT: February 3, 20XX
JC/bl

Figure 15-1, *(continued)*

4. The most efficient letter style for the ambulatory care setting is:
   a. modified block, standard
   b. full block
   c. simplified
   d. modified block, indented

5. Paper for written communications in the office should be of good quality, contain a watermark, and be:
   a. 20 pound stock
   b. 70 pound stock
   c. 50 pound stock
   d. 10 pound stock

6. A written record of what transpires during a meeting is called:
   a. agenda
   b. memoranda
   c. minutes
   d. itinerary

7. When a physician dismisses a patient due to noncompliance, a letter should be sent:
   a. express mail
   b. priority mail
   c. registered mail
   d. certified mail

8. What type of records should never be faxed?
   a. clinical
   b. administrative
   c. financial
   d. personal

CERTIFICATION REVIEW

These questions are designed to mimic the certification examinations. You can use these questions like a small "Certification Examination Study Guide," but this is not meant to take the place of the more extensive study guides. Use this portion to determine in what areas to concentrate your efforts when studying for the certification examination. Justify any "false" answers.

1. First class mail is the most common mail used. (T or F)

2. The "salutation" of a letter is the:
   a. signature
   b. greeting

   c. return address
   d. closing remark (such as: "Sincerely")
   e. the recipient's name, title, and address

3. When addressing an envelope, the proper way to list the state is:
   a. to write it out completely
   b. to abbreviate it using at least the first four letters
   c. to capitalize it using the official two-letter abbreviation
   d. any of the above as long as it is in uppercase letters and is written clearly

4. URL means:
   a. Universal Return (address) Locator
   b. Uniform Resource Locator
   c. Universal Readers Limitation
   d. Uniform Registered Locator

CASE STUDY

Ellen Armstrong, CMA, enjoys working on correspondence for Drs. Lewis and King and takes pride in her written communication skills. As an ongoing project, office manager Marilyn Johnson, CMA, asks Ellen to make suggestions for updating and revising the style manual used in the medical office for written communication guidelines. Ellen suggests the addition of a section in the style manual to discuss bias in language. Bias-free language is sensitive in applying labels to individuals or groups and uses sex-specific words and pronouns appropriately. For example, dementia is used instead of crazy or senile. Instead of using layman, consider using layperson. Apply he or she only in sex-specific usage. Marilyn and the physician–employers ask Ellen to implement the addition to the style manual.

Discuss the following:

1. Why is bias-free language an important consideration in written communications for the ambulatory care setting?
2. List other examples of biased language and give suggestions for bias-free alternatives.

SELF-ASSESSMENT

In your written communications, are you able to express yourself accurately and concisely? Able to communicate ideas effectively? Capable of proofreading and editing for content? Use this simple self-assessment to gauge your comfort and proficiency in written communications by identifying strengths and pinpointing any weak areas that could use improvement.

For each statement below, circle the corresponding letter to the response that best describes you.

1. When writing a letter, I generally feel:
   a. confident. I communicate effectively on the page and enjoy writing letters.
   b. at ease. My written communication skills are acceptable.
   c. uncomfortable. I would rather communicate verbally than through writing.

2. As far as content goes, when I am given the required information and asked to compose a letter, I:
   a. almost always understand exactly what I am being asked to communicate and am able to convey it precisely in letter form
   b. generally understand what I am being asked to communicate, but sometimes have to fine-tune my letters
   c. often have trouble understanding what I am being asked to communicate and usually have to go back and ask questions about the letter's content

3. In general, when choosing words for written correspondence, I feel:
   a. secure about my ability to select appropriate language and use medical terminology accurately
   b. pretty confident, although my general vocabulary and knowledge of medical terminology could use some improvement
   c. frustrated; I always seem to confuse words and medical terms no matter how hard I try not to

4. As far as spelling goes, I am:
   a. a top-notch speller; I always keep both a standard and medical dictionary on hand for the words I am not sure of.
   b. an adequate speller; sometimes I confuse a word here or there; I always have to proofread carefully for spelling errors
   c. a below-par speller; my letters are always littered with misspellings and someone else has to proofread my work

5. Grammatically speaking, I am:
   a. above average; I routinely find mistakes in my colleagues' work
   b. passable; I make minor mistakes but usually catch them while proofreading
   c. hopeless; people find mistakes in my work even after I have checked it twice

6. Regarding proofreader's marks, I am:
   a. highly capable of proofreading my work; if colleagues need someone to proof their work, I am first on their list
   b. an okay proofreader; I occasionally overlook a mistake, but nobody's perfect
   c. frightened; proofreading marks are just a bunch of meaningless squiggles to me

7. How would you describe your formatting skills?
   a. Exemplary. I understand all basic letter forms, and all of my letters are rigorously formatted according to correct specifications.
   b. Satisfactory. Every so often, I confuse styles or forget an annotation; but in general, all my letters are formatted correctly.
   c. Fair to nonexistent. I have trouble understanding why every letter has to be so formally constructed.

8. When adhering to office style guidelines, I:
   a. always follow the guidelines
   b. usually have no problem sticking to style guidelines; when I make a mistake, it is a rare event
   c. need improvement; my letters are frequently littered with style inconsistencies, and I do not understand the need for an office style as long as each letter is written with accurate information

9. If you had to rate your transcription skills, you would describe them as:
   a. impeccable. I make few errors and use critical thinking skills to problem-solve trouble spots before giving up and asking for help.
   b. sufficient. What I do not understand I automatically flag and ask for clarification.
   c. not as good as they should be. I hate trying to enter data from a taped voice; it is a frustrating experience.

10. Overall, I think of writing letters in the health care environment as:
   a. one of my strong suits
   b. a task that I am able to accomplish, just not one I particularly enjoy
   c. a necessary evil

Scoring: If your answers were mostly *A* responses, you have strong written communications skills and enjoy writing letters. If your responses were mostly *B*s, your written communications skills are good but could stand some improvement. Try reviewing pertinent information in this chapter to strengthen areas that need it. If your answers were mostly *C*s, you need to work on your written communication skills. Volunteer to take on as many written correspondence assignments as you can—practice may help you overcome your apprehension about writing letters and will almost certainly raise the quality of your work.

CHAPTER POST-TEST

This is similar to the Pre-Test. Perform this test without looking at the book. This is just to see how well you have understood and can recall the information presented in this chapter after you have studied it and completed the workbook exercises. You will not be graded on this portion (other than the grade you give yourself), but this is an excellent preparation for your instructor's test. You may use this Post-Test to determine what areas you need to study more. Justify any "false" answers.

1. The most commonly used of the four major letter styles in the ambulatory care setting is:
   a. full block
   b. modified block, standard
   c. facilitated block, indented
   d. simplified

2. The part of a letter that includes the return address and perhaps a logo is the:
   a. salutation
   b. inside address
   c. letterhead
   d. reference heading
   e. enclosure

3. Whenever documents are to be included in a mailed letter, the word *enclosure* should be indicated by:
   a. Enclosures
   b. Enc.
   c. 1 Enc.
   d. 2 enclosures
   e. Enclosure (2)
   f. any of the above

4. Envelopes should be addressed using a combination of uppercase and lowercase letters and with the proper punctuation. (T or F)

5. When it is desirable to send the same letter, although personalized, to many different people, a computerized feature that can be used is called:
   a. word processing letters
   b. mail merge
   c. database letters
   d. merge correspondence

6. E-mail may be used as a type of business correspondence method and is subject to the same proper use of written language as traditional mail. (T or F)

CERTIFICATION CRITERIA CHECKLIST

As you go through your education and training, keep in mind the national certification examination that you will take when you graduate. Each chapter of the textbook and workbook covers a different section of the examination criteria. To keep track of your preparation for the certification examination turn to the back of this workbook and highlight the following CMA, RMA, or CMAS certification examination criteria (if you have already highlighted them from a previous chapter, put a check mark by the criteria):

CMA

A. Medical Terminology
   2. Uses of terminology

E. Communication
   7. Receiving, organizing, prioritizing and transmitting information
   9. Fundamental writing skills

G. Data Entry
   2. Formats
   3. Proofreading

H. Equipment
   1. Equipment operation

I. Computer Concepts
   3. Computer applications

K. Screening and Processing Mail

RMA

I. General Medical Assisting Knowledge
   B. Medical Terminology
      4. Spelling

II. Administrative Medical Assisting
   C. Medical Receptionist/Secretary/Clerical
      4. (Oral and) Written communication

CMAS

8. Medical Office Management
   - Office communications

CHAPTER 16

Transcription

CHAPTER PRE-TEST

Perform this test without looking at the book. This is just to see how well you have understood and can recall the information in this chapter after you have read it, but before you have completed the workbook exercises. You will not be graded on this portion (other than the grade you give yourself). Justify any "false" answers.

1. Medical transcriptionists must have years of experience before they can do well in the field. (T or F)
2. Anyone who has computer abilities and can spell well can perform medical transcription well. (T or F)
3. Medical documents are only for the clinic and physician who generated them, so they are called "internal documents." (T or F)
4. Medical transcription is a profession that has not really undergone many changes in the last decade or so. (T or F)
5. If a medical transcriptionist cannot hear the word the dictator is saying, it is best to leave the space blank. (T or F)
6. Even though medical transcriptionists work within the medical field, because they often work alone, they do not need to be concerned with Health Insurance Portability and Accountability Act (HIPAA) regulations. (T or F)

INTRODUCTION

Many medical offices have transcription services available in the office for the physician to dictate the medical record. Those able to provide transcription services are highly skilled professionals who are in demand for their skills. The medical assistant who is able to provide these skills is in high demand. Medical transcription involves a knowledge of the equipment, including transcription machines and computers for word processing, the use of correct medical terminology for the many types of records used in the office, the ability to format documents, and good proofreading skills. The correct usage of grammar, spelling, and punctuation aids the medical assistant in demonstrating good transcription skills.

PERFORMANCE OBJECTIVES

Your career as a medical assistant may or may not include transcription, but it will certainly include medical documents. Transcription is all about medical documents such as chart notes, operative reports, history and physical examination reports, discharge summaries, emergency room summaries, radiology and pathology reports, and consultation reports, as well letters to patients and other physicians. Taking a course in transcription incorporates lessons learned in medical terminology, anatomy and physiology, pathology, word processing, English, spelling, sentence structure, grammar, proofreading, and punctuation. There is perhaps no other course that encompasses so many other course lessons. Other lessons well learned in medical transcription are less objective; for example, the lessons of striving for quality, neatness, completeness, and accuracy. Medical records are legal documents, thus perfection is the goal. Many physicians rely on the medical transcriptionist to produce perfect documents, and with this responsibility comes trust. When physicians trust that the documents are correct and accurate, they will often sign them without thoroughly proofreading them. A transcriptionist who betrays that trust puts the physician at risk legally.

Many medical clinics employ transcriptionists in the office, whereas others contract their transcription services. As a transcriptionist, you may choose to be self-employed, a contracted employee, or an employee of the clinic. Within those parameters, the actual transcription work may be performed in-house or at a remote site. The documents may be printed and brought into the office, sent in electronically for printing within the office, or, in the case of EMRs (electronic medical records), the data may be entered directly into the computer and saved in the patient's electronic chart. *The following statements are related to your learning objectives for this chapter. Fill in the blanks in the following paragraph with the appropriate term(s).*

Medical transcription is all about medical (1) ______________________. Medical transcriptionists must have a good working knowledge about medical (2) ______________________, anatomy and (3) ______________________, disease processes (4)______________________ and word processing. They must know English, (5) ______________________, (6) ______________________, (7) ______________________, and (8) ______________________. Medical documents are (9)______________________ documents; therefore, the transcriptionist must strive for (10) ______________________, (11) ______________________, (12) ______________________, and (13) ______________________.

VOCABULARY BUILDER

Find the words below that are misspelled; circle them, and then correctly spell them in the spaces provided. Then insert the correct vocabulary terms from the list that best fit the descriptions below.

athentication	discharge summary	priveliged
autapsy report	electronic	progress notes
chart notes	gross examination	proofreading
chief complaint	HIPAA	quality assurence
confidentility	history and physical	review of symptems
consultation reports	JCAHO	risk management
continuing education	magnetic tape	transcriber
correspondence	medical transcriptionist	turnaround time

current	microscopic examination	voice recognition system
digital speech standard	old	waveform audio
digitaly processed dictation	patholigy	
______________	______________	______________
______________	______________	______________
______________	______________	

1. A professional who uses word processing formats to transcribe medical records, notes, letters, and documents is called a ______________________________.
2. The part of the pathology report that describes the size and shape of a biopsy is called a ______________________________________.
3. The part of patients' hospital records that describe their entire hospital stay, progress, and condition on release is called a ____.
4. The part of the patient's medical record that contains information related to the main reason for the encounter, as well as a synopsis of the patient's previous medical information, is called the ____________________________________.
5. Reports such as History and Physicals that should be completed within 24 hours are called ___________________________ reports.
6. A type of signature that may use various computer key entries as identification is referred to as ________________________________.
7. The process of converting audio sound into a string of computer language is called _______ ____.
8. A medical report generated to describe the examinations of tissues or cells obtained through a surgery or medical procedure is the ________________ report.
9. Reports that may be completed up to 71 hours after the event are referred to as _________ ________________ reports.

Define the following terms:

1. American Association for Medical Transcription

____

____

2. Consultation report

____

____

3. Digital speech standard

____

____

4. Editing

____

____

5. Flag

____

____

6. Home-based medical transcriptionists

____

____

7. Turnaround time

____

____

8. Digital dictation

____

____

LEARNING REVIEW

1. A. List five attributes of the medical transcriptionist under each of the two major categories.

   (1) Personal attributes

   a. ______________________________________

   b. ______________________________________

   c. ______________________________________

   d. ______________________________________

   e. ______________________________________

   (2) Acquired skills developed

   a. ______________________________________

   b. ______________________________________

   c. ______________________________________

   d. ______________________________________

   e. ______________________________________

   B. Describe how the transcription machine (transcriber) differs from a simple audio recorder.

   ____

   ____

   ____

C. Correct the following paragraph:

her past medical history is postivie for the usual childhood diseases and the births of to children following normal pregnancies she has a negative pasts urgical history. she has no allergies To medications and takes tylenol for occasional headashes. She is married and has to children ages 3 and 12 months. She does not smoke or drink

D. Give two examples of each type of turnaround time report and the time of the turnaround.

STAT: (1) ______________________________

(2) ______________________________

Current: (1) ______________________________

(2) ______________________________

Old: (1) ______________________________

(2) ______________________________

2. The American Association for Medical Transcription (AAMT) began in _______.
   a. 1850
   b. 1902
   c. 1978
   d. 2000

3. Which of the following is *not* a requirement for success in the field of medical transcription?
   a. experience in the medical field
   b. keyboarding skills of 60 to 80 words per minute
   c. understanding of human anatomy
   d. knowledge of drug names and their uses

4. To take the CMT examination, the transcriptionist must have a minimum of ______ years performing medical transcription.
   a. 1
   b. 2
   c. 5
   d. 10

5. CMT recertification is accomplished through continuing education with the purpose of maintaining competency and must be completed every _____ years.
   a. 2
   b. 3
   c. 5
   d. 10

6. Radiology, pathology, and laboratory reports are usually termed as _____ to indicate the need for immediate turnaround.
   a. ASAP
   b. current
   c. old
   d. STAT

CERTIFICATION REVIEW

These questions are designed to mimic the certification examinations. You can use these questions like a small "Certification Examination Study Guide," but this is not meant to take the place of the more extensive study guides. Use this portion to determine in what areas to concentrate your efforts when studying for the certification examination. Justify any "false" answers.

1. Medical records are documents governed by laws and may be subpoenaed for review by various courts. (T or F)
2. The medical report may play a major role in substantiating injury or a malpractice claim. (T or F)
3. Joint Commission on Accreditation of Healthcare Organizations (JCAHO) allows 36 hours from admission for a history and physical report to be dictated, transcribed, and filed into the patient's medical record. (T or F)
4. When transcribing radiology or imaging reports, the date of service should be used rather than the date of dictation. (T or F)
5. Electronic signatures on medical documents are allowed by both Medicare and JCAHO. (T or F)

CASE STUDY

You are transcribing a report when you notice it is a report about your neighbor. The report states that the tests run for multiple sclerosis are positive. You had just spoken to your neighbor yesterday and she was concerned that she hadn't heard from her physician and was wondering about the results of her tests. What should you do?

SELF-ASSESSMENT

1. Access the AAMT Web site at http://www.aamt.org and click on "Certification," then "Candidate's Guide," then the "Sample Medical Transcription Related Knowledge Questions."
   A. Answer the questions to the best of your ability.
   B. Check your answers to see how well you were able to answer the questions correctly.
   C. Which transcription skills listed in the textbook were tested within these questions?
2. Do you think you would enjoy working as a transcriptionist? What about the profession appeals to you? What about the profession does not appeal to you?

CHAPTER POST-TEST

This is similar to the Pre-Test. Perform this test without looking at the book. This is just to see how well you have understood and can recall the information in this chapter after you studied it and completed the workbook exercises. You will not be graded on this portion (other than the grade you give yourself), but this is an excellent preparation for your instructor's test. You may use this Post-Test to determine what areas you need to study more. Justify any "false" answers.

1. Medical transcriptionists can do well even without a lot of experience if they are committed to exactness and quality work. (T or F)
2. Medical transcription is a job for people with good computer abilities, word processing speed; who have excellent spelling, grammar, and punctuation skills; and who care enough to do the best job possible. (T or F)
3. Medical documents are not only for the clinic and physician who generated them, they are also legal documents used by many professionals. (T or F)
4. Medical transcription is a profession that has undergone numerous changes in the last decade or so. (T or F)
5. If a medical transcriptionist cannot hear the word the dictator is saying, it is best to leave the space blank. (T or F)
6. Because medical transcriptionists work within the medical field with medical information, they need to be concerned with HIPAA regulations. (T or F)

CERTIFICATION CRITERIA CHECKLIST

As you go through your education and training, keep in mind the national certification examination that you will take when you graduate. Each chapter of the textbook and workbook covers a different section of the examination criteria. To keep track of your preparation for the certification examination, turn to the back of this workbook and highlight the following CMA, RMA, or CMAS certification examination criteria (if you have already highlighted them from a previous chapter, put a check mark by the criteria):

CMA

A. Medical Terminology
    2. Uses of terminology
F. Medicolegal Guidelines & Requirements
    2. Legislation
G. Data Entry
I. Computer Concepts
    3. Computer applications

RMA

I. General Medical Assisting Knowledge
    B. Medical Terminology
        4. Spelling
II. Administrative Medical Assisting
    C. Medical Receptionist/Secretary/Clerical
        1. Terminology
        4. (Oral and) Written communication
        6. Transcription and dictation
        8. Computer applications

CMAS

1. Medical Assisting Foundation
    - Medical terminology
3. Medical Office Clerical Assisting
    - Communication

EVALUATION OF CHAPTER KNOWLEDGE

Skills	Student Self-Evaluation Good	Average	Poor
I recognize emergency situations.	_____	_____	_____
I can explain the work of the medical transcriptionists, including attributes needed and career opportunities.	_____	_____	_____
I can describe the CMT certification process and membership in AAMT.	_____	_____	_____
I can discuss the proper ways to make corrections.	_____	_____	_____
I can describe the process of flagging.	_____	_____	_____
I can differentiate between the many types of records found in the medical office.	_____	_____	_____
I can describe turnaround time and its importance.	_____	_____	_____
I can discuss ethical and legal issues surrounding medical transcription.	_____	_____	_____

CHAPTER 17

Daily Financial Practices

CHAPTER PRE-TEST

Perform this test without looking at the book. This is just to see how well you have understood and can recall the information in this chapter after you have read it, but before you have completed the workbook exercises. You will not be graded on this portion (other than the grade you give yourself). Justify any "false" answers.

1. The management of the business details of the practice usually falls to the medical assisting staff. (T or F)
2. Every patient, regardless of insurance coverage, should be charged the same fee for the same service. (T or F)
3. You should discourage the use of credit/debit cards for medical bills. (T or F)
4. Purchase orders are to be written up when the purchase arrives. (T or F)
5. Petty cash is available for authorized use when the purchase is minor or unexpected and when a check is not necessary. (T or F)

INTRODUCTION

Ambulatory care settings depend on sound financial practices to thrive, grow, and continue to provide good patient care. To that end, medical assistants should strive to understand basic accounting and bookkeeping terms, forms, principles, and both computerized and manual systems related to these financial activities. Medical assistants should be prepared to handle a variety of financial tasks, including procedures related to accounts receivable, accounts payable, patient billing, banking, checking accounts, purchasing, and petty cash systems.

PERFORMANCE OBJECTIVES

After successful completion of this chapter you will be able to explain the importance of good communication when explaining patient fees. You will have some ideas of available options for credit arrangements for your patients and will be able to recognize when adjustments are warranted. You will be able to differentiate between manual and computerized bookkeeping systems, describe the pegboard system, and state the advantages and disadvantages of computerized bookkeeping systems. Another performance objective of this chapter is to help you be aware of and establish good working habits when working with financial records. You will be able to describe information found on and uses for the encounter form. You will be able to demonstrate a knowledge of banking procedures, including types of accounts and services, and show proficiency in preparing deposits, checks, and patient receipts and reconciling accounts. You also will be able to describe month-end activities. *The following statements are related to your learning objectives for this chapter. Fill in the blanks in the following paragraph with the appropriate term(s).*

Accounts (1) ______________________________ are all the fees that patients owe to the practice for services rendered, and accounts (2) ______________________________ are the accounts the practice owes to suppliers for supplies, services, and so forth. When explaining fees to a patient, it is best if the patient knows what to expect before the treatment. Ideally, this should be in (3) ____________________. The documentation of this discussion with Medicare and Medicaid patients is on a form called the (4) ____, or (5) __________ for short. An (6) ________________________ to a fee may be warranted for hardship cases, but remember, the same offer must be available to all patients. Patients should be encouraged to use (7) ______________________ or (8) ______________________ payments, if those payment methods are handy for them. A(n) (9) ______________________________ form is a document that goes with the patient throughout their visit and includes all the billing information on it. The traditional (10) __________________________ system of tracking the day's financial activities is quickly being replaced by (11) __________________________________ methods. There are distinct advantages and disadvantages of either method. Occasionally, there is a need for small amounts of cash for minor and unexpected expenses such as a postage due package, coffee or tea for the office, and miscellaneous other needs. This name for this reserve of cash for those purposes is called (12) __________________________.

VOCABULARY BUILDER

Find the words below that are misspelled; circle them, and then correctly spell them in the spaces provided.

accounts payible	day sheet	notary
accounts recievable	debit	payee
adjustments	dispursements	pegboard system
balance	encounter form	petty cash
cashier's check	guaranter	posting
certified check	leadger	traveler's check
credit	money market account	voucher check

______________________ ______________________ ______________________

______________________ ______________________

A. *Identify the following financial forms used in the ambulatory care setting.*

________________________ 1. Used to records individual cash transactions for minor or unexpected expenses

________________________ 2. Record of charges, payments, and adjustments for individual patients and/or family members

________________________ 3. A record of daily patient transactions used in conjunction with pegboard systems

________________________ 4. Record of services supplied and the charges and payments for those services; functions as a billing form for insurance reimbursement

B. *Identify the correct financial term or function for each definition.*

________________________ 1. Agencies that manage many private insurance plans and government-sponsored programs

________________________ 2. Small cash sum kept on hand in the office for minor or unexpected expenses

________________________ 3. Abbreviation for *received on account*

________________________ 4. Decreases the balance due

________________________ 5. The amount insurance requires patients to pay at the time of services

________________________ 6. A term for paper money

________________________ 7. A synonym for *charge slip*

________________________ 8. The acceptable abbreviation for *usual, customary, and reasonable* when referring to physician charges

________________________ 9. As a noun, this term denotes "the amount owed"; as a verb, the term means "to verify posting accuracy"

________________________ 10. Accounting function that describes the act of recording financial transactions into bookkeeping or accounting systems

________________________ 11. An increase or decrease to a patient account not due to charges incurred or payments received

________________________ 12. Accounting system that consists of day sheets, ledger cards, charge slips, and receipt forms; all forms have matching columns that align and are held in place when the system is in use

________________________ 13. Sum owed by a business for services or goods received

________________________ 14. Sum owed to a business for services or goods supplied

LEARNING REVIEW

1. Identify two work guidelines and six habits essential to creating and maintaining accurate financial records.

   A. Guidelines:

   (1) ______________________________

   (2) ______________________________

   B. Good work habits:

   (1) ______________________________

   (2) ______________________________

   (3) ______________________________

   (4) ______________________________

   (5) ______________________________

   (6) ______________________________

2. A. The checking account is the account most often used by medical assistants in the ambulatory care setting. Checking accounts are accounts that allow depositors to write checks against money placed in the account. Identify seven of the nine features that may be a part of the checking account.

   (1) ____________________ (5) ____________________

   (2) ____________________ (6) ____________________

   (3) ____________________ (7) ____________________

   (4) ____________________

   B. Administrative medical assistant Karen Ritter is responsible for assisting the office manager and accountant in performing accounts payable activities for Inner City Health Care. On September 4, she receives a $323.45 bill from RJ Medical Supply Company for blood pressure equipment the office received on August 30. Noting that the company demands payment within 30 days of billing, Karen writes a check disbursing funds to the company on September 15. The balance in the office's checking account before this check is written equals $2,610.00. Using this information, write out the check and stub below (Figure 17-1). Karen will submit the check to Susan Rice, M.D., for her signature.

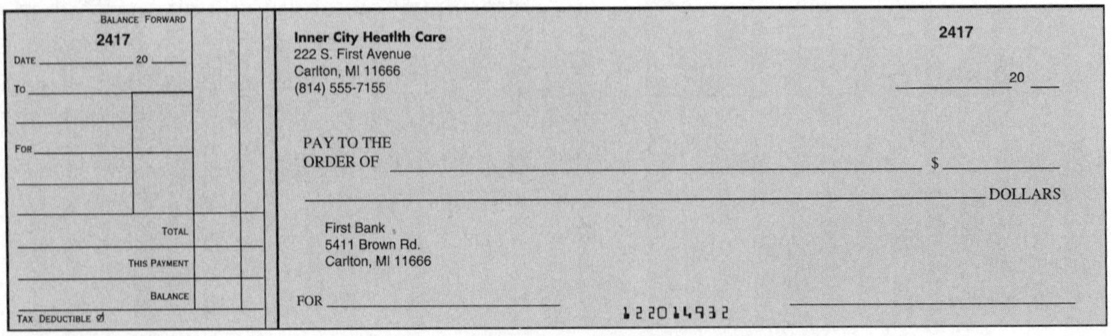

Figure 17-1

C. What are five rules to ensure that checks are properly written and recorded?

(1) ______________________________

(2) ______________________________

(3) ______________________________

(4) ______________________________

(5) ______________________________

3. A. The first rule of purchasing: Nothing is ordered or paid for without a purchase order or purchase order number. Give three reasons why it is important to ensure proper control over purchasing supplies and equipment.

(1) ______________________________

(2) ______________________________

(3) ______________________________

B. Office manager Walter Seals, CMA, is responsible for purchasing office supplies for Inner City Health Care. On September 10, Walter completes purchase order #1743 for supplies ordered from Mayflower Supply, requested by administrative medical assistant Karen Ritter. The items are taxed at 8%, and the shipping fee is prepaid. The items are billed and shipped to Inner City Health Care; the terms are net due 30 days. Complete the purchase order form (Figure 17-2).

Inner City Health Care
222 S. First Avenue
Carlton, MI 11666
(814) 555-7155

Mayflower Supply, Inc.
642 East 65th Street
Carlton, MI 11623
(814) 555-9999

2 boxes of fax paper, #62145, at $8.99 a box
5 day-view desk calendars, #24598, at $4.25 each
4 cases of copier paper, #72148, at $20.00 a box
5 boxes of highlighter pens, 12 to a box, #26773, at $3.98 a box
4 computer printer cartridges, #96187, at $49.99 each

C. When the office supplies ordered from Mayflower Supply arrive, what should be done to verify that the correct items and quantities have been received? What should be done to prepare the invoice from Mayflower Supply for payment?

____

____

____

____

____

____

4. Describe the following types of checks, which are different from checks issued from a standard business checking account.

(1) Cashier's check ______________________________

____

PURCHASE ORDER

NO. 1742

Bill To:	Ship To:	Vendor:

REQ BY	BUYER	TERMS

QTY	ITEM	UNITS	DESCRIPTION	UNIT PR	TOTAL
				SUBTOTAL	
				TAX	
				FREIGHT	
				BAL DUE	

Figure 17-2

(2) Certified check ______________________________

____

(3) Money order ______________________________

____

(4) Voucher check ______________________________

____

(5) Traveler's check ______________________________

5. Adjustments are entries made to a patient's account that do not represent charges or payments. Name three reasons why adjustments may sometimes be made to a patient's account.

(1) ______________________________

(2) ______________________________

(3) ______________________________

6. Examine the sample bank statement in Figure 17-3; then answer the following questions.

____________________ A. How many checks are not listed on the bank statement?

____________________ B. What is the total amount of these outstanding checks?

____________________ C. According to the bank statement, when was the last deposit made?

____________________ D. What was the amount of the last deposit?

____________________ E. According to Figure 17-3, what is the total of the deposits not listed on the bank statement?

____________________ F. What fees did the bank charge this month?

Summary of Account Balance — Closing Date 1/15/20XX

Account # 1257-164013 — Ending Balance $8,347.62

Beginning Balance	$7,152.18
Total Deposits and Additions	$8,643.86
Total Withdrawals	$7,433.21
Service Charge	$ 15.24

Number	Date	Amount	Number	Date	Amount
201	12/18/XX	173.82	234	1/4/XX	96.31
223*	12/18/XX	44.12	235	1/4/XX	73.48
224	12/20/XX	586.00	236	1/6/XX	325.40
225	12/21/XX	24.15	237	1/7/XX	40.00
226	12/22/XX	33.90	238	1/8/XX	66.77
228*	12/23/XX	1250.00	241*	1/9/XX	15.55
229	12/24/XX	11.75	242	1/10/XX	12.45
230	12/24/XX	19.02	243	1/10/XX	4441.25
231	1/2/XX	43.80	244	1/10/XX	64.55
232	1/3/XX	39.00			
233	1/4/XX	71.50			

*Denotes gap in check sequence

Date	Deposit Amount	Date	Deposit Amount
18-Dec	361.25	4-Jan	825.00
19-Dec	586.00	5-Jan	1286.71
20-Dec	918.21	7-Jan	608.00
21-Dec	201.00	8-Jan	811.15
2-Jan	475.00	9-Jan	1092.68
3-Jan	1478.36		

Front

1. Enter Ending Balance from the front of this statement
$ 8,347.62

2. Enter deposits not shown on this statement
$ 3,162.50

3. Subtotal (add 1 & 2)
$ 11,510.12

4. List outstanding checks or other withdrawals here

Check #	Amount
222	37.89
227	161.15
239	11.50
240	92.12
245	835.17
246	21.75
247	586.00

5. Total outstanding checks
$ 1,745.58

Balance (subtract #5 from #3)
$ 9,764.54

This should equal your checkbook balance

Back

Figure 17-3

7. A. Deposits are generally made daily. All checks to be deposited must be endorsed. Define *endorsement*. Identify the best method of endorsing checks in the ambulatory care setting and describe the benefits of using this method.

____

____

____

B. Checks received from patients and others must be inspected before preparing the checks for deposit. What guidelines should medical assistants follow in accepting and inspecting checks?

____

____

C. If a check is returned to the ambulatory care setting for insufficient funds, what procedures should be followed?

____

____

8. It is crucial to balance all financial information for each day and for the month's end. Month-end figures on the day sheet must agree with the patient ledgers. Why is it important to go through this time-consuming accounting process?

____

____

____

9. A physician's fee profile is:
   a. based on an average of all the practice's fees
   b. a continuous record of usual charges made for specific services
   c. an average of fees charged over a period of 3 months
   d. is the amount paid by insurance carriers

10. A patient encounter form:
    a. might be called a charge slip
    b. used to be called a superbill
    c. is only used in computerized systems
    d. both a and b

11. The petty cash fund is kept on hand to:
    a. make change for a patient using a large bill to pay for services
    b. make funds available for all office personnel
    c. pay for minor and incidental expenses
    d. provide funds for weekly lunches for all employees

12. When a check must be guaranteed for the amount in which it is written, a ____________ is issued.
    a. cashier's check
    b. certified check
    c. voucher check
    d. traveler's check

13. Restricting the use of a check should it be lost or stolen may be done through:
    a. reconciling
    b. balancing
    c. special endorsement
    d. blank endorsement

CERTIFICATION REVIEW

These questions are designed to mimic the certification examinations. You can use these questions like a small "Certification Examination Study Guide," but this is not meant to take the place of the more extensive study guides. Use this portion to determine in what areas to concentrate your efforts when studying for the certification examination.

1. The pegboard system of bookkeeping is sometimes called:
   a. the write-it-once system
   b. the ledger system
   c. the double-entry system
   d. the duplicated page system

2. NSF stands for:
   a. nonsufficient funds
   b. not sufficient funds
   c. not satisfactory funding
   d. negligent status of funding

3. A restrictive endorsement stamp is used to:
   a. stamp on the ledger to signify payment has been made
   b. stamp the doctor's signature to insurance forms and other documents
   c. stamp on the statement to signify you have sent a check
   d. stamp on the back of a check to signify "for deposit only"

4. When reconciling a bank statement:
   a. The reconciling should be done every month.
   b. The checkbook entries should be checked against the bank statement.
   c. The reconciling should be done daily by computer.
   d. All reconciling should be done in ink to avoid any unauthorized entries.
   e. a and b

CASE STUDY

Suzanne Berry is a new patient at the offices of Drs. Lewis and King in the Inner City Health Care. Suzanne is a single mother of two small children. Suzanne and her children are covered by medical insurance through her employer. The policy covers 80% of the usual, reasonable, and customary fees for the family's medical expenses after a $100 per person deductible, which the Berrys have already reached from expenses incurred with the family's previous health care provider. Inner City Health Care requires that patients pay for services not covered by insurance at the time of treatment. The office also charges for all scheduled office visits, unless the patient provides a 24-hour notice of cancellation. The practice accepts personal checks, major credit cards, and, under special circumstances, installment payments.

Discuss the following:

1. Take the role of office manager Marilyn Johnson, who meets with Suzanne during her first office visit, and explain the practice's policies regarding patient fees and financial obligations.
2. Suzanne asks Marilyn to clarify what she means by "usual, reasonable, and customary fees." Explain.
3. Suzanne tells Marilyn she is interested in the option of charging some larger medical fees to her credit card. What should Marilyn explain to Suzanne about the use of credit cards in the ambulatory care setting?

SELF-ASSESSMENT

1. In your personal checkbook or banking system at home, how often do you reconcile?
2. When you do reconcile, do you balance? How much time will you spend on the reconciliation to balance?

If you reconcile your bank statements on a regular basis and balance each month, congratulations! If you do not reconcile on a regular basis, start today. Gather your last bank statement. If you do not have one, call the bank and have them send you one or download one from the Internet if your bank offers Internet banking. Accept the beginning balance on the bank statement. Gather the check stubs/copies that you have written within the bank statement beginning and end dates. Check off all the checks that have gone through the bank and are listed on the statement. Add up the outstanding checks (i.e., the ones that have not gone through yet). Subtract them from the ending balance. Add in any interest you have earned for the month. Subtract any fees you have been charged. Does your amount match the bank statement? If not, go back over your math to make sure you added and subtracted correctly and fix any errors. If you still cannot balance, call the bank and ask to sit down with a representative/clerk so they can help you balance. After you balance once, the next month will be much easier.

If your bank offers Internet or online banking, and you are not using that option, consider it. Why are you not using it? Talk to a representative to be sure the online service is secure and your information is protected. If you are satisfied that it is a safe and secure service, consider taking advantage of the online option. Reconciling the monthly statements online is easy to do because the math is done for you by the computer! If you are using online banking, do you think it saves you time? Does it save you money? Is it easier than reconciling manually?

CHAPTER POST-TEST

This is similar to the Pre-Test. Perform this test without looking at the book. This is just to see how well you have understood and can recall the information presented in this chapter after you have studied it and completed the workbook exercises. You will not be graded on this portion (other than the grade you give yourself), but this is an excellent preparation for your instructor's test. You may use this Post-Test to determine what areas you need to study more. Justify any "false" answers.

1. The management of the business details is often the responsibility of the medical assisting staff. (T or F)
2. The same fees for services should be charged to every patient, regardless of whether they have insurance coverage. (T or F)
3. You should encourage the use of credit/debit cards for medical bills. (T or F)
4. Purchase orders are to be written up before the purchase is made. (T or F)
5. Petty cash is available for authorized use when the employees need cash. (T or F)

CERTIFICATION CRITERIA CHECKLIST

As you go through your education and training, keep in mind the national certification examination that you will take when you graduate. Each chapter of the textbook and workbook covers a different section of the examination criteria. To keep track of your preparation for the certification examination, turn to the back of this workbook and highlight the following CMA, RMA, or CMAS certification examination criteria (if you have already highlighted them from a previous chapter, put a check mark by the criteria):

CMA

O. Managing the Office
   2. Equipment and supply inventory

Q. Managing Practice Finances
   1. Bookkeeping systems
   4. Accounting and banking procedures

RMA

II. Administrative Medical Assisting
   B. Finance/Bookkeeping

CMAS

1. Medical Office Financial Management
   - Fundamental financial management
   - Patient accounts
   - Banking

COMPETENCY ASSESSMENT

Procedure 17-1 Recording/Posting Patient Charges, Payments, and Adjustments

Performance Objectives: To record information including services rendered, fees charged, any adjustments made, and balances pertaining to a patient's visit to the physician and the patient's account. Perform this objective within 15 minutes with a minimum score of 55 points.

Supplies/Equipment: Calculator, computer, patient's account or ledger

Charting/Documentation: Enter appropriate documentation/charting in the box.

Instructor's/Evaluator's Comments and Suggestions:

SKILLS CHECKLIST Procedure 17-1: Recording/Posting Patient Charges, Payments, and Adjustments

Name ______________________

Date ______________________

No.	Skill	Check #1 20 pts ea	Check #2 10 pts ea	Check #3 5 pts ea	Notes
1	Check patient's account before appointment to ensure it is up to date.				
2	When patient arrives, check for name, address, telephone number, and any changes in medical insurance.				
3	Fill encounter form or superbill, and attach to the patient's medical chart.				
4	When the physician completes the examination, he or she will check the procedures and diagnosis on the encounter form.				
5	Read the encounter form and calculate the total cost for procedures.				
6	Post each service as a charge or debit. Post payments received as a credit.				
7	Apply any adjustments.				
8	Determine the current balance.				
9	If recording a payment, place a restrictive endorsement on the check.				
10	Record the payment.				
11	Place cash or processed check in the appointed place.				
Student's Total Points					
Points Possible		220	110	55	
Final Score (Student's Total Points / Possible Points)					

	Notes
Start time:	
End time:	
Total time: (15 min goal)	

COMPETENCY ASSESSMENT

Procedure 17-2 Balancing Day Sheets in a Manual System

Performance Objectives: To verify that all entries to the day sheet are correct and that the totals balance. Perform this objective within 15 minutes with a minimum score of 55 points.

Supplies/Equipment: Day sheet, calculator

Charting/Documentation: Enter appropriate documentation/charting in the box.

Instructor's/Evaluator's Comments and Suggestions:

SKILLS CHECKLIST Procedure 17-2: Balancing Day Sheets in a Manual System

Name ______________________

Date ______________________

No.	Skill	Check #1 20 pts ea	Check #2 10 pts ea	Check #3 5 pts ea	Notes
1	Total columns A, B1, B2, C, and D.				
2	Proof of posting: verify that D + A − B = C.				
3	Fill encounter form or superbill, and attach to the patient's medical chart.				
4	When the physician completes the examination, he or she will check the procedures and diagnosis on the encounter form.				
5	Read the encounter form, and calculate the total cost for procedures.				
6	Post each service as a charge or debit. Post payments received as a credit.				
7	Apply any adjustments.				
8	Determine the current balance.				
9	If recording a payment, place a restrictive endorsement on the check.				
10	Record the payment.				
11	Place cash or processed check in the appointed place.				
Student's Total Points					
Points Possible		220	110	55	
Final Score (Student's Total Points / Possible Points)					
		Notes			
Start time:					
End time:					
Total time: (15 min goal)					

COMPETENCY ASSESSMENT

Procedure 17-3 Preparing a Deposit

Performance Objectives: To create a deposit slip for the day's receipts. Perform this objective within 15 minutes with a minimum score of 50 points.

Supplies/Equipment: New deposit slip, check endorsement stamp, calculator, cash and checks received for the day

Charting/Documentation: Enter appropriate documentation/charting in the box.

Instructor's/Evaluator's Comments and Suggestions:

SKILLS CHECKLIST Procedure 17-3: Preparing a Deposit

Name ______________________

Date ______________________

No.	Skill	Check #1 20 pts ea	Check #2 10 pts ea	Check #3 5 pts ea	Notes
1	Separate checks from currency.				
2	Count currency and enter amount in space provided. Gather bills in order, facing the same direction.				
3	Count all coins, and enter amount in space provided.				
4	On the back of the deposit slip, list each check separately. Include patient's name and amount of check.				
5	Total the checks listed and copy the total on the front.				
6	Verify that sum of currency, coins, and checks equals the total payments on day sheet.				
7	Attach top copy of deposit slip to deposit.				
8	Enter date and amount of the deposit on checkbook stubs.				
9	Add the amount of deposit to the checkbook balance.				
10	Deposit at the bank.				
Student's Total Points					
Points Possible		200	100	50	
Final Score (Student's Total Points / Possible Points)					

	Notes
Start time:	
End time:	
Total time: (15 min goal)	

COMPETENCY ASSESSMENT

Procedure 17-4 Reconciling a Bank Statement

Performance Objectives: To verify that the balance listed in the checkbook agrees with the balance shown by the bank. Perform this objective within 15 minutes with a minimum score of 55 points.

Supplies/Equipment: Checkbook, bank statement, calculator

Charting/Documentation: Enter appropriate documentation/charting in the box.

____

____

____

____

Instructor's/Evaluator's Comments and Suggestions:

____

____

____

____

____

____

SKILLS CHECKLIST Procedure 17-4: Reconciling a Bank Statement

Name ______________________

Date ______________________

No.	Skill	Check #1 20 pts ea	Check #2 10 pts ea	Check #3 5 pts ea	Notes
1	Make sure the balance in the checkbook is current.				
2	Subtract any service charge listed from the last balance in the checkbook.				
3	In the checkbook, check off each check listed on the statement and verify the amount against the check stub.				
4	In the checkbook, check off each deposit listed on the statement.				
5	The back of the statement contains a worksheet for balancing.				
6	Copy the ending balance from the front of the statement to the back.				
7	Go through the check stubs and record on the back of the statement any checks that have not cleared, or deposits that were not shown as received.				
8	Total the checks not cleared on the statement worksheet.				
9	Total the deposits not credited on the worksheet.				
10	Add together the statement balance and the total of deposits not credited.				
11	Subtract the total of checks not cleared. Verify with the balance in the checkbook. File the statement worksheet.				
Student's Total Points					
Points Possible		220	110	55	
Final Score (Student's Total Points / Possible Points)					

	Notes
Start time:	
End time:	
Total time: (15 min goal)	

COMPETENCY ASSESSMENT

Procedure 17-5 Balancing Petty Cash

Performance Objectives: To verify that the amount of petty cash is consistent with the beginning amount less expenditures shown on receipts. Perform this objective within 15 minutes with a minimum score of 45 points.

Supplies/Equipment: Petty cash box with cash balance, vouchers, calculator

Charting/Documentation: Enter appropriate documentation/charting in the box.

Instructor's/Evaluator's Comments and Suggestions:

SKILLS CHECKLIST Procedure 17-5: Balancing Petty Cash

Name ______________________

Date ______________________

No.	Skill	Check #1 20 pts ea	Check #2 10 pts ea	Check #3 5 pts ea	Notes
1	Count the money in the box.				
2	Total the amount of all vouchers.				
3	Subtract the amount of receipts from the original amount.				
4	When cash has been balanced, write a check only for the amount that was used.				
Check Disbursement:					
5	Sort all vouchers by account.				
6	On a sheet of paper, list the accounts.				
7	Total vouchers for each account, then record individual totals.				
8	Copy the list totals onto the "memo" portion of the stub for the replenishment check.				
9	File the list with the vouchers and receipts attached, noting the check number.				
Student's Total Points					
Points Possible		180	90	45	
Final Score (Student's Total Points / Possible Points)					

	Notes
Start time:	
End time:	
Total time: (15 min goal)	

COMPETENCY ASSESSMENT

Procedure 17-6 Recording a Nonsufficient Funds Check

Performance Objectives: To perform bookkeeping functions that keep account in proper balance. Perform this objective within 15 minutes with a minimum score of 20 points.

Supplies/Equipment: The practice's account balance, manual day sheet or computerized practice account, manual ledger or computerized patient account, NSF check

Charting/Documentation: Enter appropriate documentation/charting in the box.

Instructor's/Evaluator's Comments and Suggestions:

SKILLS CHECKLIST Procedure 17-6: Recording a Nonsufficient Funds Check

Name ________________________

Date ________________________

No.	Skill	Check #1 20 pts ea	Check #2 10 pts ea	Check #3 5 pts ea	Notes
1	Follow the office policy for notifying the patient.				
2	When the NSF check has been returned the second time, deduct the check amount from the account balance of the practice.				
3	Add the amount of the NSF check back into the patient's account or ledger.				
4	Place a brief explanation in the description column.				
Student's Total Points					
Points Possible		80	40	20	
Final Score (Student's Total Points / Possible Points)					

	Notes
Start time:	
End time:	
Total time: (15 min goal)	

EVALUATION OF CHAPTER KNOWLEDGE

Skills	Student Self-Evaluation Good	Average	Poor
I can define the key vocabulary terms in this chapter.	_____	_____	_____
I can demonstrate understanding of procedures, policies, and services.	_____	_____	_____
I understand the importance of informing patients of the office's financial policies and procedures.	_____	_____	_____
I can document various financial forms correctly.	_____	_____	_____
I understand documentation and reporting needs.	_____	_____	_____
I am able to use manual bookkeeping systems.	_____	_____	_____
I can apply computer concepts to computerized accounting systems.	_____	_____	_____
I can demonstrate the ability to manage accounts receivable.	_____	_____	_____
I can demonstrate the ability to manage accounts payable.	_____	_____	_____
I am able to establish, track, balance, and replenish a petty cash fund.	_____	_____	_____
I can write and record checks and reconcile accounts.	_____	_____	_____
I can demonstrate an understanding of purchasing procedures and the ability to prepare purchase orders.	_____	_____	_____

CHAPTER 18

Medical Insurance

CHAPTER PRE-TEST

Perform this test without looking at the book. This is just to see how well you have understood and can recall the information in this chapter after you have read it, but before you have completed the workbook exercises. You will not be graded on this portion (other than the grade you give yourself). Justify any "false" answers.

1. Managed care has simplified the patient's responsibility for payment. (T or F)
2. With managed care options, there is less emphasis on the medical assistant needing to be accurate and timely when filing insurance claims. (T or F)
3. Preexisting conditions usually require a waiting period. (T or F)
4. Coordination of benefits means that the insurance companies will take care of the paperwork. (T or F)
5. Copayment is the amount the insurance will cost the patient each month. (T or F)

INTRODUCTION

With the growing influence of managed care, many traditional insurance carriers, such as Blue Cross and Blue Shield, are joining health maintenance organizations (HMOs) and other managed care options in transforming the health care insurance industry. Students also discover the medical assistant's important role as a patient educator, helping patients understand the terms and conditions of their health insurance policies.

PERFORMANCE OBJECTIVES

After successful completion of this chapter you will be able to explain the terminology related to medical insurances. You will be able to recall several different examples of medical insurance coverage and discuss their similarities and differences. You will be familiar with several primary managed care organization models and recall the steps involved when screening patients for insurance coverage. You will know about legal and ethical issues related to medical insurance and the physician's office, including the impacts of Health Insurance Portability and Accountability Act (HIPAA) requirements. You will also be aware of the importance of obtaining referrals and preauthorizations from insurance companies before providing services and the ramifications if the referrals or preauthorizations are overlooked. *The following statements are related to your learning objectives from this chapter. Fill in the blanks in the following paragraph with the appropriate term(s).*

The term used to describe the person who is insured is (1) ____________________. The amount of money that the insured person must incur before the insurance policy begins to pay is called the (2) ____________________. Some insurance policies require that the patient pay a certain amount at the time of service. This is called the (3) ____________________. A disease or disorder the patient has before he or she opens his or her insurance policy may not be covered for a certain amount of time, because it is considered to be a (4) ____________________ condition. Sometimes insurance policies will not cover procedures and treatments either because they are considered not to be medically necessary or perhaps they have not been proved to be effective. These procedures or treatments are called (5) ____________________. Before some services are allowed, they must first be approved by the insurance company. The process for getting this approval is called (6) ____________________. Many traditional insurance policies require patients to choose one physician who will coordinate all their care. This physician is known as their PCP. PCP is an abbreviation for (7) ____________________. Some policies even limit the physicians from whom patients can seek treatment. The patients must choose their specialists from a list of approved physicians who have contracted with the insurance company. These physicians are considered to be (8) ____________________. A list of approved medications can be found on the (9) ____________________. If a medication is not on the list, the patient will have to pay more for it. Fee schedules are determined from a variety of elements, including the (10) ____________________ or practice expenses, the cost of (11) ____________________, and the (12) ____________________ for the services provided by the physician. All of these cost elements combined with the (13) ____________________ required is used to determine a fee schedule. UCR, or (14) ____________________ Fee Schedule defines the allowable fees accepted by insurance carriers. Medicare has a system called RBRVS, or (15) ____________________, in which physician's services are reimbursed based on relative value. This formula takes into consideration not only the physician's overhead expenses, the work involved, and malpractice expenses, but also a (16) ____________________ practice cost index. (17) ____________________ is a payment system used by managed care organizations in which a fixed dollar amount is reimbursed to the physician. This type of system requires the physician to practice extensive (18) ____________________ to be effective. HIPAA stands

for (19) ____
and includes several rules. One of the rules, HIPAA privacy requirements, addresses issues of (20) ______________________________. These rules state that the practice must provide the patient with a (21) ______________________________ form that outlines the provider's privacy practices. Another requirement is that the practice obtain (22) ______________________________ from the patient to use or disclose personal information. The practice must also provide the patient, on request, an accounting of any (23) ______________________ of protected information.

VOCABULARY BUILDER

Find the words below that are misspelled; circle them, and then correctly spell them in the spaces provided. Then insert the correct vocabulary terms from the list that best fit the descriptions below.

point of service plan	referral
preautherization	resourse-based relative value scale
prefered provider organization	self-insurance
primary care physician/provider	usual, customary, and reasonible
proof of eligability	Worker's Compensation insurance

______________________________ ______________________________

______________________________ ______________________________

____

1. The ____ is a doctor chosen by the patient who is the first doctor the patient sees and is responsible for making referrals for further treatment by a specialist or for hospitalization.

2. A ____ allows the enrollee to have the freedom to obtain medical care from an HMO provider or to self-refer to a non-HMO provider at a greater cost.

3. In a ____, enrollees obtain services from a network of physicians and hospitals who have contracted with the insurance company.

4. ____ was developed using values for each medical and surgical procedure based on work, practice, and malpractice costs and factoring in the regional differences.

5. ______________________________ requirement means that prior notice and approval needs to be obtained before services will be covered.

LEARNING REVIEW

1. What questions should the medical assistant ask when screening for medical insurance coverage?
   A. ______________________________
   B. ______________________________
   C. ______________________________
   D. ______________________________

2. List five measures that managed care organizations (MCOs) employ to ensure cost-effective services.
   A. ______________________________
   B. ______________________________
   C. ______________________________
   D. ______________________________
   E. ______________________________

3. What are the six MCO models in use?
   A. ______________________________
   B. ______________________________
   C. ______________________________
   D. ______________________________
   E. ______________________________
   F. ______________________________

4. List seven pieces of information that should be maintained in a log regarding preauthorization, precertification, or referral procedures for various insurance carriers.
   A. ______________________________
   B. ______________________________
   C. ______________________________
   D. ______________________________
   E. ______________________________
   F. ______________________________
   G. ______________________________

5. Identify the three common elements involved in computing a physician's fee schedule.
   A. ______________________________
   B. ______________________________
   C. ______________________________

6. Which of the following is a problem with work-related health insurance coverage?
   a. part-time employees are not usually eligible
   b. medical benefits may not transfer equally
   c. insurance companies often refuse to provide coverage for some procedures, including experimental treatments
   d. all of the above

7. The person covered under the terms of an insurance policy is called the:
   a. primary
   b. secondary
   c. beneficiary
   d. elector

8. When more than one policy covers the individual, the ________________ determines which of the policies will pay first.
   a. deductible
   b. exclusion
   c. coinsurance
   d. coordination of benefits

9. Where does one find the address to which insurance claims are to be sent?
   a. the telephone book
   b. on the back of the insurance card
   c. in the insurance provider manual
   d. none of the above

10. Blue Cross and Blue Shield are examples of a:
    a. managed care organization (MCO)
    b. health maintenance organization (HMO)
    c. preferred provider organization (PPO)
    d. traditional insurance organization

CERTIFICATION REVIEW

These questions are designed to mimic the certification examinations. You can use these questions like a small "Certification Examination Study Guide," but this is not meant to take the place of the more extensive study guides. Use this portion to determine in what areas to concentrate your efforts when studying for the certification examination. Justify any "false" answers.

1. The portion of the medical fees that the patient needs to pay at the time of services is called a:
   a. copay
   b. fee for service
   c. out of pocket expenses
   d. premium

2. The cost patients must pay each month (sometimes provided by their employers) is called the:
   a. out of pocket expenses
   b. copay
   c. premium
   d. relative value scale
3. HIPAA:
   a. is about confidentiality, patient privacy, and security of personal health information
   b. protects health insurance coverage for workers and their families when they change or lose their jobs
   c. includes national standards for electronic health care transactions
   d. establishes rules for national identifiers for providers, health plans, and employers
   e. all of the above
4. Electronic medical records have made confidentiality easier to protect. (T or F)

CASE STUDY

Lourdes Austen, a one-year survivor of breast cancer, is covered by an HMO. Lourdes's primary care physician, Dr. King, recommends that Lourdes receive a colonoscopy because she has a family history that is positive for colon cancer; medical studies have demonstrated a link between colon and breast cancers in families. Lourdes's HMO requires preauthorization before a specialist's care can be provided. Dr. King supplies the referral to a gastroenterologist who will perform the colon screening test and gives Lourdes the necessary completed referral form to take with her to her scheduled appointment.

During the colonoscopy procedure, one benign polyp is removed, and the gastroenterologist requests that Lourdes return for a follow-up examination in one week. Lourdes makes an appointment with the specialist's administrative medical assistant. When she returns one week later, the medical assistant informs Lourdes that she must have a new referral form for the office visit or the HMO will not approve payment; Lourdes will have to pay for the examination herself. "But we drove 40 minutes to get here, and no one ever told me I'd need another form for this. I thought it was all covered under the colonoscopy," Lourdes says.

Discuss the following:

1. Lourdes's HMO policy requires preauthorization. Is there anything that can be done to secure a proper referral without having to schedule another appointment for the patient or force the patient to pay for the office visit?
2. What is the role of the specialist's administrative medical assistant in this situation? Could the situation have been prevented?

SELF-ASSESSMENT

1. Take a close look at your insurance coverage. If you do not have medical insurance coverage, take a look at the coverage of a close friend or relative or choose a policy you would like to have.
   A. Does it require a copay?
   B. How much is the copay for a doctor's visit?
   C. How much is the copay for a hospital stay? Surgery?
   D. How much is the copay for medication?
   E. Does prescribed medication have to be from a formulary list?
   F. How much is the total amount you would have to pay for any given year?
2. Some people advocate doing away with health insurance for office visits and medications and just having insurance for big expenses such as catastrophic coverage. Discuss this idea with a group of at least three people. These people may be your classmates or friends/family. Write up a list of the advantages and disadvantages.
3. Some people advocate a "socialistic" method of health insurance such as Canada has. Look online for information about Canada's health care system and make a list of the advantages and disadvantages. Which way would you vote if you had a choice?

CHAPTER POST-TEST

This is similar to the Pre-Test. Perform this test without looking at the book. This is just to see how well you have understood and can recall the information presented in this chapter after you have studied it and completed the workbook exercises. You will not be graded on this portion (other than the grade you give yourself), but this is an excellent preparation for your instructor's test. You may use this Post-Test to determine what areas you need to study more. Justify any "false" answers.

1. Managed care has made the patient's responsibility for payment more complex. (T or F)
2. With managed care options, there is more emphasis on the medical assistant needing to be accurate and timely when filing insurance claims. (T or F)
3. Preexisting conditions always require a waiting period. (T or F)
4. Coordination of benefits means that the insurance companies will handle all the paperwork necessary for payment. (T or F)
5. Copayment is the amount the insurance will cost the patient's employer each month. (T or F)

CERTIFICATION CRITERIA CHECKLIST

As you go through your education and training, keep in mind the national certification examination that you will take when you graduate. Each chapter of the textbook and workbook covers a different section of the examination criteria. To keep track of your preparation for the certification examination, turn to the back of this workbook and highlight the following CMA, RMA, or CMAS certification examination criteria (if you have already highlighted them from a previous chapter, put a check mark by the criteria):

CMA

F. Medicolegal Guidelines & Requirements
   2. Legislation
   5. Physician-patient relationship

Q. Managing Practice Finances
   3. Third-party billing

RMA

II. Administrative Medical Assisting
   A. Insurance

CMAS

5. Health Care Insurance Processing, Coding and Billing
   - Insurance processing
   - Insurance billing and finances

COMPETENCY ASSESSMENT

Procedure 18-1 Screening for Insurance

Performance Objectives: To verify insurance coverage and obtain vital information required for processing and billing insurance claim forms. Perform this objective within 15 minutes with a minimum score of 25 points.

Supplies/Equipment: Patient registration forms, clipboard and black ink pen, patient's chart

Charting/Documentation: Enter appropriate documentation/charting in the box.

Instructor's/Evaluator's Comments and Suggestions:

SKILLS CHECKLIST Procedure 18-1: Screening for Insurance

Name ______________________

Date ______________________

No.	Skill	Check #1 20 pts ea	Check #2 10 pts ea	Check #3 5 pts ea	Notes
1	Ask patients to bring their insurance cards, and arrive 15–20 minutes before appointment time.				
2	Review completed patient registration form for legibility and completeness.				
3	Make front and back photocopies of patient's insurance card and attach to patient's chart.				
4	Verify proof of eligibility for Medicaid patients.				
5	Each time patient checks in, verify address and insurance coverage. Check insurance card. Determine that their primary care physician is performing the procedure and that the procedure is covered.				
Student's Total Points					
Points Possible		100	50	25	
Final Score (Student's Total Points / Possible Points)					
		Notes			
Start time:					
End time:					
Total time: (15 min goal)					

COMPETENCY ASSESSMENT

Procedure 18-2 Obtaining Referrals and Authorizations

Performance Objectives: To ascertain coverage by the insurance carrier for specific medical services, hospital admissions, inpatient or outpatient surgeries, elective procedures, or when the primary care physician elects to refer the patient to another physician. Perform this objective within 15 minutes with a minimum score of 35 points.

Supplies/Equipment: Patient's medical chart and copy of the patient's insurance card, name of the carrier contact person and telephone number, completed referral form, telephone/fax machine, pen/pencil

Charting/Documentation: Enter appropriate documentation/charting in the box.

Instructor's/Evaluator's Comments and Suggestions:

SKILLS CHECKLIST Procedure 18-2: Obtaining Referrals and Authorizations

Name ______________________________

Date ______________________________

No.	Skill	Check #1 20 pts ea	Check #2 10 pts ea	Check #3 5 pts ea	Notes
1	Collect all necessary documents and equipment.				
2	Determine the service or procedure requiring preauthorization.				
3	Complete the referral form.				
4	Proofread the completed form.				
5	Fax the completed form to the insurance carrier.				
6	Maintain a completed copy of the referral form in the patient's chart.				
7	Maintain a completed copy of the authorization number/ code in the patient's chart.				
Student's Total Points					
Points Possible		140	70	35	
Final Score (Student's Total Points / Possible Points)					
		Notes			
Start time:					
End time:					
Total time: (15 min goal)					

EVALUATION OF CHAPTER KNOWLEDGE

Skills	Student Self-Evaluation Good	Average	Poor
I can describe the history of medical insurance in this country and its evolution in recent years.	_____	_____	_____
I can define the terminology necessary to understand and submit medical insurance claims.	_____	_____	_____
I know at least five examples of medical insurance coverage.	_____	_____	_____
I can explain the significance of diagnosis-related groups.	_____	_____	_____
I am comfortable as a patient educator about insurance issues.	_____	_____	_____

CHAPTER 19

Medical Insurance Coding

CHAPTER PRE-TEST

Perform this test without looking at the book. This is just to see how well you have understood and can recall the information in this chapter after you have read it, but before you have completed the workbook exercises. You will not be graded on this portion (other than the grade you give yourself). Justify any "false" answers.

1. Medical insurance coding is a way of keeping track of the doctor's financial records. (T or F)

2. CPT stands for:
   a. Comprehensive Patient Treatments
   b. Current Procedural Terminology
   c. Curative Procedures Tried
   d. Curative Patient Treatments

3. ICD stands for:
   a. Incidental Codes of Diagnosis
   b. Internal Codes for Decisions
   c. International Codes for Diagnosis
   d. International Classifications of Diseases

4. Third party usually means the insurance company. (T or F)

5. Insurance claim forms and submissions are fairly straightforward; therefore, most anyone can perform these duties with some basic training. (T or F)

INTRODUCTION

Although managed care coverage has simplified the patient's responsibility for payment in some ways, medical assistants have the responsibility to be accurate, timely, and conscientious both in filing insurance claim forms and in understanding the conditions of individual insurance policies. Medical assisting students can use this workbook chapter to explore the role of insurance, learn insurance terminology, and apply accurate insurance coding of diagnosis and procedure codes.

PERFORMANCE OBJECTIVES

After successful completion of this chapter you will be able to explain the terminology related to medical insurance coding. You will understand the process of procedure and diagnostic coding and will be able to code a simple claim form. You will be able to explain the difference between the Centers for Medicare and Medicaid Services Form 1500 (CMS-1500) and the Uniform Bill 92 (UB92) forms, and discuss why claims follow-up is important. You will also be able to discuss legal and ethical issues related to medical coding and insurance claims processing. *The following statements are related to your learning objectives from this chapter. Fill in the blanks in the following paragraph with the appropriate term(s).*

The advent of computers has required that diagnoses and procedures be put into (1) ______________________________ format. The CPT system was developed by the (2) ______________________________________ to convert descriptions of procedures into numbers. The (3) ____ developed the ICD-9 CM to classify diseases in the same way. The current ICD-9 CM codes consist of (4) _______________________ digit codes with (5) ________________________ modifiers. (6) ____________________________________ is a way for insurance companies to reduce the reimbursement amounts if the documentation or codes are ambiguous. There are three ways this can happen: (7) ____, (8) ____, or (9) ____. Up coding, also known as (10) ____________________________, (11) ________________________, or (12) ____, occurs when the insurance carrier is deliberately billed at a higher rate service than was performed to obtain a greater reimbursement. The CPT is divided into (13) ______________________________ sections. One of the sections, called the (14) ____ section, takes every possible combination of visits into consideration and assigns each its own number. Occasionally, a service or procedure needs to be modified, so there is an optional two-digit numeric (15) ___________________________________ that can be applied as an explanation. Medicare created the (16) ____ ___________________________ system for their patients. This system has three levels. Level I uses the basic system. Level II provides codes for (17) ____________________ ____________________, (18) ____________________, and (19) ____________________. Level III codes are defined by Medicare regional (20) ____________________ carriers.

VOCABULARY BUILDER

A. *Find the words below that are misspelled; circle them, and then correctly spell them in the spaces provided.*

bindled codes
claim register
Current Procedural Terminoligy
E Codes
encounter form
explanation of benifits
fraud
Healthcare Common Procedure Coding System
insurance abuse
International Classification of Deseases
point-of-service device
U Codes
Uniform Bill

____________________ ____________________

____________________ ____________________

B. *Write the definition of the following terms or phrases.*

1. Bundled codes

____

2. Claim register

____

3. *Current Procedural Terminology (CPT)*

____

4. E Codes

____

5. Encounter form

____

6. Explanation of Benefits (EOB)

____

7. Fraud

____

8. Healthcare Common Procedure Coding System (HCPCS)

____

9. Insurance abuse

____

10. International Classification of Diseases, 9th Revision, Clinical Modifications (ICD-9-CM)

____

11. Point-of-service (POS) device

____

12. Uniform Bill (UB92)

____

13. V Codes

____

LEARNING REVIEW

1. Coding for procedures done and for visits of all kinds—office, hospital, nursing facility, home services—is found in *CPT*.

   A. *CPT* is divided into seven sections. This volume is updated annually and published by the American Medical Association. Name the seven sections.

   (1) ____________________ (5) ____________________

   (2) ____________________ (6) ____________________

   (3) ____________________ (7) ____________________

   (4) ____________________

   B. For each procedure listed, give the correct procedure code and name the *CPT* section in which the code can be found.

   1. Chemotherapy administration, infusion technique, up to 1 hour

      code: ____________________ section: ____________________

   2. Hepatitis B surface antibody

      code: ____________________ section: ____________________

   3. Simple repair of superficial wounds of scalp, neck, axillae, external genitalia, trunk or extremities (including hands and feet) 7.6 to 12.5 cm

      code: ____________________ section: ____________________

   4. Electrocardiogram, routine ECG with 12 leads; with interpretation and reports

      code: ____________________ section: ____________________

5. Hepatic venography, wedged or free, with hemodynamic evaluation, radiologic supervision, and interpretation

   code: ______________________ section: ____________________________

6. Hepatitis Be antigen (HBeAg)

   code: ______________________ section: ____________________________

7. Anesthesia for arthroscopic procedures of hip joint

   code: ______________________ section: ____________________________

2. A. Codes for diagnoses are found in the ICD-9-CM. ICD-9-CM is divided into three volumes. Specify below what information each volume contains.

   Volume I: ____

   ____

   Volume II: ____

   ____

   Volume III: ____

   ____

   B. Provide answers to the following questions:

   In which volume of the ICD would a medical assistant first look to find the diagnosis code for osteomyelitis? (1) __________________________ What is the diagnosis code for unspecified osteomyelitis of the ankle or foot? (2) ______________ Injury codes cannot stand alone, but must be accompanied by "E" Codes. What do E Codes stand for? (3) _____________________ What is the diagnosis code for obesity? (4) ____________________ "V" Codes are the last main section of Volumes I and II. What do V Codes stand for? (5) ____

   ____.

3. Errors in coding insurance claims can have far-reaching effects for both the patient and the physician. Name three effects.

   (1) ____

   ____

   (2) ____

   ____

   (3) ____

   ____

4. For each entry in the following table, insert a "D" for diagnosis or "P" for procedure on the first line. Then, enter the appropriate diagnosis or procedure code, referencing this textbook, the current revision of the ICD, or the current edition of the CPT. In the explanation column, identify whether the procedures are laboratory procedures (LAB), part of the physician's physical examination process (PE), diagnostic procedures (DP), examples of medication administration (MA), preventive measures (PM), procedures related to litigation (LEG), or rehabilitative medicine procedures (RP). For each diagnosis, give a brief definition of the patient condition or illness, consulting a medical encyclopedia if necessary.

Diagnosis/ Procedure	Entry	Code	Explanation
_____	1. Services requested after hours in addition to basic services	_____	_____
_____	2. Medicine given or taken in error	_____	_____
_____	3. Anorexia nervosa	_____	_____
_____	4. Pneumonocentesis, puncture of lung for aspiration	_____	_____
_____	5. Diabetic ketoacidosis	_____	_____
_____	6. Urinalysis; qualitative or semi-quantitative, except immunoassays, microscopic only	_____	_____
_____	7. Bruxism	_____	_____
_____	8. *Pneumocystis carinii* pneumonia	_____	_____
_____	9. Amniocentesis	_____	_____
_____	10. Epstein–Barr virus infection	_____	_____
_____	11. Gait training (includes stair climbing)	_____	_____
_____	12. Medical testimony	_____	_____
_____	13. DTP (diphtheria-tetanus-pertussis) vaccination	_____	_____
_____	14. Therapeutic or diagnostic injection (specify material injected); subcutaneous or intramuscular	_____	_____
_____	15. Narcotics affecting fetus via placenta or breast milk	_____	_____

5. Differentiate between bundled and unbundled codes.

____

____

____

6. List five common errors committed when completing insurance claim forms.
   (1) ______________________________
   (2) ______________________________
   (3) ______________________________
   (4) ______________________________
   (5) ______________________________

7. Identify seven basic elements necessary to have documented in a compliance program.
   (1) ______________________________
   (2) ______________________________
   (3) ______________________________
   (4) ______________________________
   (5) ______________________________
   (6) ______________________________
   (7) ______________________________

8. Using the number of patients enrolled in a health maintenance organization (HMO) to determine a physician's salary is called:
   a. coinsurance
   b. capitation
   c. catchment
   d. assignment

9. Part A of Medicare covers:
   a. hospice care
   b. physical therapy
   c. diagnostic tests
   d. ambulance services

10. Using an electronic device for direct communication between medical offices and a health care plan's computer is called:
    a. subrogation
    b. point of service
    c. diagnosis-related groups
    d. prospective payment

11. The most common claim form for the ambulatory setting is the:
    a. HCFA-1500
    b. HCFA-1000
    c. CMS 1500
    d. CPT 1500

12. The codes that show a patient has been seen for reasons other than sickness or injury are:
    a. S Codes
    b. D Codes
    c. V Codes
    d. X Codes

CERTIFICATION REVIEW

These questions are designed to mimic the certification examinations. You can use these questions like a small "Certification Examination Study Guide," but this is not meant to take the place of the more extensive study guides. Use this portion to determine in what areas to concentrate your efforts when studying for the certification examination.

1. What is the name of the coding system that includes codes for services provided to Medicare or Medicaid patients?
    a. HCFA
    b. CPT
    c. ICD-9
    d. HCPCS
    e. WHO

2. If a doctor believes a claim has been denied in error, which of the following is a valid course of action he or she can take?
    a. contact the assistant attorney general
    b. begin a lawsuit
    c. begin an appeal process
    d. write off the charges
    e. bill the patient

3. A Certified Professional Coder has coded a diagnosis of 670.51. What system is he or she using?
    a. CPT
    b. ICD 9
    c. ICD 10
    d. HCPCS
    e. RVS

4. In the *CPT* manual, the description of the level of E&M codes includes which of the following?
   a. complexity of the medical decision making
   b. level of history taken
   c. number of systems examined and documented
   d. new versus established patient
   e. all of the above

5. Which of the following describes Volume II of the ICD-9?
   a. known as the Tabular Index, lists all diagnostic codes in numeric order
   b. is an alphabetical listing of diagnoses.
   c. lists procedures in tabular form
   d. all of the above

CASE STUDY

Refer to the case study presented in Chapter 18 of this workbook.

Lourdes's colonoscopy required the following diagnoses and procedures. Give the correct coding for processing the insurance claim for this patient.

colonoscopy with biopsy, single or multiple________________________

flex sig (colon) ____________________________________

family history, malignant neoplasm gastrointestinal tract ________________

personal history, malignant neoplasm, breast ________________________

low-complexity office visit ______________________________

SELF-ASSESSMENT

A. Have you considered whether you would like to be an insurance coder and biller? Think about the following questions.

   1. What qualities do you possess that would make you a good candidate for a career in medical billing and coding?
   2. What qualities do you not possess but could obtain?
   3. What do you think you would like best about a position in medical coding and billing?
   4. What would be your least favorite part of the job?

B. Explore the profession of medical coding by looking on the Internet for coding organizations offering certification examinations. Differentiate between the various credentials available to coders.

CHAPTER POST-TEST

This is similar to the Pre-Test. Perform this test without looking at the book. This is just to see how well you have understood and can recall the information presented in this chapter after you have studied it and completed the workbook exercises. You will not be graded on this portion (other than the grade you give yourself), but this is an excellent preparation for your instructor's test. You may use this Post-Test to determine what areas you need to study more. Justify any "false" answers.

1. Medical insurance coding is a way of putting procedures and treatments into numeric form. (T or F)
2. CPT stands for:
   a. Comprehensive Procedural Terminology
   b. Current Procedural Terminology
   c. Complete Procedural Terminology
   d. Curative Procedural Terminology
3. ICD stands for:
   a. International Codes for Diagnosis
   b. Internal Codes for Diagnosis
   c. International Codes for Diseases
   d. International Classifications of Diseases
4. Third-party guidelines have the expectation that insurance companies will not disclose personal medical information to unauthorized persons. (T or F)
5. Insurance coding, claim forms, and submissions are complex enough that medical coders and billers need extended training and experience to do it well. (T or F)

CERTIFICATION CRITERIA CHECKLIST

As you go through your education and training, keep in mind the national certification examination that you will take when you graduate. Each chapter of the textbook and workbook covers a different section of the examination criteria. To keep track of your preparation for the certification examination, turn to the back of this workbook and highlight the following CMA, RMA, or CMAS certification examination criteria (if you have already highlighted them from a previous chapter, put a check mark by the criteria):

CMA

F. Medicolegal Guidelines & Requirements
   5. Physician–patient relationship

Q. Managing Practice Finances
   2. Coding systems

RMA

II. Administrative Medical Assisting
  A. Insurance

CMAS

5. Health Care Insurance Processing, Coding and Billing
  - Insurance coding

COMPETENCY ASSESSMENT

Procedure 19-1 Current Procedural Terminology Coding

Performance Objectives: To convert commonly accepted descriptions of medical procedures (services) and for visits of all kinds—office, hospital, nursing facility, home services—into a five-digit numeric code with two-digit numeric modifiers when required. Perform this objective within 15 minutes with a minimum score of 15 points.

Supplies/Equipment: CPT code book for the current year, copy of the encounter form and access to the patient's chart, pencil and paper

Charting/Documentation: Enter appropriate documentation/charting in the box.

Instructor's/Evaluator's Comments and Suggestions:

SKILLS CHECKLIST Procedure 19-1: Current Procedural Terminology Coding

Name ______________________

Date ______________________

No.	Skill	Check #1 20 pts ea	Check #2 10 pts ea	Check #3 5 pts ea	Notes
1	Using the CPT code book, look in the Evaluation and Management section, Office or Other Outpatient Services, New Patient. Read through until the code matching the described scenario is found.				
2	Look up Urinalysis, Routine in CPT code book index.				
3	Locate code 81002 in the Pathology and Laboratory section. Be sure the description provided matches what the physician has documented in the patient chart.				
Student's Total Points					
Points Possible		60	30	15	
Final Score (Student's Total Points / Possible Points)					

	Notes
Start time:	
End time:	
Total time: (15 min goal)	

COMPETENCY ASSESSMENT

Procedure 19-2 International Classification of Diseases, 9th Revision, Clinical Modification Coding

Performance Objectives: The ICD-9-CM code books provide a diagnostic coding system for the compilation and reporting of morbidity and mortality statistics for reimbursement purposes. Perform this objective within 15 minutes with a minimum score of 10 points.

Supplies/Equipment: Volumes 1 and 2 of the ICD-9-CM code books for the current year, copy of the encounter form and access to the patient's chart, pencil and paper

Charting/Documentation: Enter appropriate documentation/charting in the box.

Instructor's/Evaluator's Comments and Suggestions:

SKILLS CHECKLIST Procedure 19-2: International Classification of Diseases, 9th Revision, Clinical Modification Coding

Name ______________________

Date ______________________

No.	Skill	Check #1 20 pts ea	Check #2 10 pts ea	Check #3 5 pts ea	Notes
1	Using Volume II of the ICD-9-CM code books, look up the main reason or condition that brought the patient to the facility, or the specific diagnosis confirmed by test results (code 599.0).				
2	Using Volume I, look up code 599. Read all 599 listings and determine the appropriate code having the greatest level of specificity.				
Student's Total Points					
Points Possible		40	20	10	
Final Score (Student's Total Points / Possible Points)					
		Notes			
Start time:					
End time:					
Total time: (15 min goal)					

COMPETENCY ASSESSMENT

Procedure 19-3 Applying Third-Party Guidelines

Performance Objectives: To obtain written authorization to release necessary medical information to third-party payers. Perform this objective within 5 minutes with a minimum score of 10 points.

Supplies/Equipment: Patient chart, CMS-1500 claim form

Charting/Documentation: Enter appropriate documentation/charting in the box.

Instructor's/Evaluator's Comments and Suggestions:

SKILLS CHECKLIST Procedure 19-3: Applying Third-Party Guidelines

Name ______________________________

Date ______________________________

No.	Skill	Check #1 20 pts ea	Check #2 10 pts ea	Check #3 5 pts ea	Notes
1	When patient signs in, check their chart to ascertain if an "Authorization to Release Medical Information" has been signed and is currently valid.				
2	If there is no record of signature on file, have the patient sign Block 12 of the CMS-1500 form.				
Student's Total Points					
Points Possible		40	20	10	
Final Score (Student's Total Points / Possible Points)					

	Notes
Start time:	
End time:	
Total time: (5 min goal)	

COMPETENCY ASSESSMENT

Procedure 19-4 Completing a Medicare CMS-1500 Claim Form

Performance Objectives: To complete the CMS-1500 insurance claim form for Medicare for Reimbursement. Perform this objective within 30 minutes with a minimum score of 270 points.

Supplies/Equipment: Patient information, patient account or ledger card, copy of patient's insurance card, insurance claim form, computer and printer.

Charting/Documentation: Enter appropriate documentation/charting in the box.

Instructor's/Evaluator's Comments and Suggestions:

SKILLS CHECKLIST Procedure 19-4: Completing a Medicare CMS-1500 Claim Form

Name ______________________

Date ______________________

No.	Skill	Check #1 20 pts ea	Check #2 10 pts ea	Check #3 5 pts ea	Notes
1	Key in the carrier's name and address if it is not already imprinted.				
2	Complete each block as directed in the patient and insured information section.				
	Block 1 — Applicable health insurance coverage				
	Block 2 — Patient name				
	Block 3 — Birth date and sex				
	Block 5 — Mailing address and telephone number				
	Block 6 — Relationship to insured				
	Block 8 — Marital status and employment or school status				
	Blocks 9a, 9b, 9c — Completed if patient has Medigap				
	Block 10 — Indicate if condition related to work or accident				
	Block 10d — Medicaid information if appropriate				
	Block 12 — Signature of patient or representative				
3	Complete the Insured Information section:				
	Block 1a — HICN				
	Block 4 — Other insurance primary?				
	Block 7 — Insured's address and telephone number				
	Block 11— If other insurance is primary, enter group number				
	Block 11a — Insured's birth date and sex				
	Block 11b — Insured's employer's name				
	Block 11c — Primary insured's payer identification (ID) number or plan name				
	Block 11d — Blank				
	Block 13 — Signature of insured				

No.	Skill	Check #1 20 pts ea	Check #2 10 pts ea	Check #3 5 pts ea	Notes
4	Physician or supplier information:				
	Block 14 — Patient's date of illness or injury				
	Block 15 — Blank				
	Block 17 — Name of referring physician or ordering physician (if supplied)				
	Block 17a — UPIN of referring or ordering physician				
	Block 19 — Date patient last seen and UPIN of attending physician				
	Block 21 — Patient's diagnosis code				
	Block 24A — Date for each procedure, service, or supply				
	Block 24B — Place of service code				
	Block 24C — Blank for Medicare providers				
	Block 24D — CPT codes				
	Block 24E — Diagnostic codes related to the DOS and the procedures				
	Block 25 — Provider's Federal Tax ID number				
	Block 26 — Patient's account number				
	Block 27 — Accept assignment?				
	Block 31 — Signature of provider				
	Block 32 — Name and address of provider facility				
5	Complete the physician or supplier information:				
	Block 16 — Date patient is unable to work				
	Block 18 — Date medical service is furnished if related to hospitalization				
	Block 20 — Complete when billing for tests subject to price limits				
	Block 22 — Blank				
	Block 23 — Prior authorization number if required				
	Block 24F — Charge for each service				

No.	Skill	Check #1 20 pts ea	Check #2 10 pts ea	Check #3 5 pts ea	Notes
	Block 24G — Number of days or units if applicable				
	Block 24H — Blank				
	Block 24I — Blank				
	Block 24J — Blank				
	Block 24K — Pin number of provider				
	Block 28 — Total charges				
	Block 29 — Total paid by patient				
	Block 30 — Blank				
	Block 33 — Providers billing name, address, and phone number				
Student's Total Points					
Points Possible (54 steps)		1080	540	270	
Final Score (Student's Total Points / Possible Points)					

	Notes
Start time:	
End time:	
Total time: (30 min goal)	

EVALUATION OF CHAPTER KNOWLEDGE

Skills	Student Self-Evaluation Good	Average	Poor
I understand the process of procedure and diagnosis coding.	_____	_____	_____
I can code a sample claim form.	_____	_____	_____
I document accurately.	_____	_____	_____
I can explain the difference between the CMS-1500 and the UB92 forms.	_____	_____	_____
I can describe ways in which computers have altered the claims processes.	_____	_____	_____
I can discuss why claims follow-up is important to the ambulatory care setting.	_____	_____	_____
I can discuss the legal and ethical issues associated with insurance coding.	_____	_____	_____
I am comfortable as a patient educator about insurance issues.	_____	_____	_____

CHAPTER 20

Billing and Collections

CHAPTER PRE-TEST

Perform this test without looking at the book. This is just to see how well you have understood and can recall the information in this chapter after you have read it, but before you have completed the workbook exercises. You will not be graded on this portion (other than the grade you give yourself). Justify any "false" answers.

1. The Truth-in-Lending Act states:
   a. Physicians cannot charge more than 10% interest on their patient accounts.
   b. Physicians must charge interest if the account is more than 4 months past due.
   c. Physicians must notify the patients in writing if interest is to be charged on their accounts.
   d. If the physician and patient agree to an installation plan of more than four payments, the installation charge must be stated in writing.
2. The best opportunity for collection is at the time of services. (T or F)
3. Large clinics with numerous statements to send out each month will find the monthly billing cycle method to be the most efficient. (T or F)
4. A collection ratio of 80% is considered a good ratio. (T or F)

INTRODUCTION

Accurate and timely patient billing is essential to maintaining the financial health of an ambulatory care facility. Medical assistants play a vital role in managing accounts receivable. Establishing and monitoring patient billing, using either a manual or computerized system, requires attention to detail, accurate documentation, and excellent communication skills when performing duties related to the collection of outstanding debt. When performing billing and collection tasks, it is important to remember that patients have the right to choose their health care providers and should be respected as consumers.

PERFORMANCE OBJECTIVES

After successful completion of this chapter you will be able to explain the terminology related to medical billing and collections. You will be able to analyze the importance of billing accurately and billing (at least collecting copayment) at the time of services, differentiate between monthly and cycle billing, recall the components of a complete statement, analyze the importance of correct telephone collection process, and explain the process of aging accounts. You will be able to discuss the Truth-in-Lending Act, compare manual billing with computerized billing, and recall points to consider when using a collection agency. You will also be able to recall special collections problems encountered in the ambulatory care setting, describe the process of sending a collection letter, explain the ramifications of the statute of limitations, and explain the merits of a professional attitude when handling collections. *The following statements are related to your learning objectives for this chapter. Fill in the blanks in the following paragraph with the appropriate term(s).*

The ambulatory care setting's cash flow and collection process are dependent on (1) ______________________________. The (2) ______________________ status of the practice is reflected in the unpaid balance of the patient accounts. The best opportunity for collection, especially of the copayment amounts, is (3) ______________________. The (4) ______________________________ states that a practice must clearly define the charges and the interest being charged when installation payments (four or more) are being arranged with a patient. Collection letters are usually sent after (5) __________ statements have been sent to the patient with no response. When using a collection agency, the following questions should be asked: (6) ______________________________________,
(7) ____,
(8) ____,
(9) ____,
(10) ____, and
(11) ______________________________. The difference between accounts receivable ratio and collection ratio is that the (12) ______________________ refers to the speed at which the outstanding accounts are paid, and the (13) ______________ ______________________________ shows the status of the paid accounts and possible losses. Three special collection situations encountered in the ambulatory care setting are (14) ______________________, (15) ______________________, and (16) ______________________. The (17) ______________________________ defines the period in which legal action may take place.

VOCABULARY BUILDER

Find the words below that are misspelled; circle them, and then correctly spell them in the spaces provided. Then match each correct vocabulary term to its definition below.

accounts recievable ratio	collection agency	Statute of limatations
aging accounts	collection ratio	Truth-in-Lending Act
cicyle billing	monthly billing	

__________________ ____________________ ______________________

1. ________________________ A method that sends all bills at the same time each month, usually on or about the 25th day of each month
2. ________________________ A process by which accounts are determined to be overdue
3. ________________________ Also known as the Consumer Credit Protection Act of 1968; an act requiring providers of installment credits to state the charges in writing and to express the interest as an annual rate
4. ________________________ An outside establishment that collects outstanding debt
5. ________________________ Statute that defines the period of time in which legal action can take place
6. ________________________ A method of spreading billing over the whole month instead of sending bills at the end of the month
7. ________________________ The status of collections and the possible losses in a medical facility
8. ________________________ Measures the speed with which outstanding accounts are paid

LEARNING REVIEW

1. A billing efficiency report allows for careful monitoring of follow-up bills; that is, whether they were paid, if the insurance has paid, and an assessment of the patient's responsibility for payment. What five pieces of data are included in these reports from which production efficiency is calculated?

   (1) ____________________________ (4) ____________________________

   (2) ____________________________ (5) ____________________________

   (3) ____________________________

2. Identify and explain the five most common reasons some patient accounts become past due.

   (1) ____

   (2) ____

   (3) ____

   (4) ____

   (5) ____

3. A. In the pegboard system, what method is used to identify the age of accounts?

____

____

B. A written code "OD2/ 4/1" is entered on a patient ledger card. What does the code mean?

____

C. Name five criteria according to which computer programs can age accounts.

(1) ____________________ (4) ____________________

(2) ____________________ (5) ____________________

(3) ____________________

D. The computer can also generate accounts receivable reports. Name three pieces of information included on a computer-generated accounts receivable report.

(1) ____________________

(2) ____________________

(3) ____________________

4. Collection agencies generally provide two services to an ambulatory care facility. Name and describe each type of service.

(1) ____

____

(2) ____

____

5. Collection of fees when a patient has died are directed to the executor of the estate. Place a check mark next to each action below that represents a responsible action in collecting past due accounts from deceased patients' estates.

____ A. If there is no known administrator, address the statement to "Estate of (insert patient's name)" and mail to the patient's last known address.

____ B. Send an invoice via certified mail with a complete breakdown of all monies owed by the deceased patient's spouse or closest relative, noting that the survivor is responsible for making payment in full.

____ C. Wait a minimum of 10 days after the death to send a statement to the estate, out of respect for the family of the deceased.

____ D. If unsure how to proceed, contact the office's attorney or the probate court for advice on how to proceed.

6. With regard to collections, the statute of limitations is usually defined by the class of the overdue account. Name the three classes of accounts.

(1) ____________________

(2) ____________________

(3) ____________________

7. The most appropriate time to discuss fees with patients is when:
   a. services are rendered
   b. scheduling the first appointment
   c. sent by mail after services are rendered
   d. the insurance company does not pay the fee

8. The Truth-in-Lending Act is also known as the:
   a. Consumer Credit Protection Act
   b. Fair Debt Collection Practice Act
   c. Patient Bankruptcy Protection Act
   d. Accurate Billing and Collection Act

9. The charge slip is also known as the:
   a. ledger
   b. encounter form
   c. day sheet
   d. CMS-1500

10. When a patient files for bankruptcy:
    a. there is little likelihood that the debt can be collected
    b. it is best to close the account and identify the loss
    c. file a proof of claim and a copy of the account to the bankruptcy court
    d. take the account to small claims court

11. In determining how aggressive to be in debt collections, you should consider:
    a. the previous month's billing backlog
    b. production efficiency
    c. the terms of the insured's policy
    d. the value of the dollar owed

CERTIFICATION REVIEW

These questions are designed to mimic the certification examinations. You can use these questions like a small "Certification Examination Study Guide," but this is not meant to take the place of the more extensive study guides. Use this portion to determine in what areas to concentrate your efforts when studying for the certification examination. Justify any "false" answers.

1. Most states limit collections calls to between 8 AM and 8 PM. (T or F)

2. Emancipated minors are responsible for their own accounts. (T or F)

3. Collection agencies must abide by different rules than the ambulatory care center. (T or F)

4. Patients who owe money but have moved and left no forwarding address are referred to as:
   a. deadbeats
   b. skips
   c. nonpayers
   d. dead accounts

5. Statutes of limitations vary from state to state, but are usually:
   a. up to 3 years
   b. 5–10 years
   c. up to 10 years
   d. without a time limit if the account is more than a certain amount

CASE STUDY

Charles Williams, 62 years old, is a new patient of Dr. Winston Lewis at the offices of Drs. Lewis and King. On July 1, 20XX, 5 days before the patient's birthday, Charles comes to see Dr. Lewis for an appointment with a chief complaint of intermittent, irregular heartbeats or palpitations, dizziness, and chest pain. Dr. Lewis performs a comprehensive physical examination and orders several tests, including an EKG, complete blood count (CBC), and urinalysis with microscopy. The total fee for the office visit and tests is $345: $200 for the physical examination, $75 for the EKG, $25 for the urinalysis, $25 for routine venipuncture, and $20 for a CBC, which Charles pays for by check at the time of service. Charles is insured by a private carrier, All American Insurance Company, group #333210, ID number 112-45-9980, which he receives through his employer, HighTech Computer Group. Dr. Lewis asks Ellen Armstrong, CMA, to schedule a return appointment in exactly one week to go over the results of Charles's tests. Ellen schedules the appointment and prepares a charge slip for Charles's visit. She refers to his patient information sheet for the correct personal information. Charles Williams lives at 123 Greenside Street, Northborough, OH, 12346.

Complete the charge slip for Charles Williams' office visit (Figure 20-1).

SELF-ASSESSMENT

Think about a time or times when you had paid a bill late or not paid it until the following month. Without disclosing too much personal information, answer the following:

1. What was your reason(s)?
2. Did you receive an overdue notice or a phone call?
3. Which do you think would be more difficult to receive?
4. Are you likely to become defensive if the caller or notice has a threatening tone or a more understanding tone?
5. Could the tone of the notice/call leave you feeling good/bad about the event?
6. Think of ways the situation could have been handled better.
7. Will your experience affect the way you treat people who owe your clinic money?

DATE	PATIENT	SERVICE CODE	FEES CHARGE	PAID (CREDITS)	ADJ. (CREDITS)	BALANCE DUE		PREVIOUS BALANCE	NAME	RECEIPT NO.

THIS IS YOUR RECEIPT ______
AND/OR A STATEMENT OF YOUR ACCOUNT TO DATE ______

PATIENT'S NAME ☐ M ☐ F
ADDRESS
CITY STATE ZIP
RELATIONSHIP BIRTHDATE
SUBSCRIBER OR POLICY HOLDER
☐ MEDICARE ☐ MEDICAID ☐ BLUE SHIELD ☐ 65-SP.
INSURANCE CARRIER
AGREEMENT #
GROUP #

OFFICE VISITS AND PROCEDURES

99211	EST PT - MINIMAL OV	1			HOSPITAL VISIT	14	
99212	EST PT - BRIEF OV	2			EMERGENCY	15	
99213	EST PT - INTERMEDIATE OV	3			CONSULTATION	16	
99214	EST PT - EXTENDED OV	4		93000	EKG	17	
99215	EST PT - COMPREHENSIVE OV	5		93224	ELECTROCARDIOGRAPHIC MONITORING	18	
99201	NEW PT - BRIEF OV	6		93307	ECHOCARDIOGRAPHY	19	
99202	NEW PT - INTERMEDIATE OV	7		85025	CBC	20	
99203	NEW PT - EXTENDED OV	8		81000	URINALYSIS WITH MICROSCOPY	21	
99204	NEW PT - COMPLEX OV	9		36415	ROUTINE VENIPUNCTURE	22	
99205	NEW PT - COMPREHENSIVE OF	10		71020	RADIOLOGY EXAM-CHEST-2 VIEWS	23	
99238	HOSPITAL DISCHARGE	11		30300	REMOVE FOR. BODY-INTRANASAL	24	
99025	NEW PT - SURGERY PROC. PRIMARY	12				25	
	NURSING HOME VISIT	13				26	

D - OTHER SERVICES

AUTHORIZATION TO RELEASE INFORMATION: I HEREBY AUTHORIZE THE UNDERSIGNED PHYSICIAN TO RELEASE ANY INFORMATION ACQUIRED IN THE COURSE OF MY EXAMINATION OR TREATMENT.
SIGNED (PATIENT, OR PARENT IF MINOR)
______ DATE ______

NEXT APPOINTMENT ______ AT ______ AM PM
RETURN ______ DAYS ______ WEEKS ______ MONTHS

PLACE OF SERVICE ☐ OFFICE ☐ OTHER ______
DIAGNOSIS OR SYMPTOMS ______
DOCTOR'S SIGNATURE ______

L&K
LEWIS & KING, MD
2501 CENTER STREET
NORTHBOROUGH, OH 12345
03626

Figure 20-1

CHAPTER POST-TEST

This is similar to the Pre-Test. Perform this test without looking at the book. This is just to see how well you have understood and can recall the information presented in this chapter after you have studied it and completed the workbook exercises. You will not be graded on this portion (other than the grade you give yourself), but this is an excellent preparation for your instructor's test. You may use this Post-Test to determine what areas you need to study more. Justify any "false" answers.

1. The Truth-in-Lending Act states:
   a. Physicians can charge more than 10% interest on their patient accounts.
   b. Physicians can only charge interest if the account is more than 4 months overdue.
   c. Physicians must notify patients in person if interest is to be charged on their accounts.
   d. If the physician and patient agree to an installation plan of more than four payments, the installation charge must be stated in writing.
2. The best opportunity for collection is within 30 days of the time of service. (T or F)
3. Large clinics with numerous statements to send out each month will find the cycle billing method to be the most efficient. (T or F)
4. A collection ratio of 90% is considered a good ratio. (T or F)

CERTIFICATION CRITERIA CHECKLIST

As you go through your education and training, keep in mind the national certification examination that you will take when you graduate. Each chapter of the textbook and workbook covers a different section of the examination criteria. To keep track of your preparation for the certification examination turn to the back of this workbook and highlight the following CMA, RMA, or CMAS certification examination criteria (if you have already highlighted them from a previous chapter, put a check mark by the criteria):

CMA

E. Communication
   4. Professional communication and behavior

F. Medicolegal Guidelines & Requirements
   2. Legislation

Q. Managing Practice Finances
   1. Bookkeeping systems
   4. Accounting and banking procedures

RMA

II. Administrative Medical Assisting
   B. Finance/Bookkeeping

CMAS

6. Medical Office Financial Management
   - Fundamentals of financial management
   - Patient accounts

COMPETENCY ASSESSMENT

Procedure 20-1 Explaining Fees in the First Telephone Interview

Performance Objectives: To establish rapport with patients; to discuss physicians' fees; to identify patient responsibility before the first visit. Perform this objective within 15 minutes with a minimum score of 50 points.

Supplies/Equipment: Physician's fee schedule, appointment schedule, telephone

Charting/Documentation: Enter appropriate documentation/charting in the box.

Instructor's/Evaluator's Comments and Suggestions:

SKILLS CHECKLIST Procedure 20-1: Explaining Fees in the First Telephone Interview

Name ______________________________

Date ______________________________

No.	Skill	Check #1 20 pts ea	Check #2 10 pts ea	Check #3 5 pts ea	Notes
1	Place the physician's fee schedule and the appointment schedule close to the telephone.				
2	Answer call before the third ring. Identify name of the clinic and yourself.				
3	Offer assistance.				
4	Determine nature of visit, and if patient is new. Discuss possible dates for the appointment.				
5	Tell the patient you will be discussing clinic policies and will mail the Patient Information Brochure before the appointment.				
6	Ask about medical insurance. Get the identification number, name of subscriber, employer, and a telephone number of carrier.				
7	Explain that any copayment and coinsurance will be due at the time of visit.				
8	Check to see if the patient has transportation and knows how to get to the clinic. Provide directions if needed.				
9	Request that the patient arrive 15 minutes early to complete forms.				
10	After closing interview, promptly mail the Patient Information Brochure.				
Student's Total Points					
Points Possible		200	100	50	
Final Score (Student's Total Points / Possible Points)					

	Notes
Start time:	
End time:	
Total time: (15 min goal)	

COMPETENCY ASSESSMENT

Procedure 20-2 Prepare Itemized Patient Accounts for Billing

Performance Objectives: To notify patients of the fees for services rendered and collect on those accounts. Perform this objective within 20 minutes with a minimum score of 50 points.

Supplies/Equipment: Computer or typewriter, calculator, patient account of ledger cards, billing statement forms

Charting/Documentation: Enter appropriate documentation/charting in the box.

Instructor's/Evaluator's Comments and Suggestions:

SKILLS CHECKLIST Procedure 20-2: Prepare Itemized Patient Accounts for Billing

Name ______________________

Date ______________________

No.	Skill	Check #1 20 pts ea	Check #2 10 pts ea	Check #3 5 pts ea	Notes
1	Gather all accounts and ledgers with outstanding balances.				
2	Separate any accounts that are labeled as past due.				
	a. For each account, verify name and address of patient and person responsible for payment.				
	b. Place current date on statement.				
	c. Scan account information for errors.				
	d. Itemize procedures in layman's terms and indicate charges.				
	e. Identify and subtract any payments.				
	f. Calculate the unpaid balance.				
3	Discuss with the office manager and follow through on any action to be taken on past-due accounts.				
4	Place statements in envelopes and mail.				
Student's Total Points					
Points Possible (10 steps total)		200	100	50	
Final Score (Student's Total Points / Possible Points)					

	Notes
Start time:	
End time:	
Total time: (20 min goal)	

COMPETENCY ASSESSMENT

Procedure 20-3 Post/Record Adjustments

Performance Objectives: To keep track of financial adjustments. Perform this objective within 15 minutes with a minimum score of 20 points.

Supplies/Equipment: Computerized or manual bookkeeping system, patient's account, black or blue and red pen for use in manual bookkeeping system

Charting/Documentation: Enter appropriate documentation/charting in the box.

Instructor's/Evaluator's Comments and Suggestions:

SKILLS CHECKLIST Procedure 20-3: Post/Record Adjustments

Name ______________________________

Date ______________________________

No.	Skill	Check #1 20 pts ea	Check #2 10 pts ea	Check #3 5 pts ea	Notes
1	With the daily schedule of services/charges before you, enter amount received from the collection agency on a patient's account with an explanation note.				
2	Record the amount received and the explanation in the patient's account.				
3	Subtract the amount paid by the collection agency from the total charges to create the new balance.				
4	Write off this balance, indicating a zero balance on the patient's account. The difference between the amount collected and amount paid by the agency is entered as a negative adjustment on the daily sheet.				
Student's Total Points					
Points Possible		80	40	20	
Final Score (Student's Total Points / Possible Points)					

	Notes
Start time:	
End time:	
Total time: (15 min goal)	

EVALUATION OF CHAPTER KNOWLEDGE

Skills	Student Self-Evaluation Good	Average	Poor
I understand credit and collection policies and procedures.	_____	_____	_____
I understand the process of aging accounts.	_____	_____	_____
I recognize components of a complete patient statement.	_____	_____	_____
I can accurately complete a charge slip.	_____	_____	_____
I possess the ability to hold a professional telephone collection call.	_____	_____	_____
I can identify collection techniques and describe the use of each.	_____	_____	_____
I possess the ability to compose collection letters.	_____	_____	_____
I understand the importance of accounts receivable to the financial health of the ambulatory care setting.	_____	_____	_____
I know the function of credit bureaus and collection agencies.	_____	_____	_____
I can identify special collection situations and strategies for handling them.	_____	_____	_____
I can consider legal ramifications of billing and collection procedures, including the Truth-in-Lending Act, Fair Debt Collection Practices Act, small claims court, and the statute of limitations.	_____	_____	_____

CHAPTER 21

Accounting Practices

CHAPTER PRE-TEST

Perform this test without looking at the book. This is just to see how well you have understood and can recall the information in this chapter after you have read it, but before you have completed the workbook exercises. You will not be graded on this portion (other than the grade you give yourself). Justify any "false" answers.

1. Accounts receivable is the amount the physician is owed by patients. (T or F)
2. The purpose of cost analysis is to:
   a. determine the costs of each service
   b. determine the fixed costs
   c. determine the variable costs
   d. determine the total of all of the above
3. Income statements should show both profits and expenses. (T or F)
4. The W-4 Form shows the employee's withholding allowance. (T or F)

INTRODUCTION

The management of practice finances in the ambulatory care setting is one of the most important aspects in the operation of the facility. The proper management of medical facility finances includes daily financial practices, the accurate coding and processing of insurance forms, collection of accounts, and accounting practices. Accounting in the ambulatory care setting includes the collection of data on all aspects of the financial operation. If done properly, accounting can monitor the profitability of a facility and ensure that any new activities, such as computerization, result in optimum financial health. The administrative duties of medical assistants will require them to become involved in the financial operations of the ambulatory care setting. A working knowledge of accounting processes will also help medical assistants become aware of the manner in which financial realities influence workplace decisions in the ambulatory care setting, such as purchasing new equipment, hiring new employees, or implementing a facility newsletter for community outreach and patient education.

PERFORMANCE OBJECTIVES

After successful completion of this chapter you will be able to explain the terminology related to medical accounting practices used in ambulatory settings. You will be able to describe four different types of bookkeeping and accounting systems, and compare and contrast financial, managerial, and cost accounting. You will be able to explain the use and validity of the income statement, the balance sheet, the day-end summary, and the accounts receivable trial balance, as well as recall and explain useful financial ratios. You will be able to identify proper steps in accounts payable management and the impact of utilization review on reimbursement. You will also become well aware of the legal and ethical guidelines in accounting practices. *The following statements are related to your learning objectives for this chapter. Fill in the blanks in the following paragraph with the appropriate term(s).*

Accounting generates (1) ______________________________ information for the office. Although there are several different types of bookkeeping systems available to the office, most are going away from manual accounting systems and more toward (2) ______________________________ systems. (3) ______________________________ accounting provides information primarily for entities external to the clinic, such as for government. (4) ______________________________ accounting generates financial information that can enable more efficient internal control. (5) ____________________ accounting helps to determine what price the ambulatory care office is paying to perform particular services. The financial summary at the end of the day is called the (6) ____. The (7) __________________ ____ will indicate any problem between the daily journal and the ledger. Cost analysis is used to determine the costs of (8) ______________________________. (9) ______________ costs are those expenses that do not vary in total as the number of the patients vary. By contrast, the (10) ________________ __________ costs vary according to patient volume. The most commonly generated year-end report is called a (11) ________________________. A balance sheet is sometimes called a (12) ____ and is an itemized statement of (13) ________________, (14) ______________________, and the (15) ____ as of a specific date. Ratios are not difficult to calculate but can be (16) ____________________ ____________________ when using a manual system. The accounts receivable ratio measures the (17) ____, the collection ratio shows the (18) ____, and the cost ratio shows the (19) ____.

VOCABULARY BUILDER

Find the words below that are misspelled; circle them, and then correctly spell them in the spaces provided. Then match each definition below to its correct vocabulary term.

_____ 1. accounting
_____ 2. accounts payible
_____ 3. accounts recievable ratio
_____ 4. assets
_____ 5. balance sheet
_____ 6. collection ratio
_____ 7. check register
_____ 8. cost analalysis
_____ 9. cost ratio
_____ 10. cash bases of accounting
_____ 11. fixed costs
_____ 12. income statement
_____ 13. libilities
_____ 14. accrual basis of accounting
_____ 15. owner's equity
_____ 16. utilazation review
_____ 17. varieble costs

____
____
____
____
____
____
____

A. Financial statement showing net profit or loss
B. These vary in direct proportion to patient volume
C. Records and categorizes all checks written
D. The outstanding accounts receivable divided by the average monthly gross income for the past 12 months
E. A procedure that determines the cost of each service
F. An itemized statement of assets, liabilities, financial condition, and owner's equity
G. Income is recognized when the money is collected
H. These do not vary in total as the number of patients varies
I. System of monitoring the financial status of a facility and the financial results of its activities, providing information for decision making
J. Debts, financial obligations, for which one is responsible
K. The gross income divided by the amount that could have been collected, less adjustments
L. Properties of value that are owned by a business entity
M. An unwritten promise to pay a supplier for property or merchandise purchased on credit or for a service rendered
N. The amount by which business assets exceed business liabilities
O. Formula that shows the cost of a procedure or service and helps determine the financial value of maintaining certain services
P. Reports income at the time charges are generated
Q. A review of medical services before they can be performed

LEARNING REVIEW

1. There are a variety of methods used for financial management in the ambulatory care setting. Name three bookkeeping systems that are appropriate for use in a noncomputerized, or manual, environment.

   (1) ____________________

   (2) ____________________

   (3) ____________________

   Match the appropriate bookkeeping system to the following duties performed by the medical assistant.

   ____________________ A. Office manager Walter Seals, CMA, was responsible for implementing a computer system at Inner City Health Care. Before the computerized accounting program was put into effect, the urgent care center relied on a manual system of checks and balances that allowed the physician–employers to keep a firm hold on the relation between the facility's assets and the sum of liabilities and net worth.

   ____________________ B. During a temporary one-week down period in the computer system at the offices of Drs. Lewis and King while a system upgrade is installed, administrative medical assistant Ellen Armstrong completes each day's financial transactions in a daily journal, then transfers this information to the ledger through the posting process. The information will be entered into the computer once the system is up and running again.

   ____________________ C. When the patient returns the charge slip to the reception desk after an examination, Karen Ritter, CMA, carefully replaces and lines up the charge slip with the patient's name on the day sheet, then correctly inserts the ledger card under the last page of the charge slip. She proceeds to enter the total charges due and any patient payments.

2. A. Medical software packages have the ability to code information obtained in the ambulatory care setting for use in a database. When completing insurance claim forms or generating reports, the software has the capability to include the most common ____________________ and ____________________ codes. What other kinds of codes can a computerized accounting system generate that will facilitate the billing functions?

   ____

   ____

   ____

   B. The computer can also be used in the preparation of financial documents. Name four financial documents.

   (1) ____________________

   (2) ____________________

   (3) ____________________

   (4) ____________________

3. Name three ways computer service bureaus handle accounts from medical facilities.

   (1) ______________________________

   ____

   (2) ______________________________

   ____

   (3) ______________________________

   ____

4. Identify at least four steps to take to reduce the chance of embezzlement.

   (1) ______________________________

   (2) ______________________________

   (3) ______________________________

   (4) ______________________________

5. Fixed costs are expenses that do not vary in total as the number of patients seen by the medical practice grows or shrinks. Variable costs are expenses that are directly affected by patient volume.

   From the list below, identify expenses that qualify as fixed costs (FC) and those that are variable costs (VC).

   ____ 1. Interpreting laboratory test results

   ____ 2. Annual depreciation of the cost of an automatic electrocardiograph (ECG) machine

   ____ 3. Medical benefits for the office staff

   ____ 4. Purchase of reagent test strips for urinalysis

   ____ 5. Magazine subscriptions for the facility reception area

   ____ 6. Monthly telephone expenses

   ____ 7. Medical journal subscriptions for the physician–owners

   ____ 8. Purchase of a HemoCue blood glucose system

   ____ 9. Printing cost of a patient education brochure

   ____ 10. Purchase of open-shelf lateral files

   ____ 11. Adding a new position, such as a clinical medical assistant, to the office staff

   ____ 12. Property taxes on the medical facility building and grounds

   ____ 13. The monthly cost of janitorial services

   ____ 14. Purchase of disposable needle-syringe units

   ____ 15. Disposable paper gowns for patient examinations

6. To protect the practice from financial loss, physicians can purchase fidelity bonds. Name and describe the three kinds of bonds. Place a check mark in front of the one that offers the most assurance.

   (1) ____

   (2) ____

   (3) ____

7. At the offices of Drs. Lewis and King, the total accounts receivable at the end of May is $100,000 and the monthly receipts total is $75,000; the total accounts receivable at the end of June is $82,000 and the monthly receipts total is $31,000; the total accounts receivable at the end of July is $86,000 and the monthly receipts total is $20,000; the total accounts receivable at the end of August is $93,000 and the monthly receipts total is $45,000. What is the accounts receivable ratio for each month? Show your calculations in the space provided.

   May: July:

   June: August:

   Which month has the healthiest accounts receivable ratio? Why?

   ____

8. A. For the month of September, receipts at the offices of Drs. Lewis and King totaled $35,000. The Medicare/Medicaid adjustment for the month was $1,750, and the managed care adjustment was $4,500. Total charges for the month of September equaled $53,000. What is the collection ratio for the month of September? Show your calculation in the space provided.

   ____

   ____

   B. For the month of October, receipts at the offices of Drs. Lewis and King totaled $41,000. The Medicare/Medicaid adjustment for the month was $2,000, the Worker's Compensation adjustment was $750, and the managed care adjustment was $4,700. Total charges for October equaled $55,000. What is the collection ratio for the month of October? Show your calculation in the space provided.

   ____

   ____

   C. Which month has the more desirable collection ratio? Why?

   ____

9. A. A group practice of radiologists charges $225 for a routine mammogram. Total expenses related to the mammogram procedure equal $30,000 per month, and the practice performs a monthly average of 200 mammograms. What is the average cost ratio for the mammogram procedure? Show your calculations in the space provided.

   ____

   ____

B. Given the cost to patients for the mammogram procedure, is the group practice making a profit or loss on performing mammograms? What amount is the profit or loss per procedure? What amount is the profit or loss for the entire month?

____

____

10. A. Income statements reveal the cumulative profit and total expenses for each month. Monthly income and expenses are then added to arrive at year-to-date totals, which are compared with the annual budget for particular income and expense categories. Use the following information to complete the expense analysis for the first quarter office expense costs of the offices of Drs. Lewis and King. The total office expense budget for the year is $20,000 divided evenly per quarter.

Telephone expenses for January = $323.46, February = $425.93, March = $393.87

Postage and mail expenses for January = $725.45, February = $550.90, March = $601.33

Office supply expenses for January = $1,200.62, February = $325.45, March = $446.26

Yearly budget for telephone expenses = $4,000, postage and mail expenses = $8,000, office supply expenses = $8,000

Office Expenses	January	February	March	Year-to-Date	Budget for Year
Office supplies	$	$	$	$	$
Postage	$	$	$	$	$
Telephone	$	$	$	$	$
TOTALS	**$**	**$**	**$**	**$**	**$**

B. How much are the offices of Drs. Lewis and King over or under budget for quarterly office expenses? ____________________ How might the office manager use data from the budget sheet?

____

____

Why is it important to implement and track budgets for specific categories of income and expense in the ambulatory care setting?

____

____

11. Financial records should provide the following at all times:

a. salaries earned by physicians and staff

b. amount earned, owed, and collected within a given period

c. where expenses incurred in a given period

d. b and c

12. A hospital cost report for Medicare is a part of:
    a. financial accounting
    b. managerial accounting
    c. cost accounting
    d. cost analysis

13. Examples of variable costs include all of the following *except*:
    a. clinical supplies
    b. equipment costs
    c. depreciation
    d. laboratory procedures

14. The accounts receivable trial balance:
    a. tells you how much the practice owes to creditors
    b. shows any problems between the daily journal and the ledger
    c. tracks all disbursements and compares the total with the purchases
    d. uses an NCR transfer strip to copy pertinent information

15. Calculating and reviewing costs provide ambulatory care settings with:
    a. profit determining
    b. practice performance monitoring
    c. off-line batch processing
    d. a and b

CERTIFICATION REVIEW

These questions are designed to mimic the certification examinations. You can use these questions like a small "Certification Examination Study Guide," but this is not meant to take the place of the more extensive study guides. Use this portion to determine in what areas to concentrate your efforts when studying for the certification examination.

1. For the sake of accounting, a liability is:
    a. the cost of doing business
    b. considered overhead
    c. an expense
    d. a credit
    e. all of the above

2. Of the following statements, which is false?
    a. Double-entry bookkeeping is expensive.
    b. Double-entry bookkeeping is accurate.

   c. Double-entry bookkeeping is more time consuming.
   d. Double-entry bookkeeping has checks and balances in place.

3. Owner's equity is not the same as:
   a. net worth
   b. proprietorship
   c. capital
   d. accounts payable

4. Bonds may be purchased to do the following:
   a. protect the practice from embezzlement
   b. protect the practice from financial loss
   c. protect the practice from malpractice suits
   d. a and b
   e. all of the above

CASE STUDY

When the offices of Drs. Lewis and King agreed to accept individuals covered by a large managed care organization, the decision of the physician–owners was based on a complete financial analysis and projection of the expected effects the new patient load would have on the medical practice. As a result, the group practice added a second office manager and a new clinical medical assistant to the existing staff.

Discuss the following:

1. As Drs. Lewis and King absorb the new managed care patients into the practice, what can the physician–owners do to determine whether their financial analysis and projection was accurate?
2. Once the practice has assembled financial data on the effects of the new patient load, how will these data be used?
3. What beneficial effects might the addition of a clinical medical assistant have on the medical practice?

SELF-ASSESSMENT

Personal finances, as well as the finances of businesses such as ambulatory care settings, require careful planning, management, and budgeting. You can use the systems of business financial management to gain insights into your personal spending patterns and to help develop and fine-tune smart financial habits and attitudes.

For each statement, circle the response that best describes you.

1. I think saving money is:
   a. Important; I make every effort to put away a sum of money as savings on a regular basis.
   b. Great if you can find a way; I'd like to save, but I have trouble finding ways to do it.
   c. Not important right now; I have too many expenses—what I really need is a loan!

2. When planning a large purchase, such as a computer or a car, I:
   a. set a limit for spending and affordable installment payments and stick to it
   b. have a rough idea of what I can afford, but do not do any advance planning
   c. try to buy what I want and think about paying for it later

3. When considering monthly personal income and expenses, I:
   a. know exactly how much money is coming in and how much is going out to pay bills
   b. know I can cover my bills but do not keep track of exactly how much I make or spend
   c. hope for the best and if I fall short—charge it!

4. When I have extra money, I:
   a. save one third, use one third to pay off debts, and use the last third on a special purchase
   b. save half or use it to pay off debts and spend the other half on a special purchase
   c. spend it all on a special purchase

5. My checkbook is:
   a. always balanced
   b. sometimes balanced
   c. rarely balanced

6. When choosing a bank for my savings or checking, I:
   a. research interest rates, features, funds, and services carefully to find the best deal
   b. choose the bank that pays the highest interest rate
   c. just pick whatever is most convenient; banks are all the same

7. I think planning for retirement is:
   a. a priority now; the sooner you start saving, the more your money grows!
   b. important but not the most essential financial responsibility I have right now.
   c. not something I think about now—that's too far away; who can predict the future?

8. People think of me as:
   a. someone who pays attention to detail and is neat and organized
   b. someone who always manages to get the job done at the last minute
   c. someone who struggles to keep up with routine or repetitive tasks

9. I think analyzing financial data is:
   a. a smart way to assess current spending patterns and guide future spending
   b. a great thing to do if you have enough time and willpower
   c. a waste of time; besides, I just don't want to know

10. I am the kind of person who:
    a. sets short- and long-term financial goals for income and spending and works toward implementing them in a responsible way
    b. has short- and long-term financial goals but can not get around to planning for them
    c. makes financial decisions on a day-to-day basis; it is enough to deal with one day at a time

Scoring: If your answers were mostly *A* responses, congratulations! You have developed a financially responsible outlook and good recordkeeping habits. If your responses were mostly *B*s, you are thinking about financial realities and recognize the importance of a strong financial awareness. Focus on specific areas where you can improve your financial skills. If your responses were mostly *C*s, you need to work on achieving good personal financial habits. Start working on your recordkeeping skills by taking the plunge and keeping a weekly journal of expenses to see where your money goes!

CHAPTER POST-TEST

This is similar to the Pre-Test. Perform this test without looking at the book. This is just to see how well you have understood and can recall the information presented in this chapter after you have studied it and completed the workbook exercises. You will not be graded on this portion (other than the grade you give yourself), but this is an excellent preparation for your instructor's test. You may use this Post-Test to determine what areas you need to study more. Justify any "false" answers.

1. Accounts payable is the amount the physician is owed by patients. (T or F)
2. The purpose of cost analysis is to:
    a. determine the costs of each service
    b. determine the fixed costs
    c. determine the variable costs
    d. determine the total of all of the above
3. Both profits and expenses should be shown on income statements. (T or F)
4. Employees withholding allowance is recorded on the W-4 Form. (T or F)

CERTIFICATION CRITERIA CHECKLIST

As you go through your education and training, keep in mind the national certification examination that you will take when you graduate. Each chapter of the textbook and workbook covers a different section of the examination criteria. To keep track of your preparation for the certification examination turn to the back of this workbook and highlight the following CMA, RMA, or CMAS certification examination criteria (if you have already highlighted them from a previous chapter, put a check mark by the criteria):

CMA

I. Computer Concepts
   3. Computer applications

Q. Managing Practice Finances
   1. Bookkeeping systems
   4. Accounting and banking procedures
   5. Employee payroll

RMA

II. Administrative Medical Assisting
   B. Finance/Bookkeeping

CMAS

6. Medical Office Financial Management
   - Fundamentals of financial management
   - Patient accounts

COMPETENCY ASSESSMENT

Procedure 21-1 Preparing Accounts Receivable Trial Balance

Performance Objectives: A trial balance will determine if there is any problem between the daily journal and the ledger or patient accounts. Perform this objective within 20 minutes with a minimum score of 50 points.

Supplies/Equipment: Patient accounts, calculator, computer and software for computerized systems

Charting/Documentation: Enter appropriate documentation/charting in the box.

____

____

____

____

Instructor's/Evaluator's Comments and Suggestions:

____

____

____

____

____

____

SKILLS CHECKLIST Procedure 21-1: Preparing Accounts Receivable Trial Balance

Name ______________________

Date ______________________

No.	Skill	Check #1 20 pts ea	Check #2 10 pts ea	Check #3 5 pts ea	Notes
1	Pull all patient accounts that have a balance due.				
2	Enter the balance of those accounts into the calculator.				
3	Add the balances and total.				
4	Create an accounts receivable total.				
	a. Enter the accounts receivable total for the month.				
	b. Add total charges for the month. Subtotal.				
	c. Total the amount of payments received for the month.				
	d. Subtract the total payments from the total of "b" above. Subtotal.				
	e. Total the amount of the month's adjustments from the subtotal of "d" above.				
	f. Record the accounts receivable amount.				
Student's Total Points					
Points Possible (10 steps)		200	100	50	
Final Score (Student's Total Points / Possible Points)					
		Notes			
Start time:					
End time:					
Total time: (20 min goal)					

EVALUATION OF CHAPTER KNOWLEDGE

Skills	Student Self-Evaluation Good	Average	Poor
I know the importance of medical financial management in the ambulatory care setting.	_____	_____	_____
I understand and can define basic accounting terms.	_____	_____	_____
I can identify and have a working knowledge of the various accounting and bookkeeping systems.	_____	_____	_____
I understand the role computerized systems can play in the medical office.	_____	_____	_____
I recognize the challenges of converting from a manual to a computerized accounting system.	_____	_____	_____
I possess a working knowledge of cost analysis, financial records, and financial ratios.	_____	_____	_____
I understand utilization review and the importance it has in the ambulatory care setting.	_____	_____	_____
I recognize the importance of good personal and professional financial practices and habits.	_____	_____	_____

CHAPTER 22

Infection Control, Medical Asepsis, and Sterilization

CHAPTER PRE-TEST

Perform this test without looking at the book. This is just to see how well you have understood and can recall the information in this chapter after you have read it, but before you have completed the workbook exercises. You will not be graded on this portion (other than the grade you give yourself). Justify any "false" answers.

1. The single most important action you can take to avoid acquiring communicable diseases is to:
   a. not mingle with people in crowded areas
   b. wear a mask when in public
   c. wear gloves at all times
   d. wash hands frequently

2. To sanitize something literally means to:
   a. wash it well
   b. sterilize it
   c. disinfect it
   d. wipe it off

3. The difference between sterilizing and disinfecting is that sterilization gets rid of all microbes and their spores, whereas disinfection gets rid of all surface microbes, but not their spores. (T or F)

4. Epidemiology is:
   a. the study of communicable diseases only
   b. the study of diseases and other conditions and their patterns
   c. the study of *epi-*, or surfaces
   d. the study of bugs

5. The word *pathogen* means
   a. all "germs" or microorganisms
   b. bacteria and viruses only
   c. only those microorganisms that cause diseases
   d. all of the above

INTRODUCTION

During the last century, medical science, an improved standard of living, and public health measures have combined to reduce the incidence and mortality rates of infectious disease in the United States. Antibiotics and vaccines now protect much of the world from numerous ancient, deadly infectious diseases, including smallpox, measles, and tuberculosis. Because the world we live in, however, is teeming with pathogens, microorganisms that can cause disease, humankind is not, and indeed may never be, free from the threat of infectious diseases. Medical assistants who care for patients in an ambulatory care setting can help reduce the risk for infection to themselves, other health care professionals, patients, and visitors by adhering to the principles of infection control. Through the practice of medical and surgical asepsis, as well as the observance of the Centers for Disease Control and Prevention's (CDC's) Universal and Standard Precautions and Transmission-Based Precautions, medical assistants will limit the presence of infectious agents, create barriers against transmission, and decrease their own and others' risks for contracting or transmitting infectious diseases.

PERFORMANCE OBJECTIVES

After successful completion of this chapter you will be able to explain the terminology related to infection control. You will be able to describe the chain of infection and how to break the links. You will be able to define five classifications of infectious microorganisms, recall and explain the four phases our immune systems use to defend us from infectious diseases, and state the four stages of infectious diseases, as well as recall five infectious diseases, their agents of transmission, and their symptoms. After successfully finishing this chapter, you will also be aware of the Standard Precautions and will be able to give five examples of ways health care providers might be exposed to blood and other body fluids and six ways they should practice precautions. You will be able to differentiate among the three types of Transmission-Based Precautions, as well as define what they are and how they are applied. You will be able to list eight types of body fluids and give an example of each. You will also be able to describe personal protection equipment and practice proper disposal of contaminated waste. As far as sterilization, disinfection, and sanitization are concerned, you will be aware of the differences, be able to practice each method as it applies in a clinical setting, and work with the equipment and chemicals involved. *The following statements are related to your learning objective for this chapter. Fill in the blanks in the following paragraph with the appropriate term(s).*

The "chain of infection" are links/steps in the infectious process from the actual disease causing (1) ______________________, to the (2) ______________________, then to the (3) ______________________, the (4) ______________________, the (5) ______________________, and finally to the (6) ______________________.

If we break any link of the chain, we can successfully avoid the spread of the disease. Most of the "breaks" in ambulatory care occur in the transmission phase. The most effective method we, as health care workers, can use to break the transmission phase is to (7) ______________________________ frequently. Even if the transmission of disease occurs, our bodies have marvelous ways of preventing us from becoming ill. One of our first defenses is the (8) ______________________________ response. This includes the four cardinal signs: (9) ______________________, (10) ______________________, (11) ______________________, and (12) ______________________. Indications that the inflammatory response is not adequate are the accumulation of (13) ______________________, enlargement of (14) ______________________, and the possibility of (15) ______________________. Our bodies also have two main types of immune responses. One is called (16) ______________________ and does not create antibodies, the other is called (17) ______________________ and does create antibodies. Both types happen in four stages: recognition of the (18) ______________________, growth of (19) ______________________, attack against the (20) ______________________, and finally, slowdown of the immune response after (21) ______________________. Standard Precautions might best be described as a set of rules to (22) ______________________. OSHA stands for (23) ______________________ and is in place to protect the (24) ______________________. Medical asepsis is described as the use of mechanisms to destroy pathogens after they (25) ______________________. The three stages of "cleaning" surfaces, instruments, and medical equipment start with actually washing the instruments or surfaces. This washing is called (26) ______________________. The use of chemicals or boiling to further destroy microbes is called (27) ______________________. The use of chemicals or the autoclave to destroy all microbes, including their spores, is called (28) ______________________.

VOCABULARY BUILDER

A. *Find the words below that are misspelled; circle them, and then correctly spell them in the spaces provided. Then fill in the blanks in the following paragraph with the correct vocabulary term.*

contaminated	infection control	sanitization
ecorated	medical asepsis	surgical asepsis
epidemology	microorganisms	transmision
______________	______________	______________

(1) ______________________ is the study of the history, cause, and patterns of infectious diseases. Microscopic living creatures, also known as (2) ______________________, that

are capable of causing disease are called pathogens. The spread of infectious diseases can occur through direct contact, indirect contact, inhalation, ingestion, or bloodborne contact. (3) ______________________________ refers to various methods, including the CDC's Standard Precautions, health care professionals use to eliminate or reduce the risk for (4) ______________________________ of infectious microorganisms from one person to another. (5) ________________________ involves specific techniques used in the ambulatory care setting that are designed to destroy pathogens after they leave the body and to decrease the risk for spreading infection to others. (6) ________________________ is also performed in the ambulatory care setting and involves techniques designed to maintain sterile conditions during procedures to prevent pathogens from entering a patient's body during an invasive procedure.

To reduce the risk that any item, including equipment, surgical trays, and instruments, could be (7) ______________________ or exposed to microorganisms or infectious material, various sterilization techniques are used. Before instruments or other fomites are disinfected or sterilized, they must be scrubbed or cleaned to remove tissue, debris, or other impurities that may harbor pathogens, a process called (8) ____________________. Medically aseptic handwashing techniques should be performed on a regular basis to ensure the reduction of pathogens spread by the hands. To reduce the risk for chapped, (9) ________________________ skin, medical assistants can apply water-based antibacterial lotion to the hands after washing.

B. *Match the following terms with the correct definitions.*

amebic dysentery	infectious agent	pathogen
bloodborne pathogen	malaria	scabies
fomites	palliative	trichomoniasis

________________ 1. Infestation with a *Trichomonas* parasite, which may be transmitted through sexual intercourse

________________ 2. Infectious skin disease caused by the itch mite, *Sarcoptes scabiei*, which is transmitted by direct contact with infected persons

________________ 3. A pharmacologic treatment agent for a viral infection is an example of an agent that relieves only symptoms of the disease instead of curing the infection

________________ 4. A pathogen responsible for a specific infectious disease

________________ 5. Infectious intestinal disease characterized by inflammation of the mucous membrane of the colon

________________ 6. Any microorganism capable of causing disease found in blood or components of blood

________________ 7. Infectious disease caused by protozoan parasites within red blood cells; transmitted to humans by female mosquitoes

________________ 8. Substances that absorb and transmit infectious material, that is, contaminated items such as equipment

________________ 9. Any disease-producing microorganism

C. *Write a brief definition for each correct vocabulary term.*

1. Resistance ____

____

2. Vaccine ____

____

3. Antibody ____

____

4. Immunoglobulins ____

____

5. Immunity ____

____

6. Disinfection ____

____

7. Antigen ____

____

Word Search

H	P	B	F	H	X	V	L	N	O	I	T	A	Z	I	T	I	N	A	S	S	P
V	A	L	N	V	C	H	N	P	K	D	C	K	D	R	B	N	L	F	W	T	R
T	N	I	D	I	S	I	N	F	E	C	T	I	O	N	L	M	M	P	J	E	E
J	T	N	D	D	G	T	K	F	L	L	P	Q	P	N	Y	Y	V	K	M	R	V
N	I	F	E	N	R	O	B	D	O	O	L	B	G	O	S	A	L	X	M	I	E
O	B	L	T	J	T	K	L	D	I	S	E	A	S	E	C	P	H	M	D	L	N
I	I	A	A	P	A	T	H	O	G	E	N	J	T	C	K	S	R	G	L	I	T
T	O	M	N	T	C	O	N	T	R	O	L	B	I	L	M	Y	O	E	K	Z	I
C	T	M	I	A	Y	S	U	R	I	V	M	N	M	K	H	H	N	R	A	E	O
E	I	A	M	Y	I	R	R	T	J	K	E	I	V	A	P	O	L	V	C	D	N
T	C	T	A	C	T	R	V	Y	C	S	C	B	N	N	I	K	S	N	L	I	W
O	S	I	T	T	V	T	E	I	G	R	Y	D	Q	S	G	S	U	O	N	M	M
R	H	O	N	T	X	Q	T	T	O	O	W	D	S	L	N	Y	R	I	J	M	S
P	L	N	O	M	A	P	A	O	C	A	L	I	N	O	L	S	G	T	H	U	U
X	Z	H	C	T	E	S	R	U	S	A	M	O	I	X	R	Z	I	C	K	N	G
B	P	G	N	S	T	G	E	H	T	S	B	T	I	E	L	X	C	E	B	I	N
R	X	X	I	P	A	R	I	P	N	O	U	H	I	M	R	T	A	F	R	Z	U
L	K	T	J	N	G	N	P	A	S	A	C	R	L	D	E	M	L	N	J	A	F
T	N	Z	I	P	G	Q	R	Q	C	I	R	L	R	W	H	D	W	I	K	T	F
A	P	S	J	M	H	T	H	E	L	A	S	M	A	X	M	Z	I	D	M	I	Y
B	M	L	Y	N	H	F	R	N	B	R	L	Z	B	V	V	M	T	P	D	O	K
S	T	X	R	H	G	P	Y	Q	K	L	G	L	M	X	E	H	V	M	E	N	Z

antibiotics
antiseptic
asepsis
autoclave
bacteria
barriers
bloodborne
contaminated
control
disease
disinfection
epidemiology
fungus
handwashing
immunization
infection
inflammation
microscopic
microorganisms
pathogen
precautions
prevention
protection
sanitization
spread
sterilize
surgical
transmission
vaccines
virus

LEARNING REVIEW

1. The following are the common five stages of many infectious diseases. Place the stages in the proper order, starting with initial infection with a pathogen, and describe the identifying characteristics and symptoms associated with each.

   Acute Prodromal
   Declining Convalescent
   Incubation

Stage	Description
(1) ______________	______________________________
	______________________________
(2) ______________	______________________________
	______________________________
(3) ______________	______________________________
	______________________________
(4) ______________	______________________________
	______________________________
(5) ______________	______________________________
	______________________________

2. For each vaccine, identify the disease for which the vaccine provides immunity and the route of vaccine administration.

Vaccine	Disease	Route of Administration
DTP	______________	______________
HBV	______________	______________
MMR	______________	______________
Hib	______________	______________
IPV	______________	______________

3. Health care professionals use many interventions to break the chain of infection transmission. For each intervention below, identify one of the five links of infection it is intended to break.

______________________ A. Handwashing
______________________ B. Standard Precautions
______________________ C. Rapid, accurate identification of organisms
______________________ D. Aseptic technique
______________________ E. Recognition of high-risk patients
______________________ F. Isolation

________________ G. Control of excretions and secretions

________________ H. Environmental sanitation

________________ I. Treatment of underlying disease

________________ J. Airflow control

________________ K. Trash and waste disposal

________________ L. Food handling

4. A susceptible host is a person who is not resistant or immune to a pathogenic organism and is, therefore, able to contract the pathogenic organism and experience development of an infection.

   A. List the five reasons a person may be susceptible.

   (1) ________________________________

   (2) ________________________________

   (3) ________________________________

   (4) ________________________________

   (5) ________________________________

   B. Susceptibility of a person depends on several factors. For each example given, identify the correct factor of susceptibility.

   ________________ (1) Dr. Angie Esposito is physically worn down by working double shifts at Inner City Health Care. Although she loves the excitement of working intensely with patients in an urgent care setting, flu season is coming and Dr. Esposito is worried that she will succumb.

   ________________ (2) Significantly overweight and a heavy smoker, Herb Fowler is prone to colds that just will not go away; Dr. Winston Lewis is treating Herb for a case of chronic bronchitis.

   ________________ (3) Mary O'Keefe's 3-year-old son, Chris, and several other members of his play group come down with chickenpox after playing with a child infected with the disease, caused by the varicella-zoster virus.

   ________________ (4) *Pneumocystis* pneumonia is an infection common to patients who have a full-blown case of AIDS.

   ________________ (5) Jim Marshall, stressed out by the pressure to complete an architectural design ahead of schedule and on a tight budget, is depressed and angry when he gets laid up with the flu and misses two days of work.

   ________________ (6) Margaret Thomas's college-age niece is caught in an epidemic of scabies that sweeps through her dorm floor and places the students in temporary isolation until the outbreak is controlled.

______________________ (7) While vacationing at a remote spot in Mexico, Bill Schwartz eats almost a pound of shrimp at a local restaurant; the next day, he experiences severe diarrhea and vomiting. He is diagnosed with cholera, caused by the *Vibrio cholerae* bacterium harbored in the shellfish he had eaten.

5. *Immunity* is defined as the ability of the body to resist disease. Identify the correct terms or the specific form of immunity that may occur in response to specific antigens.
   A. The immune response that involves T cells and B cells to attack viruses, fungi, organ transplants, or cancer cells is called ______________________.
   B. The immune response that produces antibodies to kill pathogens and recognize them in the future is called ______________________.
   C. The immunity that follows the administration of vaccines is called ______________.
   D. The short-term immunity provided to a newborn that occurs when antibodies pass to a fetus from the mother is called ______________________.
   E. The immunity that results from contracting an infectious agent and experiencing either an acute or a subclinical infectious disease is called ______________________.
   F. The immunity achieved through administration of ready-made antibodies, such as gamma-globulin is called ______________________.

6. For each infectious disease listed below, identify the agent of transmission (virus, bacteria, fungus, etc.), at least one route of transmission, and common symptoms.
   A. AIDS

      Agent: ____

      Transmission: ____

      Symptoms: ____

      ____

      ____

      ____

   B. Tuberculosis (TB)

      Agent: ____

      Transmission: ____

      Symptoms: ____

      ____

      ____

      ____

C. Gastroenteritis

Agent: ______

Transmission: ______

Symptoms: ______

______

______

______

D. Hepatitis B

Agent: ______

Transmission: ______

Symptoms: ______

______

______

______

E. Chickenpox

Agent: ______

Transmission: ______

Symptoms: ______

______

______

______

F. Influenza

Agent: ______

Transmission: ______

Symptoms: ______

______

______

______

7. A. Describe three methods of medical asepsis used to reduce the presence of pathogens in an ambulatory care setting.

(1) ______

______

(2) ______

______

(3) ______

______

B. Place a check mark next to each statement below that represents the appropriate use of medical asepsis in the ambulatory care setting.

_________ (1) Joe Guerrero, CMA, washes his hands before performing the transfer of patient Lenore McDonell from the wheelchair to the examination table.

_________ (2) Wanda Slawson, CMA, runs a clean sheet of disposable paper over the examination table to prepare the room for the next patient. She picks up the cloth gown patient Lydia Renzi leaves unused, still in its plastic protective covering, on a chair in the examination room and places it on the examination table for the next patient to use.

_________ (3) After performing a venipuncture procedure on patient Leo McKay, Bruce Goldman, CMA, tells Leo he can just throw the gauze pad he has been holding on the venipuncture site in the trash can.

_________ (4) Anna Preciado, CMA, moving quickly to assist a patient who may be about to faint, accidentally bumps into a sterile tray of instruments, knocking some of them to the floor. The patient, who is bent over in front of Anna, picks the instruments up off the floor and places them back on the tray in the sterile field. "You dropped these," he says.

_________ (5) After assisting in the removal of an infected sebaceous cyst from a patient, clinical medical assistant Audrey Jones cleans, dresses, and bandages the wound as directed by Dr. Winston Lewis. She then disposes of all contaminated items per Occupational Safety and Health Administration (OSHA) guidelines, properly removes personal protective equipment (PPE), removes her gloves, and washes her hands.

C. For each item in part B (above) that does not reflect proper techniques of medical asepsis, explain what went wrong and how the error should be corrected.

____

____

____

____

8. ______________________ is a term used interchangeably for surgical asepsis. Living tissue surfaces, such as skin, cannot be sterilized. Name two examples of ways that skin can be rid of as many pathogens as possible before the use of a sterile covering.

(1) ____

____

(2) ____

____

9. A. For each instrument or item below, identify the method used for proper asepsis: chemical disinfection (CD), chemical sterilization (CS), or steam sterilization (SS) in an autoclave.

   Match the following equipment with the correct aseptic method.

   ______ (1) Percussion hammer
   ______ (2) Wrapped surgical instruments
   ______ (3) Stethoscopes
   ______ (4) Fiber-optic endoscopes
   ______ (5) Countertops
   ______ (6) Wheelchairs
   ______ (7) Gynecologic instruments
   ______ (8) Examination tables

   B. Why are gynecologic instruments sanitized separately from other external physical examination instruments before sterilization?

   ____

   ____

10. Identify and describe the most widely used method of sterilization in the ambulatory care setting.

    ____

    ____

    ____

    ____

11. A. List six general rules that ensure proper sterilization when using an autoclave.

    (1) ____
    (2) ____
    (3) ____
    (4) ____
    (5) ____
    (6) ____

    B. Identify the recommended requirements for effective sterilization in an autoclave.

    Temperature: ______________________
    Time for sterilization of unwrapped items: ______________________
    Time for sterilization of loosely wrapped items: ______________________
    Time for sterilization of tightly wrapped items: ______________________
    Frequency of draining of water and cleaning of autoclave: ______________________

CERTIFICATION REVIEW

These questions are designed to mimic the certification examinations. You can use these questions like a small "Certification Examination Study Guide," but this is not meant to take the place of the more extensive study guides. Use this portion to determine in what areas to concentrate your efforts when studying for the certification examination.

1. The recommended temperature for effective sterilization in an autoclave is:
   a. 212°F
   b. 250°F
   c. 150°F
   d. 220°F

2. Susceptibility to an infectious microorganism depends on all of the following *except*:
   a. number and specific types of pathogens
   b. duration of exposure to the pathogen
   c. indirect contact
   d. general physical condition

3. The body's natural way of responding when invaded by a pathogen is:
   a. inflammation
   b. septicemia
   c. immunosuppression
   d. immunization

4. The greatest natural barrier is:
   a. intact skin
   b. cilia
   c. hydrochloric acid
   d. mucous membranes

5. Specialized antibodies that can render a pathogen unable to reproduce or continue to grow are called:
   a. antigens
   b. immunoglobulins
   c. pathogenic toxins
   d. spores

CASE STUDIES

Case 1

Michelle Richards, a medical assisting intern at the Northborough Family Medical Group of Drs. Winston Lewis and Elizabeth King, attends to patient procedures and examinations under the supervision of office manager Marilyn Johnson, CMA. Although Michelle is careful to follow all infection control methods during her observations, severe dermatitis has developed on her hands. She is concerned that this condition, which has not responded to creams and lotions, is related to the latex gloves she wears during required procedures.

1. Discuss the possible causes of Michelle's symptoms.
2. Suggest a course of action that both addresses Michelle's condition and maintains the proper degree of asepsis.

Case 2

Liz Corbin, CMA, is responsible for maintaining and cleaning the autoclave at Inner City Health Care. Because this equipment is used everyday to sterilize instruments used during procedures performed at the clinic, Liz cleans the inner chamber of the autoclave daily. Once a week, she gives the autoclave a thorough cleansing.

1. Describe Liz's daily cleaning procedure.
2. Describe the weekly cleaning procedure for the autoclave.
3. Why are proper maintenance and cleaning of the autoclave important in the ambulatory care setting?

Case 3

One-year-old Marissa O'Keefe is a patient at the practice of Drs. Lewis and King. During her well-baby visit, Joe Guerrero, CMA, gives Marissa an MMR vaccine and is about to administer the scheduled fourth DTP immunization when her mother, Mary O'Keefe, voices concern about this vaccination. "I've read that the DPT shot can be dangerous and sometimes causes brain damage. Marissa had a fever after her last DPT, so I don't want to take any risks with this one. I don't think she should have this shot."

1. Should Joe administer the DPT shot to Marissa? How safe is the DPT shot? What is the *ICD-9-CM* diagnosis code for the DTP vaccination?
2. What is Joe's best therapeutic response to Mary?

SELF-ASSESSMENT

As you answer the following questions, think about how you have changed your awareness of disease prevention because of what you have learned in this chapter.

1. Are you always 100% careful to wash your hands after using the restroom?

2. How does it make you feel when you see others leaving a public restroom without washing their hands?

3. Are you always careful to wash your hands just before eating? Even if you are in a car and there is not a sink handy? What can you do in that case?

4. Besides washing your hands and avoiding direct contact with sick people, what do you suppose is the other single most important action you can take to stay healthy?

5. Do you think stress can make you sick? If so, how do you suppose that happens?

CHAPTER POST-TEST

This is similar to the Pre-Test. Perform this test without looking at the book. This is just to see how well you have understood and can recall the information presented in this chapter after you have studied it and completed the workbook exercises. You will not be graded on this portion (other than the grade you give yourself), but this is an excellent preparation for your instructor's test. You may use this Post-Test to determine what areas you need to study more. Justify any "false" answers.

1. The single most important action you can take to avoid contracting a communicable disease is to:
   a. mingle with people in crowded areas so you create immunities
   b. wear a mask when in public
   c. wear gloves at all times
   d. wash hands frequently

2. Disinfection is a way to:
   a. clean hands
   b. prepare the patient's skin for surgery
   c. clean inanimate objects, such as countertops
   d. sterilize

3. The difference between sterilizing and disinfecting is that disinfection gets rid of all microbes and their spores, whereas sterilization gets rid of all surface microbes, but not their spores. (T or F)

4. Epidemiology is:
   a. the study of communicable diseases only
   b. the study of diseases and other conditions and their patterns
   c. the study of *epi-*, or surfaces
   d. the study of bugs

5. The word *pathogen* means
   a. all "germs" or microorganisms
   b. viruses only
   c. only those microorganisms that cause diseases
   d. all of the above

CERTIFICATION CRITERIA CHECKLIST

As you go through your education and training, keep in mind the national certification examination that you will take when you graduate. Each chapter of the textbook and workbook covers a different section of the examination criteria. To keep track of your preparation for the certification examination, turn to the back of this workbook and highlight the following CMA, RMA, or CMAS certification examination criteria (if you have already highlighted them from a previous chapter, put a check mark by the criteria):

CMA

F. Medicolegal Guidelines & Requirements
   2. Legislation

R. Principles of Infection Control

S. Treatment Area
   1. Equipment preparation and operation
   2. Principles of operation (equipment)
   5. Safety precautions

RMA

III. Clinical Medical Assisting
   A. Asepsis
   B. Sterilization

CMAS

2. Basic Clinical Medical Office Assisting
   - Asepsis in the medical office

COMPETENCY ASSESSMENT

Procedure 22-1 Medical Asepsis Hand Wash

Performance Objectives: To reduce pathogens on the hands and wrists, thereby decreasing direct and indirect transmission of infectious microorganisms. Average duration is 2 minutes before beginning to work with patients, 30 seconds after each patient contact. Perform this objective within 3 minutes with a minimum score of 65 points.

Supplies/Equipment: Sink (preferably with foot-operated controls), soap (preferably liquid soap in foot-operated container; bar soap is discouraged), lotion

Charting/Documentation: Enter appropriate documentation/charting in the box.

Instructor's/Evaluator's Comments and Suggestions:

SKILLS CHECKLIST Procedure 22-1: Medical Asepsis Hand Wash

Name ______________________________

Date ______________________________

No.	Skill	Check #1 20 pts ea	Check #2 10 pts ea	Check #3 5 pts ea	Notes
1	Remove all jewelry.				
2	Prepare disposable paper towel.				
3	Never allow your clothing to touch the sink; never touch the inside of the sink with your hands.				
4	Turn on the faucet with a dry paper towel. Adjust water temperature to lukewarm. Discard paper towel.				
5	Wet hands and apply soap using a circular motion and friction; rub into a lather.				
6	Use an orange stick or brush at the first hand cleansing of each day.				
7	Rinse hands with hands pointed down and lower than elbows.				
8	Repeat soap application and lather; interlace fingers well, wash with vigorous, circular motions all parts of hands and wrists; wash for at east 1 minute or longer.				
9	Rinse well, keeping hands pointed downward.				
10	Repeat hand cleansing for the first hand cleansing of the day, or if necessary.				
11	Dry hands and wrist with disposable paper towel; do not touch towel dispenser after hand cleansing; blot instead of rubbing; if sink is not foot-operated, use a clean disposable towel to turn off water faucet.				
12	Discard paper towel in waste container.				
13	Apply lotion.				
Student's Total Points					
Points Possible		260	130	65	
Final Score (Student's Total Points / Possible Points)					

	Notes
Start time:	
End time:	
Total time: (3 min goal)	

COMPETENCY ASSESSMENT

Procedure 22-2 Removing Contaminated Gloves

Performance Objectives: To carefully remove and dispose of contaminated gloves to minimize exposure to biohazard contaminants. Perform this objective within 2 minutes with a minimum score of 35 points.

Supplies/Equipment: Biohazard waste container, contaminated gloves, soap, water, lotion

Charting/Documentation: Enter appropriate documentation/charting in the box.

Instructor's/Evaluator's Comments and Suggestions:

SKILLS CHECKLIST Procedure 22-2: Removing Contaminated Gloves

Name ______________________________

Date ______________________________

No.	Skill	Check #1 20 pts ea	Check #2 10 pts ea	Check #3 5 pts ea	Notes
1	Make a fist with the left hand. Grasp the palm of the used left glove with the right hand. Hold hands away from body and pointed downward.				
2	Turn the used left glove inside out and hold it in the right gloved hand.				
3	Holding the glove that has been removed with the hand that still has the glove on, insert two fingers of the ungloved hand between the back of the hand and the inside of the dirty glove.				
4	Turn the right dirty glove inside out over the other.				
5	Dispose of the inverted gloves into a biological waste receptacle.				
6	Wash hand thoroughly.				
7	Apply lotion.				
Student's Total Points					
Points Possible		140	70	35	
Final Score (Student's Total Points / Possible Points)					
		Notes			
Start time:					
End time:					
Total time: (2 min goal)					

COMPETENCY ASSESSMENT

Procedure 22-3 Transmission-Based Precautions: Donning a Gown, Mask, Gloves, and Cap (Isolation Technique)

Performance Objectives: To provide barriers for medical assistants to protect themselves from airborne, contact, or droplet infectious diseases when working within an inpatient setting. Perform this objective within 30 minutes with a minimum score of 95 points.

Supplies/Equipment: Disposable gowns, disposable caps, disposable masks, gloves, sink and running water, paper towels, lotion, impermeable biohazard bags, other supplies relative to client's condition

Charting/Documentation: Enter appropriate documentation/charting in the box.

____

____

____

____

Instructor's/Evaluator's Comments and Suggestions:

____

____

____

____

____

____

SKILLS CHECKLIST Procedure 22-3: Transmission-Based Precautions: Donning a Gown, Mask, Gloves, and Cap (Isolation Technique)

Name ______________________________

Date ______________________________

No.	Skill	Check #1 20 pts ea	Check #2 10 pts ea	Check #3 5 pts ea	Notes
1	Review physician orders and agency protocols relative to the type of isolation precautions.				
2	Place appropriate isolation supplies outside the patient's room and note type of isolation sign on the door (airborne, droplet, contact).				
3	Remove jewelry, laboratory coat, and other items not necessary in providing patient care.				
4	Wash hands and don disposable clothing.				
	a. Apply cap.				
	b. Apply gown.				
	c. Apply gloves.				
	d. Apply mask.				
5	Enter patient's room with all gathered supplies.				
6	Assess vital signs and perform other functions of care. Record data.				
7	Dispose of soiled articles into the biohazard bags, labeled according to content.				
8	Remove contaminated gloves, wash hands, and untie waist of gown.				
9	Remove mask. Dispose.				
10	Untie neckties of gown. Wash hands.				
11	Slip fingers of one hand inside the cuff of the other sleeve. Pull the gown over the hand, being careful not to touch the outside of the gown.				
12	Using the hand covered by the gown, pull down the gown over the other hand.				
13	Pull the gown off your arms. Hold the gown away from body and roll it into a ball with the contaminated side inside.				

No.	Skill	Check #1 20 pts ea	Check #2 10 pts ea	Check #3 5 pts ea	Notes
14	Dispose of coverings into a biohazard bag.				
15	Wash hands thoroughly, then apply lotion.				
Student's Total Points					
Points Possible (19 steps)		380	190	95	
Final Score (Student's Total Points / Possible Points)					

	Notes
Start time:	
End time:	
Total time: (30 min goal)	

COMPETENCY ASSESSMENT

Procedure 22-4 Sanitization of Instruments

Performance Objectives: To properly clean contaminated instruments to remove tissue, debris, and gross contaminations. Perform this objective within 15 minutes with a minimum score of 40 points.

Supplies/Equipment: Sink (or ultrasonic cleaner), sanitizing agent (low-sudsing detergent, approved chemical disinfectant, or blood solvent), brush, disposable paper towels, plastic apron, disposable gloves (heavy duty if cleaning sharps), goggles, biohazard waste container

Charting/Documentation: Enter appropriate documentation/charting in the box.

Instructor's/Evaluator's Comments and Suggestions:

SKILLS CHECKLIST Procedure 22-4: Sanitization of Instruments

Name ______________________

Date ______________________

No.	Skill	Check #1 20 pts ea	Check #2 10 pts ea	Check #3 5 pts ea	Notes
1	Wear disposable heavy duty gloves, goggles, and apron.				
2	Rinse the instruments in cool water and disinfectant solution as soon as possible. Rinse again under running water.				
3	If contaminated instrument must be carried to another area, place instrument in basin labeled "Biohazard."				
4	Scrub each instrument well with detergent and water; scrub under running water.				
5	Rinse well with hot water.				
6	Place instruments on muslin or paper towel.				
7	Dry instruments with muslin or disposable paper towels.				
8	Remove gloves and wash hands, then apply lotion.				
Student's Total Points					
Points Possible		160	80	40	
Final Score (Student's Total Points / Possible Points)					
		Notes			
Start time:					
End time:					
Total time: (15 min goal)					

COMPETENCY ASSESSMENT

Procedure 22-5 Chemical "Cold" Sterilization of Endoscopes

Performance Objectives: To sterilize heat-sensitive items, such as fiber-optic endoscopes, using appropriate chemical solution. Perform this objective within approximately 30 minutes (depending on the solution) with a minimum score of 55 points.

Supplies/Equipment: Chemical solution, timer, sterile water, airtight container, heavy duty gloves, sterile towels, polylined sterile drapes

Charting/Documentation: Enter appropriate documentation/charting in the box.

____

____

____

____

Instructor's/Evaluator's Comments and Suggestions:

____

____

____

____

____

____

SKILLS CHECKLIST Procedure 22-5: Chemical "Cold" Sterilization of Endoscopes

Name ______________________

Date ______________________

No.	Skill	Check #1 20 pts ea	Check #2 10 pts ea	Check #3 5 pts ea	Notes
1	Sanitize and dry instrument/scope following manufacturer's instructions.				
2	Read manufacturer's instructions regarding use of chemical sterilant.				
3	Glove with nonsterile gloves. Apply PPEs.				
4	Prepare solution according to instructions. Record the solution and ratio.				
5	Pour solution into container with a tight-fitting lid.				
6	Place scope into the solution. Begin timing.				
7	Close lid. Record date and time.				
8	Do not disturb the item until time is up.				
9	When time is up, remove the lid from the sterile water, set up the sterile field, apply the sterile towel, and lift the scope with sterile gloved hands.				
10	Using sterile gloves, hold the scope over a sink, taking care to not let it touch the sink or surrounding area; pour sterile water over and through it until completely rinsed of chemicals. Drip dry a few minutes.				
11	Place the sterile scope onto the sterile field and dry it with the sterile towels. Dispose of the towels and lay the sterile scope onto the sterile field. Cover with a sterile drape.				
Student's Total Points					
Points Possible		220	110	55	
Final Score (Student's Total Points / Possible Points)					

	Notes
Start time:	
End time:	
Total time: (30 min goal, depending on solution)	

COMPETENCY ASSESSMENT

Procedure 22-6 Wrapping Instruments for Sterilization in Autoclave

Performance Objectives: To properly wrap sanitized instruments for sterilization in an autoclave. Perform this objective within 10 minutes with a minimum score of 70 points.

Supplies/Equipment: Sanitized instruments, wrapping material (muslin or disposable wrapping paper), sterilization indicator, 2 × 2 gauze (if instrument has hinges), autoclave wrapping tape, tip protectors, permanent marker or felt-tip pen

Charting/Documentation: Enter appropriate documentation/charting in the box.

Instructor's/Evaluator's Comments and Suggestions:

SKILLS CHECKLIST Procedure 22-6: Wrapping Instruments for Sterilization in Autoclave

Name ______________________

Date ______________________

No.	Skill	Check #1 20 pts ea	Check #2 10 pts ea	Check #3 5 pts ea	Notes
1	Prepare a clean, dry, flat surface of adequate size to lay the wrapping material.				
2	Select two wraps of adequate size in which to wrap the instrument(s).				
3	Place one square of wrapping material at an angle in front of you on the flat, dry surface, with one corner pointed directly toward you.				
4	Place the sanitized instrument(s) just below the center of the wrap. Open instruments with hinges and gently place gauze or cotton in the opening. Do not close instruments. Apply tip protectors to sharp instruments.				
5	Place a sterilization indicator with the instrument(s).				
6	Bring the closest corner of the wrap up and over the article; bring tip of corner back to the folded edge. Smooth the edges. The article should be completely covered.				
7	Fold one side edge toward the center line, fan fold back to side, and crease.				
8	Repeat Step 7 for the other side.				
9	Fold the package up from the bottom.				
10	Fold the top edge down. Fold the tip back.				
11	To wrap twice, place package into center of second wrap and repeat Steps 7–10. Do not fold last tip back.				
12	Tape the autoclave tape across the point left exposed.				

No.	Skill	Check #1 20 pts ea	Check #2 10 pts ea	Check #3 5 pts ea	Notes
13	Label the tape.				
14	Placed wrapped instruments in autoclave.				
Student's Total Points					
Points Possible		280	140	70	
Final Score (Student's Total Points / Possible Points)					
		Notes			
Start time:					
End time:					
Total time: (10 min goal)					

COMPETENCY ASSESSMENT

Procedure 22-7 Sterilization of Instruments (Autoclave)

Performance Objectives: To rid instruments of all forms of microbial (microorganism) life for use in invasive procedures. Perform this objective within 45 minutes with a minimum score of 55 points.

Supplies/Equipment: Steam sterilizer (autoclave), autoclave manufacturer procedure manual, wrapped sanitized instrument package(s) with sterilization indicators placed inside the package (or unwrapped item, if removed with sterile transfer forceps)

Charting/Documentation: Enter appropriate documentation/charting in the box.

____

____

____

____

Instructor's/Evaluator's Comments and Suggestions:

____

____

____

____

____

____

SKILLS CHECKLIST Procedure 22-7: Sterilization of Instruments (Autoclave)

Name ______________________

Date ______________________

No.	Skill	Check #1 20 pts ea	Check #2 10 pts ea	Check #3 5 pts ea	Notes
1	Check water level in autoclave, and add distilled water, if necessary.				
2	Depending on the autoclave, turn knob to fill, allow chamber to fill. Turn knob to next position.				
3	Load package(s) into autoclave.				
4	Close autoclave door and seal. Turn on autoclave; set temperature and pressure (or, depending on the autoclave, set to sterilize).				
5	When temperature dial indicates 250°F, and 15 lbs of pressure, begin exposure time and set timer.				
6	After completion of the cycle, exhaust steam pressure from the autoclave.				
7	Open the door 1 inch after the pressure gauge indicates zero pressure and temperature has decreased to at least 212°F.				
8	Allow the contents to completely dry.				
9	Remove wrapped contents with dry, clean hands and store in clean, dry area.				
10	Remove unwrapped contents with sterile transfer forceps.				
11	Items not to be used as sterile may be handled with clean hands and stored in a clean, dry area.				
Student's Total Points					
Points Possible		220	110	55	
Final Score (Student's Total Points / Possible Points)					

	Notes
Start time:	
End time:	
Total time: (45 min goal)	

EVALUATION OF CHAPTER KNOWLEDGE

	Student Self-Evaluation		
Skills	Good	Average	Poor
I can define key vocabulary terms correctly.	_____	_____	_____
I can identify and understand the importance of infection control in the ambulatory care setting.	_____	_____	_____
I observe Universal and Standard Precautions.	_____	_____	_____
I can define the five classifications of infectious organisms.	_____	_____	_____
I can describe the four stages of infectious diseases.	_____	_____	_____
I can state and describe the four phases of immune response.	_____	_____	_____
I understand the purpose of timely sanitization of contaminated instruments.	_____	_____	_____
I can identify four methods of sterilization.	_____	_____	_____
I can define both surgical and medical asepsis.	_____	_____	_____
I can perform competent wrapping technique and proper operation of the autoclave.	_____	_____	_____

CHAPTER 23

Taking a Medical History, the Patient's Chart, and Methods of Documentation

CHAPTER PRE-TEST

Perform this test without looking at the book. This is just to see how well you have understood and can recall the information in this chapter after you have read it, but before you have completed the workbook exercises. You will not be graded on this portion (other than the grade you give yourself). Justify any "false" answers.

1. To diagnose is to give a name to the condition or disease a patient has. (T or F)
2. Subjective statements are those statements that could be described as "opinion." (T or F)
3. When a patient "complains" of something, he or she is:
   a. just whining
   b. filing a law suit
   c. explaining his or her symptoms
   d. gossiping
4. Once a medical assistant has asked a patient whether he or she has any allergies, and the information has been recorded, the medical assistant does not need to keep asking. (T or F)
5. If a disease is familial, that means it is communicable to close family members living in the same house. (T or F)

INTRODUCTION

The patient's medical history is an invaluable tool in helping the physician treat the patient effectively. When taking or updating patient medical histories, the medical assistant must be as thorough and accurate in documentation as possible, while remaining respectful of the patient's emotional needs and right to privacy. Therapeutic communication skills, including, but not limited to, active listening, recognizing nonverbal cues, and adapting communication to the patient's ability to understand, are essential to the process of obtaining accurate and complete patient medical documentation.

PERFORMANCE OBJECTIVES

After successful completion of this chapter you will be able to explain the terminology related to taking a medical history, creating and maintaining a patient chart, and methods of documentation. You will be able to define the parts of a medical history, identify and use effective methods to interact with your patients, and in doing so, obtain a good medical history from the patient. You will also be able to accurately and completely chart/document medical information in the patient's record using either the SOAP method or problem-oriented medical record (POMR) method. You will have the skills to be sensitive to the cultural diversity of your patients and will be able to explain methods of showing cultural sensitivity. You will know why the medical record is so important and also will be able to explain the areas of concern regarding Health Insurance Portability and Accountibility Act (HIPAA) and medical information. *The following statements are related to your learning objectives for this chapter. Fill in the blanks in the following paragraph with the appropriate term(s).*

One of the most important skills a medical assistant can obtain and cultivate is the skill of interviewing patients to obtain an accounting of their (and their family's) past medical treatments, surgeries, illnesses, and habits. This accounting is called a (1) ______________________. After the patient has completed a Medical History Form, the medical assistant will begin the patient interview for particular pieces of information such as allergies and (2) ______________________, with the physician completing the interview to ascertain in-depth information about the current illnesses. The patient chart is a (3) ______________________ document that is a collection of confidential patient information. Therefore, it is critical that the information in the patient medical record/chart be (4) ______________________, (5) ______________________, (6) ______________________, and (7) ______________________. As always, the medical assistant should continuously be aware of and sensitive to cultural differences and other issues that might hinder (8) ______________________. Parts of the medical history include the patients' (9) ______________________; the patients' present (10) ______________________; their past (11) ______________________; their (12) ______________________ history, which includes information about conditions they may have inherited; and their (13) ______________________ history, which includes hobbies, sexual activities, drinking and smoking habits, and their marital status. The physician then performs an organized, predictable, total body examination that is documented under the title of (14) ______________________. When charting information, organized methods are used. One is called the SOAP method and includes (15) ______________________, (16) ______________________, (17) ______________________, and (18) ______________________ information. Another popular method used when the patient has more than one physician using the chart is called the (19) ______________________________.

VOCABULARY BUILDER

Find the words below that are misspelled; circle them, and then correctly spell them in the spaces provided. Then match the correct vocabulary terms from the list that best fit the descriptions below.

A. allergy's
B. chart
C. chief complaint
D. clinical diagnosus
E. famileal
F. objective sign
G. problem-orientated medical record (POMR)
H. SOAP
I. source-oriented medical record (SOMR)
J. subjective complaint
K. differential diagnosis

______________________ ______________________

______________________ ______________________

____ 1. The main reason the patient comes to the doctor

____ 2. Diseases or conditions with genetic links such as breast and colon cancers, coronary artery disease, diabetes mellitus, and hypertension

____ 3. Mary O'Keefe calls Dr. King's office to schedule an emergency appointment and tells Ellen Armstrong, CMA, that her 3-year-old son Chris awakened during the night with a high fever and extreme pain in his right ear

____ 4. Dr. King examines 3-year-old Chris O'Keefe's right ear with an otoscope and observes that the ear is inflamed; the ear is also draining

____ 5. When a 19-year-old young woman comes into Inner City Health Care with extreme abdominal pain localized to the lower right quadrant, vomiting, slight fever, and loss of appetite, Dr. Whitney orders a CBC, a urinalysis, and an abdominal ultrasound to distinguish between possible diagnoses of acute appendicitis or an ovarian cyst that has become twisted.

____ 6. Dr. Whitney confirms a diagnosis of acute appendicitis for the female emergency patient, based on subjective and objective information from the patient's history, the findings of the physical examination, and the results of the laboratory tests ordered

____ 7. A patient's file of medical history and treatment, kept by the physician

____ 8. A traditional form of charting that consists of a chronologic set of notes for each visit, beginning with the patient's first visit

____ 9. Charting method that lists patient data in the following order: Subjective/Objective/Assessment/Plan

____ 10. An acquired abnormal immune response to a substance (allergen) that does not normally cause a reaction

____ 11. The most efficient way of recording chart notes, especially in multiphysician clinics or practices

LEARNING REVIEW

1. 3/10/XX CC: NVD × 4 days. T > 100°F × 2 days. Loss of appetite.

   Decode this chart note. ____

   A mistake is made in the chart note above: three days should be listed instead of four. Using proper procedure, correct the chart note.

2. Every physician/patient interview is a cross-cultural one. List four questions a medical assistant might ask while taking a medical history that will help bridge social and cultural beliefs to obtain accurate information about a patient's condition that the physician will need to give proper care and treatment.

   (1) ____
   (2) ____
   (3) ____
   (4) ____

3. List the eight possible characteristics of chief complaints.

   (1) ____________________ (5) ____________________
   (2) ____________________ (6) ____________________
   (3) ____________________ (7) ____________________
   (4) ____________________ (8) ____________________

4. Decode each component of Figure 23-1. Put all information into lay terms and write out all abbreviations.

A.	7/15/20XX	
B.	CC: lower abdominal pain × 1 wk $\bar{c}$ $\uparrow$ malaise.	
C.	Wt. 135 Ht. 5′5″ T 99.8°F R 19 P 78 regular BP 134/82	
D.	Pt describes $\uparrow$ urge to urinate $\bar{c}$ burning sensation on urination; pressure in abdomen; lack of energy.	
E.	Past Med Hist	freq. UTIs dx Type II diabetes mellitus 1987; Rx Glynase 3 mg tab qd quit smoking 20 yrs ago weight $\downarrow$ 10lbs in last 2 yrs.
F.	Allergies	no known
G.	Family Hist	no Δ
H.	Habits	< 2 glasses wine per wk no smoking, regular exercise

Figure 23-1

A. ______________________________
B. ______________________________
C. ______________________________
D. ______________________________
E. ______________________________
F. ______________________________
G. ______________________________
H. ______________________________

5. After the history is taken by the medical assistant, the physician will perform a review of systems (ROS). In addition to the patient's general state of health, list 10 body systems the physician will assess during the ROS.

(1) ______________________ (6) ______________________
(2) ______________________ (7) ______________________
(3) ______________________ (8) ______________________
(4) ______________________ (9) ______________________
(5) ______________________ (10) ______________________

6. Communicating across the life span may mean:
   a. helping a parent cope with a child who is being treated
   b. seeing a child without a parent when the parent is upset
   c. making certain the parent accompanies a teenager or older adult
   d. a and b

7. The medical history form includes the social history, medical history, family history, review of systems, and:
   a. insurance information
   b. chief complaint
   c. physician's history
   d. diagnosis and prognosis

8. Primary administrative information includes the patient's full name, telephone numbers, insurance information, and:
   a. addresses
   b. date of birth
   c. vital signs
   d. a and b

9. The CCR, or Continuity of Care Record:
   a. ensures that a minimum standard of information is to be shared with other providers
   b. will have no effect on the amount of errors made in the patient's chart
   c. is being established by the American Academy of Gerontologists
   d. can only be completed by physicians

CERTIFICATION REVIEW

These questions are designed to mimic the certification examinations. You can use these questions like a small "Certification Examination Study Guide," but this is not meant to take the place of the more extensive study guides. Use this portion to determine in what areas to concentrate your efforts when studying for the certification examination. Justify any "false" answers.

1. Which is not a component of SOAP charting?
   a. subjective information
   b. assessment of symptoms
   c. symptoms
   d. plan for treatment
2. POMR stands for:
   a. privacy of medical records
   b. problem-oriented medical records
   c. payment of medical resources
   d. parts of medical records
3. Charts (medical records) belong to the physician, and nobody has a right to see them without a court order. (T or F)
4. Abbreviations of medical terms can be confusing from institution to institution, so JCAHO has actually created a list of "forbidden" abbreviations. (T or F)

CASE STUDY

Nancy Catalina is a new patient of Dr. Esposito's at Inner City Health Care. Nancy, an 88-year-old Italian-born woman, comes to see Dr. Esposito at the urging of her granddaughter Leslie, who has set up the appointment for her. Nancy's primary care physician of 35 years has just retired; her only criteria for a new physician is that the physician must be of Italian descent.

When scheduling the appointment, Leslie notes to Liz Corbin, CMA, her grandmother's medical history of mild angina pectoris, high blood pressure, hiatal hernia, and rheumatoid arthritis. On the day of the examination, Liz questions Nancy directly about her medical history. Nancy talks extensively about her aches and pains, moving back and forth in time between current problems and problems that took place as far back as 40 years ago. In each case, a gentle reminder from her granddaughter brings Nancy back to a discussion of her present physical condition. On each reminder, Nancy acknowledges the difference between past and current events and admits she had gotten off track, although this is not readily apparent from her answers to Liz. It is clear that Leslie's knowledge of her grandmother's life and medical history makes it possible for Liz to distinguish between events in Nancy's past and events in her present, guiding her back to the task at hand, which is taking a current medical history for the patient's permanent record.

Discuss the following:

1. What communications skills will Liz need to use to get the most accurate information from Nancy?
2. What can the manner in which this patient relates information reveal about her?
3. What effect does Nancy's granddaughter have on the process of taking the medical history? Is the effect beneficial or disruptive?

SELF-ASSESSMENT

Think about when you go to work as a medical assistant and try to answer the following questions. Be as self-reflective as you can.

1. When you are asked to complete a Medical History Form, what are some of the emotions that you experience? Do you *dread* the work (especially if you aren't feeling well)? Are you *concerned* that you will not know all the answers, have all the dates and numbers, and so on? Are you *frustrated* because you have filled out so many forms already? Are you ever *embarrassed* about some of the questions? Do you feel *guilty* that you will not answer some of the questions honestly? Do you *feel stupid* if you do not understand all the questions? Do you *feel hindered* because you did not bring your glasses or you have a sprained wrist or are too sick to fill out the form? Think of other feelings you have that are not listed here.

2. Whenever a patient sees a new doctor or has not been in to the doctor for a while, or even on a periodic basis, a new Medical History Form needs to be filled out. There is always paperwork to complete. Can you think of a better/easier/more efficient way to update patient information? Could computers make the job easier? What do you think will happen in the future?

3. Remember your feelings when you ask your patients to fill out the Medical History Forms, and be sensitive to their needs. How might you assist them, without dedicating time away from your other duties?

POST-TEST

This is similar to the Pre-Test. Perform this test without looking at the book. This is just to see how well you have understood and can recall the information presented in this chapter after you have studied it and completed the workbook exercises. You will not be graded on this portion (other than the grade you give yourself), but this is an excellent preparation for your instructor's test. You may use this Post-Test to determine what areas you need to study more. Justify any "false" answers.

1. To diagnose means to predict the outcome of a disease or condition. (T or F)

2. Objective statements are those statements that could be described as "opinion." (T or F)

3. When a patient "denies" something, he or she is:
   a. just whining
   b. not being truthful
   c. explaining his or her symptoms
   d. trying to blame someone else

4. Once a medical assistant has asked a patient whether he or she has any allergies, and the information has been recorded, the medical assistant needs to keep asking them at every office visit. (T or F)

5. If a disease is familial, that means it has a pattern of occurring within families and blood relations. (T or F)

CERTIFICATION CRITERIA CHECKLIST

As you go through your education and training, keep in mind the national certification examination that you will take when you graduate. Each chapter of the textbook and workbook covers a different section of the examination criteria. To keep track of your preparation for the certification examination, turn to the back of this workbook and highlight the following CMA, RMA, or CMAS certification examination criteria (if you have already highlighted them from a previous chapter, put a check mark by the criteria):

CMA

E. Communication
   2. Recognizing and responding to verbal and nonverbal communication
   4. Professional communication and behavior
   5. Evaluating and understanding communication
   6. Interviewing techniques

F. Medicolegal Guidelines & Requirements
   3. Documenting/reporting

J. Records Management
   5. Medical records

T. Patient Preparation and Assisting the Physician
   1. Performing telephone and in-person screening

U. Patient History Interview

RMA

II. Administrative Medical Assisting
    C. Medical Receptionist/Secretarial/Clerical
        4. Oral and written communications
        5. Records and chart management

CMAS

2. Basic Clinical Medical Office Assisting
    - Basic health history interview
    - Basic charting

COMPETENCY ASSESSMENT

Procedure 23-1 Taking a Medical History

Performance Objectives: To obtain a medical history from a patient new to the practice. Perform this objective within 25 minutes with a minimum score of 40 points.

Supplies/Equipment: Patient medical history form, clipboard, pen

Charting/Documentation: Enter appropriate documentation/charting in the box.

Instructor's/Evaluator's Comments and Suggestions:

SKILLS CHECKLIST Procedure 23-1: Taking a Medical History

Name ____________________

Date ____________________

No.	Skill	Check #1 20 pts ea	Check #2 10 pts ea	Check #3 5 pts ea	Notes
1	Introduce yourself to the patient. Confirm the identity of the patient and escort him or her to the examination room.				
2	Make eye contact and use positive body language to put the patient at ease.				
3	Explain the purpose and importance of obtaining the information, ask questions, get as much pertinent information as possible.				
4	Ask questions clearly, being sure the patient understands. Ask about allergies.				
5	Repeat patient answers when needed to confirm. Be specific when documenting.				
6	Write legibly with dark blue or black ink.				
7	Recheck form to be sure parts are complete. Add additional information as provided; make sure all information is accurate and legible.				
8	Prepare the patient for the review of systems and the physical examination as needed.				
Student's Total Points					
Points Possible		160	80	40	
Final Score (Student's Total Points / Possible Points)					

	Notes
Start time:	
End time:	
Total time: (25 min goal)	

EVALUATION OF CHAPTER KNOWLEDGE

Skills	Student Self-Evaluation		
	Good	Average	Poor
I understand the necessity and function of the medical history in patient treatment.	____	____	____
I can define the parts of the medical history.	____	____	____
I can identify and use effective methods of interacting with patients.	____	____	____
I can obtain a medical history from a patient.	____	____	____
I can explain different methods of charting/documentation.	____	____	____
I can define SOAP and relate the function of this charting approach.	____	____	____
I understand issues of cultural sensitivity in taking a medical history.	____	____	____
I can adapt communication to individuals' abilities to understand.	____	____	____
I perform within ethical boundaries.	____	____	____
I exhibit therapeutic communications skills.	____	____	____
I document accurately.	____	____	____
I can serve as a liaison between the physician and others.	____	____	____

CHAPTER 24

Vital Signs and Measurements

CHAPTER PRE-TEST

Perform this test without looking at the book. This is just to see how well you have understood and can recall the information in this chapter after you have read it, but before you have completed the workbook exercises. You will not be graded on this portion (other than the grade you give yourself). Justify any "false" answers.

1. Patient weight is measured to determine only how much fat the patient has. (T or F)
2. A normal pulse rate is between 60 and 100 for adults. (T or F)
3. A normal respiration rate is between 12 and 20 for adults. (T or F)
4. Blood pressure is the amount of pressure that is exerted on the inside of the veins. (T or F)
5. High blood pressure is also called hypertension. (T or F)
6. High blood pressure is always caused by inactivity and diet. (T or F)

INTRODUCTION

One of the primary tasks of medical assistants is measuring patients' vital signs. The vital or cardinal signs—temperature, pulse, respiration (TPR), and blood pressure (BP)—are important indicators of general health and must be measured and recorded with care. Because every individual's normal vital signs are different from those of every other person, the initial visit at any medical practice is usually used to record the patient's baseline vital signs. The baseline gives medical professionals an idea of what is normal for that patient and provides a point of comparison for use during future visits. For this reason, accuracy is especially important when recording vital signs at each patient's first visit. Medical assistants need to recognize factors that may influence the results of vital signs. Weight and height measurements may also be taken as further indications of the patient's condition. Aseptic techniques must be observed when taking patients' vital signs.

PERFORMANCE OBJECTIVES

After successful completion of this chapter you will be able to explain the terminology related to vital signs and body measurements, you will be able to accurately measure height and weight, head and chest circumference, temperature, pulse rate, respirations, and blood pressures. You will recognize and know what causes abnormal temperatures, pulse rates, respiration rates, and blood pressures; what some of the treatments are; and the prognosis of conditions related to abnormal vital signs. *The following statements are related to your learning objectives for this chapter. Fill in the blanks in the following paragraph with the appropriate term(s).*

(1) ________________ is a collective term that includes temperature, pulse, respirations, and blood pressures. An increase in body temperature may be caused by (2) ________________, increased (3) ________________, or (4) ________________ intake, exposure to (5) ________________, (6) ________________, (7) ________________ that increase metabolism, (8) ________________, severe (9) ________________, and (10) ________________. A decrease in body temperature may result from (11) ________________, decreased (12) ________________, (13) ________________, a depressed (14) ________________, exposure to (15) ____________, drugs that (16) ________________ and (17) ________________. Temperature may be taken in several ways. The most common routes for the ambulatory care setting are (18) ________________, (19) ________________, and (20) ________________. For environmental concerns, we have eliminated the use of (21) ________________ thermometers in medical settings, and we should encourage our patients to switch to (22) ________________ thermometers. Febrile means (23) ________________. There are (24) ________________ main sites for measuring pulse on the body. The most accessible (and therefore the most commonly used) site in ambulatory care is the (25) ________________ site. The term used to describe a rapid pulse rate is (26) ________________; a slow rate is termed (27) ________________. The medical term meaning difficulty with breathing is (28) ________________. When measuring blood pressure, it is important not to allow the gauge to move faster than (29) ________________ ________________. The American Heart Association currently suggests the best blood pressure for adults is (30) ________________.

VOCABULARY BUILDER

Find the words below that are misspelled; circle them, and then correctly spell them in the spaces provided. Insert one of the following correct vocabulary terms into each sentence describing a clinical situation.

apnea	eupnea	rales
arhymia	frenulum	rhoncki
baseline	hyperpnea	stertorious
bradicardia	hypertension	stridor
bradipnea	hyperventalation	systole
Cheyne–Stokes	hypotension	tachycardia
diastole	hypoventilation	tachypnea
dyspnea	orthopnea	wheezes
emphasema	pyrexia	____________
____________	____________	____________
____________	____________	____________

1. Maria Jover comes to the office of Drs. Lewis and King reporting that she cannot breathe when she lies down. Joe Guerrero, CMA, notes ____________ on her chart.
2. Winston Lewis, MD, warns Herb Fowler that he is at risk for ____________, a chronic pulmonary condition that causes destruction of air sacs in the lungs, if he does not quit smoking.
3. Liz Corbin, CMA, writes ____________ on Annette Samuel's chart when she counts the patient's respiration rate at 45 breaths per minute.
4. "I'm so tired lately; I barely have the energy to get out of bed," Martin Gordon tells Audrey Jones, CMA, when he comes in for a regular examination. Audrey suspects moderate ____________ and immediately takes Martin's blood pressure.
5. As Bruce Goldman, CMA, measures young Henry Hansen's respiration rate, he hears the bubbling, crackling sound known as ____________ each time Henry inhales.
6. Wanda Slawson, CMA, is taking Edith Leonard's temperature orally. She is careful to insert the thermometer under Edith's tongue, just beside her ____________
7. Marissa O'Keefe is rushed to see Elizabeth King, MD, after swallowing a coin. Dr. King can clearly hear a crowing ____________ when the toddler tries to inhale, so she knows that the obstruction is in the upper airway.
8. At a scheduled examination, Lenny Taylor's pulse is recorded at a regular 40 beats per minute: ____________ .
9. Rhoda Au seems nervous and agitated during her first visit to Inner City Health Care, and Bruce Goldman, CMA, notes her respiration rate at more than 35 breaths per minute. To ease her ____________ , he speaks to Rhoda calmly and has her breathe into a paper bag.

10. Bruce Goldman, CMA, can hear a distinct snoring sound in the throat called ________________________, when he measures Leo McKay's respiration rate.
11. Jim Marshall's blood pressure is a high 180/88 when Joe Guerrero, CMA, measures it. 180 is the ______________.
12. Dr. Winston Lewis takes careful note of Mr. Marshall's 160/100 blood pressure reading and discusses with him the dangers of ________________________ and the possible need of medication to control this condition.
13. Abigail Johnson's breathing is noticeably labored at one of her checkups. Joe Guerrero, CMA, notes this ________________________ on her chart.
14. Three-year-old Chris O'Keefe has had what seems to be a persistent chest cold for weeks. Audrey Jones, CMA, hears high-pitched ________________________ when he exhales, leading Dr. Winston Lewis to consider asthma instead.
15. David Kipperley visits Inner City Health Care for a persistent choking problem, but Wanda Slawson, CMA, notices that his breathing is shallow and his respiration rate is 10 breaths per minute. She alerts James Whitney, MD, to this ________________________ .
16. Audrey Jones, CMA, is happy to note that Lenore McDonnell's normal respiration indicates ________________________ .
17. Dottie Tate's breath sounds are all normal, but her respiration is very slow—only 8 or 9 breaths per minute. This ________________________ worries Liz Corbin, CMA, so she alerts Dr. King immediately and notes it prominently on Dottie's chart.
18. While checking John O'Keefe's pulse, Joe Guerrero, CMA, notes a decided ____________________: a premature contraction or PVC.
19. Bill Schwartz is suffering from a persistent cough. Bruce Goldman, CMA, can hear a distinct snoring sound in the lungs when his listens to Bill's labored breathing. Dr. Ray Reynolds confirms that this ________________________ respiration may be related to the problem.
20. Juanita Hansen's resting pulse rate is 120 beats per minute. This ________________________ concerns Susan Rice, MD, who orders a series of cardiac tests to try to find its cause.
21. Louise Kipperley comes to the clinic with a high fever. Wanda Slawson, CMA, confirms Louise's fast and deep respiratory rate, remembering that ________________________ is commonly seen in feverish patients.

LEARNING REVIEW

1. Body temperature can be affected by many factors. An alteration in body temperature may be a sign of disease or it may be normal for the person being examined.

   A. How is body heat produced? What part of the brain maintains the balance between the body's heat production and heat loss?

   ____

   ____

B. List five processes that cause a body to lose heat. Then match each one to the example that best describes it.

___ 1. ______________________________ ___ 4. ______________________________

___ 2. ______________________________ ___ 5. ______________________________

___ 3. ______________________________

a. Ellen Armstrong, CMA, climbs into a cold bed on a February night.

b. Anna Preciado, CMA, enjoys a good aerobic workout, which produces a full-body sweat.

c. On a trip to New York City, Bruce Goldman, CMA, attends a taping of the *Late Show with David Letterman*, known for its cold studio temperatures.

d. Karen Ritter, CMA, uses a portable fan to get through a temporary breakdown in the air-conditioning system on a July day at Inner City Health Care.

e. Liz Corbin, CMA, performs her daily routine of yoga breathing exercises.

C. List three factors that may increase body temperature.

(1) ______________________________

(2) ______________________________

(3) ______________________________

D. List three factors that may decrease body temperature.

(1) ______________________________

(2) ______________________________

(3) ______________________________

E. What is a synonym for *fever?* ______________________________ Read sentences a, b, and c below, and determine which type of fever each is describing. Write the type and the corresponding letter in the spaces provided.

___ 1. ______________________________

___ 2. ______________________________

___ 3. ______________________________

a. The patient's temperature fluctuates from 99° to 100° to 99°F.

b. The patient's temperature fluctuates from 99° to 98.4° to 99.3°F.

c. The patient's temperature fluctuates from 99.8° to 100°F for a period of two days.

2. A. Fill in the normal range of blood pressure for each of the following life stages.

Infant ______________________________

Child, age 6 ______________________________

Child, age 10 ______________________________

Adolescent, age 16 ______________________________

Adult ______________________________

B. How can each of the following factors affect a patient's blood pressure?

Blood volume ______________________________

Peripheral resistance ______________________________

Vessel elasticity ______________________________

Condition of the heart muscle ______________________________

Name four other factors that can affect blood pressure.

(1) ____________________ (3) ____________________

(2) ____________________ (4) ____________________

C. What is the name of the sounds heard during blood pressure measurement?

____________________ The sounds have five distinct phases. The act of listening for the sounds is called ____________________. Identify each phase and explain what is happening in the body during that phase and what kind of sound is heard.

____________ (1) This phase may be used to record the diastolic pressure in children and in those patients in whom a tapping sound is heard to zero.

____

____

____________ (2) This phase occurs as the blood pressure cuff deflates.

____

____

____________ (3) This phase is recorded as the diastolic pressure.

____

____

____________ (4) This phase begins with the first sound heard and is used to determine the systolic reading of the blood pressure.

____

____

____________ (5) If earlier phases are missed, this phase may be erroneously recorded as the systolic pressure.

____

____

3. A. Define hypertension. What are the four types of hypertension?

____

____

____

(1) ____________________ (3) ____________________

(2) ____________________ (4) ____________________

B. Define hypotension. What are three possible causes of hypotension?

____

____

____

(1) ______________________

(2) ______________________

(3) ______________________

4. Fill in the normal pulse rate range for each of the following life stages.

Birth ______________________

Infant, age < 1 year ______________________

Child, age 1–7 ______________________

Child, age > 7 ______________________

Adult ______________________

5. Describe each of the following common pulse abnormalities.

Bradycardia ______________________

Tachycardia ______________________

PVC ______________________

Sinus arrhythmia ______________________

6. Identify the name of each common pulse site described below and match the site to its proper location on the body in Figure 24-1 by placing the correct letter in the spaces provided.

A. The site most commonly used for blood pressure readings.

____

____

B. The site used for leg blood pressure measurements to monitor circulation.

____

____

C. The site commonly used for infant pulse rates.

____

____

D. The site used in emergencies and when performing cardiopulmonary resuscitation (CPR).

____

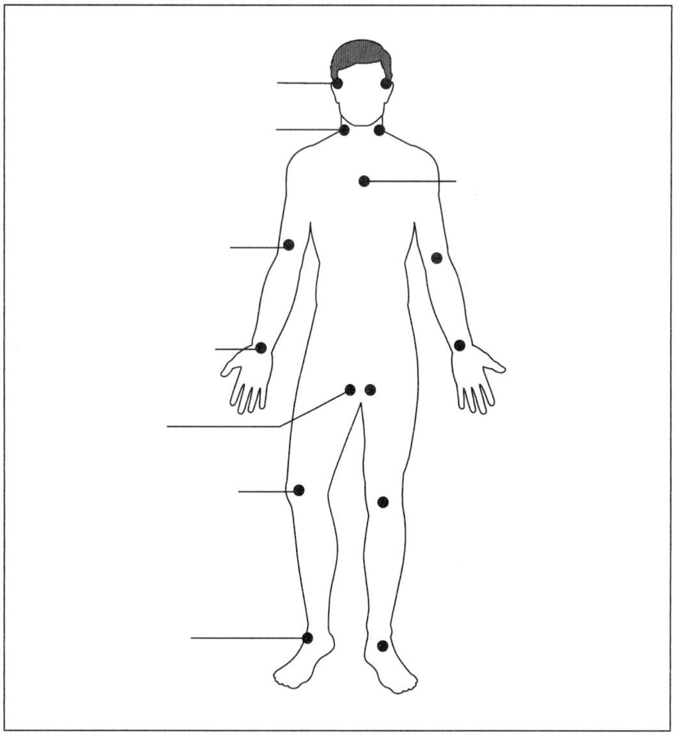

Figure 24-1

E. The site used to control circulation or monitor bleeding from the head and scalp.

____

F. The site used to monitor lower limb circulation.

____

G. The site most commonly used to take a pulse rate.

____

H. The site used to control bleeding in the thigh.

____

7. Fill in the normal range of respiratory rates for each of the following life stages

   Infant ____________________

   Child, age 1–7 ____________________

   Adult ____________________

8. List the five abnormal breath sounds that may be heard during a check of the vital signs. Briefly describe how each may be recognized.

   A. ____

   B. ____

   C. ____

   D. ____

   E. ____

9. A. What are the four characteristics of the pulse? Define each.

   (1) ____

   (2) ____

   (3) ____

   (4) ____

   B. What are the three characteristics of respiration? Define each.

   (1) ____

   (2) ____

   (3) ____

   C. What is the normal ratio relation of respiration to the pulse rate? ________________

   D. Determine how your pulse and respiration rates change during different physical activities. Chart your own pulse and respiration rates for each of the following activities.

   (1) After 3 minutes at rest, seated in a straight-backed chair, feet resting on the floor, and hands resting on the thighs.

   ____

(2) After 3 minutes of marching in place at a comfortable pace.

____

(3) After 3 minutes of strong aerobic activity, such as jumping jacks or jogging in place.

____

(4) Note the variations in the characteristics of the pulse and respiration as your body moved from rest to strong activity.

____

____

(5) Calculate the ratio of respiration to pulse for your resting, active, and aerobic rates listed earlier. Show your calculations in the spaces provided.

Rest Active Aerobic

____

10. An aural temperature is taken in the:
    a. mouth
    b. ear
    c. axilla
    d. rectum

11. When obtaining a pulse rate from the fifth intercostal space at the midclavicular line on the left, it may be referred to as the ______________ pulse:
    a. femoral
    b. temporal
    c. brachial
    d. apical

12. A normal respiratory rate is referred to as:
    a. orthopnea
    b. bradypenia
    c. bradycardia
    d. eupnea

13. Malignant hypertension is:
    a. borderline
    b. below normal
    c. life threatening
    d. within normal limits

CERTIFICATION REVIEW

These questions are designed to mimic the certification examinations. You can use these questions like a small "Certification Examination Study Guide," but this is not meant to take the place of the more extensive study guides. Use this portion to determine in what areas to concentrate your efforts when studying for the certification examination.

1. Which of the following is not a routine a body measurement?
   a. chest circumference
   b. head circumference
   c. ankle circumference
   d. height
2. In converting inches to feet, which of the following is true?
   a. 62 inches is 5 feet, 2 inches
   b. 62 inches is 6 feet, 2 inches
   c. 62 inches is 6 feet exactly
   d. 62 inches is 5 feet, 6 inches
3. When converting Fahrenheit to Celsius, which of the following is the correct formula?
   a. Fahrenheit temperature minus 32 multiplied by 5/9
   b. Fahrenheit temperature multiplied by 5/9 minus 32
   c. Fahrenheit temperature plus 32 multiplied by 5/9
   d. Fahrenheit temperature multiplied by 9/5 plus 32
4. What is considered a normal pulse and respiration rate for an adult?
   a. pulse of 52, respiration of 20
   b. pulse of 80, respiration of 24
   c. pulse of 66, respiration of 16
   d. pulse of 20, respiration of 60
   e. both b and c are normal
5. Which of the following is not a requirement to obtain accurate blood pressure?
   a. The cuff should be the proper size.
   b. The cuff should be placed correctly over the radial artery.
   c. The arm should be at heart level.
   d. The deflation should not be faster than 2 to 4 ml/sec per heartbeat.
   e. All of the above are correct.

CASE STUDIES

As a medical assistant, you can expect to take patients' vital signs as a regular part of your responsibilities. You will have to make decisions about the equipment and methods used to take these measurements and answer patients' questions about each procedure. For each of the following scenarios, discuss the following:

1. What measurement method and site is the medical assistant most likely to use in this case, and why?
2. What is the medical assistant's best therapeutic response to the patient?

Case 1

Wayne Elder lives near Inner City Health Care in a group home for developmentally delayed adults. Wayne has a history of colds and ear infections in both ears. He visits the clinic one morning with dizziness and pain in his right ear. As Wanda Slawson, CMA, prepares to take Wayne's temperature, she learns that he drank a cup of hot coffee just before walking to the clinic. Wayne Elder asks, "How come you need to know what I ate? It's my ear that hurts."

Case 2

Henry Hansen is rushed to Inner City Health Care unconscious. He is bleeding profusely from a cut on his head. "He fell down the stairs," sobs Henry's mother, Juanita. Administrative medical assistant Karen Ritter alerts Dr. James Whitney, one of the clinic physicians, and calls 911 to summon emergency services personnel. The first thing clinical medical assistant Bruce Goldman does, after determining that Henry is breathing, is to take Henry's pulse. "What are you doing?" Juanita, who is almost hysterical now, screams. "Why aren't you waking him up?"

Case 3

Abigail Johnson, who suffers from many of the problems of advancing age, including diabetes mellitus, is an older adult patient of Elizabeth King, MD. A friendly woman, Abigail has a good rapport with everyone in the office—all of whom, she says, are "just like family"—and is eager to please the staff. One winter day she comes in with possible flu symptoms.

When Audrey asks Abigail to prepare for a weight measurement, Abigail says, "Oh, do we have to do that today? I'm just not up to it. Besides, I don't want to know how much I weigh right now. When I feel better, then I'll focus on losing more weight. You understand how I feel, don't you?"

SELF-ASSESSMENT

A. As you respond to the following questions, think of how your experiences will affect how you treat your patients.

1. Think of the last time you had your height and weight measured. Did you have enough privacy to make you feel comfortable?

2. When you had your blood pressure taken, did the medical assistant share your measurements with you? Did you feel comfortable asking questions?

3. Has any health care provider ever discussed any of your vital signs or body measurements with you? Why or why not? Have you been informed of risk factors related to your health that may have affected your vital signs or body measurements?

B. Do you still have mercury thermometers in your home? If so, call your local health department to find out where to take them for disposal, and then obtain an electronic or digital version for future use. How do you think your patients will feel when you encourage them to do the same? Write out exactly what you will say to them to convince them of the importance of replacing all mercury thermometers with a safer alternative.

POST-TEST

This is similar to the Pre-Test. Perform this test without looking at the book. This is just to see how well you have understood and can recall the information presented in this chapter after you have studied it and completed the workbook exercises. You will not be graded on this portion (other than the grade you give yourself), but this is an excellent preparation for your instructor's test. You may use this Post-Test to determine what areas you need to study more. Justify any "false" answers.

1. Patient weight is measured sometimes to determine how much water the patient is retaining. (T or F)
2. A normal pulse rate is between 80 and 100 for adults. (T or F)
3. A normal respiration rate is between 16 and 20 for adults. (T or F)
4. Blood pressure is the amount of pressure that is exerted on the inside of the arteries. (T or F)
5. High blood pressure is also called hyportension. (T or F)
6. High blood pressure can be decreased by increasing activity, dietary changes, medications, and picking your parents better. (T or F)

CERTIFICATION CRITERIA CHECKLIST

As you go through your education and training, keep in mind the national certification examination that you will take when you graduate. Each chapter of the textbook and workbook covers a different section of the examination criteria. To keep track of your preparation for the certification examination, turn to the back of this workbook and highlight the following CMA, RMA, or CMAS certification examination criteria (if you have already highlighted them from a previous chapter, put a check mark by the criteria):

CMA

S. Treatment Area
   2. Principles of operation (equipment)

T. Patient Preparation and Assisting the Physician
   2. Vital signs

RMA

III. Clinical Medical Assisting
   D. Vital Signs and Mensurations

CMAS

2. Basic Clinical Medical Office Assisting
   - Vital signs and measurements

COMPETENCY ASSESSMENT

Procedure 24-1 Measuring an Oral Temperature Using an Electronic Thermometer

Performance Objectives: To obtain an oral temperature. Perform this objective within 5 minutes with a minimum score of 90 points.

Supplies/Equipment: Electronic thermometer, probe covers, biohazard waste container

Charting/Documentation: Enter appropriate documentation/charting in the box or in the patient's chart/medical record.

Instructor's/Evaluator's Comments and Suggestions:

SKILLS CHECKLIST Procedure 24-1: Measuring an Oral Temperature Using an Electronic Thermometer

Name ______________________________

Date ______________________________

No.	Skill	Check #1 20 pts ea	Check #2 10 pts ea	Check #3 5 pts ea	Notes
1	Wash hands and follow Standard Precautions.				
2	Assemble equipment.				
3	Identify patient.				
4	Determine if the patient has ingested hot or cold drinks or food, or has been smoking within the previous half hour.				
5	Explain the procedure.				
6	Select blue (oral) probe.				
7	Cover with probe cover.				
8	Insert under the tongue to either side of the mouth.				
9	Instruct the patient to close mouth without placing teeth on thermometer.				
10	Leave in place until the beep is heard.				
11	Rechecks pulse and breathing every few minutes.				
12	Remove thermometer after appropriate time has elapsed.				
13	Read the results on the display window.				
14	Discard probe cover.				
15	Replace thermometer in the base holder.				
16	Wash hands.				
17	Record temperature.				
18	Document procedure.				
Student's Total Points					
Points Possible		360	180	90	
Final Score (Student's Total Points / Possible Points)					
		Notes			
Start time:					
End time:					
Total time: (5 min goal)					

COMPETENCY ASSESSMENT

Procedure 24-2 Measuring an Aural Temperature Using a Tympanic Thermometer

Performance Objectives: To obtain an aural temperature using a tympanic thermometer. Perform this objective within 5 minutes with a minimum score of 65 points.

Supplies/Equipment: Tympanic thermometer, covers or ear speculum, biohazard waste container

Charting/Documentation: Enter appropriate documentation/charting in the box or in the patient's chart/medical record.

Instructor's/Evaluator's Comments and Suggestions:

SKILLS CHECKLIST Procedure 24-2: Measuring an Aural Temperature Using a Tympanic Thermometer

Name ______________________

Date ______________________

No.	Skill	Check #1 20 pts ea	Check #2 10 pts ea	Check #3 5 pts ea	Notes
1	Wash hands and follow Standard Precautions.				
2	Assemble equipment.				
3	Identify patient.				
4	Explain the procedure.				
5	Place cover on thermometer.				
6	Set thermometer to start.				
7	Place probe into ear canal and activate.				
8	Wait until the temperature is displayed.				
9	Remove from the ear.				
10	Discard cover into waste container.				
11	Wash hands.				
12	Replace thermometer.				
13	Record temperature.				
Student's Total Points					
Points Possible		260	130	65	
Final Score (Student's Total Points / Possible Points)					

	Notes
Start time:	
End time:	
Total time: (5 min goal)	

COMPETENCY ASSESSMENT

Procedure 24-3 Measuring a Rectal Temperature Using a Digital Thermometer

Performance Objectives: To obtain a rectal temperature using a digital thermometer. Perform this objective within 5 minutes with a minimum score of 90 points.

Supplies/Equipment: Digital thermometer with red probe (rectal), probe cover, lubricating jelly, gloves, biohazard waste container

Charting/Documentation: Enter appropriate documentation/charting in the box.

Instructor's/Evaluator's Comments and Suggestions:

SKILLS CHECKLIST Procedure 24-3: Measuring a Rectal Temperature Using a Digital Thermometer

Name ______________________

Date ______________________

No.	Skill	Check #1 20 pts ea	Check #2 10 pts ea	Check #3 5 pts ea	Notes
1	Wash hands and glove. Follow Standard Precautions.				
2	Assemble equipment.				
3	Identify patient.				
4	Explain the procedure.				
5	Remove clothing from the waist down, drape as necessary.				
6	Position patient in Sims' position.				
7	Place prove cover on red (rectal) probe.				
8	Lubricate with lubricating jelly.				
9	Spread buttock; gently insert thermometer into the rectum past the sphincter (1.5 inches) for adult.				
10	Hold buttocks together while holding the thermometer.				
11	Hold in place until the beep is heard.				
12	Read results.				
13	Remove from rectum.				
14	Discard probe cover.				
15	Replace thermometer in the base holder.				
16	Remove gloves, place in biohazard container, and wash hands.				
17	Offer tissue to patient; assist with dressing as necessary.				
18	Record on the patient chart labeled with "(R)."				
Student's Total Points					
Points Possible		360	180	90	
Final Score (Student's Total Points / Possible Points)					

	Notes
Start time:	
End time:	
Total time: (5 min goal)	

COMPETENCY ASSESSMENT

Procedure 24-4 Measuring an Axillary Temperature

Performance Objectives: To obtain an axillary temperature using a digital thermometer. Perform this objective within 5 minutes with a minimum score of 75 points.

Supplies/Equipment: Digital thermometer, cover/sheath, waste container, patient chart

Charting/Documentation: Enter appropriate documentation/charting in the box or in the patient's chart/medical record.

Instructor's/Evaluator's Comments and Suggestions:

SKILLS CHECKLIST Procedure 24-4: Measuring an Axillary Temperature

Name ______________________________

Date ______________________________

No.	Skill	Check #1 20 pts ea	Check #2 10 pts ea	Check #3 5 pts ea	Notes
1	Wash hands and follow Standard Precautions.				
2	Assemble equipment; place sheath on thermometer.				
3	Identify patient.				
4	Explain the procedure.				
5	Ask patient to remove clothing to provide access to axilla.				
6	Gown as necessary to maintain patient modesty and warmth.				
7	Wipe axillary area with dry towel or towelette to remove moisture.				
8	Place thermometer in axilla.				
9	Ask patient to fold arm against chest or abdomen.				
10	Leave in place until thermometer beeps.				
11	Carefully remove.				
12	Discard sheath.				
13	Read temperature.				
14	Wash hands.				
15	Document temperature in patient's record, indicating axillary (Ax) temperature.				
Student's Total Points					
Points Possible		300	150	75	
Final Score (Student's Total Points / Possible Points)					

	Notes
Start time:	
End time:	
Total time: (5 min goal)	

COMPETENCY ASSESSMENT

Procedure 24-5 Measuring an Oral Temperature Using a Disposable Oral Strip Thermometer

Performance Objectives: To obtain an oral temperature. Perform this objective within 3 minutes with a minimum score of 90 points.

Supplies/Equipment: Oral strip thermometer, gloves, biohazard waste container, patient chart

Charting/Documentation: Enter appropriate documentation/charting in the box or in the patient's chart/medical record.

____

____

____

____

Instructor's/Evaluator's Comments and Suggestions:

____

____

____

____

____

____

SKILLS CHECKLIST Procedure 24-5: Measuring an Oral Temperature Using a Disposable Oral Strip Thermometer

Name ______________________________

Date ______________________________

No.	Skill	Check #1 20 pts ea	Check #2 10 pts ea	Check #3 5 pts ea	Notes
1	Wash hands and follow Standard Precautions.				
2	Assemble equipment.				
3	Identify patient.				
4	Position the patient in a comfortable position.				
5	Determine if the patient has ingested hot or cold drinks or food, or has been smoking within the previous half hour.				
6	Explain the procedure.				
7	Apply gloves.				
8	Insert disposable oral strip thermometer under the tongue to the side of the frenulum.				
9	Instruct the patient to close mouth tightly.				
10	Leave in place for 60 seconds (or follow manufacturer's instructions).				
11	Remove thermometer after appropriate time has elapsed.				
12	Wait 10 seconds to read the dots (follow manufacturer's instructions).				
13	Read the temperature.				
14	Discard strip in biohazard container.				
15	Remove gloves and discard in biohazard container.				
16	Wash hands.				
17	Record temperature.				
18	Document the procedure.				
Student's Total Points					
Points Possible		360	180	90	
Final Score (Student's Total Points / Possible Points)					

	Notes
Start time:	
End time:	
Total time: (3 min goal)	

COMPETENCY ASSESSMENT

Procedure 24-6 Measuring a Radial Pulse

Performance Objectives: To obtain a pulse rate. Perform this objective within 3 minutes with a minimum score of 50 points.

Supplies/Equipment: Watch or clock with a second hand, patient chart

Charting/Documentation: Enter appropriate documentation/charting in the box or in the patient's chart/medical record.

Instructor's/Evaluator's Comments and Suggestions:

SKILLS CHECKLIST Procedure 24-6: Measuring a Radial Pulse

Name ______________________

Date ______________________

No.	Skill	Check #1 20 pts ea	Check #2 10 pts ea	Check #3 5 pts ea	Notes
1	Wash hands.				
2	Identify patient.				
3	Explain the procedure.				
4	Position the patient with the wrist resting on either a table or on his or her lap.				
5	Locate radial pulse with the pads of your first three fingers. Do not use thumb.				
6	Gently compress the radial artery enough to feel the pulse.				
7	Count pulsations for 1 full minute or 30 seconds, then multiply by 2.				
8	Note any irregularities in rhythm, volume, and characteristics.				
9	Wash hands.				
10	Record the pulse in the patient chart following the temperature, noting any irregularities.				
Student's Total Points					
Points Possible		200	100	50	
Final Score (Student's Total Points / Possible Points)					

	Notes
Start time:	
End time:	
Total time: (3 min goal)	

COMPETENCY ASSESSMENT

Procedure 24-7 Taking an Apical Pulse

Performance Objectives: To obtain an apical pulse rate. Perform this objective within 15 minutes with a minimum score of 75 points.

Supplies/Equipment: Stethoscope, watch with second hand, alcohol wipes, disinfectant

Charting/Documentation: Enter appropriate documentation/charting in the box or in the patient's chart/medical record.

Instructor's/Evaluator's Comments and Suggestions:

SKILLS CHECKLIST Procedure 24-7: Taking an Apical Pulse

Name ______________________

Date ______________________

No.	Skill	Check #1 20 pts ea	Check #2 10 pts ea	Check #3 5 pts ea	Notes
1	Wash hands.				
2	Assemble equipment.				
3	Wipe earpiece with alcohol wipes; allow to dry completely.				
4	Identify patient.				
5	Explain the procedure.				
6	Assist patient in disrobing as needed, removing clothing from waist up.				
7	Provide a gown or drape for patient modesty and warmth.				
8	Position the patient in a supine position.				
9	Locate the fifth intercostal space, midclavicular, left of sternum.				
10	Place stethoscope on the site and listen for the lub-dup sound of the heart.				
11	Count the pulse for 1 minute.				
12	Assist the patient to sit up and dress.				
13	Wash hands.				
14	Wipe ear pieces, diaphragm, and tubing of stethoscope with disinfectant.				
15	Record the pulse in the patient chart following the temperature, noting any irregularities.				
Student's Total Points					
Points Possible		300	150	75	
Final Score (Student's Total Points / Possible Points)					

	Notes
Start time:	
End time:	
Total time: (15 min goal)	

COMPETENCY ASSESSMENT

Procedure 24-8 Measuring the Respiration Rate

Performance Objectives: To obtain the repiratory rate of a patient. Perform this objective within 5 minutes with a minimum score of 35 points.

Supplies/Equipment: Watch with a second hand, patient chart

Charting/Documentation: Enter appropriate documentation/charting in the box or in the patient's chart/medical record.

____

____

____

____

Instructor's/Evaluator's Comments and Suggestions:

____

____

____

____

____

____

SKILLS CHECKLIST Procedure 24-8: Measuring the Respiration Rate

Name ______________________

Date ______________________

No.	Skill	Check #1 20 pts ea	Check #2 10 pts ea	Check #3 5 pts ea	Notes
1	Wash hands.				
2	Identify patient.				
3	Position the patient comfortably.				
4	Watch the rise and fall of the chest wall or shoulders. Record for 60 seconds, or record for 30 seconds then multiply by 2.				
5	Note the depth and the rhythm and breath sounds while counting.				
6	Wash hands.				
7	Record the respirations and any irregularities.				
Student's Total Points					
Points Possible		140	70	35	
Final Score (Student's Total Points / Possible Points)					

	Notes
Start time:	
End time:	
Total time: (5 min goal)	

COMPETENCY ASSESSMENT

Procedure 24-9 Measuring Blood Pressure

Performance Objectives: To obtain an accurate blood pressure. Perform this objective within 5 minutes with a minimum score of 105 points.

Supplies/Equipment: Stethoscope, blood pressure cuff (sphygmomanometer), disinfectant wipes, patient chart

Charting/Documentation: Enter appropriate documentation/charting in the box or in the patient's chart/medical record.

____

____

____

____

Instructor's/Evaluator's Comments and Suggestions:

____

____

____

____

____

____

SKILLS CHECKLIST Procedure 24-9: Measuring Blood Pressure

Name ______________________

Date ______________________

No.	Skill	Check #1 20 pts ea	Check #2 10 pts ea	Check #3 5 pts ea	Notes
1	Wash hands.				
2	Assemble equipment.				
3	Disinfect stethoscope.				
4	Identify patient.				
5	Explain the procedure.				
6	Position the patient comfortably with the arm at heart level.				
7	Bare the upper arm. Remove the arm from the sleeve if necessary.				
8	Palpate the brachial artery.				
9	Securely center the bladder of the cuff on the upper arm at least 2 inches above the antecubital space.				
10	Position the stetoscope diaphragm over the brachial artery in the antecubital space. Hold into position. Do not allow the diaphragm to go under the edge of the cuff.				
11	Inflate the cuff smoothly and quickly to just above the patient's normal systolic pressure (or about 160).				
12	Deflate the cuff at a rate of 2 mm per heartbeat.				
13	Listen for the Korotkoff sounds, Phase I.				
14	Continue deflating the cuff, noting Korotkoff phases.				
15	Note when all sounds disappear.				
16	Continue deflating the cuff at the same rate for at least another 10 mm after all sounds have disappeared.				
17	The cuff may be deflated quickly and completely.				
18	Remove the cuff.				
19	Disinfect the stethoscope.				
20	Wash hands.				
21	Record the respirations and any irregularities.				
Student's Total Points					
Points Possible		420	210	105	
Final Score (Student's Total Points / Possible Points)					

	Notes
Start time:	
End time:	
Total time: (5 min goal)	

COMPETENCY ASSESSMENT

Procedure 24-10 Measuring Height

Performance Objectives: To obtain the height of a patient. Perform this objective within 15 minutes with a minimum score of 55 points.

Supplies/Equipment: Scale with measuring bar, patient chart

Charting/Documentation: Enter appropriate documentation/charting in the box or in the patient's chart/medical record.

Instructor's/Evaluator's Comments and Suggestions:

SKILLS CHECKLIST Procedure 24-10: Measuring Height

Name ______________________________

Date ______________________________

No.	Skill	Check #1 20 pts ea	Check #2 10 pts ea	Check #3 5 pts ea	Notes
1	Wash hands.				
2	Identify patient.				
3	Explain the procedure.				
4	Instruct the patient to remove his or her shoes and stand on the scale with his or her back to the measuring bar. Have him or her look straight ahead and keep his or her head level.				
5	Assist the patient onto the scale.				
6	Lower the measuring bar until it rests firmly on his or her head.				
7	Assist the patient stepping off the scale. Allow him or her to sit and put on shoes.				
8	Read the height measurement.				
9	Lower the measuring bar to its original position.				
10	Wash hands.				
11	Record the height.				
Student's Total Points					
Points Possible		220	110	55	
Final Score (Student's Total Points / Possible Points)					

	Notes
Start time:	
End time:	
Total time: (15 min goal)	

COMPETENCY ASSESSMENT

Procedure 24-11 Measuring Adult Weight

Performance Objectives: To obtain the weight of a patient. Perform this objective within 5 minutes with a minimum score of 65 points.

Supplies/Equipment: Scale with balance beam or digital scale, patient chart

Charting/Documentation: Enter appropriate documentation/charting in the box or in the patient's chart/medical record.

____

____

____

____

Instructor's/Evaluator's Comments and Suggestions:

____

____

____

____

____

____

SKILLS CHECKLIST Procedure 24-11: Measuring Adult Weight

Name ______________________

Date ______________________

No.	Skill	Check #1 20 pts ea	Check #2 10 pts ea	Check #3 5 pts ea	Notes
1	Wash hands.				
2	Identify patient.				
3	Explain the procedure.				
4	Place a paper towel on the scale.				
5	Instruct the patient to remove heavy objects from his or her pockets.				
6	Instruct the patient to remove his or her shoes and jacket and step onto the scale.				
7	Move the weight on the 50 lb bar to the estimate number.				
8	Slowly slide the upper weight on the bar until the tip of the bar is balanced.				
9	Read the weight by adding the two measurements together.				
10	Assist the patient off the scale.				
11	Provide a chair for him or her to put on his or her shoes.				
12	Return the weights to zero.				
13	Wash hands.				
Student's Total Points					
Points Possible		260	130	65	
Final Score (Student's Total Points / Possible Points)					

	Notes
Start time:	
End time:	
Total time: (5 min goal)	

EVALUATION OF CHAPTER KNOWLEDGE

Skills	Student Self-Evaluation Good	Average	Poor
I can define and describe key terms relating to temperature, pulse, respiration, and blood pressure readings.	____	____	____
I understand normal and abnormal body temperatures, as well as factors that affect temperature.	____	____	____
I can identify various types of thermometers and know procedures for their care, storage, and use.	____	____	____
I know anatomic locations of pulse sites and procedures for obtaining pulse rate at each one.	____	____	____
I can identify normal and abnormal pulse rates, including common arrhythmias.	____	____	____
I understand the procedure for obtaining respiration rate.	____	____	____
I can identify normal and abnormal respiration rates and breath sounds.	____	____	____
I have the ability to use blood pressure equipment and understand measurement procedures.	____	____	____
I can identify normal and abnormal blood pressure readings, including factors that affect it.	____	____	____
I can accurately measure blood pressure.	____	____	____
I understand procedures for obtaining height and weight measurements.	____	____	____
I have the ability to accurately record all measurements on the patient's chart.	____	____	____

CHAPTER 25

The Physical Examination

CHAPTER PRE-TEST

Perform this test without looking at the book. This is just to see how well you have understood and can recall the information in this chapter after you have read it, but before you have completed the workbook exercises. You will not be graded on this portion (other than the grade you give yourself).

1. (Palpation) (Palpitation) is when the patient can feel his or her heartbeat. (circle the correct one)

2. Which of the following is not a method used during a physical examination?
   a. percussion
   b. menstruation
   c. manipulation
   d. auscultation

3. Which is a component of a routine physical examination?
   a. what the patient looks like
   b. how the patient walks
   c. if the patient has bad breath
   d. all of the above

4. Which of the following is not a position used in physical examinations of patients?
   a. lithotomy
   b. supine
   c. dorsal recumbent
   d. reverse Trendelenburg

5. Choose the correct spelling of the instrument used to examine the inside of the eyeball.
   a. opthalmoscope
   b. optomescope
   c. ophthalmoscope
   d. otoscope

INTRODUCTION

The medical assistant assists the physician in the physical examination of patients, commonly performing duties related to patient preparation and examination room preparation and maintenance. Medical assisting students can use this workbook chapter to explore the standard routine of a physical examination and the standard sequence of events that occur during the examination, allowing for variations due to physician preference, type of practice, and the patient's chief complaint. By assisting the physician with efficiency and accuracy, medical assistants make vital contributions to physicians' abilities to make accurate diagnoses and formulate treatment plans based on patients' medical histories, physical examinations, and accurate results of laboratory tests and diagnostic procedures. Medical assistants observe aseptic technique and standard precautions as required during physical examinations. At all times, appropriate empathy and respect for the patient are shown.

PERFORMANCE OBJECTIVES

After successful completion of this chapter you will be able to explain to a patient what to expect during a physical examination by a physician. You will be familiar with all the equipment and supplies needed during a physical examination and how to use and care for them, what types of assessments the doctor will perform, and all the components of the routine physical examination. You will also know what your role as a medical assistant will be in preparing the patient for the examination, getting the room and supplies ready, and assisting the physician during the examination. *The following statements are related to your learning objectives for this chapter. Fill in the blanks in the following paragraph with the appropriate term(s).*

There are basically six methods used by the physician to examine the human body. They are (1) ____________________ or ____________________, (2) ____________________, (3) ____________________, (4) ____________________, (5) ____________________, and (6) ____________________. In preparation for the physical examination, the patient may be placed in a variety of positions, depending on the examination needed. Some of these positions are (7) ____________________, (8) ____________________, (9) ____________________, (10) ____________________, (11) ____________________, (12) ____________________, and (13) ____________________. The tape measure, percussion hammer, and tuning fork are all equipment used during the (14) ____________________. The basic components of the physical examination are to observe and assess patients' general appearance, their gait, their stature and posture, their body movements, their nutritional health, as well as their (15) ______________________, (16) ____________________________, and (17) ____________________________. When physicians perform the physical examination, they will follow a certain sequence, usually starting at the (18) ______________ and progressing through the body.

VOCABULARY BUILDER

Find the words below that are misspelled; circle them, and then correctly spell them in the spaces provided. Then identify the correct vocabulary terms most appropriate for each example below from a patient's physical examination.

ataxia	pallor	vertigo
bruits	piorrhea	vertiligo
cyanosis	schleroderma	
jaundice	symmetry	
labirynthitis	tinnitus	____________________
________________	______________________	____________________

______________________________ 1. During a physical examination of Louise Kipperley, a 48-year-old woman, Dr. Esposito checks Louise's face for tight and atrophied skin.

______________________________ 2. Leo McKay comes to Inner City Health Care with mouth pain. Dr. Reynolds examines Leo's mouth for dental hygiene and for this condition, which is the discharge of pus from the gums around the teeth.

______________________________ 3. Medical assistant Liz Corbin observes the gait of Geraldine Potter, a 36-year-old woman diagnosed with multiple sclerosis. Geraldine's gait is lurching and unsteady, with her feet widely placed.

______________________________ 4. Annette Samuels is diagnosed with hepatitis B virus (HBV) by Dr. Mark Woo. Annette contracted the virus from an infected needle used to pierce her navel. Among Annette's symptoms, noted by Dr. Woo during the physical examination, was a distinct yellowing of Annette's skin and the whites of her eyes.

______________________________ 5. Lenny Taylor, an older adult man with Alzheimer's disease, is brought to Inner City Health Care by his son George. Apparently, Lenny had gotten lost in a park near his home and had been wandering for hours in the cold. Dr. Whitney observes a bluish color in the beds of Lenny's fingernails and toenails and on his lips, tongue, and the mucous membranes lining the inside of his mouth.

______________________________ 6. After performing a routine venipuncture procedure on patient Rhoda Au, Bruce Goldman, CMA, notices that all color has drained from Rhoda's face.

_______________ 7. Abigail Johnson's 28-year-old granddaughter Lucy comes in for an examination with Dr. King after observing white patches of depigmentation on her hand. "Is this what Michael Jackson had?" she asks Dr. King.

_______________ 8. While performing a complete physical examination on patient Rowena Lawrence, Dr. King listens for abnormal sounds from vital organs while auscultating her abdomen.

_______________ 9. During a routine physical examination of Lenore McDonnell, a young woman confined to a wheelchair, Dr. Lewis checks for the correspondence in size, shape, and position of body parts on opposite sides of her body.

_______________ 10. Mary O'Keefe brings her 3-year-old son, Chris, to see Dr. King when he exhibits a high fever and pain in his ear. The toddler, diagnosed with otitis media, keeps placing his hands over his ears and crying, "Mommy, stop noise."

_______________ 11. Rowena Lawrence's 6-year-old daughter, Felicia, diagnosed with a case of the mumps, returns with her mother for a reexamination with Dr. Lewis when the child experiences a sensation that the room is spinning, caused by inflammation of the labyrinth.

_______________ 12. While taking Susan O'Donnell's blood (venipuncure procedure), she described the room as spinning and felt light-headed.

LEARNING REVIEW

1. Match the correct method of examination used by a physician to the entry below that best describes it.

auscultation	observation or inspection
manipulation	palpation
mensuration	percussion

_______________ A. On his physical examination of Charles Williams, Dr. Winston Lewis looks at the patient to assess his general health, posture, body movements, skin, mannerisms, and care in grooming while verbally reviewing Charles's medical history with him.

_______________ B. Dr. Mark Woo uses a stethoscope to listen to the bowel sounds that accompany peristalsis.

_______________ C. Dr. King performs range of motion exercises on patient Margaret Thomas, who is suspected of having Parkinson's disease.

_______________ D. Dr. Rice taps Edith Leonard's chest to feel and hear the hollow quality expected from clear lungs.

_____________________ E. During Marissa O'Keefe's well-baby visit, chest and head circumference measurements are recorded in the patient's medical record.

_____________________ F. When Leo McKay comes to Inner City Health Care with acute stomach pains, Dr. Reynolds feels his stomach and abdomen for irregularities in size, texture, and condition of vital organs.

2. For each procedure listed below, identify the most likely examination position that will be required during the physician's examination. Use a medical encyclopedia for reference, if necessary.

_____________________________ A. Urinary catheterization

_____________________________ B. Auscultation for audible bowel sounds that are a normal part of the digestive process

_____________________________ C. Colposcopy to observe the cervix under magnified illumination for evidence of precancerous cells, followed by a cone biopsy for laboratory analysis

_____________________________ D. Internal hemorrhoids are examined through the use of a proctoscope

_____________________________ E. Percutaneous renal biopsy to aid in diagnosis of a suspected case of glomerulonephritis

_____________________________ F. An ECG is performed on an older adult woman with angina pectoris

_____________________________ G. A variation of this position is used for patients experiencing shock

_____________________________ H. Proctoscopy to investigate a suspected case of proctitis, inflammation of the rectum

3. Identify each entry below as a piece of medical equipment (ME), a laboratory procedure (LP), a part of the human body (BP), or a patient illness or condition (PI). Then identify the correct component or sequence of the physical examination to which the entry relates.

	Component or Sequence of Physical Examination
____ A. Sphygmomanometer	______________________________
____ B. Aphonia	______________________________
____ C. Lymph nodes	______________________________
____ D. Edema	______________________________
____ E. Anal fissures	______________________________
____ F. Emphysema	______________________________
____ G. Pharyngeal mirrors	______________________________
____ H. Scrotum	______________________________
____ I. Areola	______________________________
____ J. Electrocardiography	______________________________

____ K. Kyphosis ________________________________

____ L. Dysphasia ________________________________

____ M. Urinalysis ________________________________

____ N. Achilles tendon ________________________________

____ O. Tympanic membrane ________________________________

4. Symmetry would be noted by using the following method of assessment:
   a. auscultation
   b. palpation
   c. percussion
   d. observation

5. Another term used for the supine position or the position assumed when lying face up is:
   a. dorsal recumbent
   b. horizontal recumbent
   c. lithotomy
   d. Sims'

6. Orthostatic hypotension occurs as:
   a. blood pressure decreases
   b. blood pressure increases
   c. blood pressure normalizes
   d. pulse increases

7. The preferred position for administration of an enema or rectal suppositories would be the:
   a. Trendelenburg
   b. supine
   c. prone
   d. Sims'

8. Determining the amount of flexion and extension of a patient's extremities would be which form of assessment?
   a. mensuration
   b. palpation
   c. manipulation
   d. percussion

CERTIFICATION REVIEW

These questions are designed to mimic the certification examinations. You can use these questions like a small "Certification Examination Study Guide," but this is not meant to take the place of the more extensive study guides. Use this portion to determine in what areas to concentrate your efforts when studying for the certification examination.

1. A patient having a examination of the abdomen should be placed in which position?
   a. supine
   b. prone
   c. lithotomy
   d. Sims'

2. Listening to the patient's chest as he or she breathes is called:
   a. auscultation
   b. percussion
   c. inspection
   d. palpation

3. The process of inspection is also called:
   a. percussion
   b. measuration
   c. observation
   d. palpitations

4. Which of the following is *not* a piece of equipment needed in the examination room?
   a. goose neck lamp
   b. Mayo tray
   c. red bag waste container
   d. adjustable stool

5. Which of the following is *not* a word used to describe skin color?
   a. jaundice
   b. cyanosis
   c. bruits
   d. pallor

CASE STUDY

Rowena Lawrence brings her 5-year-old son, Bobby, to Inner City Health Care with a suspected case of the mumps contracted from his sister Felicia. As Bruce Goldman, CMA, helps the child remove his clothing, leaving only his underwear on, the child becomes increasingly fearful and begins to cry. Rowena's gentle reprimand to "hush up and do what you're told" makes the boy cry harder. It is obvious that the child is uncomfortable and feverish.

Discuss the following:

1. What can the medical assistant do to calm the child and make him more comfortable?
2. What should be Bruce's therapeutic response?

SELF-ASSESSMENT

Think about the last time you went to the doctor. As you answer the following questions and remember your personal experiences, think about how your experience will affect the way you treat your patients in the future. If you have no personal experiences, try to imagine how you would feel and react.

1. Did you have to undress at all? How did that feel? Did you get cold or feel a bit awkward?
2. When you had your blood pressure taken, did the cuff cause pain or discomfort as it got tighter? Did you say something to the medical assistant? Do you think most people speak up when they are uncomfortable?
3. Have you ever noticed a sick patient in a public place? What were the clues that told you the patient was sick? Do you think your skills of observation will be enhanced after you complete this chapter?

POST-TEST

This is similar to the Pre-Test. Perform this test without looking at the book. This is just to see how well you have understood and can recall the information presented in this chapter after you have studied it and completed the workbook exercises. You will not be graded on this portion (other than the grade you give yourself), but this is excellent preparation for your instructor's test. You may use this Post-Test to determine what areas you need to study more.

1. (Palpation) (Palpitation) is when the doctor feels the patient's abdomen. (circle the correct one)
2. Which of the following is not a method used during a physical examination?
   a. percussion
   b. manipulation
   c. auscultation
   d. symmetry
3. Which is a component of a routine physical examination?
   a. what the patient looks like
   b. how the patient walks
   c. if the patient has bad breath
   d. the patient's test results

4. Which of the following is not a position used in physical examinations of patients?
   a. lithotomy
   b. reverse Trendelenburg
   c. prone
   d. dorsal recumbent

5. Choose the correct spelling of the instrument used to examine the inside of the eyeball.
   a. opthalmoscope
   b. ophthalmoscope
   c. optalmascope
   d. otoscope

CERTIFICATION CRITERIA CHECKLIST

As you go through your education and training, keep in mind the national certification examination that you will take when you graduate. Each chapter of the textbook and workbook covers a different section of the examination criteria. To keep track of your preparation for the certification examination turn to the back of this workbook and highlight the following CMA, RMA, or CMAS certification examination criteria (if you have already highlighted them from a previous chapter, put a check mark by the criteria):

CMA
S. Treatment Area
  4. Preparing/maintaining treatment areas
T. Patient Preparation and Assisting the Physician
  3. Examinations
  4. Procedures
  5. Explanation and instructions
  6. Instruments, supplies and equipment

RMA
III. Clinical Medical Assisting
  E. Physical Examinations

CMAS
2. Basic Clinical Medical Office Assisting
  • Examination preparation

COMPETENCY ASSESSMENT

Procedure 25-1 Positioning Patient in the Supine Position

Performance Objectives: To safely and properly assist patient into supine position for examination of anterior surface of the body from head to toe. Perform this procedure within 15 minutes with a minimum score of 45 points.

Supplies/Equipment: Drape, gown

Charting/Documentation: Enter appropriate documentation/charting in the box.

Instructor's/Evaluator's Comments and Suggestions:

SKILLS CHECKLIST Procedure 25-1: Positioning Patient in the Supine Position

Name ______________________________

Date ______________________________

No.	Skill	Check #1 20 pts ea	Check #2 10 pts ea	Check #3 5 pts ea	Notes
1	Wash hands.				
2	Assemble supplies.				
3	Assist patient to sit on end of table.				
4	Assist patient to lie back on table as you pull out the table extension. Support patient's back while extending foot of table.				
5	Cover patient with drape from shoulders to ankles.				
6	Place small pillow under patient's head.				
7	Upon completion of a procedure, assist patient to sitting position.				
8	Push table extension back into place while supporting patient's feet.				
9	Once patient is stable (check color of skin and pulse), give further instructions as required.				
Student's Total Points					
Points Possible		180	90	45	
Final Score (Student's Total Points / Possible Points)					

	Notes
Start time:	
End time:	
Total time: (15 min goal)	

COMPETENCY ASSESSMENT

Procedure 25-2 Positioning Patient in the Dorsal Recumbent Position

Performance Objectives: To safely and properly assist patient to dorsal recumbent position for catheterization or pelvic, head, neck, chest, abdominal, or lower limb examination. Perform this procedure within 15 minutes with a minimum score of 45 points.

Supplies/Equipment: Drape, gown

Charting/Documentation: Enter appropriate documentation/charting in the box.

Instructor's/Evaluator's Comments and Suggestions:

SKILLS CHECKLIST Procedure 25-2: Positioning Patient in the Dorsal Recumbent Position

Name ______________________

Date ______________________

No.	Skill	Check #1 20 pts ea	Check #2 10 pts ea	Check #3 5 pts ea	Notes
1	Wash hands.				
2	Assist patient to sit on end of table.				
3	Assist patient to lie back on table as you pull out the table extension. Support patient's back while extending foot of table.				
4	Assist patient to bend knees and place feet flat on the surface of the table. Push in foot extension.				
5	Cover patient with drape from shoulders to ankles.				
6	Place small pillow under patient's head.				
7	Upon completion of a procedure, assist patient to sitting position. Push table extension back into place while supporting patient's feet.				
8	Have patient sit at end of table for a few minutes.				
9	Once patient is stable (check color of skin and pulse), give further instructions as required.				
Student's Total Points					
Points Possible		180	90	45	
Final Score (Student's Total Points / Possible Points)					

	Notes
Start time:	
End time:	
Total time: (15 min goal)	

COMPETENCY ASSESSMENT

Procedure 25-3 Positioning Patient in the Lithotomy Position

Performance Objectives: To safely and properly assist patient in lithotomy position for genital or pelvic examination or for urinary catheterization. Perform this procedure within 15 minutes with a minimum score of 65 points.

Supplies/Equipment: Drape, gown

Charting/Documentation: Enter appropriate documentation/charting in the box.

Instructor's/Evaluator's Comments and Suggestions:

SKILLS CHECKLIST Procedure 25-3: Positioning Patient in the Lithotomy Position

Name ______________________

Date ______________________

No.	Skill	Check #1 20 pts ea	Check #2 10 pts ea	Check #3 5 pts ea	Notes
1	Wash hands.				
2	Have patient disrobe from waist down and put on gown.				
3	Assist patient to sit on end of table. Cover patient's lap and legs with drape.				
4	Assist patient to lie back on table as you support patient's back while extending foot of table.				
5	Position and lock stirrups.				
6	Have patient slide down on table. Have patient move as close to edge of examination table as possible.				
7	Assist patient to bend knees and assist her in placing feet in stirrups. Move drape to diamond shape to ensure privacy.				
8	Place small pillow under patient's head.				
9	Upon completion of procedure, extend foot extension of table.				
10	Place feet on extension and assist patient to slide toward head of table.				
11	Assist patient to sitting position.				
12	Have patient sit at end of table for a few minutes.				
13	Once patient is stable (check color of skin and pulse), give further instructions as required.				
Student's Total Points					
Points Possible		260	130	65	
Final Score (Student's Total Points / Possible Points)					

	Notes
Start time:	
End time:	
Total time: (15 min goal)	

COMPETENCY ASSESSMENT

Procedure 25-4 Positioning Patient in the Fowler's Position

Performance Objectives: To safely and properly assist patient into the Fowler's position for examination of upper body and head; often used for patient with cardiovascular or respiratory problems. Perform this procedure within 15 minutes with a minimum score of 55 points.

Supplies/Equipment: Drape, gown

Charting/Documentation: Enter appropriate documentation/charting in the box.

Instructor's/Evaluator's Comments and Suggestions:

SKILLS CHECKLIST Procedure 25-4: Positioning Patient in the Fowler's Position

Name ______________________

Date ______________________

No.	Skill	Check #1 20 pts ea	Check #2 10 pts ea	Check #3 5 pts ea	Notes
1	Wash hands.				
2	Provide gown and assist to disrobe if necessary.				
3	Assist patient to sit on end of table. Cover patient's lap and legs with drape.				
4	Assist patient to slide back on table leaning against the back rest, which has been raised slightly.				
5	Support patient's feet while extending foot of table.				
6	Position head of table at a 90-degree angle (45-degree angle for Semi-Fowler's)				
7	Place pillow under patient's knees for comfort.				
8	Cover patient with drape from shoulders to ankles.				
9	Upon completion of procedure, replace foot extension.				
10	Have patient sit at end of table for a few minutes.				
11	Once patient is stable (check color of skin and pulse), give further instructions as required.				
Student's Total Points					
Points Possible		220	110	55	
Final Score (Student's Total Points / Possible Points)					

	Notes
Start time:	
End time:	
Total time: (15 min goal)	

COMPETENCY ASSESSMENT

Procedure 25-5 Positioning Patient in the Knee-Chest Position

Performance Objectives: To safely and properly assist patient in knee-chest position for examination of the rectum, sigmoid colon, and in some instances the vagina. Perform this procedure within 15 minutes with a minimum score of 55 points.

Supplies/Equipment: Drape, gown

Charting/Documentation: Enter appropriate documentation/charting in the box.

Instructor's/Evaluator's Comments and Suggestions:

SKILLS CHECKLIST Procedure 25-5: Positioning Patient in the Knee-Chest Position

Name ______________________

Date ______________________

No.	Skill	Check #1 20 pts ea	Check #2 10 pts ea	Check #3 5 pts ea	Notes
1	Wash hands.				
2	Have patient completely undress. Provide gown.				
3	Instruct patient to sit on end of table with drape over lap and legs.				
4	Instruct patient to lie back on table while you support patient's back and extend foot of table.				
5	Assist patient to turn onto abdomen by turning toward you. Support patient by placing your left hand on patient's back and guide patient toward you. Adjust drape.				
6	Assist patient to rise to knees while bending at hips to place chest on table, keeping covered with drape.				
7	Arms are bent to side of head with hands under head.				
8	If this position is uncomfortable, have patient rest on elbows. Adjust drape from shoulders to ankles, creating a triangle or diamond shape.				
9	Upon completion of procedure, assist patient to lie flat on abdomen, then turn onto the back toward you, and then return to sitting position.				
10	Have patient sit at end of table for a few minutes.				
11	Once patient is stable (check color of skin and pulse), give further instructions as required.				
Student's Total Points					
Points Possible		220	110	55	
Final Score (Student's Total Points / Possible Points)					

	Notes
Start time:	
End time:	
Total time: (15 min goal)	

COMPETENCY ASSESSMENT

Procedure 25-6 Positioning Patient in the Prone Position

Performance Objectives: To safely and properly assist patient into the prone position for examination of posterior aspect of the body including the back, spine, or legs. Perform this procedure within 15 minutes with a minimum score of 45 points.

Supplies/Equipment: Drape, gown

Charting/Documentation: Enter appropriate documentation/charting in the box.

Instructor's/Evaluator's Comments and Suggestions:

SKILLS CHECKLIST Procedure 25-6: Positioning Patient in the Prone Position

Name ______________________

Date ______________________

No.	Skill	Check #1 20 pts ea	Check #2 10 pts ea	Check #3 5 pts ea	Notes
1	Wash hands.				
2	Have patient undress. Provide gown.				
3	Assist patient to sit on end of table. Place drape over lap and legs.				
4	Assist patient to lie back on table while you support patient's back and extend foot of table.				
5	Assist patient to turn toward you, then onto abdomen being careful to stay in center of table to avoid a fall. Place pillow under feet and head.				
6	Adjust patient drape from shoulders to ankles.				
7	Upon completion of procedure, assist patient to lie flat on abdomen, then turn onto the back toward you, and then return to sitting position.				
8	Have patient sit at end of table for a few minutes.				
9	Once patient is stable (check color of skin and pulse), give further instructions as required.				
Student's Total Points					
Points Possible		180	90	45	
Final Score (Student's Total Points / Possible Points)					

	Notes
Start time:	
End time:	
Total time: (15 min goal)	

COMPETENCY ASSESSMENT

Procedure 25-7 Positioning Patient in the Sims' Position

Performance Objectives: To safely and properly assist patient into Sims' position for rectal examination, rectal temperature, proctoscopy, sigmoidoscopy, for an enema, and, in some instances, for vaginal examination. Perform this procedure within 15 minutes with a minimum score of 55 points.

Supplies/Equipment: Drape, gown

Charting/Documentation: Enter appropriate documentation/charting in the box.

Instructor's/Evaluator's Comments and Suggestions:

SKILLS CHECKLIST Procedure 25-7: Positioning Patient in the Sims' Position

Name ______________________

Date ______________________

No.	Skill	Check #1 20 pts ea	Check #2 10 pts ea	Check #3 5 pts ea	Notes
1	Wash hands.				
2	Have patient undress. Provide gown.				
3	Assist patient to sit on end of table. Place drape over lap and legs.				
4	Assist patient to lie back on table while you support patient's back and extend foot of table.				
5	Assist patient to turn toward you onto the left side with left arm behind body, placing body weight on chest. Adjust drape.				
6	Assist patient to slightly flex left knee and flex right knee to a 90-degree angle for support.				
7	Right arm is bent in front of body with hand toward head at an angle to provide support.				
8	Adjust drape from shoulders to ankles creating triangle or diamond shape.				
9	Upon completion of procedure, instruct patient to turn toward you, onto back, and then to sitting position.				
10	Have patient sit at end of table for a few minutes.				
11	Once patient is stable (check color of skin and pulse), give further instructions as required.				
Student's Total Points					
Points Possible		220	110	55	
Final Score (Student's Total Points / Possible Points)					

	Notes
Start time:	
End time:	
Total time: (15 min goal)	

COMPETENCY ASSESSMENT

Procedure 25-8 Assisting with a Complete Physical Examination

Performance Objectives: To assist physician in a complete physical examination. Perform this objective within 30 minutes with a minimum score of 200 points.

Supplies/Equipment: Balance beam or digital scale, patient gown, drape, thermometer, stethoscope, sphygmomanometer, alcohol wipes, examination lights, otoscope, tuning fork, ophthalmoscope, penlight, nasal speculum, tongue depressor, percussion hammer, tape measure, cotton balls, safety pin, gloves, tissues, lubricant, emesis basin, gauze sponges, specimen bottle and slides and requisition form, biohazard waste container

Charting/Documentation: Enter appropriate documentation/charting in the box.

Instructor's/Evaluator's Comments and Suggestions:

SKILLS CHECKLIST Procedure 25-8: Assisting with a Complete Physical Examination

Name ______________________

Date ______________________

No.	Skill	Check #1 20 pts ea	Check #2 10 pts ea	Check #3 5 pts ea	Notes
1	Wash hands.				
2	Assemble equipment.				
3	Place instruments/supplies in easily accessible sequence for physician use.				
4	Greet and identify patient. Introduce yourself.				
5	Explain procedure to patient.				
6	Review medical history with patient.				
7	Take and record patient vital signs, visual acuity, and hearing test results.				
8	Obtain a urine specimen.				
9	Obtain all required blood samples.				
10	Perform electrocardiogram if directed by physician.				
11	Provide patient with appropriate gown and drape.				
12	Assist patient to disrobe completely; explain where the opening of the gown is to be placed.				
13	Assist patient in sitting at the end of the table; drape patient across lap and legs.				
14	Inform physician when patient is ready.				
15	When the physician arrives, remain by the patient ready to assist patient and physician.				
16	Position patient into a sitting or supine position for the head, throat, eye, ear, and neck examination.				
17	Turn off lights for retinal examination if instructed.				
18	Hand the physician instruments as required.				
19	The sitting position will be maintained for auscultation of the chest and heart.				

No.	Skill	Check #1 20 pts ea	Check #2 10 pts ea	Check #3 5 pts ea	Notes
20	Assist the patient into a supine position and drape for examination of the chest.				
21	Maintain a quiet atmosphere to enhance the ability of the physician in hearing heart and lung sounds.				
22	Position patient into supine position and drape for abdominal examinations and examination of extremities.				
23	Gynecologic examination may then be performed. Position patient and assist physician appropriately.				
24	If rectal examination is necessary, assist patient into Sims' position.				
25	Place patient into prone position for examination of posterior aspect of body.				
26	Upon completion of the examination, assist patient to a sitting position and allow patient to sit at end of table for a few minutes.				
27	Assure patient stability (check color of skin, pulse) before allowing patient to stand up.				
28	Assist patient in dressing as needed; provide privacy.				
29	Chart any notes or patient instructions per physician orders.				
30	Escort patient to physician's office for discussion of examination results.				
31	Apply disposable gloves.				
32	Dispose of gown and drape into biohazard waste container.				
33	Dispose of contaminated materials into biohazard container.				
34	Remove table paper and dispose into biohazard waste container.				
35	Disinfect counters and examination table with a solution of 10% bleach or other appropriate disinfectant.				

No.	Skill	Check #1 20 pts ea	Check #2 10 pts ea	Check #3 5 pts ea	Notes
36	Clean, disinfect, or sterilize reusable instruments as appropriate.				
37	Remove gloves, discard into biohazard waste container.				
38	Wash hands.				
39	Replace table paper and equipment in preparation for the next patient.				
40	Document the procedure.				
Student's Total Points					
Points Possible		800	400	200	
Final Score (Student's Total Points / Possible Points)					

	Notes
Start time:	
End time:	
Total time: (30 min goal)	

EVALUATION OF CHAPTER KNOWLEDGE

Skills	Student Self-Evaluation Good	Average	Poor
I understand six methods used in physical examinations.	_____	_____	_____
I can demonstrate the ability to place patients in eight positions used for physical examinations.	_____	_____	_____
I understand draping techniques and the importance of patient's privacy.	_____	_____	_____
I can identify instruments and supplies necessary for examination of various body parts.	_____	_____	_____
I can identify basic components of the physical examination.	_____	_____	_____
I can identify the sequence followed during a routine physical examination.	_____	_____	_____
I can recall the method of examination, instruments used, and positions for examination of at least eight body parts.	_____	_____	_____
I understand quality-control techniques and guidelines.	_____	_____	_____
I do observe all Standard Precautions and apply principles of aseptic technique.	_____	_____	_____
I document accurately, maintaining medical records and completing requisition forms.	_____	_____	_____
I know how to prepare the patient for the procedure.	_____	_____	_____
I can respect the patient and attend to the patient's emotional needs during physical examination.	_____	_____	_____
I can prepare and maintain examination and treatment areas.	_____	_____	_____

CHAPTER 26

Obstetrics and Gynecology

CHAPTER PRE-TEST

Perform this test without looking at the book. This is just to see how well you have understood and can recall the information in this chapter after you have read it, but before you have completed the workbook exercises. You will not be graded on this portion (other than the grade you give yourself). Justify any "false" answers.

1. Obstetrics has to do with pregnancy and delivery, and gynecology has to do with female reproductive issues. (T or F)
2. Which of the following are addressed during the initial prenatal visit and examination?
   a. genetic diseases/conditions in the family
   b. kidney and heart diseases/conditions and diabetes
   c. nutritional deficiencies
   d. all of the above
3. During pregnancy, which of the following is potentially dangerous?
   a. rapid weight gain
   b. visual changes
   c. hypertension
   d. chill, fever
   e. all of the above
4. It is recommended that pelvic examinations and Papanicolaou (Pap) smears be performed on all women older than 20 years (or at the onset of sexual activity) on an annual basis. (T or F)

5. Because the physician will perform the breast examination during the annual physical, it is not important for women to perform breast self-examinations on themselves. (T or F)

6. The Pap smear is designed to detect which type of cancer?
   a. cervical
   b. vaginal
   c. ovarian
   d. all of the above
   e. a and b only

INTRODUCTION

In the office of an obstetrician/gynecologist, the medical assistant assists the physician with the care and treatment of the female patient. The medical assistant must possess knowledge of the female anatomy, diseases and disorders that can affect the female during both nonpregnant and pregnant states, and the tests and treatments that may be encountered in the office. Promotion of health and prevention of disease are also important for the health of the patient, and the medical assistant plays an important role in the education of the patient during her life span.

PERFORMANCE OBJECTIVES

After successful completion of this chapter you will be able to explain the terminology related to obstetrics and gynecology. In the area of obstetrics, you will know the importance of early and frequent prenatal care and what is included in each prenatal examination. You will be able to cite at least a dozen conditions/diseases that can adversely affect a pregnant woman and her child. You will know why tests such as ultrasound and amniocentesis are performed, you will be able to list and explain six different types of abortions, and you will be able to explain the stages of labor and what happens during the postpartum phase. In the area of gynecology, you will be able to list and explain several common disorders/conditions and diseases that can affect women, including sexually transmitted diseases and their associated tests and treatments used. You will also know how to educate female patients about how to better care for their bodies. You will be able to teach a woman how to perform a breast self-examination, and you will be able to educate patients about menopause and also contraception methods. *The following statements are related to your learning objectives for this chapter. Fill in the blanks in the following paragraph with the appropriate term(s).*

During the first prenatal visit, a thorough (1) ______________________ and (2) ______________________ examination is performed. This will include (3) ______________, (4) ______________, (5) ______________ and (6) ______________________ examinations. (7) ______________________ measurements are taken to ascertain if the pelvis is adequate for (8) ______________ delivery. At the monthly or weekly visits that follow, the medical assistant will take the patient's (9) ______________________, test her (10) ______________________ and (11) ______________________, and educate her about (12) ______________, (13) ______________________, and (14) ______________, preparing for (15) ________________________________, and any other patient education or problem solving as directed by the physician. During the pregnancy, potentially serious conditions can develop. The symptoms you must teach your patients to be aware of, and alert you to, include rapid (16) ________________________________, (17) ________________________, (18) ________________________________ (which you will detect during her visit), (19) ________________________ and (20) ________________________ (other than the usual, which is to be expected), (21) ________________________, (22) ________________________________, abdominal (23) ______________, (24) ________________________, one-sided (25) ________________________ or (26) ________________________ pain, and (27) ______________ or (28) ______________________. Even though we think of abortion as being an elective surgery, any loss of the fetus is called an abortion. If it is elective, it is called a (29) ____________________ abortion, whereas if it happens unplanned, it is called a (30) ________________ abortion (or miscarriage). The (31) ____________________ period is the 4 to 6 weeks immediately after the delivery. During routine gynecologic visits, the woman will be taught how to perform (32) ________________________________ examinations on a monthly basis. As a part of the gynecologic examinations, the (33) ________________________ will be performed, which is a screening tool for cervical and vaginal cancer, but not ovarian cancer. Some of the more common diseases and disorders that affect women are (34) ________________________________, (35) ________________________, (36) ________________________________, (37) ________________________, (38) ________________________________, and PID or (39) ________________________________. Some of the diagnostic tests and treatments the medical assistant will be assisting with in the gynecologic setting include (40) __________________, which is using a magnifying lens to closely examing cervical tissue, (41) ________________________, (42) ________________________________, which is a freezing of the cervix, (43) ______________________, using a scope, and (44) ________________________________, sometimes referred to as a D & C. Some of the more common STDs or (45) ________________________________ that affect women are (46) __________________, (47) ______________________, (48) ____________________________, and (49) ____________________.

VOCABULARY BUILDER

Find the words below that are misspelled; circle them, and then correctly spell them in the spaces provided. Then fill in the blanks in the following paragraph with the correct vocabulary terms from the list.

abortion	effacement	parturation
amniocentesis	gestation	pelvic inflammatory disease
Braxton–Hicks	gonorrhea	placenta abruptio
cervical punch biopsy	human papilloma virus	placenta previa
colposcopy	hysterosalpingogram	preeclampsia
cryosurgery	Lamaze	primigravida
dialation	lochia	puerperium
dismenorrhea	multigravida	sickle cell anemia
dyspareunia	neonatal	Tay–Sachs
eclampsia	nullipara	trichomoniasis
ectopic	oxytocin	

____________________ ___________________________

____

1. Discharge from the uterus of blood, mucus, and tissue during the period after childbirth is called ____________________________.
2. The period of development from conception to birth is called __________________________.
3. Any pregnancy that occurs outside of the uterus is called _____________________.
4. A __________________________ is a visual examination of vaginal and cervical tissues using a type of microscope with a magnifying lens and powerful lights.
5. ____ is an infection of the uterus, fallopian tubes, and adjacent pelvic structures.
6. A term that means "painful menses" is __________________________________.
7. _______________________ occurs when the placenta implants itself low in the uterus and partially or completely covers the cervical os.
8. _____________________________ is the term given to a woman who has not carried a pregnancy to birth.
9. Two types of sexually transmitted diseases are __________________________, which is caused by bacteria, and _________________________________, which is caused by a virus.
10. _______________________________________ is an invasion of a protozoa, often transmitted through sexual contact.

LEARNING REVIEW

1. A. Identify each part of the female reproductive system in Figure 26-1. Describe each part and its function in the spaces provided. Use your medical dictionary and anatomy resources if needed.

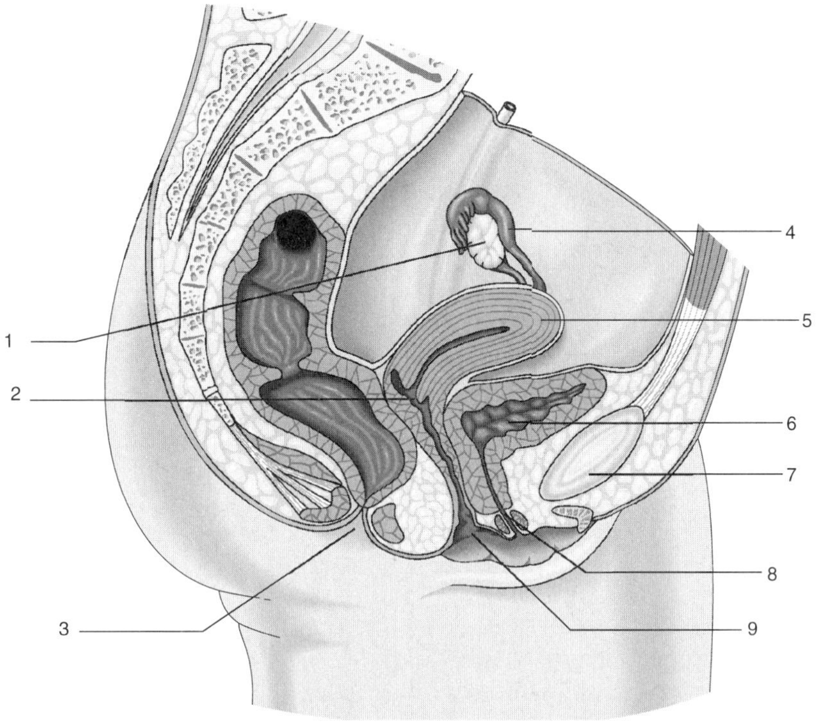

Figure 26-1

1. Part: ______________________
   Function: ______________________
2. Part: ______________________
   Function: ______________________
3. Part: ______________________
   Function: ______________________
4. Part: ______________________
   Function: ______________________
5. Part: ______________________
   Function: ______________________
6. Part: ______________________
   Function: ______________________
7. Part: ______________________
   Function: ______________________
8. Part: ______________________
   Function: ______________________
9. Part: ______________________
   Function: ______________________

B. Match each female condition or disease to its description.

______ 1. PID

______ 2. Menopause

______ 3. Endometriosis

______ 4. Ovarian cancer

______ 5. Ovarian cysts

______ 6. Dysmenorrhea

A. Malignant cells found in the ovaries

B. Painful menstruation

C. Period of time that marks permanent cessation of menstrual activity

D. Inflammatory disease of the pelvis involving some or all of the reproductive organs, usually transmitted sexually

E. Painful condition characterized by endometrial cells adhering to tissues and organs outside of the uterus

F. Cysts located on the ovaries

C. The chart below lists complications of pregnancy. Fill in the description, symptoms, and treatments that correspond to the complication.

Complication	Description	Symptoms	Treatment
Abortion/Interruption of pregnancy:			
1. Spontaneous			
2. Complete			
3. Missed			
4. Incomplete			
5. Threatened			
6. Induced			

Eclampsia			
Preeclampsia			
Gestational diabetes			
Hyperemesis gravidarum			
Placenta previa			
Placenta abruptio			

D. The obstetric history includes the total number of pregnancies and the number of live births. For each history, give the number of pregnancies and the number of live births.

(1) Gravida 3 Para 1 Abortion 1: ______________________________

(2) Gravida 6 Para 4 Abortion 0: ______________________________

(3) Gravida 3 Para 1 Abortion 2: ______________________________

2. What branch of medicine treats the mother and fetus through all stages of labor, delivery, and postpartum?
   a. gynecology
   b. prenatal care
   c. obstetrics
   d. puerperium

3. Which of the following is a sign/symptom of preeclampsia?
   a. hypertension
   b. rapid weight gain
   c. headache
   d. all of the above

4. A potentially life-threatening disorder during pregnancy that is characterized by hypertension, edema, and proteinuria and may put both the mother and fetus in danger is:
   a. placenta previa
   b. placenta abruptio
   c. eclampsia
   d. gestational diabetes

5. Breast self-examination should be performed:
   a. monthly
   b. 2 to 3 days after mensus
   c. every 2 weeks
   d. yearly

6. The gynecologic disease in which an infection is caused by a microorganism that may lead to infertility or ectopic pregnancy if not treated is:
   a. endometriosis
   b. Bartholin gland infection
   c. menopause
   d. pelvic inflammatory disease

CERTIFICATION REVIEW

These questions are designed to mimic the certification examinations. You can use these questions like a small "Certification Examination Study Guide," but this is not meant to take the place of the more extensive study guides. Use this portion to determine in what areas to concentrate your efforts when studying for the certification examination.

1. Which of the following are types of abortions?
   a. spontaneous, complete, incomplete, interrupted, medical
   b. miscarriage, threatened, induced, voluntary, medical
   c. induced, spontaneous, postpartum, complete, medical
   d. complete, threatened, incomplete, induced, missed, spontaneous
   e. interrupted, complete, induced, medical, voluntary

2. During a prenatal visit, the urine is tested for which two substances?
   a. drugs, including alcohol, and glucose
   b. infection and glucose
   c. glucose and protein
   d. bilirubin and protein

3. Which of the following are not tests/procedures performed on pregnant women?
   a. ultrasound
   b. amniocentesis

c. chorionic villi sampling
d. alpha fetal protein
e. colonoscopy

4. LMP means:
   a. localized medical practices
   b. last menstrual period
   c. localized menstrual pain
   d. limited medical plan
   e. last medical prenatal (examination)

5. A prenatal condition that causes sudden weight gain, an increase in blood pressure, and proteinuria is called:
   a. toxemia
   b. preeclampsia
   c. hyperemesis
   d. gestational diabetes
   e. a and b

6. A painful condition characterized by tissue from the inside of the uterus adhering to the organs outside the uterus is called:
   a. preeclampsia
   b. endometriosis
   c. metrometriosis
   d. menopause
   e. pelvic inflammatory disease

7. Bartholin glands:
   a. contain mucus for lubrication of the vagina
   b. can become inflamed and infected
   c. are situated on both sides of the vaginal orifice
   d. are similar to the male's Cowper glands
   e. all of the above

8. Chlamydia, condylomata, HIV, and gonorrhea are all:
   a. complications of pregnancy
   b. diagnosed during the Pap smear and pelvic examination
   c. sexually transmitted
   d. curable
   e. diagnosed through blood tests

CASE STUDY

In the office, the physician instructs you that a Pap smear and pelvic examination will be done on Mrs. Smith in Room 1. What is your role in assisting these procedures?

SELF-ASSESSMENT

Think about the last time you went to your physician for an examination. As you answer the following questions and remember your personal experiences think about how your experiences will affect the way you treat your patients in the future. If you have no personal experiences, try to imagine how you would feel and react. All of the following situations may be discussed in small groups with your classmates.

1. Which questions were you asked the last time you went to your physician for a pelvic examination? Try to think of five.

2. When the physician came into the room, were you dressed and in the examination room? Were you undressed and sitting on the examination table? Were you undressed and lying down? Were you undressed and lying down in the lithotomy position? Which of the previous scenarios would make you the most comfortable? Which would make you the most uncomfortable?

3. How comfortable are you with discussing private information with your physician? How about with your medical assistant? Are you more comfortable with one or the other? Why do you suppose you would be?

POST-TEST

This is similar to the Pre-Test. Perform this test without looking at the book. This is just to see how well you have understood and can recall the information presented in this chapter after you have studied it and completed the workbook exercises. You will not be graded on this portion (other than the grade you give yourself), but this is an excellent preparation for your instructor's test. You may use this Post-Test to determine what areas you need to study more. Justify any "false" answers.

1. Obstetrics has to do with female issues, and gynecology has to do with pregnancy. (T or F)

2. Which of the following are addressed during the initial prenatal visit and examination?
   a. genetic diseases/conditions in the family
   b. kidney and heart diseases/conditions and diabetes
   c. nutritional deficiencies
   d. all of the above

3. During pregnancy, which of the following is potentially dangerous?
   a. rapid weight gain
   b. visual changes
   c. hypertension
   d. chill, fever
   e. all of the above

4. It is recommended that pelvic examinations and Pap smears be performed on all women older than 25 years (or at the onset of sexual activity) on an annual basis. (T or F)

5. Even though the physician will perform the breast examination during the annual physical, it is still important for women to be performing breast self-examinations on themselves. (T or F)

6. The Pap smear is designed to detect which type of cancer?
   a. cervical
   b. ovarian
   c. vaginal
   d. breast
   e. all of the above
   f. a and c only

CERTIFICATION CRITERIA CHECKLIST

As you go through your education and training, keep in mind the national certification examination that you will take when you graduate. Each chapter of the textbook and workbook covers a different section of the examination criteria. To keep track of your preparation for the certification examination, turn to the back of this workbook and highlight the following CMA, RMA, or CMAS certification examination criteria (if you have already highlighted them from a previous edition, put a check mark by the criteria):

CMA
A. Medical Terminology
B. Anatomy and Physiology
E. Communication
    3. Patient instruction
P. Office Policies and Procedures
    2. Patient education
T. Patient Preparation and Assisting the Physician
    3. Examinations
    4. Procedures
V. Collecting and Processing Specimens; Diagnostic Testing

RMA
I. General Medical Assisting Knowledge
    A. Anatomy and Physiology
    B. Medical Terminology
    F. Patient Education
III. Clinical Medical Assisting
    E. Physical Examinations
    L. Laboratory Procedures

CMAS
1. Medical Assisting Foundation
    • Medical terminology
    • Anatomy and physiology
2. Basic Clinical Medical Office Assisting
    • Examination preparation

COMPETENCY ASSESSMENT

Procedure 26-1 Assisting with Routine Prenatal Visits

Performance Objectives: To monitor the progress of the pregnancy. Perform this objective within 20 minutes with a minimum score of 85 points.

Supplies/Equipment: Disposable gloves, patient gown, scale, tape measure, sphygmomanometer, stethoscope, Doppler fetoscope, coupling agent and supplies as needed, urine specimen container, urinalysis chemical testing reagent strip, biohazard waste container

Charting/Documentation: Enter appropriate documentation/charting in the box.

Instructor's/Evaluator's Comments and Suggestions:

SKILLS CHECKLIST Procedure 26-1: Assisting with Routine Prenatal Visits

Name ______________________________

Date ______________________________

No.	Skill	Check #1 20 pts ea	Check #2 10 pts ea	Check #3 5 pts ea	Notes
1	Wash hands.				
2	Set up equipment.				
3	Identify patient and explain procedure.				
4	Obtain urine specimen.				
5	Measure blood pressure.				
6	Weigh patient.				
7	Have patient disrobe from waist down; put on gown, opening in the front.				
8	In laboratory, test urine specimen.				
9	Assist patient onto examination table and drape her.				
10	Assist physician with examination as required.				
11	After examination, assist patient to sitting position and assess her color and pulse.				
12	Provide instructions and clarify physician's orders as needed.				
13	Apply gloves, discard disposable supplies, and disinfect equipment.				
14	Remove gloves.				
15	Wash hands.				
16	Clean and repare room for next patient.				
17	Record information in patient's chart/medical record.				
Student's Total Points					
Points Possible		340	170	85	
Final Score (Student's Total Points / Possible Points)					

	Notes
Start time:	
End time:	
Total time: (20 min goal)	

COMPETENCY ASSESSMENT

Procedure 26-2 Instructing Patient in Breast Self-Examination

Performance Objectives: To properly instruct a woman in the procedure for performing a breast self-examination. Perform this objective within 20 minutes with a minimum score of 30 points.

Supplies/Equipment: Breast model, breast self-examination brochure, mirror is useful

Charting/Documentation: Enter appropriate documentation/charting in the box.

Instructor's/Evaluator's Comments and Suggestions:

SKILLS CHECKLIST Procedure 26-2: Instructing Patient in Breast Self-Examination

Name ______________________________

Date ______________________________

No.	Skill	Check #1 20 pts ea	Check #2 10 pts ea	Check #3 5 pts ea	Notes
1	Using a patient information brochure, instruct the patient on the proper method to perform a breast self-examination (see brochure or text procedure for details).				
2	Discuss the ideal positioning, time of the month, frequency, methods, and the pattern to follow while examining the breasts.				
3	Help her determine a day each month that will be conductive for her to perform the examination.				
4	Answer any questions she has and give her your number to call if she needs further instructions.				
5	Provide her with additional educational materials and resources that are approved by your physician.				
6	Have her report any abnormalities to you or the physician immediately.				
Student's Total Points					
Points Possible		120	60	30	
Final Score (Student's Total Points / Possible Points)					

	Notes
Start time:	
End time:	
Total time: (20 min goal)	

COMPETENCY ASSESSMENT

Procedure 26-3 Assisting with Pelvic Examination and Pap Test (Conventional and Thin Prep® Methods)

Performance Objectives: To assist the physician in collecting cervical cells for laboratory analysis for early detection of malignant cells of the cervix, to assess the health of the reproductive organs, and to detect diseases leading to early diagnosis and treatment. Perform this objective within 25 minutes with a minimum score of 115 points.

Supplies/Equipment: Nonsterile gloves (two or three pair), vaginal speculum, warm water or warming light, light source, drape sheet and patient gown, tissues, vaginal lubricant, laboratory requisition, urine specimen container and urine testing supplies, biohazard waste container, adjustable stool for physician, supplies for the Pap test according to the method used. (For ThinPrep Pap: cervical spatula, brush and broom, ThinPrep container with solution. For conventional Pap test: microscope slides, fixative and specimen bottle, cervical spatula, and cytology brush.)

Charting/Documentation: Enter appropriate documentation/charting in the box.

Instructor's/Evaluator's Comments and Suggestions:

SKILLS CHECKLIST Procedure 26-3: Assisting with Pelvic Examination and Pap Test (Conventional and Thin Prep® Methods)

Name ______________________

Date ______________________

No.	Skill	Check #1 20 pts ea	Check #2 10 pts ea	Check #3 5 pts ea	Notes
1	Wash hands and assemble necessary supplies near patient.				
2	Request that patient empty her bladder.				
3	Provide patient with a gown. Request that she completely undress and don the gown, opening in front.				
4	Explain the procedure.				
5	Instruct patient to sit at end of table. Drape the patient for privacy. If performing the conventional Pap test, label the frosted end of the slide to include the patient's name and site of specimen collection.				
6	Assist the patient into the lithotomy position. Patient's knees should be relaxed and thighs rotated out as far as comfortable. Drape for privacy and warmth.				
7	Encourage patient to breathe slowly and deeply through the mouth during the examination.				
8	Warm speculum.				
9	Hand speculum, cervical spatula, cytology brush, and broom to the physician as needed.				
10	Apply gloves.				
11	If performing conventional Pap test, hold slide for the physician to apply smear of exfoliated cells, one for each specimen site. Label slides according to site. Spray fixative over each slide within 10 seconds at a distance of about 6 inches. Allow to dry for at least 10 minutes.				
12	If performing ThinPrep® Pap test, remove the cap from the ThinPrep® solution, when the cervical cells have been obtained on the broom, vigorously swish the broom in the solution until all cells have been deposited.				

No.	Skill	Check #1 20 pts ea	Check #2 10 pts ea	Check #3 5 pts ea	Notes
13	Place lubricant on the physician's gloved fingers without touching the gloves.				
14	Assist the physician as needed during the rest of the examination.				
15	Assist the patient to wipe genitalia and perineal area.				
16	Help the patient to a seated position, allowing her to rest for a while. Check her pulse and skin color.				
17	Discard disposable supplies. If stainless steel speculum was used, soak in cool water in preparation for later sanitization and sterilization.				
18	Remove gloves and wash hands.				
19	Assist the patient to sit up and get down off the table as needed.				
20	Instruct the patient to dress. Inform the patient of how and when test results will be reported.				
21	Prepare laboratory requisition form completely and properly. Place slides into slide container (conventional Pap), and place container into biohazard specimen bag. Place requisition into outside pocket of bag. Send to laboratory.				
22	Wash hands.				
23	Document in the patient's chart that test is performed and slide has been sent to reference laboratory.				
Student's Total Points					
Points Possible		460	230	115	
Final Score (Student's Total Points / Possible Points)					

	Notes
Start time:	
End time:	
Total time: (25 min goal)	

COMPETENCY ASSESSMENT

Procedure 26-4 Wet Prep/Wet Mount and Potassium Hydroxide (KOH) Prep

Performance Objectives: To test a vaginal area and determine the cause of vaginitis. The wet prep/wet mount tests for yeast, bacteria, and trichomonas; the KOH prep tests for fungi. Perform this objective within 25 minutes with a minimum score of 70 points.

Supplies/Equipment: Cotton-tipped applicator, small test tube, normal saline (0.5 ml, or a few drops), two microscope slides and coverslips, 10% potassium hydroxide (KOH; 0.5 ml, or a few drops), two microscope slides and coverslips, microscope, vaginal speculum, patient drape, gloves, other equipment as necessary for a vaginal examination.

Charting/Documentation: Enter appropriate documentation/charting in the box.

Instructor's/Evaluator's Comments and Suggestions:

SKILLS CHECKLIST Procedure 26-4: Wet Prep/Wet Mount and Potassium Hydroxide (KOH) Prep

Name ______________________

Date ______________________

No.	Skill	Check #1 20 pts ea	Check #2 10 pts ea	Check #3 5 pts ea	Notes
1	Prepare the patient for a pelvic examination.				
2	Place several drops of normal saline into a small test tube.				
3	Using the cotton-tipped applicator, the physician obtains a sampling of discharge from the vagina and hands it to the medical assistant.				
4	Rinse the swab in the test tube containing saline, pressing the cotton tip against the inside of the test tube to express all the specimen.				
5	Dispose of the cotton-tipped applicator into a biohazard container.				
6	Apply a drop on a microscope slide and cover. Hand the slide to the physician for the microscopy examination.				
7	Assist the patient back to a sitting position. Instruct her to dress; offer to assist if needed.				
8	In the laboratory, the physician will view the slide for yeast, bacteria, and trichomonas.				
9	After performance of the wet prep/wet mount, apply a few drops of KOH into the remaining solution in the test tube; place a drop on a fresh slide and cover.				
10	The physician will perform a microscopic examination for fungi.				
11	Dispose of all slides and the test tube into a sharps container.				
12	Disinfect the laboratory area and equipment.				

No.	Skill	Check #1 20 pts ea	Check #2 10 pts ea	Check #3 5 pts ea	Notes
13	Return to the patient and assist as needed.				
14	Chart the procedure and document the test as needed.				
Student's Total Points					
Points Possible		280	140	70	
Final Score (Student's Total Points / Possible Points)					
		Notes			
Start time:					
End time:					
Total time: (25 min goal)					

COMPETENCY ASSESSMENT

Procedure 26-5 Amplified DNA ProbeTec Test for Chlamydia and Gonorrhea

Performance Objectives: To test a vaginal specimen for diagnosis of chlamydia and gonorrhea, and to use as a screening tool for pregnant women. Perform this objective within 25 minutes with a minimum score of 55 points.

Supplies/Equipment: Amplified DNA ProbeTec Kit (pink), vaginal speculum, patient drape, gloves, laboratory requisition, biohazard specimen transport bag, other equipment as necessary for a vaginal examination

Charting/Documentation: Enter appropriate documentation/charting in the box.

Instructor's/Evaluator's Comments and Suggestions:

SKILLS CHECKLIST Procedure 26-5: Amplified DNA ProbeTec Test for Chlamydia and Gonorrhea

Name ______________________

Date ______________________

No.	Skill	Check #1 20 pts ea	Check #2 10 pts ea	Check #3 5 pts ea	Notes
1	Prepare the patient for a pelvic examination.				
2	Hand the large swab to the physician.				
3	Discard the large swab into the biohazard waste container.				
4	Hand the small Mini-tip Culturette Swab to the physician.				
5	After specimen is retained, immediately place the swab into the transport tube and recap.				
6	If using the ProbeTec Wet Transport tube, break off the tip of the swab into the liquid before recapping.				
7	Place specimen into biohazard specimen transport bag.				
8	Remove gloves and wash hands.				
9	Assist patient as needed.				
10	Complete requsition and place it into the outside pocket of the specimen transport bag.				
11	Document.				
Student's Total Points					
Points Possible		220	110	55	
Final Score (Student's Total Points / Possible Points)					

	Notes
Start time:	
End time:	
Total time: (25 min goal)	

EVALUATION OF CHAPTER KNOWLEDGE

Skills	Student Self-Evaluation Good	Average	Poor
I can explain the procedures the patient will encounter during obstetric visits, from the initial prenatal visit through the postpartum period.	_____	_____	_____
I can describe tests and procedures the patient may encounter during prenatal visits.	_____	_____	_____
I can explain common complications of pregnancy.	_____	_____	_____
I can demonstrate the procedure for a breast examination.	_____	_____	_____
I can identify equipment used during the gynecologic examination.	_____	_____	_____
I can demonstrate positioning for the gynecologic examination.	_____	_____	_____
I can explain gynecologic diseases and conditions.	_____	_____	_____
I can explain diagnostic tests used to detect diseases of the female reproductive system.	_____	_____	_____

CHAPTER 27

Pediatrics

CHAPTER PRE-TEST

Perform this test without looking at the book. This is just to see how well you have understood and can recall the information in this chapter after you have read it, but before you have completed the workbook exercises. You will not be graded on this portion (other than the grade you give yourself). Justify any "false" answers.

1. Pediatrics deals with birth through adolescence. (T or F)
2. Toddlers are:
   a. children from birth to 2 years old
   b. children from about 1 to about 3 years old
   c. children from the time they are able to walk until they are in kindergarten
   d. children from about 2 to 5 years old
3. Measurements of babies consist of length, weight, chest circumference, and head circumference. (T or F)
4. Normal childhood immunizations include which of the following?
   a. DTaP, MMR, Hib, and HIV
   b. tetanus, DTaP, MMR, and IPV
   c. IPV, MMR, DTaP, Hib, and HBV
   d. HBV, Hib, pertussis, and HAV
   e. both c and d
5. The preferred site for injections for a child younger than 2 years is:
   a. the vastus lateralis
   b. the gluteus medius

c. the deltoid
d. any of the above is acceptable

6. Normal pulse and respiration for an 8-year-old child is:
   a. pulse of 80, respiration of 30
   b. pulse of 80, respiration of 12
   c. pulse of 120, respiration of 20
   d. pulse of 86, respiration of 18
   e. none of the above

INTRODUCTION

Patients at a certain age need specialized care. Medical assistants assist the physician with many clinical procedures that are an integral component of specialty examinations such as those used with the pediatric patient. Medical assistants who are employed in a pediatric office will need additional skills and ongoing training to stay proficient in the most current technologies and treatments used to provide quality care to patients. This workbook chapter should be used by students to become familiar with appropriate clinical procedures in pediatrics, including taking vital signs and measurement of infants.

PERFORMANCE OBJECTIVES

After successful completion of this chapter you will be able to explain the terminology related to pediatrics. You also will be able to obtain childhood vital signs and body measurements and will be able to plot a child's physical development on a graph. You will be knowledgeable about stages of development for children as they grow. You will be intimately aware of which immunizations are required for infants and children, as well as suggested immunizations. You will be able to list and explain several common disorders/conditions and diseases that can affect children, including the most common symptoms and treatments; and you will know how to screen for visual and auditory impairments. *The following statements are related to your learning objectives for this chapter. Fill in the blanks in the following paragraph with the appropriate term(s).*

During a routine examination, the medical assistant should measure the infant's (1) ________________ and (2) ________________, (3) ________________, and (4) ________________. The infant's growth should be recorded on a graph called a (5) ________________, as well as in the chart notes. There are many different theories on growth and (6) ________________; each theory focuses on a particular aspect of development and its principles, strengths, and weaknesses. The medical assistant will apply an inclusive approach to each (7) ________________ child. Common childhood immunizations given before the age of 2 years are (8) ________________, (9) ________________, (10) ________________, (11) ________________, (12) ________________, (13) ________________, and (14) ________________. Disorders that affect children can run anywhere from the common (15) ________________ and the common ear infection called (16) ________________________, to the more serious breathing problem of (17) ________________________. One serious condition that is affecting more and more children every year is child abuse. You, as a medical assistant, need to work with other members of the health care team to be aware of common signs of abuse. Some injuries to note are (18) ______________________________, (19) ______________________________, (20) ______________________________, (21) ______________________________, (22) ______________________________, (23) ______________________________, (24) ____________________________, and (25) ______________________. Also, routine (26) ____________________________________ are often missed by neglectful or abusive parents. If abuse is suspected, there are specific steps to be taken.

VOCABULARY BUILDER

Find the words below that are misspelled; circle them, and then correctly spell them in the spaces provided.

blood preasure	myringotomy	phynelketonuria
circumfrence	pediatrics	tonsilitis
fontanelle	pediculosis	vacination

________________ ________________ ________________

________________ ________________

Define the following vocabulary terms:

Exudate ____

____

Myringotomy ____

____

Suppurative ____

____

Tympanostomy ____

____

Otitis media ____

____

Tonsillitis ____

____

Pediculosis ____

____

LEARNING REVIEW

Mary O'Keefe has called for an emergency appointment for her 3-year-old son, Chris, for an examination with Dr. King, because he awakened during the night with a high fever and severe pain in his right ear, which is draining.

1. Ellen Armstrong, CMA, must prepare the examination room for the patient. Based on Chris's symptoms, what equipment will Ellen want to assemble for Dr. King's physical examination of Chris? List the equipment in the order it will most likely be used in the examination.

____

____

____

____

2. When Mary O'Keefe arrives with her son, Ellen takes them to examination room 2 and prepares the patient for Dr. King's physical examination. Ellen tells Mary that Dr. King will be examining Chris's ear and may want to take some laboratory tests. Ellen takes and records the child's vital signs:

   T 102.1°F; P 115 (AP) bounding, sinus arrhythmia; R 28; 76/42/0, rt. arm, sitting.

   A. Explain the meaning and significance of each vital sign measurement, including the method and equipment used.

   Temperature: ____

   Pulse: ____

   Respiration: ____

   Blood pressure: ____

   B. Chris is fussy and disagreeable, but not uncooperative, while Ellen takes his vital signs. What can a medical assistant do to facilitate the measurement of a fussy child's vital signs?

   ____

   ____

3. Ellen assists Dr. King with the physical examination of the patient. After assessing the vital sign measurements taken by the medical assistant, Dr. King examines Chris's ear and lungs. A swab of fluid discharge is taken from the patient's ear. What is the role of the medical assistant during the physician's examination of this patient?

____

____

____

____

4. Dr. King makes a clinical diagnosis of otitis media for this patient and orders laboratory testing to be performed on the patient's specimen.

   A. What criteria are necessary for a physician to make a clinical diagnosis?

   ___

   B. What is otitis media? Why are children more likely at risk for this condition? How is otitis media commonly treated? What patient education can the health care team offer? (Consult a medical reference or encyclopedia for help in answering this question.)

   ___

   ___

CERTIFICATION REVIEW

These questions are designed to mimic the certification examinations. You can use these questions like a small "Certification Examination Study Guide," but this is not meant to take the place of the more extensive study guides. Use this portion to determine in what areas to concentrate your efforts when studying for the certification examination.

1. The head circumference of a newborn should range between:
   a. 12.5 and 14.5 inches
   b. 14.5 and 16.5 inches
   c. 16.5 and 18.5 inches
   d. 18.5 and 20.5 inches

2. The axillary temperature is taken:
   a. in the rectum
   b. in the mouth
   c. in the armpit
   d. in the ear

3. The respiratory rate of a 1-year-old child should range between _____ breaths per minute.
   a. 20 and 30
   b. 20 and 40
   c. 16 and 20
   d. 12 and 20

4. Otitis media is:
   a. an inflammation of the middle ear
   b. an infestation of parasitic lice
   c. spasms of the bronchi
   d. an infection of the tonsils

CASE STUDY

The following is a true story of a young boy (about age 8 years) who presented to the urologist with testicular torsion. Background information includes testicles that are suspended in the scrotal sac by the vas deferens tube. Occasionally, a testicle can become twisted, causing circulation to become compromised. The testicle swells, becomes extremely painful, and can quickly become necrotic from lack of blood supply. When this occurs, the solution is surgery. Either the testicle is removed (if it has become damaged), or it is surgically tacked into place. The other testicle is also tacked into place, so it does not occur on the other side in the future. In this case, the young boy started crying when he was told that he needed to go to the surgery center, that the doctor would put him to sleep and then would fix his testicle, and that when he woke up he would feel a lot better. The child was inconsolable. Why do you think he was so upset?

a. He was scared of the pain.

b. He was afraid of what would happen.

c. He was embarrassed.

d. Other ______________________________

Discuss this situation with your classmates, either in small groups or as a whole class, and see what other reasons for the patient's reaction you can gather. The answer will be revealed to you by your instructor after your discussion. The answer was revealed to me when I sat down with the boy and asked him exactly what frightened him. I was planning to reassure him that it would not hurt because he would be asleep during the procedure. I had assumed that his real concern was the pain. When you learn the reason this child was afraid, you need to remember not to assume that you already know the cause and also remember to talk and listen to the patient.

SELF-ASSESSMENT

As you respond to the following questions, think of how your experiences will affect how you treat your patients.

1. Think of your first memory of going to the doctor's office or getting any medical treatment. Think of how you felt from what you can remember. You may have more than one vivid memory, or you may have to think really hard to come up with any memories. Maybe your memories are not at a hospital or doctor's office; that is, maybe you received medical care from your parents, grandparents, or a neighbor. Your memories might not be exactly accurate, but they are a child's perception, and the feelings are real. This awareness can help you interact well with your young patients. Circle all of the words from the following list that come to mind as you take this mental journey back in time (if you have more than one incident to remember, use different colored inks to circle the words). You may even add a couple of your own descriptors if necessary.

helpless	embarrassed	alone
afraid of pain	relieved	excited
pain	guilty	afraid of being punished
happy with the attention	loved	safe
invaded	angry	afraid of what was happening
dizzy	powerless	afraid of the blood
stupid	______________	______________

Each of our memories will be different, and we will all have different feelings about them. Try to keep this in mind as you treat your young patients. Try to respect what feelings they have and strive to make them comfortable. Reasure them as much as you can.

POST-TEST

This is similar to the Pre-Test. Perform this test without looking at the book. This is just to see how well you have understood and can recall the information presented in this chapter after you have studied it and completed the workbook exercises. You will not be graded on this portion (other than the grade you give yourself), but this is an excellent preparation for your instructor's test. You may use this Post-Test to determine in what areas you need to study more. Justify any "false" answers.

1. Pediatrics is the practice of medicine with children from birth through age 14. (T or F)
2. Toddlers are children from:
   a. about 1 to 3 years old
   b. birth to 2 years old
   c. the time they are able to walk until they are in kindergarten
   d. about 2 to 5 years old
3. Measurements of babies consist of chest circumference, head circumference, length, and weight. (T or F)
4. Normal childhood immunizations include of which of the following:
   a. MMR, tetanus, DTaP, and IPV
   b. Hib, DTaP, MMR, and HIV
   c. IPV, MMR, DTaP, Hib, and HBV
   d. HBV, Hib, pertussis, and HAV
   e. both c and d
5. The preferred site for injections for a child younger than 2 years is:
   a. the vastus lateralis
   b. the gluteus medius
   c. the deltoid
   d. any of the above sites are acceptable
6. Normal pulse and respiration for a child who is 8 years old is:
   a. respiration of 30, pulse of 80
   b. respiration of 18, pulse of 86
   c. respiration of 12, pulse of 80
   d. respiration of 20, pulse of 120
   e. none of the above

CERTIFICATION CRITERIA CHECKLIST

As you go through your education and training, keep in mind the national certification examination that you will take when you graduate. Each chapter of the textbook and workbook covers a different section of the examination criteria. To keep track of your preparation for the certification examination, turn to the back of this workbook and highlight the following CMA, RMA, or CMAS certification examination criteria (if you have already highlighted them from a previous chapter, put a check mark by the criteria):

CMA

E. Communication
  1. Adapting communication to an individual's ability to understand

T. Patient Preparation and Assisting the Physician
  2. Vital signs
  3. Examinations

V. Collecting and Processing Specimens; Diagnostic Testing

W. Preparing and Administering Medications
  1. Pharmacology
  4. Maintaining medication and immunization records

RMA

I. General Medical Assisting Knowledge
  F. Patient Education

III. Clinical Medical Assisting
  D. Vital Signs and Mensurations
  E. Physical Examinations
  F. Clinical Pharmacology

CMAS

2. Basic Clinical Medical Office Assisting
  - Vital signs and measurements
  - Examination preparation
  - Basic pharmacology

COMPETENCY ASSESSMENT

Procedure 27-1 Maintaining Immunization Records

Performance Objectives: To establish and maintain a record of childhood immunizations. Perform this objective within 15 minutes with a minimum score of 25 points.

Supplies/Equipment: Medication note of vaccine ordered and administered, vial of vaccine administered, child's Vaccine Administration Record, patient chart, pen

Charting/Documentation: Enter appropriate documentation/charting in the box.

Instructor's/Evaluator's Comments and Suggestions:

SKILLS CHECKLIST Procedure 27-1: Maintaining Immunization Records

Name ______________________

Date ______________________

No.	Skill	Check #1 20 pts ea	Check #2 10 pts ea	Check #3 5 pts ea	Notes
1	Give the parent the most recent copy of the Vaccine Information Statement (VIS).				
2	After administering the vaccine, document the procedure in the patient's medical record and in his or her Vaccine Record.				
3	Using the medication note and the vaccine vial, fill out the Vaccine Record according to which vaccine you administered. Note the headings, type of vaccine, date given (month, day, year), dose, route, site, vaccine lot number, and manufacturer. Make a notation as to which VIS was given, the date it was given, and your signature.				
4	File the clinic copy and give the parent the patient's copy.				
5	Document steps taken.				
Student's Total Points					
Points Possible		100	50	25	
Final Score (Student's Total Points / Possible Points)					

	Notes
Start time:	
End time:	
Total time: (15 min goal)	

COMPETENCY ASSESSMENT

Procedure 27-2 Measuring the Infant: Weight, Length, Head, and Chest Circumference

Performance Objectives: To obtain an accurate measurement of an infant's weight, length, head circumference, and chest circumference. Perform this objective within 30 minutes with a minimum score of 150 points.

Supplies/Equipment: Infant scale, paper protector, flexible nonstretchy measuring tape, straight-edge ruler, measuring board (optional), patient's medical record including a growth chart, pen, biohazard waste container, drape or towel

Charting/Documentation: Enter appropriate documentation/charting in the box.

____

____

____

____

Instructor's/Evaluator's Comments and Suggestions:

____

____

____

____

____

____

SKILLS CHECKLIST Procedure 27-2: Measuring the Infant: Weight, Length, Head, and Chest Circumference

Name ______________________

Date ______________________

No.	Skill	Check #1 20 pts ea	Check #2 10 pts ea	Check #3 5 pts ea	Notes
Measuring Weight					
1	Wash hands. Explain the procedure to the parents.				
2	Undress the infant (including the diaper).				
3	Place all weights to left of scale to check balance.				
4	Place a clean paper drape or towel on scale; check balance of scale for accuracy, being sure to compensate for the weight of the towel.				
5	Gently place infant on the scale on his or her back. Place own hand slightly above the infant to ensure safety.				
6	Place the bottom weight to its highest measurement that will not cause the balance to drop to the bottom edge.				
7	Slowly move upper weight until the balance bar rests in the center of the indicator. Read the infant's weight while he or she is lying still.				
8	Return both weights to their resting position to the extreme left.				
9	Gently remove infant and assist parent to apply diaper as needed.				
10	Discard used protective paper drape or towel.				
11	Sanitize scale.				
12	Wash hands (if examination is complete).				
13	Document results on growth chart, patient's chart, and parent's booklet, if available. Connects dots from previous examination with a straight edge to complete graph.				
Measuring Length					
1	Wash hands. Explain procedure to parents.				
2	Remove infant's shoes.				
3	Gently place infant on his or her back on the examination table. If a measuring board is being used, hold infant's head against the				

No.	Skill	Check #1 20 pts ea	Check #2 10 pts ea	Check #3 5 pts ea	Notes
	headboard at zero and the heel against the footboard. If using a measuring tape, hold the head steady and mark the top of the head on the table paper. Gently walk your hands down the body of the infant to the heel, ensuring that the head does not shift and the paper is not wrinkling. Keeping the leg straight, mark the end of the heel on the table paper.				
4	Gently remove the infant and return to parents. Measure the distance between the head mark and the heel mark. Read the length in inches and centimeters.				
5	Wash hands (if examination is complete).				
6	Document on the growth chart and in the medical record.				
Measuring Head Circumference					
1	Wash hands and explain procedure to parents.				
2	Establish rapport with infant.				
3	Place measuring tape snug around the forehead at the widest part.				
4	Read the measurement.				
5	Return the child to the parent. Wash hands (if examination is complete).				
6	Document the measurements in the medical record and on the growth chart.				
Measuring Chest Circumference					
1	Wash hands and explain the procedure to the parents.				
2	Use one thumb to hold the tape measure at the zero mark against the infant's chest at the midsternal area.				
3	Read measurement to the nearest 0.01 cm.				
4	Wash hands.				
5	Document the results.				
Student's Total Points					
Points Possible (30 steps)		600	300	150	
Final Score (Student's Total Points / Possible Points)					

	Notes
Start time:	
End time:	
Total time: (30 min goal)	

COMPETENCY ASSESSMENT

Procedure 27-3 Taking an Infant's Rectal Temperature with a Digital Thermometer

Performance Objectives: To obtain a rectal temperature using a digital thermometer. Perform this objective within 15 minutes with a minimum score of 100 points.

Supplies/Equipment: Digital thermometer (red probe) and probe cover, lubricating jelly, 4 × 4 gauze sponges, gloves, biohazard waste container

Charting/Documentation: Enter appropriate documentation/charting in the box.

Instructor's/Evaluator's Comments and Suggestions:

SKILLS CHECKLIST Procedure 27-3: Taking an Infant's Rectal Temperature with a Digital Thermometer

Name ______________________________

Date ______________________________

No.	Skill	Check #1 20 pts ea	Check #2 10 pts ea	Check #3 5 pts ea	Notes
1	Wash hands.				
2	Assemble equipment.				
3	Identify the patient.				
4	Explain the procedure to the parent(s).				
5	Remove the infant's diaper.				
6	Position the infant in a prone or supine position, having parent or another medical assistant safeguard.				
7	Place sheath on the thermometer.				
8	Lubricate the tip of the thermometer.				
9	Apply gloves.				
10	Spread the infant's buttocks, then insert the thermometer gently into the rectum past the sphincter. For an infant, this is 0.5 inch.				
11	Hold buttocks together while holding the thermometer. If necessary, restrain the infant.				
12	Hold the thermometer in place until the beep is heard.				
13	Remove the thermometer from the rectum.				
14	Note the temperature reading.				
15	Remove the probe cover by ejecting it into a biohazard waste container.				
16	Remove gloves; discard in biohazard waste container.				
17	Wash hands.				
18	Wipe probe with antiseptic and replace the thermometer on holder base.				

No.	Skill	Check #1 20 pts ea	Check #2 10 pts ea	Check #3 5 pts ea	Notes
19	Assist the parent in dressing the infant as necessary.				
20	Record in the patient's chart as a rectal temperature.				
Student's Total Points					
Points Possible		400	200	100	
Final Score (Student's Total Points / Possible Points)					

	Notes
Start time:	
End time:	
Total time: (15 min goal)	

COMPETENCY ASSESSMENT

Procedure 27-4 Taking an Apical Pulse on an Infant

Performance Objectives: To obtain an apical pulse rate. Perform this objective within 15 minutes with a minimum score of 80 points.

Supplies/Equipment: Stethoscope, watch with second hand, alcohol wipes

Charting/Documentation: Enter appropriate documentation/charting in the box.

Instructor's/Evaluator's Comments and Suggestions:

SKILLS CHECKLIST Procedure 27-4: Taking an Apical Pulse on an Infant

Name ______________________

Date ______________________

No.	Skill	Check #1 20 pts ea	Check #2 10 pts ea	Check #3 5 pts ea	Notes
1	Wash hands.				
2	Assemble equipment.				
3	Identify the patient.				
4	Explain the procedure to the parent(s).				
5	Assist in undressing the infant, if necessary.				
6	Provide a drape for the infant, if necessary for warmth				
7	Position the infant in a supine position or seated in the parent's lap.				
8	Locate the fifth intercostals space, midclavicular line, left of sternum.				
9	Places warmed stethoscope on the site and listen for the lub-dup sound of the heart.				
10	Count the pulse for 1 minute; each lub-dub equals one heartbeat.				
11	Wash hands.				
12	Record the pulse in the infant's chart with the designation of "(AP)" to denote the apical method of obtaining the pulse.				
13	Note any arrhythmias.				
14	Assist the patient and parents as needed.				
15	Clean the earpieces and diaphragm of the stethoscope with alcohol wipes.				
16	Wash hands again.				
Student's Total Points					
Points Possible		320	160	80	
Final Score (Student's Total Points / Possible Points)					

	Notes
Start time:	
End time:	
Total time: (15 min goal)	

COMPETENCY ASSESSMENT

Procedure 27-5 Measuring Infant's Respiration Rate

Performance Objectives: To measure the infant's respiration rate. Perform this objective within 15 minutes with a minimum score of 35 points.

Supplies/Equipment: Watch with second hand

Charting/Documentation: Enter appropriate documentation/charting in the box.

Instructor's/Evaluator's Comments and Suggestions:

SKILLS CHECKLIST Procedure 27-5: Measuring Infant's Respiration Rate

Name ______________________

Date ______________________

No.	Skill	Check #1 20 pts ea	Check #2 10 pts ea	Check #3 5 pts ea	Notes
1	Wash hands.				
2	Identify the patient.				
3	Position the infant in a supine position.				
4	Place hand on the infant's chest to feel the rise and fall of the chest wall for 1 minute.				
5	Note depth, rhythm, and breath sounds while counting.				
6	Wash hands.				
7	Record the respiration rate in patient's chart, noting irregularities and sounds.				
Student's Total Points					
Points Possible		140	70	35	
Final Score (Student's Total Points / Possible Points)					
		Notes			
Start time:					
End time:					
Total time: (15 min goal)					

COMPETENCY ASSESSMENT

Procedure 27-6 Obtaining a Urine Specimen from an Infant or Young Child

Performance Objectives: To obtain a specimen of urine from an infant or a young child. Perform this objective within 20 minutes with a minimum score of 65 points.

Supplies/Equipment: Urine collection bag, laboratory request form, gloves, washcloth, soap, water, towel, biohazard waste container

Charting/Documentation: Enter appropriate documentation/charting in the box.

Instructor's/Evaluator's Comments and Suggestions:

SKILLS CHECKLIST Procedure 27-6: Obtaining a Urine Specimen from an Infant or Young Child

Name ______________________

Date ______________________

No.	Skill	Check #1 20 pts ea	Check #2 10 pts ea	Check #3 5 pts ea	Notes
1	Wash and glove hands.				
2	Assemble equipment.				
3	Identify the patient and explain the procedure to the parent(s).				
4	Instruct the parent to remove the diaper.				
5	Wash and dry perineal area.				
6	Apply the collection bag, secure with adhesive tabs.				
7	Replace the diaper carefully.				
8	Frequently check the bag for urine.				
9	Remove the bag carefully after the specimen has been collected.				
10	Prepare the specimen as required. Send to the laboratory in a specimen container with a requisition, or process the specimen in the physician's office laboratory.				
11	Remove gloves and discard in biohazard waste container.				
12	Wash hands.				
13	Record collection in the patient's chart.				
Student's Total Points					
Points Possible		260	130	65	
Final Score (Student's Total Points / Possible Points)					

	Notes
Start time:	
End time:	
Total time: (20 min goal)	

EVALUATION OF CHAPTER KNOWLEDGE

Skills	Student Self-Evaluation		
	Good	Average	Poor
I understand the growth and development stages of the pediatric patient.	____	____	____
I understand the immunization schedule and the preventable diseases specific to the pediatric population.	____	____	____
I can demonstrate the ability to measure weight, height, head circumference, and chest circumference of the pediatric patient.	____	____	____
I can demonstrate the ability to obtain accurate vital signs from the pediatric patient.	____	____	____
I can prepare the pediatric patient for examination.	____	____	____
I observe all Standard Precautions and apply principles of aseptic technique.	____	____	____

CHAPTER 28

Male Reproductive System

CHAPTER PRE-TEST

Perform this test without looking at the book. This is just to see how well you have understood and can recall the information in this chapter after you have read it, but before you have completed the workbook exercises. You will not be graded on this portion (other than the grade you give yourself).

1. The most common disease afflicting men older than 50 years is:
   a. prostate cancer
   b. benign prostatic hypertrophy (BPH)
   c. epididymitis
   d. testicular cancer

2. ED stands for:
   a. erectile disorder
   b. erectile dysfunction
   c. elemental disease
   d. epididymal disorder

3. Which of the following is *not* a sexually transmitted disease (STD) that afflicts men?
   a. genital herpes
   b. chlamydia
   c. gonorrhea
   d. epididymis

4. Vasectomy consists of:
   a. dissection of the seminal vesicles
   b. dissection of the vas deferens
   c. dissection of the testicles
   d. removal of the epididymis

INTRODUCTION

Medical assistants must have a fundamental knowledge of the male reproductive system when assisting the physician with examinations and procedures related to the male system. Medical assisting students can use this chapter to test themselves in the knowledge of the reproductive system of the male, including familiarity with diseases and treatments that they may encounter in the ambulatory center.

PERFORMANCE OBJECTIVES

After successful completion of this chapter you will be able to define the terms related to the male reproductive system, as well as the most common diseases and disorders, and their symptoms, diagnostic tests, and treatments. You will be familiar with the anatomy and physiology of the male reproductive system. You will also understand the importance of health promotion and prevention of diseases that afflict men. You will be able to assist men in understanding the importance of and the process of testicular self-examination on a regular basis. You will know how to assist the physician in surgical and other procedures related to the male reproductive system. *The following statements are related to your learning objectives for this chapter. Fill in the blanks in the following paragraph with the appropriate term(s).*

The male reproductive system consists of a pair of (1) ________________ suspended in the (2) ____________________ in which sperm and (3) ______________________ are produced. The scrotum can contract and relax to help regulate the (4) ____________________________ of the testes for optimum (5) ______________________________. The male reproductive system is closely related to the male (6) ______________________ system, which explains why diseases and disorders of one system will probably affect the other. A disease in which the prostate gland becomes enlarged is called (7) ____. A disease in which the prostate becomes inflamed is called (8) ___________________________. Cancer of the (9) ________________________ is the leading cause of cancer death in men after lung and colon cancer. The PSA test is a (10) ___________________ test. PSA stands for (11) _____________________________. The PSA test is specifically related to the activity of the (12) _______________________ gland. A (13) ______________ must be performed to definitively diagnose cancer of the prostate. A condition in which the epididymis becomes inflamed is called (14) ______________________. It is usually caused by (15) ______________________. (16) ______________________ is a disease usually caused by poor hygiene in uncircumcised men. In severe cases, (17) ______________________ may be necessary. Treatment of male infertility will depend on the (18) ____________. If the reason is a blockage, (19) ______________________ is indicated. If the reason is an infection, (20) ______________________ will be prescribed. Other reasons may not be treatable, and (21) ______________________ may be attempted to conceive. ED or (22) ______________________, also called impotence, occurs with the inability to achieve or maintain an erection. Sometimes the cause is (23) ______________________; other times it is physical. Treatment is based on the (24) ______________________ of the dysfunction. (25) ______________________ is the name of the surgical procedure that is performed if sterilization is desired. It involves the dissection of the (26) ______________________ on both sides.

VOCABULARY BUILDER

Find the words in Column A below that are misspelled; circle them, and then correctly spell them in the spaces provided. Then match the following correct vocabulary terms listed in Column A with their corresponding definitions listed in Column B.

Column A

A. Chriptorchidism
B. Intervenous pyelogram
C. Orchiectomy
D. Residual
E. Retention
F. Transluminator
G. Transureteral resection

____
____
____
____

Column B

_____ 1. Urine held in the bladder; inability to empty the bladder
_____ 2. Amount of urine remaining in bladder immediately after voiding; seen with hyperplasia of prostate
_____ 3. Undescended testicle
_____ 4. X-ray of the kidneys, ureter, and bladder using a contrast medium
_____ 5. Instrument used to inspect a cavity or organ by passing a light through the walls
_____ 6. Removal of prostate tissue using a device inserted through the urethra
_____ 7. Surgical excision of a testicle

LEARNING REVIEW

1. Identify each part of the male reproductive system in Figure 28-1. Describe each part and its function in the space provided. Then, using the textbook, a medical dictionary, or the Internet, list one common disorder that would adversely affect the part described.

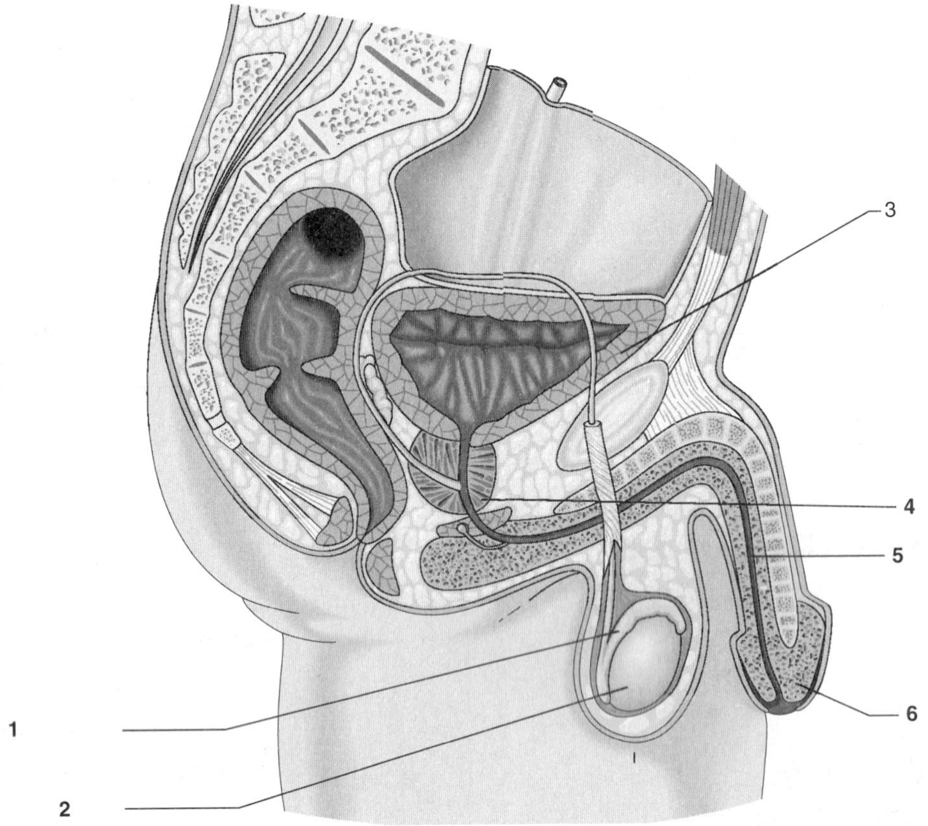

Figure 28-1

(1) Part: ______________________________

Common disorder: ______________________________

(2) Part: ______________________________

Common disorder: ______________________________

(3) Part: ______________________________

Common disorder: ______________________________

(4) Part: ______________________________

Common disorder: ______________________________

(5) Part: ______________________________

Common disorder: ______________________________

(6) Part: ______________________________

Common disorder: ______________________________

2. Which is a common symptom of benign hypertrophic prostate gland?
   a. the inability to empty the bladder
   b. a diminished flow of urine
   c. difficulty with starting to urinate
   d. all of the above

3. The third leading cause of cancer deaths among men is:
   a. testicular cancer
   b. lung cancer
   c. prostate cancer
   d. none of the above

4. The best way to determine that a patient has prostate cancer is by a(n):
   a. biopsy of the prostate
   b. PSA blood test
   c. rectal examination
   d. x-ray

5. Which of the following is not a sexually transmitted disease?
   a. hyperplasia
   b. gonorrhea
   c. syphilis
   d. chlamydia

6. PSA tests should be performed:
   a. monthly
   b. biannually
   c. annually
   d. every 6 months

CERTIFICATION REVIEW

These questions are designed to mimic the certification examinations. You can use these questions like a small "Certification Examination Study Guide," but this is not meant to take the place of the more extensive study guides. Use this portion to determine in what areas to concentrate your efforts when studying for the certification examination. Justify any "false" answers.

1. Testicular cancer is one of the leading causes of death in men younger than:
   a. 25
   b. 60
   c. 40
   d. 50

2. Male individuals from the onset of puberty should examine their testicles every:
   a. 6 months
   b. year
   c. month
   d. 3 months

3. BPH is a condition of the prostate. It stands for:
   a. benign prostatic hypertrophy
   b. benign prostatic hyperplasia
   c. beginning prostate hyperactivity
   d. benign prostate hyperactivity

4. Because of the latest discoveries in medications, ED can always be cured. (T or F)

5. Which of the following STDs is *not* treated with antibiotics?
   a. chlamydia
   b. gonorrhea
   c. syphilis
   d. genital herpes
   e. none of the above

CASE STUDY

Mr. Jones, a 75-year-old patient, has just been diagnosed with prostatic cancer. The physician has explained what is to be expected, but he is upset and asks you for your help in understanding the disease and treatment. How will you help him?

SELF-ASSESSMENT

How do you think you will feel when assisting with a genitourinary examination or procedure on a male patient? Do you think it will be easier if the patient is much younger or much older than you are? Do you think older medical assistants feel more comfortable assisting with these types of examinations, regardless of their professional experience? Do you think you will become more comfortable with time? Do you think your male patient is also uncomfortable?

After giving these questions some thought, answer the following questions. Discuss your ideas with other students. Discuss your ideas with male friends, family members, or classmates to gain more perspectives.

1. Do you think your behavior or attitude will have anything to do with your patient's comfort level?

2. What might you do to make yourself more comfortable during a male genitourinary examination/procedure?

3. What might you do to make your patient more comfortable?

4. What would you do if a patient became "suggestive" or made a lewd comment directed toward you?

POST-TEST

This is similar to the Pre-Test. Perform this test without looking at the book. This is just to see how well you have understood and can recall the information presented in this chapter after you have studied it and completed the workbook exercises. You will not be graded on this portion (other than the grade you give yourself), but this is an excellent preparation for your instructor's test. You may use this Post-Test to determine what areas you need to study more.

1. In men older than 50 years, a common disease condition is:
   a. prostate cancer
   b. BPH
   c. epididymitis
   d. testicular cancer

2. ED stands for:
   a. erectile dysfunction
   b. erectile disorder
   c. erectile disease
   d. epididymal disorder

3. Which of the following is an STD that afflicts men?
   a. chlamydia
   b. balanitis
   c. Peyronie's
   d. epididymis

4. The dissection of the vas deferens is called a:
   a. vas-deferenectomy
   b. vasotomy
   c. vasectomy
   d. deferenectomy

CERTIFICATION CRITERIA CHECKLIST

As you go through your education and training, keep in mind the national certification examination that you will take when you graduate. Each chapter of the textbook and workbook covers a different section of the examination criteria. To keep track of your preparation for the certification examination, turn to the back of this workbook and highlight the following CMA, RMA, or CMAS certification examination criteria (if you have already highlighted them from a previous chapter, put a check mark by the criteria):

CMA

A. Medical Terminology
B. Anatomy and Physiology
E. Communication
    3. Patient instruction
P. Office Policies and Procedures
    2. Patient education
T. Patient Preparation and Assisting the Physician
    3. Examinations
    4. Procedures
V. Collecting and Processing Specimens; Diagnostic Testing

RMA

I. General Medical Assisting Knowledge
    A. Anatomy and Physiology
    B. Medical Terminology
    F. Patient Education
III. Clinical Medical Assisting
    E. Physical Examinations
    I. Laboratory Procedures

CMAS

1. Medical Assisting Foundation
    - Medical terminology
    - Anatomy and physiology
2. Basic Clinical Medical Office Assisting
    - Examination preparation

COMPETENCY ASSESSMENT

Procedure 28-1 Instructing Patient in Testicular Self-Examination

Performance Objectives: To provide a patient with the correct procedure for performing testicular self-examination. Perform this objective within 15 minutes with a minimum score of 35 points.

Supplies/Equipment: Testicular self-examination card, anatomy illustration

Charting/Documentation: Enter appropriate documentation/charting in the box.

____

____

____

____

Instructor's/Evaluator's Comments and Suggestions:

____

____

____

____

____

____

SKILLS CHECKLIST Procedure 28-1: Instructing Patient in Testicular Self-Examination

Name ______________________

Date ______________________

No.	Skill	Check #1 20 pts ea	Check #2 10 pts ea	Check #3 5 pts ea	Notes
1	Identify yourself and explain the procedure.				
2	Explain that the patient should examine his testicles in a warm shower.				
3	Instruct the patient to examine each testicle separately with both hands.				
4	Instruct him to place the index and middle fingers underneath the testicle and the thumbs on top. Roll the testicle gently between the fingers.				
5	Instruct him how to locate the epididymis and to look for swelling or changes in the scrotal area.				
6	Provide an anatomy chart to him that illustrates the testes and epididymis. Provide him with a testicular self-examination card and encourage the patient to report any unusual findings to you or the physician immediately.				
7	Document your patient education.				
Student's Total Points					
Points Possible		140	70	35	
Final Score (Student's Total Points / Possible Points)					

	Notes
Start time:	
End time:	
Total time: (15 min goal)	

EVALUATION OF CHAPTER KNOWLEDGE

Skills	Student Self-Evaluation Good	Average	Poor
I understand the importance of health promotion and prevention of disease with the male patient.	____	____	____
I can explain testicular self-examination.	____	____	____
I can describe common disorders and diseases of the male reproductive system.	____	____	____
I can identify signs and symptoms of the various disorders and diseases of the male reproductive system.	____	____	____
I can describe common diagnostic tests and procedures used in the male reproductive system.	____	____	____

CHAPTER 29

Gerontology

CHAPTER PRE-TEST

Perform this test without looking at the book. This is just to see how well you have understood and can recall the information in this chapter after you have read it, but before you have completed the workbook exercises. You will not be graded on this portion (other than the grade you give yourself). Justify any "false" answers.

1. Older adults are healthier today than they were a generation ago. (T or F)
2. Chronic diseases are just a part of what will happen as we age. (T or F)
3. To be old is to be sick, weak, and confused. (T or F)
4. Every system in the body undergoes changes as people age. (T or F)
5. The senses of sight, hearing, taste, and smell diminish with age. (T or F)
6. There is not much a person can do to counteract the effects of aging. (T or F)

INTRODUCTION

The care of the older adult patient is becoming more apparent as society ages. Over the next 30 years, the population will continue to grow older. The body systems go through many changes, which can lead to problems with health. There are societal biases that occur, leading to psychological difficulties in older adults. Medical assistants must be knowledgeable about the needs of the aged, including their societal, psychological, and physical needs. They also must be able to communicate well with older adults and identify special issues, such as elder abuse, and special needs, such as vision and hearing impairments.

PERFORMANCE OBJECTIVES

After successful completion of this chapter you will be able to explain the terminology related to geriatrics. You will understand the normal aging processes and the stereotyping that can sometimes present as discrimination. You will have learned to be sensitive to the myths about aging and to be aware of the changes that do occur with aging. You will know how to help aging patients stay healthy and how to prevent some of the complications that can come with age-related disorders. You will have skills to communicate effectively with your aging patients, especially the hearing and visually impaired. You will also be aware of challenges and successful techniques to use when working with memory-impaired patients. *The following statements are related to your learning objectives for this chapter. Fill in the blanks in the following paragraph with the appropriate term(s).*

(1) ________________ is the branch of medicine that encompasses older adults and their special needs. Aging is (2) ______________________ and universal. There is no (3) _____________________ specific to aging. Some functional changes are related to (4) _____________, (5) ______________, and (6) _______________ resources. (7) ______________ structure, (8) _________________, and (9) _______________ all play a part. Some of the factors that can influence an individual's degree of aging are smoking, misuse of chemicals such as (10) __________________________ or other (11) ________________________, type of (12) ______________________, and (13) __________________________________. Visual changes may occur because of (14) __________________________ production of (15) ____________________. (16) ____________________ loss is not uncommon. This occurs over a period of years. (17) __________________ and (18) ______________________ may also diminish, making food less appealing. This can lead to (19) ___________ of weight, and the person can even become (20) _________________________. Skin changes can also occur, and hair (21) ____________ or thinning of the hair can be a problem. The brain shrinks in size, causing some loss of (22) ________________ for some but not all people. Often, older adults have less (23) ________________ strength and are less (24) _______________________. Lung capacity can decrease, and blood vessels can undergo changes. Other changes in other systems can occur, but all in all, today's older adults are more (25) ______________________ and healthier than ever before. Knowing about the changes that can occur in older adults can help patients and their health care providers eliminate or forestall complications. There are many techniques the (26) ___________________________ can do to communicate more effectively with older adults. You should talk (27) _______________________ and (28) ____________________, while keeping the tone (29) ________________. Keep instructions (30) ____________________. Listen carefully and treat all people with respect.

VOCABULARY BUILDER

Find the words from Column A that are misspelled; circle them, and then correctly spell them in the spaces provided. Then match the following correct vocabulary terms listed in Column A with their corresponding definitions listed in Column B.

Column A

A. Arterialsclerosis
B. Dementia
C. Geriatrics
D. Incontinance
E. Macular degeneration
F. Pernicous anemia
G. Presbycusis
H. Residule urine
I. Transient ischemic attack

____

____

____

____

Column B

_____ 1. The branch of medicine that deals with older adults

_____ 2. Disease marked by degeneration of the macular area of the retina of the eye

_____ 3. Progressive loss of hearing ability caused by the normal aging process

_____ 4. Temporary loss of blood to the brain, causing strokelike symptoms

_____ 5. Urine remaining in the bladder after urination

_____ 6. Loss of the ability to retain urine in the bladder

_____ 7. Disorder involving the stomach that causes a deficiency of red blood cells

_____ 8. Decrease in cognitive abilities, especially memory impairment, often associated with Alzheimer's and Parkinson's diseases

_____ 9. Disease that leads to thickening, hardening, and loss of elasticity of the arteries

LEARNING REVIEW

Identification of System Problems

1. A. List two problems that might occur with each system as people age.

   1. Vision and hearing: (a) ______________________________
      (b) ______________________________
   2. Taste and smell: (a) ______________________________
      (b) ______________________________
   3. Integumentary system: (a) ______________________________
      (b) ______________________________
   4. Nervous system: (a) ______________________________
      (b) ______________________________
   5. Musculoskeletal system: (a) ______________________________
      (b) ______________________________
   6. Respiratory system: (a) ______________________________
      (b) ______________________________

7. Cardiovascular system: (a) ______________________
(b) ______________________

8. Gastrointestinal system: (a) ______________________
(b) ______________________

9. Urinary system: (a) ______________________
(b) ______________________

10. Reproductive system: (a) ______________________
(b) ______________________

B. List five ways to improve communication with the geriatric patient.
(1) ______________________
(2) ______________________
(3) ______________________
(4) ______________________
(5) ______________________

2. Why is gerontology becoming more recognized?
   a. The population is decreasing.
   b. The population is increasing.
   c. The average life span is decreasing.
   d. The average life span is increasing.

3. The progressive loss of hearing ability caused by the normal aging process is called:
   a. senility
   b. presbycusis
   c. deafness
   d. audio deficiency

4. Why does food become less appealing as one ages, often decreasing the desire to eat and causing weight loss?
   a. taste buds decrease in size
   b. taste buds increase in size
   c. teeth deteriorate
   d. acid indigestion

5. The nervous system is affected by aging, resulting in all of the following *except*:
   a. insomnia
   b. problems with balance
   c. increased pain sensation
   d. problems with temperature regulation

6. The buildup of plaque in blood vessels is called:
   a. incontinence
   b. heart attack
   c. arteriosclerosis
   d. cardiopulmonary dysfunction

CERTIFICATION REVIEW

These questions are designed to mimic the certification examinations. You can use these questions like a small "Certification Examination Study Guide," but this is not meant to take the place of the more extensive study guides. Use this portion to determine in what areas to concentrate your efforts when studying for the certification examination. Justify any "false" answers.

1. When giving instructions to older adults, it always a good idea to (circle all that apply):
   a. speak really loud
   b. write it down clearly and in a large print
   c. have patients repeat the instructions back to you if you think they did not understand completely
   d. a and b
   e. all of the above

2. When going over medications with geriatric patients, it is helpful for them to bring all their medications with them in their original containers. (T or F)

3. If you suggest memory joggers (such as use of a calendar for appointments and making lists) to your geriatric patients, you will insult their intelligence. (T or F)

4. Dementia can include:
   a. memory loss
   b. confusion
   c. aggression and agitation
   d. a and b only
   e. all of the above

5. Every system in the body is going to be affected by aging. (T or F)

6. Older adult patients have a heightened sense of pain compared with younger patients. (T or F)

CASE STUDIES

Case 1

Sam Jones, 84 years old, has been examined by the physician and is ready to leave the office. Mr. Jones tells you he is having trouble remembering to take the many medications the doctor has given him and that is why he forgets to take them. As the medical assistant, what can you tell Mr. Jones that will help him in taking his medications?

Case 2

Sandy Jones, the granddaughter of Sam Jones, has come to the office with her grandfather because she is concerned about his health. She tells you that she is concerned at the recent weight loss of her grandfather, but knows it is because of his not eating well. Mr. Jones is 84 years old and lives alone. How will you respond to Miss Jones?

SELF-ASSESSMENT

Without looking in the textbook, list 15 adjectives that describe older adults. Then list 15 adjectives that describe young adults. As you make your list, consider your personal biases toward older adults. Consider the differences in the two lists and think of why you chose those descriptors. When you are finished, discuss your lists with classmates. Share stories about people in your lives who are extraordinarily healthy and happy as they age. Think about the prejudices and assumptions you carry toward aging patients. Try to remember these as you work with those patients. It might be a good idea to create a list of tips to remember about geriatrics and keep it posted by your workstation.

POST-TEST

This is similar to the Pre-Test. Perform this test without looking at the book. This is just to see how well you have understood and can recall the information presented in this chapter after you have studied it and completed the workbook exercises. You will not be graded on this portion (other than the grade you give yourself), but this is an excellent preparation for your instructor's test. You may use this Post-Test to determine what areas you need to study more. Justify any "false" answers.

1. Older adults are less healthy today than they were a generation ago. (T or F)
2. Chronic diseases do not have to be a normal part of aging. (T or F)
3. Memory loss is Alzheimer's. (T or F)
4. Few changes occur as people age. (T or F)
5. As people age, their senses of sight, hearing, taste, and smell will diminish. (T or F)
6. There is much a person can do to counteract the effects of aging. (T or F)

CERTIFICATION CRITERIA CHECKLIST

As you go through your education and training, keep in mind the national certification examination that you will take when you graduate. Each chapter of the textbook and workbook covers a different section of the examination criteria. To keep track of your preparation for the certification examination, turn to the back of this workbook and highlight the following CMA, RMA, or CMAS certification examination criteria (if you have already highlighted them from a previous chapter, put a check mark by the criteria):

CMA

C. Psychology
   2. Developmental stages of the life cycle
   3. Hereditary, cultural and environmental influences on behavior

E. Communication
   1. Adapting communication to an individual's ability to understand
   3. Patient instruction
   4. Professional communication and behavior
   5. Evaluating and understanding communication

RMA

I. General Medical Assisting Knowledge
   E. Human Relations
   F. Patient Education

CMAS

1. Medical Assisting Foundation
   - Professionalism
2. Basic Clinical Medical Office Assisting
   - Basic health history interview

EVALUATION OF CHAPTER KNOWLEDGE

	Student Self-Evaluation		
Skills	Good	Average	Poor
I can explain expected physiologic changes that occur as part of the aging process.	_____	_____	_____
I can explain functional changes that can occur with aging.	_____	_____	_____
I can describe prevention techniques for complications arising from age-related disorders.	_____	_____	_____
I can explain myths about aging.	_____	_____	_____
I can explain communication techniques to use with older adults.	_____	_____	_____

CHAPTER 30

Examinations and Procedures of Body Systems

CHAPTER PRE-TEST

Perform this test without looking at the book. This is just to see how well you have understood and can recall the information in this chapter after you have read it, but before you have completed the workbook exercises. You will not be graded on this portion (other than the grade you give yourself). Justify any "false" answers.

1. Urinary catheterization is performed only in hospitals during surgeries. (T or F)
2. When performing a urinalysis, the specimen is automatically checked for drugs. (T or F)
3. Instillation and irrigation mean the same thing. (T or F)
4. A barium swallow is used to examine:
   a. the entire large intestine
   b. the stomach and the entire small intestine
   c. the stomach and part of the small intestine
   d. the esophagus, the stomach, the small and large intestines
5. To test visual acuity, the patient must be able to recognize the letters of the English alphabet. (T or F)
6. Medical assistants do not remove casts. (T or F)
7. Pulse oximetry is a way of counting the pulse at the wrist to determine the heart rate. (T or F)

INTRODUCTION

Patients with symptoms specific to a particular body system or body part need specialized care. Medical assistants assist the physician with many clinical procedures that are integral components of specialty examinations. Medical assistants who are employed in a specialist's office or a setting that treats a variety of patient problems will need additional skills and ongoing training to stay proficient in the most current technologies and treatments used to provide quality care to patients. Medical assisting students should use this workbook chapter to become familiar with specialties and body system examinations and with the appropriate clinical procedures in urology; the respiratory system; the musculoskeletal, neurologic, special senses, and circulatory systems; blood and lymph; and the integumentary system.

PERFORMANCE OBJECTIVES

After successful completion of this chapter you will be familiar with many patient examinations, techniques, equipment, and supplies needed. You will be able to perform many diagnostic tests related to specific conditions and diseases. You will know new methods of educating patients in preparation for examinations and diagnostic tests and also teaching them how to care for themselves after procedures and tests. You will also know how to care for your patients and assist the physician during specialty examinations, procedures, and diagnostic tests. This chapter also reexamines skills related to asepsis, sterile techniques, patient interaction and communications, vital signs, and patient assessments that were learned in other chapters. *The following statements are directly related to your learning objectives for this chapter. Fill in the blanks in the following paragraph with the appropriate term(s).*

As new diagnostic tests and treatment procedures are developed, the medical assistant may refine (1) ________________ skills and (2) ________________ new ones to be (3) ________________ and (4) ________________ and to provide the most (5) ________________, up-to-date (6) ________________ care to our patients. Patients with symptoms related to specific body systems need (7) ________________ care. The most common test to diagnose urinary system disorders is the (8) ________________. You will learn this procedure in Chapter 42. One of the ways to obtain a urine specimen for testing is through urinary (9) ________________. An IVP, which stands for (10) ________________, is used to examine the kidneys, ureters, and bladder using x-rays and an injection of an iodine-based (11) ________________ medium. A (12) ________________ procedure uses a lighted scope to visualize the interior of the bladder and the urethra. Urine may also be tested for illegal use or abuse of (13) ________________, which is a test that legally requires a signed (14) ________________ form from the patient. The digestive system has many diseases and disorders that may need to be (15) ________________ through special testing and procedures. Symptoms of digestive system disorders may include (16) ________________, (17) ________________, (18) ________________, (19) ________________,

(20) ______________________________, (21) ______________________________,
(22) ___________________________, (23) ________________________________,
(24) ______________________________, (25) ____________________________,
(26) ___________________________, and (27) ___________________________.
A peptic ulcer, if found in the stomach, is called a (28) ________________________ ulcer. An ulcer is an example of a digestive system disorder. Sometimes, gastric ulcers are caused by bacteria called (29) ______________________________. When a lighted fiberoptic scope, called an (30) ______________________________, is used to view the inside of the digestive organs, it is named after the organ it is examining. For example, the scope used to examine the esophagus, stomach, and duodenum is called an EGD or (31) ____________________________ ____________________. An endoscope used to view the inside of the colon or large intestine is called an (32) __________________________________, whereas the sigmoid portion of the colon is viewed with a shorter endoscope called a (33) _______________________________. Sometimes, the doctor will want to test a patient's stool for hidden (34) _______________ blood. This test requires a sample of stool that is tested using a chemical called a (35) ____________________. When testing the sharpness or (36) _________________ of a patient's vision. A distance of (37) ___________ feet is marked off for the patient to stand at while viewing the (38) ___________________________ eye chart. If a patient reads the chart well at the 20/40 line, that indicates the patient is seeing at (39) _________________ feet what normal vision would see at (40) ___________________ feet. This result indicates that the patient needs to see an (41) _________________________ or optometrist for further testing and perhaps prescription corrective glasses/contacts. The test most commonly performed for testing color vision uses the (42) ___________________________ plates. The ear will often become impacted with ear wax, called (43) ______________________, and the physician will recommend an ear flushing, called ear (44) _____________________________, to remove the wax. The medical assistant will always be aware of patient safety when performing this procedure. The respiratory system is all important to (45) _______________________________. We will sometimes use a test called a (46) _______________________ to measure air capacity, (47) ______________________________, and (48) ____________________________ of the lungs. These tests are called pulmonary (49) _______________________ tests or PFT. Pulse (50) ___________________________ is a test that determines the amount of oxygen saturated in the patient's blood. It consists of placing a small (51) _____________________ or clip onto the patient's finger, toe, (52) _________________________________, or (53) ______________________________. Musculoskeletal disorders consist of pain, strain, sprain, deformities, inflammation, diseases, and bone fractures. The most common disorder in this system is (54) __________________________________. Diagnostic procedures for fractures involve the use of (55) ______________________________ and visual examination

techniques. Examination of the neurologic system is performed in conjunction with the (56) ______________________________, but it can also be performed separately if the patient is exhibiting signs or symptoms such as (57) ______________, (58) ______________, (59) ______________, (60) ______________________________, or (61) ______________________.

VOCABULARY BUILDER

Find the words in Column A that are misspelled; circle them, and then correctly spell them in the spaces provided. Then match each of the correct vocabulary terms listed below to its proper definition.

Column A

______ 1. Erythemia
______ 2. Demyelination
______ 3. Comedome
______ 4. Carbuncle
______ 5. Bronchi
______ 6. Biopsy
______ 7. Auricle
______ 8. Aphasia
______ 9. Alveoli
______ 10. Akinesia
______ 11. Vescicle
______ 12. Spirometer
______ 13. Ossicle
______ 14. Opthalmoscope
______ 15. Ocluder
______ 16. Obturator
______ 17. Nebulizer
______ 18. Lesion
______ 19. Hydronephrosis
______ 20. Gate

____
____
____
____
____

Column B

A. Complete or partial loss of muscle movement
B. Air sacs in the lungs
C. The absence or impairment of the ability to communicate through speech
D. The portion of the external ear that is not connected to the head
E. Obtaining a representative tissue sample for microscopic examination
F. The two main branches leading from the trachea to the lungs
G. An inflammation of the skin and deeper tissues that terminates in slough and suppuration
H. The typical small lesion of acne vulgaris
I. Destruction or removal of the myelin sheath
J. A form of macule showing diffused redness of the skin
K. A manner of walking
L. A collection of urine in the renal pelvis caused by obstructed outflow forming a cyst
M. A wound, an injury, or any pathologic change in body tissue
N. A device for producing a fine spray
O. A device used to close up or obstruct
P. A device used to close or block a canal, vessel, or passage of the body
Q. A device for examining the interior of the eye
R. A small bone such as the malleus, incus, and stapes
S. An instrument used to measure and record the volume of inhaled and exhaled air
T. Small raised skin lesion containing fluid

LEARNING REVIEW

1. Bacteria that reach the urinary tract through the blood are called ____________ infection.
   a. homogenous
   b. hematogenous
   c. ascending
   d. descending

2. High levels of nitrogenous waste in the blood may result in:
   a. polyuria
   b. oliguria
   c. uremia
   d. pyuria

3. A sigmoidoscopy is a diagnostic examination of the:
   a. ear
   b. bladder
   c. colon
   d. eye

4. Guaiac slides are used to detect:
   a. occult blood in the stool
   b. the type of bacteria found in otitis media
   c. thrush of the mucous membranes of the mouth
   d. cholelithiasis

5. A diagnostic test done to determine the presence of stones, duct obstruction, or inflammation of the gallbladder is called a:
   a. barium enema
   b. barium swallow
   c. cholecystogram
   d. gastroscopy

CERTIFICATION REVIEW

These questions are designed to mimic the certification examinations. You can use these questions like a small "Certification Examination Study Guide," but this is not meant to take the place of the more extensive study guides. Use this portion to determine in what areas to concentrate your efforts when studying for the certification examination. Justify any "false" answers.

1. Common symptoms of urinary tract diseases and disorders are:
   a. dysuria, proteinuria, hematuria, and dysphagia
   b. dysuria, frequency, oliguria, and urinary suppression
   c. hematuria, pain, frequency, and headache
   d. frequency, hematuria, backache, and dysuria

2. Cystitis is another name for what disorder?
   a. kidney cysts
   b. gall bladder disease
   c. multiple cysts of the breasts or other area
   d. bladder infection

3. UTI means:
   a. urinary tract infection
   b. urinary tract inflammation
   c. urinary tract involvement
   d. urinary treatment initiated

4. The medical term meaning "hidden" is:
   a. cult
   b. occult
   c. crypt
   d. retro

5. Which of the following is an eating disorder?
   a. bulimia
   b. anorexia nervosa
   c. diverticulosis
   d. Crohn's disease
   e. a and b

6. The medical condition of having an increase in intraocular pressure is called:
   a. glaucoma
   b. retinal detachment
   c. cataract
   d. macular degeneration

7. Ear lavage or irrigation is performed for:
   a. impacted sebum
   b. impacted cerumen
   c. impacted lacrimal glands
   d. otitis media

8. The leading cause of blindness in the United States is:
   a. retinal detachment
   b. cataract
   c. glaucoma
   d. diabetes

9. Cholecystectogram is a test for:
   a. kidney stones
   b. diseases of the gall bladder
   c. diseases of the blood vessels
   d. gastrointestinal disorders

10. Which of the following is *not* determined by a chest radiograph?
    a. bronchitis
    b. pneumonia
    c. pharyngitis
    d. tuberculosis

11. The type of arthritis that is considered an autoimmune disease is osteoarthritis. (T or F)

12. In the musculoskeletal systems, strain and sprain mean the same thing. (T or F)

13. Which of the following cardiovascular diseases may require a bypass surgery?
    a. myocardial infarction
    b. pericarditis
    c. thrombophlebitis
    d. coronary artery disease

14. Which of the following cardiovascular diseases may be treated with antibiotics?
    a. thrombophlebitis
    b. pericarditis
    c. angina pectoris
    d. valve stenosis

15. Which of the following diseases is caused by a lack of dopamine?
    a. epilepsy
    b. depression
    c. Reye's syndrome
    d. Parkinson's disease

16. Shingles is a type of:
    a. herpes
    b. psoriasis
    c. dermatitis
    d. acne

17. The type of disease in which the white blood cells become prolific is:
    a. anemia
    b. infectious mononucleosis
    c. leukemia
    d. lymphedema

CASE STUDY

Mary O'Keefe has called for an emergency appointment for her 3-year-old son, Chris, for an examination with Dr. King, because he awakened during the night with a high fever and severe pain in his right ear, which is draining.

1. Ellen Armstrong, CMA, must prepare the examination room for the patient. Based on Chris's symptoms, what equipment will Ellen want to assemble for Dr. King's physical examination of Chris? List the equipment in the order it will most likely be used in the examination.

   ____

   ____

   ____

   ____

2. When Mary O'Keefe arrives with her son, Ellen takes them to examination room 2 and prepares the patient for Dr. King's physical examination. Ellen tells Mary that Dr. King will be examining Chris's ear and may want to take some laboratory tests. Ellen takes and records the child's vital signs:

   T 102.1°F; P 115 (AP) bounding, sinus arrhythmia; R 28; 76/42/0, rt. arm, sitting.

   A. Explain the meaning and significance of each vital sign measurement, including the method and equipment used.

      Temperature: ____

      Pulse: ____

Respiration: ______________________________

Blood pressure: ______________________________

B. Chris is fussy and disagreeable, but not uncooperative, while Ellen takes his vital signs. What can a medical assistant do to facilitate the measurement of a fussy child's vital signs?

____

____

3. Ellen assists Dr. King with her physical examination of the patient. After assessing the vital sign measurements taken by the medical assistant, Dr. King examines Chris's ear and lungs. A swab of fluid discharge is taken from the patient's ear. What is the role of the medical assistant during the physician's examination of this patient?

____

____

____

____

4. Dr. King makes a clinical diagnosis of otitis media for this patient and orders laboratory testing to be performed on the patient's specimen.

A. What criteria are necessary for a physician to make a clinical diagnosis?

____

B. What is otitis media? Why are children more likely at risk for this condition? How is otitis media commonly treated? What patient education can the health care team offer? (Consult a medical reference or encyclopedia for help in answering this question.)

____

____

SELF-ASSESSMENT

Think of a time when you or a close family member had to go to the physician's office and then go through a diagnostic procedure or test for a medical disorder or a disease. Fill in the following outline with as much information as you can remember.

1. What were the patient's symptoms? Try to list two or three symptoms.
2. Describe how the disease started? (Suddenly? Gradually, Over time? Related to an injury?)
3. Did the patient go to the emergency department or to the physician's office first?
4. Did the physician, or his or her staff, clearly explain the test or procedure to the patient or the patient's family?
5. What were some of the feelings that you had during the process? List two or three feelings.

6. Could the medical assistant or doctor have reassured you better or kept you better informed, or did they do a good job of answering your questions and meeting your needs and the needs of the patient?

7. How will your experience influence your interaction with your patients when you are assisting with a diagnostic test or procedure? What will you pay special attention to that you might not have if you had not had the experience describe above?

CHAPTER POST-TEST

This is similar to the Pre-Test. Perform this test without looking at the book. This is just to see how well you have understood and can recall the information presented in this chapter after you have studied it and completed the workbook exercises. You will not be graded on this portion (other than the grade you give yourself), but this is an excellent preparation for your instructor's test. You may use this Post-Test to determine what areas you need to study more. Justify any "false" answers.

1. Urinary catheterization often is performed in clinics, hospitals, and surgery centers. (T or F)

2. When performing a routine urinalysis, the specimen is not checked for drugs. (T or F)

3. Instillation and irrigation are different procedures. (T or F)

4. A barium swallow is used to examine:
   a. the esophagus, the stomach, the small and large intestines
   b. both the small and the large intestines
   c. the stomach and the entire small intestine
   d. the stomach and part of the small intestine

5. To test visual acuity, the patient does not need to recognize the letters of the English alphabet. (T or F)

6. Medical assistants often remove casts. (T or F)

7. Pulse oximetry is used to determine the oxygen saturation of the blood in a noninvasive way. (T or F)

CERTIFICATION CRITERIA CHECKLIST

As you go through your education and training, keep in mind the national certification examination that you will take when you graduate. Each chapter of the textbook and workbook covers a different section of the examination criteria. To keep track of your preparation for the certification examination, turn to the back of this workbook and highlight the following CMA, RMA, or CMAS certification examination criteria (if you have already highlighted them from a previous chapter, put a check mark by the criteria):

CMA

A. Medical Terminology
B. Anatomy and Physiology
R. Principles of Infection Control
S. Treatment Area
T. Patient Preparation and Assisting the Physician
    3. Examinations
V. Collecting and Processing Specimens; Diagnostic Testing
    5. Vision
    6. Hearing
    7. Respiratory Testing

RMA

I. General Medical Assisting Knowledge
    A. Anatomy and Physiology
    B. Medical Terminology
III. Clinical Medical Assisting
    A. Asepsis
    E. Physical Examinations
    I. Laboratory Procedures

CMAS

1. Medical Assisting Foundation
    - Medical terminology
    - Anatomy and physiology
2. Basic Clinical Medical Office Assisting
    - Asepsis in the medical office
    - Examination preparation

COMPETENCY ASSESSMENT

Procedure 30-1 Obtaining a Urine Sample for Drug Screening

Performance Objectives: To obtain a urine specimen from a patient for drug testing. Perform this procedure within 20 minutes with a minimum score of 65 points.

Supplies/Equipment: Urine drug kit (provide at least two choices), gloves, biohazard waste container, forms, permanent pen

Charting/Documentation: Enter appropriate documentation/charting in the box.

Instructor's/Evaluator's Comments and Suggestions:

SKILLS CHECKLIST Procedure 30-1: Obtaining a Urine Sample for Drug Screening

Name ______________________

Date ______________________

No.	Skill	Check #1 20 pts ea	Check #2 10 pts ea	Check #3 5 pts ea	Notes
1	Ask the patient for photo ID, have him or her sign consent form, and keep copies of all.				
2	Wash hands and explain procedure.				
3	Supply two kits and have patient choose which test to use.				
4	Have patient remove unnecessary outer garments, empty pockets, and wash and dry his or her hands.				
5	Instruct patient to collect minimum of 40 ml urine in the container.				
6	Glove. Test and record the temperature of the urine, volume, and any contamination.				
7	Label specimen and have patient initial lid.				
8	Seal specimen kit bag and have patient initial.				
9	Secure sample in a locked container until pickup.				
10	Collector and donor affirm and sign procedure steps.				
11	Remove gloves. Dispose of into biohazard waste.				
12	Wash hands.				
13	Document procedure in patient's chart.				
Student's Total Points					
Points Possible		260	130	65	
Final Score (Student's Total Points / Possible Points)					

	Notes
Start time:	
End time:	
Total time: (20 min goal)	

COMPETENCY ASSESSMENT

Procedure 30-2 Performing a Urinary Catheterization on a Female Patient

Performance Objectives: To obtain a sterile urine specimen for analysis, to measure post-void residual, or to relieve urinary retention. Perform this procedure within 25 minutes with a minimum score of 175 points.

Supplies/Equipment: Catheter kit containing needed supplies, sterile gloves, antiseptic cleansing solution, waxed bag or nearby biohazard bag, lubricant, sterile cotton balls, forceps and Betadine® or Betadine® swabs, sterile urine cup, sterile 2 × 2 gauze, sterile absorbent pad, tissue, sterile catheter as ordered, laboratory requisition, biohazard specimen transfer bag if needed

Charting/Documentation: Enter appropriate documentation/charting in the box.

Instructor's/Evaluator's Comments and Suggestions:

SKILLS CHECKLIST Procedure 30-2: Performing a Urinary Catheterization on a Female Patient

Name ______________________

Date ______________________

No.	Skill	Check #1 20 pts ea	Check #2 10 pts ea	Check #3 5 pts ea	Notes
1	Identify the patient and explain the procedure.				
2	Instruct the patient to breathe slowly and try to relax during the procedure.				
3	Wash hands and assemble supplies.				
4	Place catheter kit onto clean, dry Mayo tray.				
5	Provide adequate lighting.				
6	Have patient undress from the waist down. Provide a patient drape.				
7	Position patient so she is lying on her back with her feet together and knees relaxed apart.				
8	Arrange the drape so that only her genital area is exposed.				
9	Touching only the edges, open the outer wrapping of the kit using sterile technique. The wrapping can provide the sterile field.				
10	Touching only the corners, place the sterile absorbent pad under the patient's buttocks. Empty contents of the kit container onto the sterile field, touching only the outside of the container.				
11	Ask patient to keep her knees apart.				
12	Wash hands and apply sterile gloves.				
13	Pour Betadine® over the cotton balls in one of the compartments of the container, or open the Betadine® swabs.				
14	Open the urine container.				
15	Apply sterile lubricant to the tip of the catheter. You may place lubricant onto the 2 × 2 gauze squares first.				

No.	Skill	Check #1 20 pts ea	Check #2 10 pts ea	Check #3 5 pts ea	Notes
16	Remind patient to relax. Using nondominant hand, spread the labia apart. With sterile dominant hand, use forceps to cleanse the genitalia with the Betadine®-soaked cotton balls, or use the Betadine® swabs. Use three separate swipes, discarding each cotton ball/swab after each swipe. Discard each after use into nearby (within reach) waxed or biohazard bag. Discard forceps if used. Continue to hold labia apart.				
17	Place sterile catheter tray between patient's legs, touching only the sterile surface of the tray, and take great care not to contaminate sterile dominant hand/glove. Pick up sterile catheter holding it 3 to 4 inches from lubricated tip. Let the other end rest in a sterile compartment of the kit tray between the patient's legs.				
18	Gently insert the catheter into urinary meatus approximately 6 inches or until urine begins to flow.				
19	Interrupt urine flow by clamping or crimping the catheter.				
20	Place end of catheter into sterile specimen cup if a sample is needed. If sample is not needed, you may discard it later.				
21	Collect specimen by unclamping or uncrimping the catheter and collecting about 60 ml.				
22	Allow the remaining urine to flow into the original container until it stops.				
23	Remove catheter gently and slowly.				
24	Dry area with tissue.				
25	Tighten the lid on the urine specimen container.				
26	Remove procedure items. Remove gloves, wash hands.				
27	Position the patient for comfort.				
28	Assist the patient to sit up.				
29	Help patient to sit on the edge of the table. Check her color and pulse.				

No.	Skill	Check #1 20 pts ea	Check #2 10 pts ea	Check #3 5 pts ea	Notes
30	Apply gloves. Discard disposable items according to OSHA guidelines.				
31	If collecting a specimen for analysis, label the container.				
32	Assist the patient from the examination table. Offer tissues and sink for washing her hands.				
33	Clean room and table. Remove gloves and dispose of into biohazard waste container.				
34	Wash hands.				
35	Document the procedure in the patient's chart. Include amount of urine removed. If sample is to be sent to laboratory, complete laboratory requisition form and place specimen into transfer bag. Place requisition in outer pocket of bag. Seal and send.				
Student's Total Points					
Points Possible		700	350	175	
Final Score (Student's Total Points / Possible Points)					

	Notes
Start time:	
End time:	
Total time: (25 min goal)	

COMPETENCY ASSESSMENT

Procedure 30-3 Performing a Urinary Catheterization on a Male Patient

Performance Objectives: To obtain a sterile urine specimen for analysis or to relieve urinary retention. Perform this procedure within 25 minutes with a minimum score of 135 points.

Supplies/Equipment: Catheter kit containing needed supplies, sterile gloves, antiseptic cleansing solution, waxed bag or nearby biohazard bag, lubricant, sterile cotton balls, forceps and Betadine® or Betadine® swabs, tissues, sterile urine cup, sterile 2 × 2 gauze, sterile absorbent pad, tissue, sterile catheter as ordered, laboratory requisition, biohazard specimen transfer bag if needed

Charting/Documentation: Enter appropriate documentation/charting in the box.

____

____

____

____

Instructor's/Evaluator's Comments and Suggestions:

____

____

____

____

____

____

SKILLS CHECKLIST Procedure 30-3: Performing a Urinary Catheterization on a Male Patient

Name ______________________

Date ______________________

No.	Skill	Check #1 20 pts ea	Check #2 10 pts ea	Check #3 5 pts ea	Notes
1	Identify the patient and explain the procedure.				
2	Instruct the patient to breathe slowly and to try to relax during the procedure.				
3	Wash hands and assemble supplies.				
4	Place catheter kit onto clean, dry Mayo tray near the patient.				
5	Provide adequate lighting.				
6	Have patient undress from the waist down. Provide a patient drape.				
7	Position patient so he is lying on his back.				
8	Arrange the drape so that only his external genitalia is exposed.				
9	Touching only the edges, open the outer wrapping of the kit using sterile technique. The wrapping can provide the sterile field.				
10	Touching only the corners, place the sterile absorbent pad on the patient's lap, under the patient's penis. Empty contents of the kit container onto the sterile field, touching only the outside of the container.				
11	Wash hands and apply sterile gloves.				
12	Open fenestrated drape and, using sterile technique, place fenestration over the penis.				
13	Empty contents of kit onto the sterile field. Set the container near the patient, taking care to maintain sterility of inside of container.				
14	Apply sterile lubricant to the tip of the catheter. You may place lubricant onto the 2 × 2 gauze squares first. Pour Betadine® over the cotton balls in one of the compartments of the container or open the Betadine® swabs.				

No.	Skill	Check #1 20 pts ea	Check #2 10 pts ea	Check #3 5 pts ea	Notes
15	Using nondominant hand, hold the penis below the glans. In uncircumcised males, the skin must be pulled back to expose the meatus. This must be done with the nondominant hand to keep the dominant hand sterile.				
16	With sterile dominant hand, use forceps to cleanse the meatus with the Betadine®-soaked cotton balls or use the Betadine® swabs. Discard each after use into nearby (within reach) waxed or biohazard bag. Discard forceps if used. Continue to hold foreskin down.				
17	Using the dominant sterile hand, pick up sterile catheter holding it 3 to 4 inches from lubricated tip. Let the other end rest in a sterile compartment of the kit container. Holding the penis upright and straight, insert the lubricated catheter into urinary meatus approximately 6 inches or until urine begins to flow.				
18	Obtain a specimen in the sterile cup if needed. Interrupt urine flow by clamping or crimping the catheter. Place end of catheter into sterile specimen cup if a sample is needed. If sample is not needed, you may discard it later. Collect about 60 ml urine.				
19	After urine flow ceases, remove catheter gently and slowly.				
20	Dry area with tissue. Remove gloves, wash hands.				
21	Position the patient for comfort; assist patient to sit up. Check his color and pulse.				
22	Reglove. Discard disposable items according to OSHA guidelines.				
23	If collecting a specimen for analysis, label the container.				
24	Assist the patient from the examination table. Offer tissues and sink for washing his hands.				
25	Clean room and table. Remove gloves and dispose of into biohazard waste container.				
26	Wash hands.				

No.	Skill	Check #1 20 pts ea	Check #2 10 pts ea	Check #3 5 pts ea	Notes
27	Document the procedure in patient's chart. Include amount of urine removed. If sample is to be sent to laboratory, complete laboratory requisition form and place specimen into transfer bag. Place requisition in outer pocket of bag. Seal and send.				
Student's Total Points					
Points Possible		540	270	135	
Final Score (Student's Total Points / Possible Points)					

	Notes
Start time:	
End time:	
Total time: (25 min goal)	

COMPETENCY ASSESSMENT

Procedure 30-4 Fecal Occult Blood Test

Performance Objectives: To teach the patient how to properly obtain a fecal specimen, and then return it to the office for testing. To test feces for occult blood in the Physician's Office Laboratory. Perform this procedure within 15 minutes with a minimum score of 85 points.

Supplies/Equipment: *Obtaining the specimen:* An occult slide test kit containing three slides, six applicators, envelope, and instructions. *Testing the specimen:* Prepared slides from the patient, occult blood developer from same manufacturer, gloves, biohazard waste container.

Charting/Documentation: Enter appropriate documentation/charting in the box.

Instructor's/Evaluator's Comments and Suggestions:

SKILLS CHECKLIST Procedure 30-4: Fecal Occult Blood Test

Name ______________________

Date ______________________

No.	Skill	Check #1 20 pts ea	Check #2 10 pts ea	Check #3 5 pts ea	Notes
Teaching the Patient How to Obtain the Specimens					
1	Check expiration date of occult slides.				
2	Identify the patient.				
3	Fill out the information on the front except the date collected.				
4	Explain the collection procedure. The patient will need to:				
	a. Keep the slides at room temperature away from direct sunlight.				
	b. When ready to obtain a specimen, date the front and open each slide from the front.				
	c. Using one of the applicators, obtain a sample of stool and smear it lightly onto the first section.				
	d. Repeat for the other section using a different applicator and taking the sample from a different area of the stool.				
	e. Dispose of the applicators carefully.				
	f. Allow to dry for a few hours, then close the flap.				
	g. Check the information and date on the front.				
	h. Repeat the procedure with the next two bowel movements on subsequent days.				
5	Provide the patient with the envelope into which to place the finished slides. Caution the patient not to mail the slides, but rather return them personally.				
6	Record that the test kit and instructions were provided to the patient.				

No.	Skill	Check #1 20 pts ea	Check #2 10 pts ea	Check #3 5 pts ea	Notes
Testing the Slides					
1	Apply gloves.				
2	Check the expiration date of the chemical developer.				
3	Lay a paper towel on a clean, dry surface. Lay the slides on the towel. Provide adequate lighting. Open the back of the slides.				
4	Apply 2 drops of developer on the slide (following manufacturer's instructions).				
5	Interpret the results between 30 and 60 seconds (following manufacturer's instructions).				
6	Note a positive reaction—any blue coloring at any place on the slide.				
7	Perform the quality-control procedure by placing 1 drop on each of the positive and negative control samples. Ensure the quality of both the slides and the developer.				
8	Dispose of all supplies according to OSHA guidelines. Disinfect the area.				
9	Remove gloves and dispose of into biohazard waste container.				
10	Wash hands.				
11	Document the results in patient's chart.				
Student's Total Points					
Points Possible (17 steps total)		340	170	85	
Final Score (Student's Total Points / Possible Points)					

	Notes
Start time:	
End time:	
Total time: (15 min goal)	

COMPETENCY ASSESSMENT

Procedure 30-5 Performing Visual Acuity Testing Using a Snellen Chart

Performance Objectives: To perform a visual screening test to determine a patient's distance visual acuity. Perform this procedure within 15 minutes with a minimum score of 45 points.

Supplies/Equipment: Snellen eye chart (appropriate for age and language ability) placed at eye level without glare on it, occluder, pointer, disinfectant wipes

Charting/Documentation: Enter appropriate documentation/charting in the box.

Instructor's/Evaluator's Comments and Suggestions:

SKILLS CHECKLIST Procedure 30-5: Performing Visual Acuity Testing Using a Snellen Chart

Name ______________________

Date ______________________

No.	Skill	Check #1 20 pts ea	Check #2 10 pts ea	Check #3 5 pts ea	Notes
1	Wash hands and assemble equipment.				
2	Prepare the area to be well lit with no distractions or glare and with a distance of 20 feet between the chart and the patient.				
3	Introduce yourself, identify the patient, and explain the procedure. Test with corrective lens worn unless otherwise directed by the physician.				
4	Instruct the patient to stand behind the 20-foot mark and cover the left eye with the occluder. Instruct her to keep her left eye open under the occluder and not to apply pressure to the eye.				
5	Stand near the chart and point to Row 3, instructing the patient to read each letter with the right eye, verbally identifying each letter as it is read. If the patient is unable to read line 3, go to the next larger line (line 2) to start.				
6	Record the results at the smallest line the patient is able to read correctly with fewer than two errors. Vision will be recorded for the right eye, the left eye, and both eyes.				
7	Record the patient's reaction during the test, such as extreme squinting, leaning forward, or tearing.				
8	When finished with testing the right eye, test the left eye, and then both eyes.				
9	Disinfect the occluder, wash hands, and record the procedure.				
Student's Total Points					
Points Possible		180	90	45	
Final Score (Student's Total Points / Possible Points)					

	Notes
Start time:	
End time:	
Total time: (15 min goal)	

COMPETENCY ASSESSMENT

Procedure 30-6 Measuring Near Visual Acuity

Performance Objectives: To measure the near vision of a patient. Perform this procedure within 15 minutes with a minimum score of 70 points.

Supplies/Equipment: Visual acuity eye chart, occluder, disinfectant wipes

Charting/Documentation: Enter appropriate documentation/charting in the box.

Instructor's/Evaluator's Comments and Suggestions:

SKILLS CHECKLIST Procedure 30-6: Measuring Near Visual Acuity

Name ______________________

Date ______________________

No.	Skill	Check #1 20 pts ea	Check #2 10 pts ea	Check #3 5 pts ea	Notes
1	Wash hands.				
2	Introduce yourself and identify the patient.				
3	Explain the procedure to the patient and provide him or her with an occluder. Test with corrective lens worn unless otherwise directed by the physician.				
4	Position the patient comfortably.				
5	Hold the near vision card 14 inches from the patient (use a measuring tape).				
6	Have the patient lightly cover the left eye with the occluder. Explain to the patient that he or she is not to close the right eye under the occluder or press on the right eye with the occluder.				
7	Have the patient read the paragraphs printed on the card.				
8	Once the patient has reached the line where more than two mistakes are made, note the visual acuity for that eye. Allow the patient to repeat the line for accuracy.				
9	Repeat the process to measure the left eye.				
10	Repeat the process for both eyes.				
11	Record the results in the patient chart. Results are charted 14/14 for normal near vision.				
12	Disinfect the occluder.				
13	Wash hands.				
14	Record the results.				
Student's Total Points					
Points Possible		280	140	70	
Final Score (Student's Total Points / Possible Points)					

	Notes
Start time:	
End time:	
Total time: (15 min goal)	

COMPETENCY ASSESSMENT

Procedure 30-7 Performing Color Vision Test Using the Ishihara Plates

Performance Objectives: To assess a patient's ability to distinguish between the colors red and green. Perform this procedure within 15 minutes with a minimum score of 20 points.

Supplies/Equipment: Ishihara color plates

Charting/Documentation: Enter appropriate documentation/charting in the box.

Instructor's/Evaluator's Comments and Suggestions:

SKILLS CHECKLIST Procedure 30-7: Performing Color Vision Test Using the Ishihara Plates

Name ______________________

Date ______________________

No.	Skill	Check #1 20 pts ea	Check #2 10 pts ea	Check #3 5 pts ea	Notes
1	Wash hands and assemble the chair and Ishihara plates in a well-lit, quiet room. Introduce yourself and identify the patient.				
2	Hold each plate 30 inches (75 cm) from the patient and tilted slightly so the plate is right within the line of the patient's vision.				
3	Record the number given by the patient on each plate.				
4	Assess the patient's readings and record in the patient's chart.				
Student's Total Points					
Points Possible		80	40	20	
Final Score (Student's Total Points / Possible Points)					

	Notes
Start time:	
End time:	
Total time: (15 min goal)	

COMPETENCY ASSESSMENT

Procedure 30-8 Performing Eye Instillation

Performance Objectives: To treat eye infections, soothe irritations, anesthetize, or dilate pupils. Perform this procedure within 10 minutes with a minimum score of 75 points.

Supplies/Equipment: Sterile eye dropper, sterile ophthalmic medication as ordered by the physician, sterile cotton balls, sterile gloves, tissue or gauze

Charting/Documentation: Enter appropriate documentation/charting in the box.

____

____

____

____

Instructor's/Evaluator's Comments and Suggestions:

____

____

____

____

____

____

SKILLS CHECKLIST Procedure 30-8: Performing Eye Instillation

Name ______________________

Date ______________________

No.	Skill	Check #1 20 pts ea	Check #2 10 pts ea	Check #3 5 pts ea	Notes
1	Wash hands.				
2	Assemble supplies using sterile technique.				
3	Check the medication order carefully including the expiration date. Read the label three times.				
4	Introduce yourself and identify the patient.				
5	Explain the procedure to the patient and inform him or her that instillation may temporarily blur his vision.				
6	Position the patient in a sitting position or lying down.				
7	Instruct the patient to stare at a fixed spot during instillation of the drops/ointment.				
8	Prepare the medication. Apply gloves.				
9	Have the patient look up and expose the lower conjunctiva of the affected eye by using fingers and a gauze square or tissue.				
10	Place the number of drops ordered in the center of the lower conjunctival sac or a thin line of ointment in the lower surface, being careful not to touch the eyelid, eyeball, or the eyelashes with the tip of the medication applicator. If using a multi-dose medication, be extremely careful to prevent contamination of the applicator. If this is a single-dose medication, discard it after using.				
11	Have the patient close the eye and roll the eyeball to distribute the medication.				
12	Blot excess medication from eyelids with tissue from inner to outer canthus. Do not rub or wipe.				
13	Dispose of supplies according to OSHA guidelines.				

No.	Skill	Check #1 20 pts ea	Check #2 10 pts ea	Check #3 5 pts ea	Notes
14	Wash hands.				
15	Document the procedure in patient's chart.				
Student's Total Points					
Points Possible		300	150	75	
Final Score (Student's Total Points / Possible Points)					

	Notes
Start time:	
End time:	
Total time: (10 min goal)	

COMPETENCY ASSESSMENT

Procedure 30-9 Performing Eye Patch Dressing Application

Performance Objectives: To apply a sterile eye patch. Perform this procedure within 10 minutes with a minimum score of 45 points.

Supplies/Equipment: Sterile eye patch(s) (some physicians request double layer), tape

Charting/Documentation: Enter appropriate documentation/charting in the box.

Instructor's/Evaluator's Comments and Suggestions:

SKILLS CHECKLIST Procedure 30-9: Performing Eye Patch Dressing Application

Name ______________________________

Date ______________________________

No.	Skill	Check #1 20 pts ea	Check #2 10 pts ea	Check #3 5 pts ea	Notes
1	Wash hands and assemble supplies.				
2	Identify patient.				
3	Explain the procedure.				
4	Position the patient in a sitting or supine position.				
5	Instruct the patient to close both eyes during the application of the eye patch. Open eye patch package using sterile technique.				
6	Apply the eye patch(es) by touching only the outside of the patch. Allow the inside to remain sterile.				
7	Secure the patch(es) with tape placed diagonally from mid-forehead to below the ear. Tape should allow for no shifting of the patch or gapping.				
8	Wash hands.				
9	Document the procedure and supply verbal and written instructions to the patient. Assess that the patient has a ride home.				
Student's Total Points					
Points Possible		180	90	45	
Final Score (Student's Total Points / Possible Points)					

	Notes
Start time:	
End time:	
Total time: (10 min goal)	

COMPETENCY ASSESSMENT

Procedure 30-10 Performing Eye Irrigation

Performance Objectives: To irrigate the patient's eye to remove foreign debris, cleanse of discharge, remove chemicals, or apply antiseptic. Perform this procedure within 15 minutes with a minimum score of 85 points.

Supplies/Equipment: Sterile irrigation solution as ordered by physician, sterile bulb syringe (rubber), kidney-shaped basin to catch irrigation solution, sterile cotton balls, sterile gloves, biohazard waste container, towel, pillow

Charting/Documentation: Enter appropriate documentation/charting in the box.

Instructor's/Evaluator's Comments and Suggestions:

SKILLS CHECKLIST Procedure 30-10: Performing Eye Irrigation

Name ______________________

Date ______________________

No.	Skill	Check #1 20 pts ea	Check #2 10 pts ea	Check #3 5 pts ea	Notes
1	Wash hands and assemble supplies.				
2	Identify patient.				
3	Explain the procedure to the patient.				
4	Position the patient in a supine position.				
5	Check expiration date on the solution bottle.				
6	Check label three times. Warm solution to body temperature.				
7	Tilt head toward affected eye; place towel on patient's shoulder.				
8	Place basin beside the affected eye.				
9	Apply sterile gloves.				
10	Moisten two to three cotton balls with irrigation solution and clean the eyelids and eyelashes of affected eye, wiping from inner to outer canthus.				
11	Expose the lower conjunctiva by separating the eyelid with index finger and thumb.				
12	Have patient stare at a fixed spot.				
13	Irrigate the affected eye with sterile solution by resting the bulb on the bridge of the nose. Allow solution to flow from inner to outer canthus. Do not touch the eye or surrounding area with the tip of the bulb.				
14	After irrigation, dry the eyelid and eyelashes with sterile cotton balls.				
15	Discard supplies in biohazard container if discharge or exudate is present.				
16	Remove gloves.				
17	Wash hands and document procedure.				
Student's Total Points					
Points Possible		340	170	85	
Final Score (Student's Total Points / Possible Points)					

	Notes
Start time:	
End time:	
Total time: (15 min goal)	

COMPETENCY ASSESSMENT

Procedure 30-11 Performing Audiometry

Performance Objectives: To assist in testing a patient for hearing loss. Perform this procedure within 20 minutes with a minimum score of 60 points.

Supplies/Equipment: Audiometer with headphones, quiet room

Charting/Documentation: Enter appropriate documentation/charting in the box.

Instructor's/Evaluator's Comments and Suggestions:

SKILLS CHECKLIST Procedure 30-11: Performing Audiometry

Name ______________________

Date ______________________

No.	Skill	Check #1 20 pts ea	Check #2 10 pts ea	Check #3 5 pts ea	Notes
1	Wash hands and assemble equipment and supplies.				
2	Prepare quiet room.				
3	Identify the patient and explain the procedure.				
4	Position patient in a comfortable sitting position.				
5	Have patient put on head phones. The procedure is done on each ear separately.				
6	If the medical assistant has been trained to perform the procedure, the physician will authorize the medical assistant to perform the audiometry. The audiometer is started at a low frequency. The patient will indicate when a sound is heard while the medical assistant plots it on the graph.				
7	The frequencies generally increase until completed.				
8	The other ear is checked in the same manner.				
9	The results are given to the physician for interpretation.				
10	Equipment is cleaned following manufacturer's instructions.				
11	Wash hands.				
12	Document procedure in patient's chart.				
Student's Total Points					
Points Possible		240	120	60	
Final Score (Student's Total Points / Possible Points)					

	Notes
Start time:	
End time:	
Total time: (20 min goal)	

COMPETENCY ASSESSMENT

Procedure 30-12 Performing Ear Irrigation

Performance Objectives: To remove impacted cerumen, discharge, or foreign materials from the ear canal as directed by the physician. Perform this procedure within 25 minutes with a minimum score of 110 points.

Supplies/Equipment: Irrigation solution as ordered by the physician warmed to 98.6°F to 103°F, ear syringe or bulb or ear irrigation equipment, kidney-shaped basin or ear irrigation basin, larger basin for warmed solution, towel, cotton balls, tissues, otoscope

Charting/Documentation: Enter appropriate documentation/charting in the box.

Instructor's/Evaluator's Comments and Suggestions:

SKILLS CHECKLIST Procedure 30-12: Performing Ear Irrigation

Name ______________________

Date ______________________

No.	Skill	Check #1 20 pts ea	Check #2 10 pts ea	Check #3 5 pts ea	Notes
1	Wash hands and assemble equipment.				
2	Identify patient.				
3	Explain the procedure and inform the patient that during the procedure, a minimal amount of discomfort and dizziness may be experienced. Be sure the physician has examined the ear before irrigation.				
4	Place the patient in a sitting position and use an otoscope to visualize the affected ear.				
5	Cleanse the outer ear with a wet cotton ball moistened with irrigation solution.				
6	Gently pull the auricle upward and back to straighten the ear canal.				
7	Tilt the patient's head slightly forward and to the affected side.				
8	Place towel on the patient's shoulder on the affected side.				
9	Place the ear basin under the affected ear and have the patient hold the basin in place.				
10	If using medication, check label of solution three times for correctness and also check the expiration date.				
11	Pour solution into a basin and fill the syringe with the warmed irrigation solution as prescribed. If using plain warm water, fill the irrigation syringe/bulb as needed. Flush warm water through the tubing/syringe several times to warn the tubing and equipment.				
12	Straighten the external auditory canal for adults by pulling back and upward on the auricle.				

No.	Skill	Check #1 20 pts ea	Check #2 10 pts ea	Check #3 5 pts ea	Notes
13	Gently insert the syringe tip into the affected ear. Do not insert too deeply. Do not occlude external auditory canal. Direct the flow upward toward roof of canal. Check with patient about any discomfort or pain. Do not continue if pain is present.				
14	Repeat the irrigation, allowing the solution to drain from the ear and noting the return. Allow for free flow of return each time. Stop if the patient feels any discomfort.				
15	Dry the outer ear and visualize the inner ear with the otoscope to verify the procedure has removed or dislodged the foreign material or cerumen.				
16	Notify the physician the procedure has been completed.				
17	When the procedure has been completed, remove the ear basin and towel.				
18	Have patient lie on the affected side on examination table, or tilt head to the affected side for ear to continue draining.				
19	Provide tissue to the patient to catch any further drainage. Insert cotton balls into ear canal if directed by physician.				
20	Dispose of supplies.				
21	Wash hands.				
22	Document procedure in patient's chart, noting return and amount. Provide instructions to the patient to report any pain or dizziness and not to insert foreign objects into the ear canal.				
Student's Total Points					
Points Possible		440	220	110	
Final Score (Student's Total Points / Possible Points)					

	Notes
Start time:	
End time:	
Total time: (25 min goal)	

COMPETENCY ASSESSMENT

Procedure 30-13 Performing Ear Instillation

Performance Objectives: To soften impacted cerumen, fight infection with antibiotics, or relieve pain. Perform this procedure within 15 minutes with a minimum score of 65 points.

Supplies/Equipment: Otic medication as prescribed by the physician, sterile ear dropper, cotton balls, gloves

Charting/Documentation: Enter appropriate documentation/charting in the box.

Instructor's/Evaluator's Comments and Suggestions:

SKILLS CHECKLIST Procedure 30-13: Performing Ear Instillation

Name ______________________

Date ______________________

No.	Skill	Check #1 20 pts ea	Check #2 10 pts ea	Check #3 5 pts ea	Notes
1	Wash hands and assemble supplies.				
2	Identify patient.				
3	Explain the procedure.				
4	Position the patient to either lie on unaffected side or to sitting position with head tilted toward the unaffected ear.				
5	Check the otic medication three times against the physician's order and assess the expiration date.				
6	Draw up the prescribed amount of medication.				
7	Gently pull the top of the ear upward and back (adult) or pull ear downward and backward (child).				
8	Instill prescribed dose of medication (number of drops) by squeezing rubber bulb on dropper into the affected ear.				
9	Have patient maintain the position for about 5 minutes to retain medication.				
10	When instructed by the physician, insert moistened cotton ball into external ear canal for 15 minutes.				
11	Dispose of supplies.				
12	Wash hands.				
13	Document the procedure and any patient reaction.				
Student's Total Points					
Points Possible		260	130	65	
Final Score (Student's Total Points / Possible Points)					

	Notes
Start time:	
End time:	
Total time: (15 min goal)	

COMPETENCY ASSESSMENT

Procedure 30-14 Assisting with Nasal Examination

Performance Objectives: To assist the physician with the nasal examination when looking for polyps, engorged superficial blood vessels, and to assist in the possible removal of a foreign object. Perform this procedure within 20 minutes with a minimum score of 45 points.

Supplies/Equipment: Nasal speculum, hands-free light source, gloves, kidney basin, bayonet forceps

Charting/Documentation: Enter appropriate documentation/charting in the box.

Instructor's/Evaluator's Comments and Suggestions:

SKILLS CHECKLIST Procedure 30-14: Assisting with Nasal Examination

Name ______________________

Date ______________________

No.	Skill	Check #1 20 pts ea	Check #2 10 pts ea	Check #3 5 pts ea	Notes
1	Wash hands and assemble supplies.				
2	Identify patient.				
3	Explain the procedure to the patient.				
4	Place the patient in a sitting position.				
5	Reassure the patient.				
6	Hand the physician equipment and supplies as needed.				
7	When the examination/treatment is completed, clean equipment and dispose of supplies per OSHA guidelines.				
8	Wash hands.				
9	Document procedure noting foreign object if applicable, document any instructions given to patient, and assist in scheduling a surgical appointment for polyp removal if needed, according to physician's orders.				
Student's Total Points					
Points Possible		180	90	45	
Final Score (Student's Total Points / Possible Points)					

	Notes
Start time:	
End time:	
Total time: (20 min goal)	

COMPETENCY ASSESSMENT

Procedure 30-15 Cautery Treatment of Epistaxis

Performance Objectives: To assist the physician with the nasal examination when looking for polyps or engorged superficial blood vessels and to assist with the removal of foreign object, or to treat epistaxis. Perform this procedure within 20 minutes with a minimum score of 55 points.

Supplies/Equipment: Nasal speculum; hands-free light source; gloves; kidney basin; bayonet forceps; for treatment of epistaxis: epinephrine, silver nitrate applicators, cotton balls, cotton-tipped applicators, small syringe and large gauge needle, small med cup, local anesthetic, antibiotic ointment as ordered by physician

Charting/Documentation: Enter appropriate documentation/charting in the box.

Instructor's/Evaluator's Comments and Suggestions:

SKILLS CHECKLIST Procedure 30-15: Cautery Treatment of Epistaxis

Name ______________________________

Date ______________________________

No.	Skill	Check #1 20 pts ea	Check #2 10 pts ea	Check #3 5 pts ea	Notes
1	Wash hands and assemble supplies.				
2	Identify patient.				
3	Explain the procedure to the patient.				
4	Place the patient in a sitting position for foreign object removal and lying position for cautery. Give the patient a catch basin and tissues.				
5	Assist the physician as needed. Reassure the patient.				
6	Hand the physician supplies as needed. For epistaxis treatment, withdraw 1 to 2 ml xylocaine from vial and squirt it into small medicine cup. Cotton-tipped applicators are dipped into the anesthetic for application to the nasal membrane. The friable blood vessel is then cauterized with application of the silver nitrate.				
7	Warn the patient that it may sting and be prepared for the patient to sneeze. Support the patient as needed.				
8	Instruct the patient on post-operative care: Do not blow nose or otherwise irritate or disturb the scab that is forming.				
9	Clean equipment and dispose of supplies per OSHA guidelines.				
10	Wash hands.				
11	Document procedure noting foreign object removed if applicable, document any instructions given to patient, and assist in scheduling a surgical appointment for polyp removal if needed, according to physician's orders.				
Student's Total Points					
Points Possible		220	110	55	
Final Score (Student's Total Points / Possible Points)					

	Notes
Start time:	
End time:	
Total time: (20 min goal)	

COMPETENCY ASSESSMENT

Procedure 30-16 Performing Nasal Instillation

Performance Objectives: To provide medication to the nasal tissues as ordered by the physician. Perform this procedure within 15 minutes with a minimum score of 60 points.

Supplies/Equipment: Medication as ordered by physician, medicine dropper (sterile), tissues

Charting/Documentation: Enter appropriate documentation/charting in the box.

Instructor's/Evaluator's Comments and Suggestions:

SKILLS CHECKLIST Procedure 30-16: Performing Nasal Instillation

Name ______________________

Date ______________________

No.	Skill	Check #1 20 pts ea	Check #2 10 pts ea	Check #3 5 pts ea	Notes
1	Wash hands and assemble supplies.				
2	Identify patient.				
3	Explain the procedure to the patient.				
4	Place the patient with the head lower than the shoulders, either lying down or tilted back if sitting.				
5	Draw medication into dropper after checking medication three times and checking expiration date.				
6	Place the dropper over the center of the affected nostril. Do not touch the inside of the nostril.				
7	Repeat the procedure for the other nostril if required. Dispose of dropper and recap medication container using sterile technique.				
8	Instruct the patient to remain in position for 5 minutes.				
9	Provide tissues to the patient when the patient returns to a normal sitting position.				
10	Dispose of the supplies per OSHA guidelines.				
11	Wash hands.				
12	Document the procedure. Include the medication ordered, number of drops, and which nostril.				
Student's Total Points					
Points Possible		240	120	60	
Final Score (Student's Total Points / Possible Points)					

	Notes
Start time:	
End time:	
Total time: (15 min goal)	

COMPETENCY ASSESSMENT

Procedure 30-17 Administer Oxygen by Nasal Cannula for Minor Respiratory Distress

Performance Objectives: To provide a low dose of concentrated oxygen to a patient during periods of respiratory distress. Perform this procedure within 15 minutes with a minimum score of 60 points.

Supplies/Equipment: Portable oxygen tank with stand, disposable nasal cannula with connecting tube, flow meter, pressure regulator

Charting/Documentation: Enter appropriate documentation/charting in the box.

____

____

____

____

Instructor's/Evaluator's Comments and Suggestions:

____

____

____

____

____

____

SKILLS CHECKLIST Procedure 30-17: Administer Oxygen by Nasal Cannula for Minor Respiratory Distress

Name ______________________

Date ______________________

No.	Skill	Check #1 20 pts ea	Check #2 10 pts ea	Check #3 5 pts ea	Notes
1	Wash hands and assemble supplies.				
2	Identify the patient and explain the procedure. Teach the patient about cannula positioning, clearing the cylinder valve, and precautions around oxygen use.				
3	Open the cylinder one full turn counterclockwise.				
4	Check the pressure gauge.				
5	Attach the nasal cannula to the tubing, and then to the flow meter.				
6	Adjust the flow rate according to the physician's order.				
7	Check for oxygen flow through the cannula.				
8	Place the tips of cannula into the patient's nostrils no more than 1 inch.				
9	Adjust the tubing around the patient's ears and secure it under the chin.				
10	Answer the patient's questions.				
11	Wash hands.				
12	Document the procedure.				
Student's Total Points					
Points Possible		240	120	60	
Final Score (Student's Total Points / Possible Points)					

	Notes
Start time:	
End time:	
Total time: (15 min goal)	

COMPETENCY ASSESSMENT

Procedure 30-18 Instructing Patient in Use of Metered Dose Nebulizer

Performance Objectives: To instruct a patient in the correct use of a handheld nebulizer, a device that delivers a fine mist of medication with or without the use of oxygen to the respiratory tract including the lungs. Perform this procedure within 20 minutes with a minimum score of 65 points.

Supplies/Equipment: Handheld nebulizer containing medication ordered by the physician

Charting/Documentation: Enter appropriate documentation/charting in the box.

Instructor's/Evaluator's Comments and Suggestions:

SKILLS CHECKLIST Procedure 30-18: Instructing Patient in Use of Metered Dose Nebulizer

Name ______________________________

Date ______________________________

No.	Skill	Check #1 20 pts ea	Check #2 10 pts ea	Check #3 5 pts ea	Notes
1	Wash hands and assemble equipment.				
2	Identify patient.				
3	Check medication order three times.				
4	Demonstrate the use of the equipment to the patient, and then have the patient repeat the demonstration.				
5	Instruct the patient to sit upright and to exhale fully.				
6	Holding the nebulizer, close the mouth, lips, and teeth around the mouthpiece.				
7	Tilting the head back, instruct the patient to take a deep breath and at the same time push the bottle against the mouthpiece.				
8	Instruct the patient to continue to inhale until the lungs are full.				
9	Remove the mouthpiece and exhale slowly.				
10	Repeat Steps 5 through 8 if the physician has ordered more than one dose.				
11	Check patient for adverse reactions.				
12	Wash hands.				
13	Document that the patient was given instructions and has demonstrated to you the use of the nebulizer.				
Student's Total Points					
Points Possible		260	130	65	
Final Score (Student's Total Points / Possible Points)					

	Notes
Start time:	
End time:	
Total time: (20 min goal)	

COMPETENCY ASSESSMENT

Procedure 30-19 Spirometry Testing

Performance Objectives: To prepare a patient for a spirometry to obtain optimum test results. Perform this procedure within 20 minutes with a minimum score of 55 points.

Supplies/Equipment: Spirometer, disposable mouthpiece

Charting/Documentation: Enter appropriate documentation/charting in the box.

____

____

____

____

Instructor's/Evaluator's Comments and Suggestions:

____

____

____

____

____

____

SKILLS CHECKLIST Procedure 30-19: Spirometry Testing

Name ______________________________

Date ______________________________

No.	Skill	Check #1 20 pts ea	Check #2 10 pts ea	Check #3 5 pts ea	Notes
1	Wash hands and assemble equipment.				
2	Identify patient.				
3	Explain the procedure and equipment to the patient. Allow the patient to breathe into the machine to become acquainted with the equipment.				
4	Place the patient in a comfortable position. Loosen tie or collar.				
5	Instruct the patient not to bend at the waist when blowing into the mouthpiece.				
6	Reinforce the inhalation process (deep breaths to fill the lungs to maximum capacity).				
7	Instruct the patient to continue blowing into the mouthpiece until instructed to stop.				
8	Be supportive and encouraging throughout the test.				
9	Wash hands.				
10	Attend to patient's needs.				
11	Place the test results on the patient's chart after being reviewed by the physician. Document the procedure.				
Student's Total Points					
Points Possible		220	110	55	
Final Score (Student's Total Points / Possible Points)					

	Notes
Start time:	
End time:	
Total time: (20 min goal)	

COMPETENCY ASSESSMENT

Procedure 30-20 Pulse Oximetry

Performance Objectives: To measure arterial oxyhemoglobin saturation within seconds, using an external sensor. Perform this procedure within 5 minutes with a minimum score of 75 points.

Supplies/Equipment: Pulse oximeter, sensor, soap and water, alcohol wipes, nail polish remover (if needed)

Charting/Documentation: Enter appropriate documentation/charting in the box.

Instructor's/Evaluator's Comments and Suggestions:

SKILLS CHECKLIST Procedure 30-20: Pulse Oximetry

Name ______________________________

Date ______________________________

No.	Skill	Check #1 20 pts ea	Check #2 10 pts ea	Check #3 5 pts ea	Notes
1	Wash hands and assemble equipment.				
2	Identify patient.				
3	Explain the procedure and equipment to the patient.				
4	Select a site for the sensor. The finger is commonly used.				
5	If the patient has poor circulation, use another site such as the bridge of the nose, ear lobe, or forehead.				
6	Clean the site with alcohol. Remove nail polish if needed. Wash with soap and water.				
7	Apply sensor.				
8	Connect sensor to oximeter with a sensor cable.				
9	Turn on oximeter. A tone and a pulse fluctuation can be heard. Adjust volume.				
10	Set the alarms that alert medical assistant to levels either too high or too low.				
11	Check the pulse manually and compare with the oximeter. Readings should agree.				
12	Note results according to the manufacturer's instructions.				
13	Notify physician of abnormal results (less than 95%).				
14	Document procedure noting the type of sensor being used, the site of application, and the results.				
15	When the oximeter is not in use, plug it in to save the battery. When in use, cover the sensor with a towel or keep it from direct sunlight, which could interfere with the reading.				
Student's Total Points					
Points Possible		300	150	75	
Final Score (Student's Total Points / Possible Points)					

	Notes
Start time:	
End time:	
Total time: (5 min goal)	

COMPETENCY ASSESSMENT

Procedure 30-21 Assisting with Plaster Cast Application

Performance Objectives: To assist the physician in cast application. Perform this procedure within 25 minutes with a minimum score of 90 points.

Supplies/Equipment: Plaster bandage rolls or synthetic cast rolls (For small arm cast, use two to three 2- or 3-inch rolls. For short leg cast, use two to three 3- to 4-inch rolls. For long leg cast, use three to four 4- to 6-inch rolls.), container of warm water that is lined with plastic or cloth to catch loose plaster, stockinette (3-inch width for arms, 4- 6-inch width for legs, etc.), Webril padding rolls, bandage scissors, gloves, walking heel if needed, lotion if using synthetic casting

Charting/Documentation: Enter appropriate documentation/charting in the box.

Instructor's/Evaluator's Comments and Suggestions:

SKILLS CHECKLIST Procedure 30-21: Assisting with Plaster Cast Application

Name ______________________

Date ______________________

No.	Skill	Check #1 20 pts ea	Check #2 10 pts ea	Check #3 5 pts ea	Notes
1	Identify the patient and explain the procedure.				
2	Answer any questions about the injury or cast application.				
3	Wash hands and assemble the equipment and supplies.				
4	Position the patient in a sitting position or as required by the physician.				
5	Put on gloves and drape patient and area around the procedure.				
6	Clean and dry the area to be casted as directed by the physician. Chart any areas of bruising, redness, or open wounds.				
7	Pad bony prominence with sponge rubber (optional). Follow physician's directions.				
8	Provide the correct width and length of stockinette for the area on which cast is being applied. Physician may request the medical assistant to apply the stockinette.				
9	Provide physician with correct width of Webril padding rolls.				
10	When the physician is ready, hold on to the end of the plaster cast roll and dip it into the container of water for 5 seconds. Remove from water and gently squeeze to remove excess water. Hand to the physician. If using synthetic casting material (fiberglass), no water is used, but lotion may be applied to physician's gloved hands to keep resin from sticking to gloves.				
11	Assist with the application of the cast material as requested by the physician.				
12	Reassure patient as needed.				
13	After the application, clean any plaster off patient, review cast care instructions, and provide written instructions for cast care and exercises as directed by the physician.				

No.	Skill	Check #1 20 pts ea	Check #2 10 pts ea	Check #3 5 pts ea	Notes
14	Let plaster in basin settle to the bottom before pouring off the water. Be cautious to keep plaster from going down the drain. Wipe basin clean of residual plaster into the waste container using a paper towel. If using synthetic casting material, do not let the resin touch the sink, countertop, or examination table. Dispose of inner core carefully.				
15	Clean work area.				
16	Remove gloves and wash hands.				
17	Schedule patient for next appointment to have cast checked.				
18	Document the procedure.				
Student's Total Points					
Points Possible		360	180	90	
Final Score (Student's Total Points / Possible Points)					

	Notes
Start time:	
End time:	
Total time: (25 min goal)	

COMPETENCY ASSESSMENT

Procedure 30-22 Assisting with Cast Removal

Performance Objectives: Removal of a cast. Perform this procedure within 20 minutes with a minimum score of 70 points.

Supplies/Equipment: Cast cutter, cast spreader, bandage scissors, bag for disposing of cast materials, drape

Charting/Documentation: Enter appropriate documentation/charting in the box.

Instructor's/Evaluator's Comments and Suggestions:

SKILLS CHECKLIST Procedure 30-22: Assisting with Cast Removal

Name ______________________

Date ______________________

No.	Skill	Check #1 20 pts ea	Check #2 10 pts ea	Check #3 5 pts ea	Notes
1	Wash hands.				
2	Drape patient and area.				
3	Explain the cast removal process to the patient. Assure the patient that the saw will not cut the skin.				
4	Make two cuts, one down each side. With a marker, draw one line down the medial side and one line down the lateral side. These are your cutting lines. If removing an arm cast, also cut the small area between the thumb and index finger.				
5	Begin cutting at the top by pressing down on the saw, not allowing the saw to stay in one place. You will be making circular-type motions: down, toward you or away, then up. Keep the saw moving.				
6	When pressing down with the saw, stop and pull upward as soon as you feel the saw go through the cast and onto the Webril padding. After the procedure, provide written instructions for postcare.				
7	When the cast is cut into two pieces, place the closed cast spreader into the space. Spread and hold the cast apart with the cast spreader while cutting through the Webril and stockinette with the cast scissors. Take care not to press on any tender areas.				
8	When the cast and padding is completely cut into two pieces, remove the cast without traumatizing the limb.				
9	Assist as the physician examines the limb.				
10	If the fracture is determined to be healed, assist the patient to wash the limb, apply lotion in a gentle rub, and caution the patient not to scratch the tender skin.				

No.	Skill	Check #1 20 pts ea	Check #2 10 pts ea	Check #3 5 pts ea	Notes
11	Reassure the patient that skin color and muscle will improve with therapy.				
12	Clean equipment and room.				
13	Wash hands.				
14	Document cast removal and appearance of body part from which cast was removed.				
Student's Total Points					
Points Possible		280	140	70	
Final Score (Student's Total Points / Possible Points)					

	Notes
Start time:	
End time:	
Total time: (20 min goal)	

COMPETENCY ASSESSMENT

Procedure 30-23 Assisting the Physician during a Lumbar Puncture or Cerebrospinal Fluid Aspiration

Performance Objectives: To assemble supplies and position the patient for removal of cerebrospinal fluid (CSF), from the lumbar area, which will be sent to the laboratory for analysis. Perform this procedure within 30 minutes with a minimum score of 115 points.

Supplies/Equipment: Drape; xylocaine 1–2%; syringe and needle for anesthetic; sterile gloves; disposable sterile lumbar puncture tray to include: skin antiseptic with applicator, adhesive bandage, spinal puncture needle, three to four test tubes with secure tops, laboratory requisition, specimen transport bag, patient drape, manometer, laboratory requisition, examination light, gauze sponges

Charting/Documentation: Enter appropriate documentation/charting in the box.

___

___

___

___

Instructor's/Evaluator's Comments and Suggestions:

___

___

___

___

___

___

SKILLS CHECKLIST Procedure 30-23: Assisting the Physician during a Lumbar Puncture or Cerebrospinal Fluid Aspiration

Name ______________________________

Date ______________________________

No.	Skill	Check #1 20 pts ea	Check #2 10 pts ea	Check #3 5 pts ea	Notes
1	Reinforce physician's explanation of the procedure and answer patient's questions.				
2	Verify the patient has signed a consent form.				
3	Have patient empty his or her bladder and bowel.				
4	Wash hands and set up sterile field for physician.				
5	Cleanse the puncture site with antiseptic soap and water. Rinse.				
6	Position the patient in lateral recumbent position with his or her back at the edge of the examination table.				
7	Drape the patient.				
8	Have the patient draw the knees up to the abdomen, grasp onto knees, and flex chin on chest.				
9	Assist as the physician swabs the puncture site with antiseptic.				
10	Assist as the physician drapes the area with the sterile fenestrated drape.				
11	Assist physician to aspirate anesthetic.				
12	Help the patient maintain this position until the needle has been inserted into spinal canal. This is usually better accomplished while standing in front of the patient and holding his or her head and back of knees.				
13	Remind the patient to breathe evenly and not to hold breath or talk, which could interfere with the pressure reading.				
14	At the physician's direction, have the patient straighten his or her legs. Assist as needed while the physician reads the manometer.				
15	Assist as the physician collects spinal fluid.				

No.	Skill	Check #1 20 pts ea	Check #2 10 pts ea	Check #3 5 pts ea	Notes
16	After the procedure has been completed, the physician will apply an adhesive bandage. The patient is placed in prone position for 2 to 3 hours or as directed.				
17	Apply gloves. Cap specimens tightly.				
18	Label samples with patient name, date, and CSF #1, #2, and #3.				
19	Send the labeled specimen to the laboratory in the specimen bag with requisition. Store in incubator until picked up.				
20	Clean area.				
21	Remove gloves.				
22	Wash hands.				
23	Document procedure.				
Student's Total Points					
Points Possible		460	230	115	
Final Score (Student's Total Points / Possible Points)					

	Notes
Start time:	
End time:	
Total time: (30 min goal)	

COMPETENCY ASSESSMENT

Procedure 30-24 Assisting the Physician with a Neurologic Screening Examination

Performance Objectives: To determine a patient's neurologic status. Perform this procedure within 20 to 30 minutes with a minimum score of 25 points.

Supplies/Equipment: Percussion hammer, safety pin or sensory wheel, material for odor identification, cotton ball, tuning fork, flashlight, tongue blade, ophthalmoscope

Charting/Documentation: Enter appropriate documentation/charting in the box.

____

____

____

____

Instructor's/Evaluator's Comments and Suggestions:

____

____

____

____

____

____

SKILLS CHECKLIST Procedure 30-24: Assisting the Physician with a Neurologic Screening Examination

Name ______________________

Date ______________________

No.	Skill	Check #1 20 pts ea	Check #2 10 pts ea	Check #3 5 pts ea	Notes
1	Wash hands.				
2	While taking the patient's medical history, observe level of awareness, memory, cognition, and mood.				
3	Assist while the physician checks reflexes using the percussion hammer.				
4	Assist while the physician checks the patient's sensory abilities, recognition of simple items, and cranial nerves; performs finger to nose test; and checks the ability to run the heel down the opposite shin. Assist the patient as needed during and after the examination.				
5	Document the procedure in patient's chart.				
Student's Total Points					
Points Possible		100	50	25	
Final Score (Student's Total Points / Possible Points)					

	Notes
Start time:	
End time:	
Total time: (20–30 min goal)	

EVALUATION OF CHAPTER KNOWLEDGE

Skills	Student Self-Evaluation Good	Average	Poor
I can describe how to perform urinary catheterization on a female patient.	_____	_____	_____
I can state proper protocol when collecting urine for drug screening.	_____	_____	_____
I can describe patient preparation for occult blood testing.	_____	_____	_____
I can discuss patient instructions for the upper gastrointestinal series, a barium enema, and a cholescystogram.	_____	_____	_____
I can differentiate between an instillation and an irrigation of the eye and ear.	_____	_____	_____
I can discuss the different types of visual acuity tests and how to use each appropriately.	_____	_____	_____
I can explain the medical assistant's role when assisting with audiometry.	_____	_____	_____
I can describe how to teach a patient to perform a nasal irrigation.	_____	_____	_____
I can teach a patient the proper use of a metered dose nebulizer.	_____	_____	_____
I can discuss the role of the medical assistant during spirometry.	_____	_____	_____
I can explain the medical assistant's role in cast application and cast removal and the patient teaching guidelines for cast care.	_____	_____	_____
I can list items required by the physician for a neurologic examination and explain the medical assistant's role in assisting in the examination.	_____	_____	_____
I can identify patient education information for sputum collections.	_____	_____	_____
I can explain oxygen administration using a nasal cannula.	_____	_____	_____
I can apply principles of aseptic technique and observe standard precautions for infection control.	_____	_____	_____
I can properly prepare patients for procedures.	_____	_____	_____
I can perform selected tests that assist the physician with diagnosis and treatment.	_____	_____	_____
I can perform oximetry.			
I can exhibit therapeutic communications skills in interaction with patients and attend to patients' emotional needs.	_____	_____	_____
I can communicate at the level proper for the receiver's ability to understand.	_____	_____	_____

CHAPTER 31

Assisting with Office/Ambulatory Surgery

CHAPTER PRE-TEST

Perform this test without looking at the book. This is just to see how well you have understood and can recall the information in this chapter after you have read it, but before you have completed the workbook exercises. You will not be graded on this portion (other than the grade you give yourself). Justify any "false" answers.

1. The anesthesia used in ambulatory care surgery is different from anesthesias used in major surgeries. (T or F)

2. *Dressing* and *bandage* are different words that mean the same thing. (T or F)

3. *Inflammation* means infection. (T or F)

4. The signs of inflammation are:
   a. redness, drainage, pain, and swelling
   b. redness, pain, and swelling
   c. redness, pain, swelling, and tenderness
   d. redness, pain, swelling, and warmth

5. A sterile item is free from all microorganisms and their spores. (T or F)

6. Only major surgeries require the patient to sign an Informed Consent Form. (T or F)

7. Patients must be told all the things that can go wrong in a surgery and what their options are if they choose not to have surgery. (T or F)

INTRODUCTION

Surgery is often performed in the ambulatory care setting by a physician with the help of a medical assistant. Medical assistants must be knowledgeable about surgical asepsis and sterile principles, surgical instruments, suture materials, surgical supplies and equipment, and basic surgery setups. Medical assistants should also know how to prepare patients for minor surgery, provide patient care, and assist the physician during common minor surgical procedures performed in the ambulatory care setting.

PERFORMANCE OBJECTIVES

After successful completion of this chapter you will be familiar with minor office surgery and how it differs from major surgery. You will know about surgical asepsis and how it differs from medical asepsis, as discussed in Chapter 22. You will be able to list several rules for maintaining sterile areas. You will be familiar with various sizes and types of suture material and suture needles, and what each might be used for. You will be able to identify many surgical instruments and describe their uses and how to care for them. You will be able to select the most appropriate types of dressings and bandages for a given situation and will be able to demonstrate proper application of each type. You will be familiar with a number of local anesthetics and will be able to explain when it is and when it is not appropriate to use epinephrine in local anesthetics. You will be able to list preoperative instructions for patient preparations, as well as postoperative care instructions for the patient and the caregiver. Regarding sterile procedures, you will be able to apply sterile gloves, set up a sterile surgical tray, assist in office surgery, and work within sterile boundaries. In this chapter you will also become familiar with alternative treatments to traditional surgeries and recognizing when each modality might or might not be appropriate. *The following statements are related to your learning objectives for this chapter. Fill in the blanks in the following paragraph with the appropriate term(s).*

Ambulatory/office surgery differs from major surgery not only in (1) ________________, but in the (2) ________________, (3) ________________ and (4) ________________, and (5) ________________ needed. Surgical asepsis uses practices known as (6) ________________. Handcleansing for medical asepsis is defined as removing pathogens from the hands (7) ________________, whereas handwashing for surgical asepsis is the removal of as many microorganisms as possible (8) ________________. When maintaining sterile areas, there are certain rules or (9) ________________ to follow. For instance, all items must be held above (10) ________________. Do not turn (11) ________________ on a sterile field. Do not cough, (12) ________________, or (13) ________________ over a sterile field. The word *suture*, when used as a verb, means (14) ________________; when used as a noun, the word is describing the (15) ________________ used. When suture material is used to tie, it is called (16) ________________. The verb for tying is to (17) ________________. Suture comes in many sizes and types, with 6–0 being the (18) (smallest/largest). The smaller sutures are used for delicate tissues, as on the (19) ________________ or (20) ________________, and the larger sizes are used for tougher areas that need more reinforcement. Suture can be made of many materials such as (21) ______________, (22) ______________, (23) ______________, (24) ______________, and (25) ______________. Some sutures are made to dissolve. These are termed (26) ______________ sutures. Instruments used in surgery are often categorized according to their functions. The cutting category contains (27) ______________ and (28) ______________. The grasping/clamping category contains (29) ______________, (30) ______________, (31) ______________, and (32) ______________. A third category, dilating and probing instruments, contains the (33) ______________, (34) ______________, (35) ______________, (36) ______________, and (37) ______________. Instruments that do not fit into these categories are often referred to as (38) ______________ instruments. Immediately after instruments are used, they should be soaked in a solution of (39) ______________ water and (40) ______________ detergent. Immediately after sanitization, instruments should be thoroughly (41) ______________ and (42) ______________ to prevent spotting and water damage. This is also a good time to examine instruments for (43) ______________, (44) ______________, and (45) ______________. The main difference between dressings and bandages is that (46) ______________ are sterile and are applied directly to the wound, whereas (47) ______________ are applied on top. Bandages are used to keep (48) ______________ in place, to provide (49) ______________ and (50) ______________, and to (51) ______________. One of the most common injectible (52) ______________ ______________ used in ambulatory care is xylocaine. It, and other injectible anesthetics, are often available combined with a chemical called (53) ______________, which causes vasoconstriction and is used to reduce blood flow to an area. It should never be used on (54) ______________, (55) ______________, (56) ______________, or (57) ______________ because of circulatory complications that can occur. When preparing a patient for surgery, it is important to go over any special instructions. They may need to modify their (58) ______________; adjust (59) ______________; acquire special (60) ______________; adjust their personal, home, and (61) ______________ situations; obtain (62) ______________ from their insurance; and prepare for the (63) ______________ period. Postoperative instructions should be (64) ______________ and (65) ______________ by the patient.

VOCABULARY BUILDER

A. *Find the words in Column A that are misspelled; circle them, and then correctly spell them in the spaces provided. Then match each of the vocabulary terms below with its correct definition.*

Column A

_____ 1. Inflamation

_____ 2. Ephinephrine

_____ 3. Ligature

_____ 4. Sodium hydroxide

_____ 5. Hibeclens®

_____ 6. Anestesia

_____ 7. Betadine®

_____ 8. Silver nitrate

_____ 9. Isopryl alcohol

_____ 10. Hydrogen proxide

_____ 11. Strictures

_____ 12. Tetnus

_____ 13. Surgical asepsis

____

____

____

____

____

____

Column B

A. The trade name for povidone-iodine, a topical anti-infective

B. A toxic preparation important as a germicide and local astringent

C. Partial or complete loss of sensation, with or without loss of consciousness

D. A hormone secreted by the adrenal medulla in response to stimulation of the sympathetic nervous system

E. A condition free from germs, infection, and any form of life

F. A narrowing or constriction of the lumen of a tube, duct, or hollow organ

G. Trade name for chlorhexidine gluconate

H. A thread or wire for tying a blood vessel or other structure to constrict or fasten it

I. The nonspecific immune response that occurs in reaction to any type of bodily injury

J. NaOH, a caustic antacid used in detergents and other commercial compounds

K. An acute infectious disease of the central nervous system (CNS) caused by an exotoxin

L. A clean, flammable liquid used in medical preparations for external use

M. In aqueous solution, it is used as a mild antiseptic, germicide, and cleansing agent

B. *Match the vocabulary words below with their correct definitions.*

_____ 1. Allergies

_____ 2. Antibacterial

_____ 3. Approximate

_____ 4. Bandage

_____ 5. Cautery

_____ 6. Contamination

_____ 7. Dressings

_____ 8. Infection

_____ 9. Informed consent

_____ 10. Liquid nitrogen

_____ 11. Mayo stand/instrument tray

_____ 12. Ratchets

_____ 13. Surgery cards

_____ 14. Suture

_____ 15. Swaged/Atraumatic

A. To bring together the edges of a wound

B. A written reference for surgeries and procedures

C. Gauze or other material applied directly to a wound to absorb secretions and for protection

D. When a surgical needle is attached to a length of suture material

E. Surgical material or thread; may describe the act of sewing with the surgical material and needle

F. Being sensitive to a normally harmless substance that causes an autoimmune reaction

G. An invasion of pathogens into living tissue

H. A voluntary agreement to have a procedure or surgery after a patient has been informed about the risks and benefits

I. A portable metal tray table used for setting up sterile fields for minor surgery and procedures

J. Capable of destroying bacteria

K. Commonly and incorrectly referred to as "dry ice," it is a volatile freezing agent used to destroy unwanted tissue such as warts

L. The locking mechanisms on the handles of many surgical instruments

M. The destruction of tissue by burning

N. Gauze or other material applied over dressing to protect and immobilize

O. To make something unclean, often used to describe a sterile area being made "unsterile" or exposing a clean area to a pathogenic substance

LEARNING REVIEW

1. An acceptable border between a sterile and a nonsterile area is:
   a. 1 inch
   b. 2 inches
   c. 4 inches
   d. 5 inches

2. The preferred length for suture material because it is manageable yet long enough to complete most suture procedures is:
   a. 10 inches
   b. 8 inches
   c. 12 inches
   d. 18 inches

3. Suture material that is used when more time is needed for healing is coated with:
   a. magnesium
   b. chromion
   c. calcium
   d. iodine

4. Application of a caustic chemical or destructive heat that burns tissue is called:
   a. cryotherapy
   b. evisceration
   c. approximation
   d. cauterization

5. Locking mechanism located between the rings of the handles of surgical instruments that is used for locking the instrument is called the:
   a. serration
   b. box-lock
   c. ratchet
   d. probe

6. Identify each entry below as an example that follows strict sterile principles or an example in which the sterile area, field, or tray is contaminated by writing "sterile" or "contaminated" in the spaces provided.

____________________ A. Bruce Goldman, CMA, collects used instruments handed to him by Dr. Mark Woo during a minor surgical procedure to excise an infected sebaceous cyst by placing the instruments in a separate container or area out of view of the patient.

____________________ B. Ellen Armstrong, CMA, sets up a sterile field for a minor surgical procedure. After setting up the field, she remembers that a sterile solution is required and leaves the room to obtain the solution to be poured into a sterile cup.

____________________ C. Wanda Slawson, CMA, removes a dressing from a wound on a patient's arm and reaches over the sterile field to discard the used dressing in a biohazard waste container she has placed on the other side of the sterile field that she set up for the procedure.

____________________ D. Patient Edith Leonard will not stop talking and asking questions as Liz Corbin, CMA, removes sutures from a small wound on Edith's arm sustained during a recent fall. The medical assistant is careful to time her responses to Edith so she is not talking when she is working directly over the sterile field.

____________________ E. Anna Preciado, CMA, applies sterile gloves in preparation to assist Dr. Lewis with a minor surgical procedure. During the procedure, she comforts the patient and assists the physician as required. When Anna's hands are not in use, she keeps them down at her sides, careful not to touch her gloved hands to her clothing or any other nonsterile item.

For each previous example that represents a contamination of a sterile area, field, or tray, describe what went wrong and also the correct sterile guidelines for each circumstance.

____

____

____

____

7. Identify each action that follows as an action appropriate to medical aseptic hand washing technique (MAH) or surgical aseptic hand washing technique (SAH).

_____ A. Do not apply lotion

_____ B. Glove for protection

_____ C. 2- to 3-minute duration

_____ D. Scrub nails with brush and clean under each nail with cuticle stick

_____ E. Apply lotion

_____ F. Wash hands, wrists, and forearms to the elbows

_____ G. Hands held down during rinsing

_____ H. 2- to 5-minute duration

CERTIFICATION REVIEW

These questions are designed to mimic the certification examinations. You can use these questions like a small "Certification Examination Study Guide," but this is not meant to take the place of the more extensive study guides. Use this portion to determine in what areas to concentrate your efforts when studying for the certification examination. Justify any "false" answers.

1. Surgical instruments that have opposing cutting edges are classified as:
   a. hemostats
   b. probes
   c. forceps
   d. scissors
   e. scalpels
2. Surgical instruments that have ratchets are used for:
   a. cutting
   b. clamping
   c. probing
   d. exploring
   e. opening
3. Suture material may also be called ligature. (T or F)
4. The word *ligature* means "to tie." (T or F)

5. Thumb forceps may also be called:
   a. pickups
   b. towel clamps
   c. hemostats
   d. Allis forceps

6. Tissue forceps have teeth, dressing forceps do not. (T or F)

7. Epinephrine causes blood vessels to dilate. (T or F)

CASE STUDY

Audrey Jones, CMA, will assist Dr. Lewis in suturing a long, deep, gaping laceration in Lenore McDonnell's leg, sustained when she fell while performing a wheelchair transfer from a car to the sidewalk on her campus. Audrey must prepare the examination room and assemble a sterile surgical tray for the physician's suturing procedure.

1. From the selection that follows, identify each instrument by name. In the spaces provided, give a brief description of each instrument's use. Then choose which instruments Audrey might need to prepare a sterile surgical tray for Dr. Lewis's suturing of the lacerated wound by placing an X in the appropriate boxes.

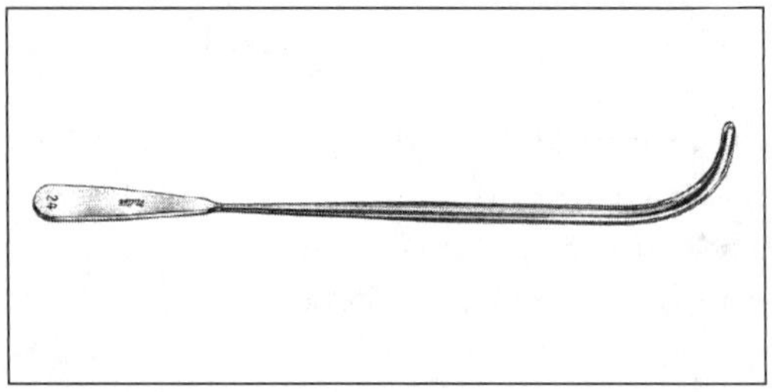

☐ A. ______________________________

Purpose: ______________________________

____

____

____

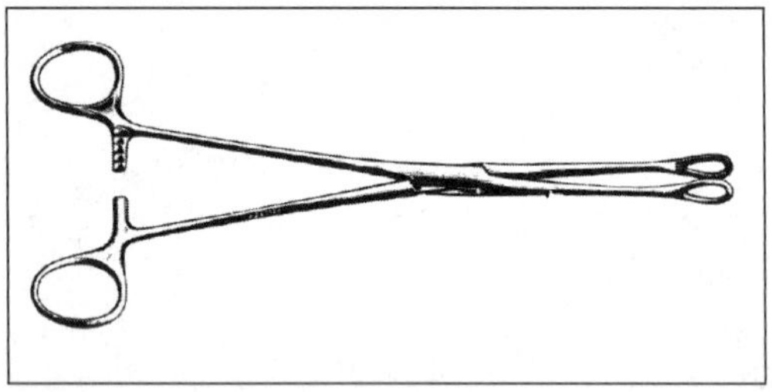

☐ B. ______________________________

Purpose: ______________________________

____

____

____

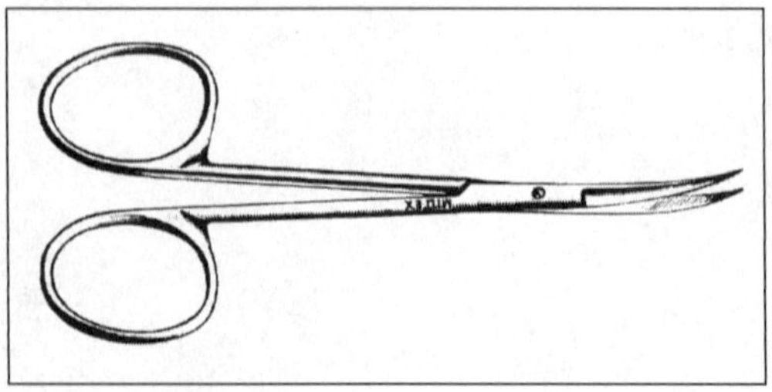

☐ C. ______________________________

Purpose: ______________________________

____

____

____

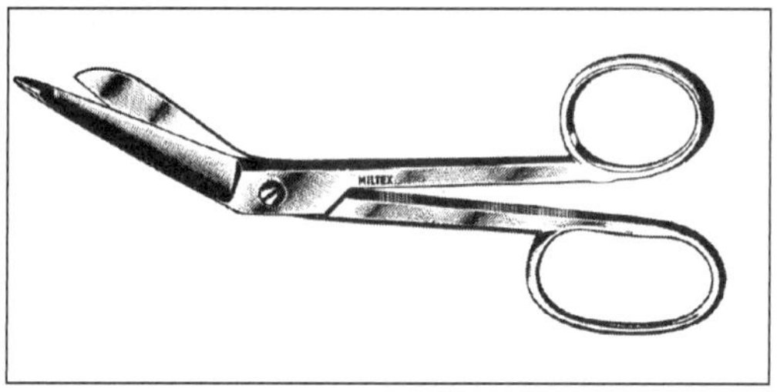

☐ D. ______________________________

Purpose: ______________________________

____

____

____

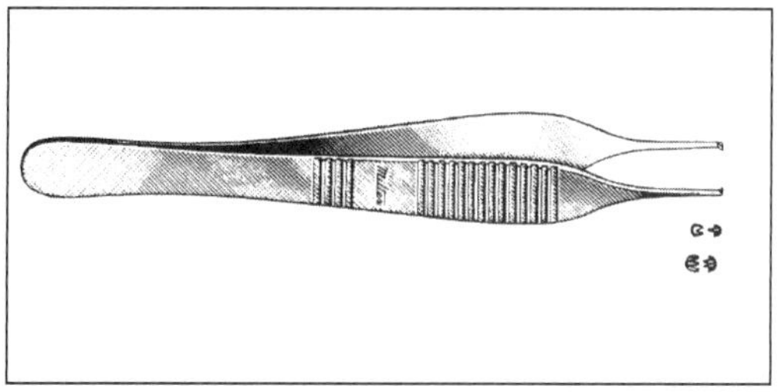

☐ E. ______________________________

Purpose: ______________________________

____

____

____

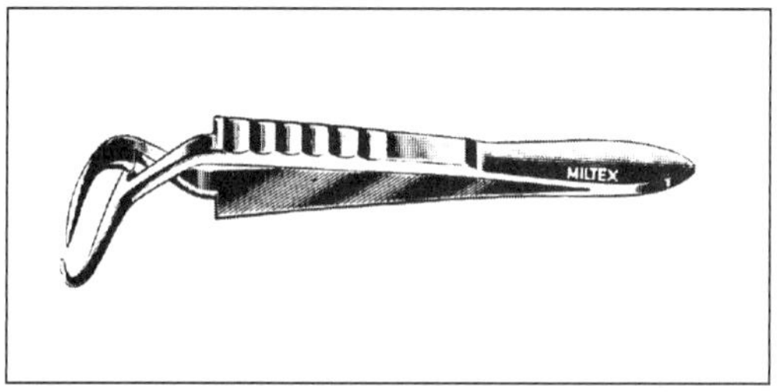

☐ F. ______________________________

Purpose: ______________________________

____

____

____

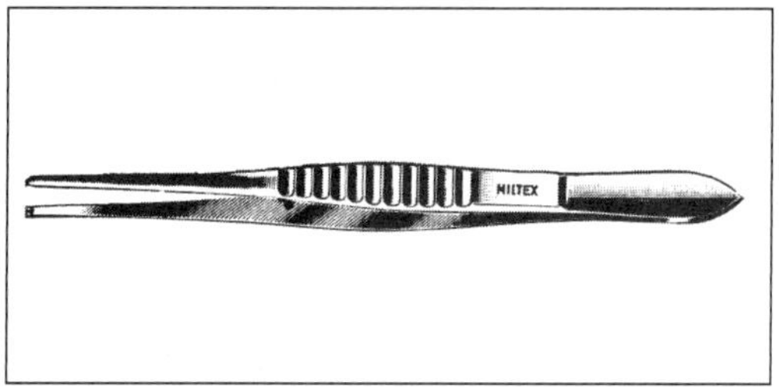

☐ G. ______________________________

Purpose: ______________________________

____

____

____

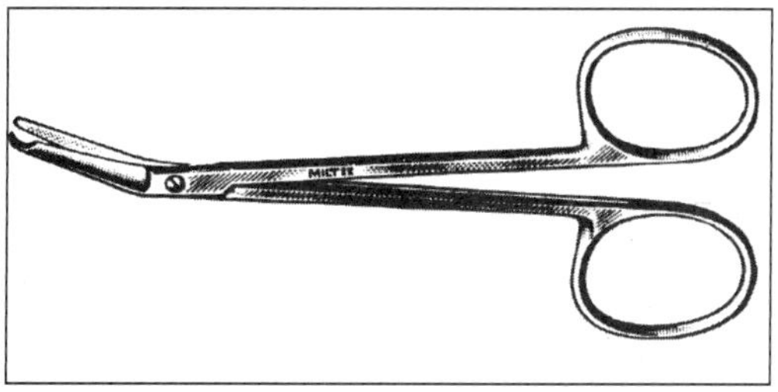

☐ H. ______________________________

Purpose: ______________________________

____

____

____

2. What other equipment will Audrey need to place on the sterile surgical tray to assist the physician in suturing of the lacerated wound? ______________________________

____

What supplies will be needed for the side table? ______________________________

____

When Lenore McDonnell returns to the physician's office to have sutures removed from her leg, Dr. Lewis checks the wound for the degree of healing and instructs Audrey Jones, CMA, to remove the sutures.

3. From the selection of instruments shown in exercise 1, which four will Audrey require for the suture removal procedure?

   ______________________ ______________________

   ______________________ ______________________

4. What other equipment and supplies will Audrey assemble?

   ____

   ____

   ____

5. What technique will Audrey use to perform the removal of the sutures?

   ____

   ____

   ____

6. After removing the sutures, what additional patient care will Audrey give? Why?

   ____

   ____

   ____

SELF-ASSESSMENT

Think of a time when you or a family member experienced a surgical event. If you have not had a personal surgical experience, interview a friend or family member and gather answers to the following questions.

1. Did the doctor or his or her staff explain the procedure clearly?
2. Were your questions answered to your satisfaction?
3. What was of greatest concern to you (financial concerns, pain, recovery, results, etc.)?
4. Did the recovery go as expected?
5. Were the results what you expected?
6. What could have made the experience better?

CHAPTER POST-TEST

This is similar to the Pre-Test. Perform this test without looking at the book. This is just to see how well you have understood and can recall the information presented in this chapter after you have studied it and completed the workbook exercises. You will not be graded on this portion (other than the grade you give yourself), but this is an excellent preparation for your instructor's test. You may use this Post-Test to determine what areas you need to study more. Justify any "false" answers.

1. Anesthetics used in ambulatory care surgery are different from anesthetics used in major surgeries. (T or F)
2. Dressings and bandages differ in that bandages are sterile and dressings are not. (T or F)
3. Inflamed wounds are always infected. (T or F)
4. The cardinal signs of inflammation are:
   a. redness, pain, swelling, and tenderness
   b. redness, drainage, pain, and swelling
   c. redness, pain, and swelling
   d. redness, pain, swelling, and warmth
5. A sterile item is free from all viruses and their spores. (T or F)
6. Patients are only required to sign an Informed Consent Form if they are having major surgery. (T or F)
7. Patients must be told, in writing, all the things that can go wrong in a surgery and what other options they have, besides surgery. (T or F)

CERTIFICATION CRITERIA CHECKLIST

As you go through your education and training, keep in mind the national certification examination that you will take when you graduate. Each chapter of the textbook and workbook covers a different section of the examination criteria. To keep track of your preparation for the certification examination, turn to the back of this workbook and highlight the following CMA, RMA, or CMAS certification examination criteria (if you have already highlighted them from a previous chapter, put a check mark by the criteria):

CMA

R. Principles of Infection Control

S. Treatment Area

    1. Equipment preparation and operation

    4. Preparing/maintaining treatment areas

T. Patient Preparation and Assisting the Physician

    6. Instruments, supplies and equipment

RMA

III. Clinical Medical Assisting
   A. Asepsis
   B. Sterilization
   C. Instruments
   F. Clinical Pharmacology
   G. Minor Surgery

CMAS

2. Basic Clinical Medical Office Assisting
   - Asepsis in the medical office
   - Examination preparation
   - Basic pharmacology

COMPETENCY ASSESSMENT

Procedure 31-1 Applying Sterile Gloves

Performance Objectives: Because hands cannot be sterilized, everyone performing sterile procedures must wear sterile gloves. This procedure provides direction on how to apply sterile gloves without compromising sterility. Perform this procedure within 15 minutes with a minimum score of 50 points.

Supplies/Equipment: Packaged pair of sterile gloves of appropriate size; flat, clean, dry surface

Charting/Documentation: Enter appropriate documentation/charting in the box.

____

____

____

____

Instructor's/Evaluator's Comments and Suggestions:

____

____

____

____

____

____

SKILLS CHECKLIST Procedure 31-1: Applying Sterile Gloves

Name ______________________

Date ______________________

No.	Skill	Check #1 20 pts ea	Check #2 10 pts ea	Check #3 5 pts ea	Notes
1	Remove rings and watch. Wash hands using surgical asepsis.				
2	Inspect glove package for tears or stains.				
3	Place the glove package on a clean, dry, flat surface above waist level.				
4	Peel open the package, taking care not to touch the sterile inner surface of the package. Do not allow the gloves to slide beyond the sterile inner border.				
5	The gloves should be positioned with the cuffs toward you, the palms up, and the thumbs pointing outward.				
6	With the index finger and thumb of the nondominant hand, grasp the inner cuffed edge of the opposite glove. Pick the glove straight up off the surface without dragging the fingers over any nonsterile surface.				
7	With the palm up on the dominant hand, slide the hand into the glove. Do not allow the outside of the glove to come in contact with anything.				
8	With the gloved hand, pick up the remaining glove for the other hand by slipping all four fingers under the outside of the cuff.				
9	With the palm up, slip the second hand into the glove. Maintain tension on the glove. The gloved thumb should be held straight away (like hitchhiking) so it does not touch the nonsterile arm.				
10	Adjust the gloves on the hands as needed. Do not touch nonsterile surfaces with the gloved hands.				
Student's Total Points					
Points Possible		200	100	50	
Final Score (Student's Total Points / Possible Points)					

	Notes
Start time:	
End time:	
Total time: (15 min goal)	

COMPETENCY ASSESSMENT

Procedure 31-2 Setting Up and Covering a Sterile Field

Performance Objectives: To lay a sterile field onto a Mayo tray suitable for surgery or a sterile procedure, and to cover the sterile tray with another sterile drape. Perform this procedure within 15 minutes with a minimum score of 50 points.

Supplies/Equipment: Disposable sterile polylined field drapes or sterile towels (two), Mayo instrument tray/stand positioned above the waist with stem to the right, at right angle to the counter

Charting/Documentation: Enter appropriate documentation/charting in the box.

____

____

____

____

Instructor's/Evaluator's Comments and Suggestions:

____

____

____

____

____

____

SKILLS CHECKLIST Procedure 31-2: Setting Up and Covering a Sterile Field

Name ______________________

Date ______________________

No.	Skill	Check #1 20 pts ea	Check #2 10 pts ea	Check #3 5 pts ea	Notes
1	Wash hands.				
2	Sanitize and disinfect a Mayo instrument tray. Check that the tray is above waist level and the stem is to the right.				
3	Select disposable sterile field drape and place the package on a clean, dry, flat surface at right angle to the Mayo stand.				
4	Open the package, exposing the fan-folded drape. Ensure that the cut corners are toward you.				
5	With thumb and forefinger, grasp the top cut corner without touching the rest of the drape and pick the drape up high enough to prevent it from dragging across any nonsterile area.				
6	Holding drape above waist level and away from your body, allow it to unfold naturally. Do not shake. Grasp another corner so both corners along one edge are being held.				
7	Keep the drape above your waist and away from your body; reach over the Mayo tray with the drape. Do not allow the drape to touch anything.				
8	Gently pull the drape or towel toward you as it is laid onto the tray. Do not touch or reach over the sterile field. If adjustments are needed, walk around the tray or reach under, touching only the edges.				
9	After setting the instruments and supplies on the tray, it must be covered.				

No.	Skill	Check #1 20 pts ea	Check #2 10 pts ea	Check #3 5 pts ea	Notes
10	To cover with a second sterile drape or towel, follow Steps 3 through 6. Then, instead of pulling the drape toward you as outlined in Steps 7 and 8, which would necessitate reaching over the tray, apply the cover drape by holding it up in front of the tray, line up the lower edges, and carefully ease the drape over the tray.				
Student's Total Points					
Points Possible		200	100	50	
Final Score (Student's Total Points / Possible Points)					

	Notes
Start time:	
End time:	
Total time: (15 min goal)	

COMPETENCY ASSESSMENT

Procedure 31-3 Opening Sterile Packages of Instruments and Supplies and Applying Them to a Sterile Field

Performance Objectives: To open sterile packages of surgical instruments and supplies and place them onto a sterile field using sterile technique. Perform this procedure within 20 minutes with a minimum score of 50 points.

Supplies/Equipment: Mayo instrument tray draped with a sterile field, sterile gloves, wrapped-twice sterile surgical instruments, prepackaged sterile surgical supplies

Charting/Documentation: Enter appropriate documentation/charting in the box.

____

____

____

____

Instructor's/Evaluator's Comments and Suggestions:

____

____

____

____

____

____

SKILLS CHECKLIST 31-3: Opening Sterile Packages of Instruments and Supplies and Applying Them to a Sterile Field

Name ______________________

Date ______________________

No.	Skill	Check #1 20 pts ea	Check #2 10 pts ea	Check #3 5 pts ea	Notes
1	Assemble supplies.				
2	Wash hands and set up sterile field as described in Procedure 31-2.				
3	Position twice-wrapped package of surgical instruments on palm of nondominant hand with outer envelope flap on top.				
4	Grasping the taped end of the top flap, open the first flap away from you. Do not touch the inside of the flap.				
5	Grasping just the folded back tips of the side flaps, pull the right-sided flap to the right. Then pull the left-sided flap to the left, taking care not to reach over the package.				
6	Pull the last flap toward you by grasping the folded back tip, taking care not to touch the inner contents of the package.				
7	Gather all of the loose edges together to obtain a snug covering over your nondominant hand. Close your covered thumb over the inner package and carefully apply the inner package to the sterile field.				
8	Open peel-apart packages using sterile technique by grasping both edges of the flaps and pulling them apart in a rolling apart motion, keeping both hands together. The sterile item should be exposed gradually between the two edges. The sterile inner contents may then be offered to the sterile-gloved physician or applied to the sterile field using a flipping motion or positioned upside down over the field and released.				

No.	Skill	Check #1 20 pts ea	Check #2 10 pts ea	Check #3 5 pts ea	Notes
9	Apply sterile gloves and arrange instruments and supplies on the tray in an organized and logical manner according to the physician's preference.				
10	Apply the sterile cover as described in Procedure 31-2.				
Student's Total Points					
Points Possible		200	100	50	
Final Score (Student's Total Points / Possible Points)					
		Notes			
Start time:					
End time:					
Total time: (20 min goal)					

COMPETENCY ASSESSMENT

Procedure 31-4 Pouring a Sterile Solution into a Cup on a Sterile Field

Performance Objectives: To pour a sterile solution into a cup on a sterile tray in a sterile manner. Perform this procedure within 5 minutes with a minimum score of 45 points.

Supplies/Equipment: Covered sterile surgical tray with a sterile cup in upper right corner, container of sterile scrub solution (as ordered)

Charting/Documentation: Enter appropriate documentation/charting in the box.

Instructor's/Evaluator's Comments and Suggestions:

SKILLS CHECKLIST Procedure 31-4: Pouring a Sterile Solution into a Cup on a Sterile Field

Name ______________________

Date ______________________

No.	Skill	Check #1 20 pts ea	Check #2 10 pts ea	Check #3 5 pts ea	Notes
1	Wash hands.				
2	Transport the covered surgical tray to the surgical area before pouring solution.				
3	Read the label of the solution container three times and check expiration date.				
4	Remove the cap from the solution container, taking care not to touch the inner surface of the cap. Place the cap upside down on the counter surface. When cap is held in hand, hold it right side up.				
5	Read the label again to assure accuracy. Place palm over label to protect the label from stains. Cleanse the lip by pouring a small amount into a bowl, cup, or sink that is outside the sterile field.				
6	Carefully pull back the upper right corner of the tray cover to expose the cup.				
7	Approaching from the corner of the tray and using the cleansed side of the lip of the container, pour the needed amount of solution into the sterile cup. Take care not to splash.				
8	Replace the corner of the drape cover using sterile technique.				
9	Replace the cap of the solution container using sterile technique.				
Student's Total Points					
Points Possible		180	90	45	
Final Score (Student's Total Points / Possible Points)					

	Notes
Start time:	
End time:	
Total time: (5 min goal)	

COMPETENCY ASSESSMENT

Procedure 31-5 Assisting with Office/Ambulatory Surgery

Performance Objectives: To maintain sterility during surgical procedures. Perform this procedure within 30 minutes with a minimum score of 135 points.

Supplies/Equipment: *On Mayo stand:* sterile field and cover drapes (two), gauze sponges, scalpel (handle and blade), operating scissors, thumb forceps, hemostats (curved and straight), dressing forceps, suture pack, needle holder, skin retractor, transfer forceps. *May be on sterile field or on the side (physician preference):* fenestrated drape, needles and syringe for anesthesia, prep bowl/cup, Betadine® solution. *On counter or side table:* Sterile gloves in package, labeled biopsy containers with formalin, laboratory requisition, anesthesia vial, alcohol wipes, dressings, tape, bandages, biohazard container, extra gauze in sterile package

Charting/Documentation: Enter appropriate documentation/charting in the box.

Instructor's/Evaluator's Comments and Suggestions:

SKILLS CHECKLIST Procedure 31-5: Assisting with Office/Ambulatory Surgery

Name ______________________________

Date ______________________________

No.	Skill	Check #1 20 pts ea	Check #2 10 pts ea	Check #3 5 pts ea	Notes
1	Check room for equipment, readiness, and cleanliness.				
2	Wash hands.				
3	Set up side table of nonsterile items.				
4	Perform surgical asepsis hand cleansing.				
5	Set up sterile field on a Mayo stand or on a clean, dry, flat surface.				
6	Add sterile items.				
7	Apply sterile gloves. Arrange instruments according to use. Remove gloves.				
8	Cover the sterile field with a sterile drape if not being used immediately.				
9	Identify patient, explain the procedure, and position the patient.				
10	Prepare the patient's skin.				
11	Remove the sterile cover from the sterile field as the physician applies sterile gloves.				
12	Assist the physician as necessary, being certain to follow the principles of surgical asepsis:				
	a. Hold the vial for the physician to withdraw anesthetic.				
	b. Adjust the tray and stool for the physician.				
	c. Assure good light source.				
	d. Comfort and support the patient as needed.				
	e. Assist the physician as needed.				
	f. Hand instruments to the physician and receive used instruments as needed (must have sterile glove on one hand).				
	g. If needed, hold biopsy container to receive specimen. Maintain sterility of specimen, container, and lid.				
	h. Assist with dressing the site if needed.				
13	Assist patient as necessary.				

No.	Skill	Check #1 20 pts ea	Check #2 10 pts ea	Check #3 5 pts ea	Notes
14	The specimen container must be covered tightly; labeled with the patient's name, date, type and source of specimen; and placed in the biohazard specimen transport bag. The requisition is to be completed and placed into the outer pocket of the transport bag.				
15	Wearing appropriate personal protective equipment (PPE), clean surgical or examination room.				
	a. Dispose of used gauze into biohazard container and sharps into sharps container.				
	b. Rinse used instruments in cool water, soak in enzymatic cleaner, sanitize, dry, wrap, and sterilize.				
	c. Gloves and other PPE should be disposed of into biohazard container.				
16	Wash hands.				
17	Document in the patient's record that the specimen was sent to the laboratory.				
Student's Total Points					
Points Possible (27 steps total)		540	270	135	
Final Score (Student's Total Points / Possible Points)					
		Notes			
Start time:					
End time:					
Total time: (30 min goal)					

COMPETENCY ASSESSMENT

Procedure 31-6 Dressing Change

Performance Objectives: To remove a wound dressing, clean the wound and apply a dry, sterile dressing. Perform this procedure within 20 minutes with a minimum score of 110 points.

Supplies/Equipment: *On the sterile field:* Several sterile gauze sponges and other dressing material as needed, sterile bowl/cup with Betadine® solution or prepared sterile Betadine swap sticks, sterile dressing forceps, sterile sponge forceps. *On counter side area:* Nonsterile gloves, sterile gloves in package, container of sterile water, sterile cotton-tipped applicators in package, sterile adhesive strips, antibacterial ointment/cream as ordered, tape, sponge forceps, bandage scissors, waterproof waste bag, biohazard waste container

Charting/Documentation: Enter appropriate documentation/charting in the box.

____

____

____

____

Instructor's/Evaluator's Comments and Suggestions:

____

____

____

____

____

____

SKILLS CHECKLIST Procedure 31-6: Dressing Change

Name ____________________

Date ____________________

No.	Skill	Check #1 20 pts ea	Check #2 10 pts ea	Check #3 5 pts ea	Notes
1	Wash hands.				
2	Prepare sterile field. Add gauze sponges, bowl, and forceps.				
3	Position a waterproof bag away from the sterile area.				
4	Pour Betadine® solution into sterile bowl or use swab sticks.				
5	Identify the patient and explain the procedure.				
6	Reassure and comfort the patient as needed.				
7	Loosen tape on dressing, or cut off bandage.				
8	Put on nonsterile gloves or use forceps.				
9	Carefully remove bandage, then place it in biohazard waste container. Do not pass over sterile field.				
10	Remove dressing, taking care not to stress the wound. If stuck to the wound, wet with sterile water, allow to soak, then remove dressing. Note type and amount of drainage present.				
11	Place used dressing into waterproof bag without touching inside or outside of bag.				
12	Assess wound and note any drainage or signs of infection. Remove and discard gloves into waterproof bag.				
13	Wash hands.				
14	Apply sterile gloves.				
15	Clean the wound with antiseptic solution as ordered.				
16	Dispose of used gauze in waterproof bag.				
17	Using sterile cotton-tipped applicators, apply ointment/cream to the wound as ordered. Using sterile forceps, apply sterile gauze sponge(s) to wound.				

No.	Skill	Check #1 20 pts ea	Check #2 10 pts ea	Check #3 5 pts ea	Notes
18	Remove gloves and dispose of in waterproof bag or into biohazard waste.				
19	Secure dressing with adhesive tape, roller bandage, or elastic bandage. Splint if needed as ordered.				
20	Dispose of waterproof bag in biohazard container.				
21	Wash hands.				
22	Document the procedure and describe wound appearance and healing progress.				
Student's Total Points					
Points Possible		440	220	110	
Final Score (Student's Total Points / Possible Points)					
		Notes			
Start time:					
End time:					
Total time: (20 min goal)					

COMPETENCY ASSESSMENT

Procedure 31-7 Wound Irrigation

Performance Objectives: To irrigate a wound to remove the accumulation of excessive exudates that impairs and delays healing. Perform this procedure within 20 minutes with a minimum score of 105 points.

Supplies/Equipment: Sterile gloves, sterile irrigation kit, sterile dressing material, waterproof pad, sterile solution (according to doctor's orders), nonsterile gloves, waterproof waste bag

Charting/Documentation: Enter appropriate documentation/charting in the box.

____

____

____

____

Instructor's/Evaluator's Comments and Suggestions:

____

____

____

____

____

____

SKILLS CHECKLIST Procedure 31-7: Wound Irrigation

Name ______________________

Date ______________________

No.	Skill	Check #1 20 pts ea	Check #2 10 pts ea	Check #3 5 pts ea	Notes
1	Check physician's order. Select the solution.				
2	Identify the patient. Explain the procedure.				
3	Wash hands.				
4	Position patient for comfort and access to site. Provide good lighting.				
5	Protect area under site with absorbent pad.				
6	Apply nonsterile gloves, remove the dressing, and dispose into waterproof waxed bag.				
7	Note the wound's appearance, color, amount of discharge, and odor of discharge.				
8	Remove and discard gloves into biohazard container.				
9	Wash hands.				
10	Maintain sterile technique and open sterile irrigation tray and the dressings. Use the inner kit wrapping as a sterile field.				
11	Pour the irrigation solution into the sterile container.				
12	Apply sterile gloves.				
13	Place the sterile drainage basin at the edge of the wound.				
14	Fill the irrigating syringe with the solution and wash the wound.				
15	Continue to wash the wound until the solution runs clear and the wound appears cleaned.				
16	Dry the wound edges with sterile gauze.				
17	Reassess the wound.				
18	Apply a sterile dressing.				
19	Remove gloves and dispose of them into biohazard container.				

No.	Skill	Check #1 20 pts ea	Check #2 10 pts ea	Check #3 5 pts ea	Notes
20	Wash hands.				
21	Document.				
Student's Total Points					
Points Possible		420	210	105	
Final Score (Student's Total Points / Possible Points)					

	Notes
Start time:	
End time:	
Total time: (20 min goal)	

COMPETENCY ASSESSMENT

Procedure 31-8 Preparation of Patient Skin before Surgery

Performance Objectives: To remove as many microorganisms as possible from the patient's skin before surgery. Perform this procedure within 20 minutes with a minimum score of 100 points.

Supplies/Equipment: Absorbent pad, sterile drapes (two), one fenestrated drape if doctor prefers, disposable skin prep kit (includes antiseptic soap, several sponges, razor, and a container for water), sterile water, antiseptic solution (as ordered), sterile bowl, sterile gloves (two pair)

Charting/Documentation: Enter appropriate documentation/charting in the box.

Instructor's/Evaluator's Comments and Suggestions:

SKILLS CHECKLIST Procedure 31-8: Preparation of Patient Skin before Surgery

Name ____________________

Date ____________________

No.	Skill	Check #1 20 pts ea	Check #2 10 pts ea	Check #3 5 pts ea	Notes
1	Wash hands.				
2	Assemble the supplies.				
3	Identify the patient.				
4	Explain the procedure. Check for signed consent forms.				
5	Provide good lighting.				
6	Position patient for comfort and access to site.				
7	Wash hands.				
8	Protect area under site with absorbent pad.				
9	Apply sterile gloves or use sterile transfer forceps.				
10	Open kit.				
11	Apply antiseptic soap with gauze sponges, beginning in center of operative site and moving in concentric circles outward.				
12	Discard used sponges as used.				
13	Using razor and holding skin taut, shave hair away from operative site following hair growth pattern.				
14	When hair has been removed, scrub again in circular motion for 2 to 5 minutes.				
15	Rinse shave area with sterile water and pat dry with sterile gauze.				
16	Remove and discard absorbent pad, gauze sponges, disposable prep kit and gloves.				
17	Wash hands.				
18	Using sterile technique, place sterile towel/drape under operative site.				
19	Cover the site with another sterile drape. Instruct the patient not to touch the area.				

No.	Skill	Check #1 20 pts ea	Check #2 10 pts ea	Check #3 5 pts ea	Notes
20	Pour antiseptic solution into bowl for physician to apply with sterile gauze. Drape with fenestrated drape according to physician's preference.				
Student's Total Points					
Points Possible		400	200	100	
Final Score (Student's Total Points / Possible Points)					
		Notes			
Start time:					
End time:					
Total time: (20 min goal)					

COMPETENCY ASSESSMENT

Procedure 31-9 Suturing of Laceration or Incision Repair

Performance Objectives: To set up and assist with the procedure of suturing a wound. Perform this procedure within 20 minutes with a minimum score of 95 points.

Supplies/Equipment: *On the sterile tray:* syringe and needle for anesthetic, hemostats (curved), Adson with teeth or thumb tissue forceps, needle holder with cutting edge or plain needle holder and curved iris scissors, suture pack (suture material and needle, sized and typed according to physician's preference), gauze sponges. *On counter:* anesthetic as ordered by the physician, dressings, bandages, tape, splint/brace/sling (optional), sterile gloves in package.

Charting/Documentation: Enter appropriate documentation/charting in the box.

____

____

____

____

Instructor's/Evaluator's Comments and Suggestions:

____

____

____

____

____

____

SKILLS CHECKLIST Procedure 31-9: Suturing of Laceration or Incision Repair

Name ______________________________

Date ______________________________

No.	Skill	Check #1 20 pts ea	Check #2 10 pts ea	Check #3 5 pts ea	Notes
1	Wash hands.				
2	Identify the patient and explain the procedure. Check for signed consent forms.				
3	Reassure and comfort the patient as needed.				
4	Assess the cause of wound and its severity. Determine allergies and last tetanus booster. Identify health concerns and possible complications (current meds). Soak wound in antiseptic solution as ordered. Clean and dry wound. Position patient comfortably, lying down.				
5	Assist the physician as needed.				
6	Support the patient as needed.				
Give Postoperative Care					
7	Apply sterile gloves				
8	Clean area around the wound and dry wound.				
9	Dress and bandage the wound, and splint the area following physician's preference.				
10	Remove gloves.				
11	Wash hands.				
12	Check patient's vital signs.				
13	Explain wound care to the patient (and caregiver) and provide written instructions, symptoms of infection, and after-hours' phone number.				
14	Assist the patient with any concerns or questions.				
15	Arrange for follow-up appointment and medication as ordered.				
16	Don personal protective equipment (PPE).				
17	Dispose of used supplies according to OSHA guidelines, clean room, sanitize instruments, and sterilize for reuse.				

No.	Skill	Check #1 20 pts ea	Check #2 10 pts ea	Check #3 5 pts ea	Notes
18	Wash hands.				
19	Document the procedure including patient education.				
Student's Total Points					
Points Possible		380	190	95	
Final Score (Student's Total Points / Possible Points)					
		Notes			
Start time:					
End time:					
Total time: (20 min goal)					

COMPETENCY ASSESSMENT

Procedure 31-10 Sebaceous Cyst Excision

Performance Objectives: To remove an inflamed or infected sebaceous cyst or to remove a sebaceous cyst that is not inflamed or infected but is located on an area of the body where the cyst is unsightly or where it may become irritated from rubbing. Perform this procedure within 20 minutes with a minimum score of 105 points.

Supplies/Equipment: *On sterile field:* Syringe and needle for anesthesia, iris scissors (curved), mosquito hemostat (curved), scalpel blade and handle, tissue forceps (two), suture material with needle, needle holder, Mayo scissors (curved). *On the counter:* skin prep supplies, extra sterile gauze (in package), fenestrated drape in package, antiseptic solution as ordered, gloves (sterile in package and nonsterile), personal protective equipment, anesthesia as directed, sterile dressing in package, bandages, tape, biohazard waste container, alcohol pledgets, sterile culture tube, requisition and transport bag (optional).

Charting/Documentation: Enter appropriate documentation/charting in the box.

Instructor's/Evaluator's Comments and Suggestions:

SKILLS CHECKLIST Procedure 31-10: Sebaceous Cyst Excision

Name ______________________

Date ______________________

No.	Skill	Check #1 20 pts ea	Check #2 10 pts ea	Check #3 5 pts ea	Notes
1	Wash hands.				
2	Identify patient and explain the procedure.				
3	Reassure and comfort the patient as needed.				
4	Determine any known allergies and last tetanus booster.				
5	Check for signed consent form.				
6	Identify any health concerns to avoid complications, check medications.				
7	Position the patient comfortably, lying down.				
8	Perform the skin preparation as directed.				
9	Wear appropriate PPE. Include goggles if cyst is infected.				
10	Assist physician with the anesthesia by holding the vial while the physician withdraws the appropriate amount of anesthesia. Continue to assist while physician excises the cyst and sutures the site.				
11	Support patient during surgery.				
Give Postoperative Care					
12	Apply sterile gloves.				
13	Clean area around wound.				
14	Dress and bandage the wound.				
15	Dispose of items appropriately. Remove gloves.				
16	Wash hands.				
17	Check the patient's vital signs.				
18	Explain wound care and provide written instructions. Include symptoms of infection.				
19	Assist the patient with questions or concerns.				

No.	Skill	Check #1 20 pts ea	Check #2 10 pts ea	Check #3 5 pts ea	Notes
20	Arrange for follow-up appointment and medication.				
21	Document the procedure and that the culture was sent to laboratory if appropriate.				
Student's Total Points					
Points Possible		420	210	105	
Final Score (Student's Total Points / Possible Points)					

	Notes
Start time:	
End time:	
Total time: (20 min goal)	

COMPETENCY ASSESSMENT

Procedure 31-11 Incision and Drainage of Localized Infection

Performance Objectives: To assist with the incision and drainage of an abscess (localized infection). Perform this procedure within 25 minutes with a minimum score of 105 points.

Supplies/Equipment: *On sterile tray:* syringe/needle for anesthesia; instruments as determined by physician: scalpel blade and handle, tissue forceps (two), thumb dressing forceps, Mayo scissors (curved), iris scissors (curved), mosquito hemostat (curved), gauze sponges (many), fenestrated drape, antiseptic solution in sterile cup. *On side area:* skin prep supplies, gloves (sterile unopened and nonsterile), personal protective equipment (PPE), anesthesia as directed, sterile dressing unopened, bandages, tape, culture container, requisition and transport bag (optional), biohazard waste container, extra gauze sponges unopened, iodoform gauze wicking, alcohol pledgets, antiseptic solution.

Charting/Documentation: Enter appropriate documentation/charting in the box.

Instructor's/Evaluator's Comments and Suggestions:

SKILLS CHECKLIST Procedure 31-11: Incision and Drainage of Localized Infection

Name ______________________

Date ______________________

No.	Skill	Check #1 20 pts ea	Check #2 10 pts ea	Check #3 5 pts ea	Notes
1	Wash hands.				
2	Identify patient and explain the procedure.				
3	Reassure and comfort the patient as needed.				
4	Determine any known allergies and last tetanus booster.				
5	Check for signed consent form.				
6	Identify any health concerns to avoid possible complications.				
7	Position the patient comfortably, lying down.				
8	Put on PPE, including goggles.				
9	Perform the skin preparation as directed.				
10	Assist physician with the anesthesia by holding the vial while the physician withdraws the appropriate amount of anesthesia.				
11	Support patient during surgery.				
Give Postoperative Care					
12	Apply sterile gloves.				
13	Clean area around wound.				
14	Dress and bandage the wound. Use extra thicknesses for absorption of drainage/exudates.				
15	Dispose of items according to OSHA guidelines. Remove gloves.				
16	Wash hands.				
17	Check the patient's vital signs.				
18	Explain wound care and provide written instructions. Explain to watch for symptoms of infection.				
19	Assist the patient with questions or concerns.				
20	Arrange for follow-up appointment and medication.				
21	Document the procedure.				
Student's Total Points					
Points Possible		420	210	105	
Final Score (Student's Total Points / Possible Points)					

	Notes
Start time:	
End time:	
Total time: (25 min goal)	

COMPETENCY ASSESSMENT

Procedure 31-12 Aspiration of Joint Fluid

Performance Objectives: To remove excess synovial fluid from a joint after injury. Perform this procedure within 20 minutes with a minimum score of 115 points.

Supplies/Equipment: *On surgical field:* syringe/needle for anesthesia (size and gauge as directed), syringe/needle for drainage (size and gauge as directed), sturdy hemostat or needle driver (to remove needle from syringe), gauze sponges (many, sterile), sterile basin for aspirated fluid, fenestrated drape (optional). *On side counter:* skin prep supplies, gloves (sterile, in package and nonsterile), personal protective equipment (PPE), anesthesia as directed, cortisone medication as directed, culture tube, specimen container, pathology requisition, biohazard specimen transfer bag, alcohol swabs, dressings, bandages, tape, biohazard waste container

Charting/Documentation: Enter appropriate documentation/charting in the box.

Instructor's/Evaluator's Comments and Suggestions:

SKILLS CHECKLIST Procedure 31-12: Aspiration of Joint Fluid

Name ______________________

Date ______________________

No.	Skill	Check #1 20 pts ea	Check #2 10 pts ea	Check #3 5 pts ea	Notes
1	Wash hands.				
2	Identify patient and explain the procedure.				
3	Reassure and comfort the patient as needed.				
4	Determine any known allergies and last tetanus booster.				
5	Check for signed consent form.				
6	Identify any health concerns.				
7	Position the patient comfortably, lying down.				
8	Put on PPE, including goggles.				
9	Perform the skin preparation unless the physician prefers to do it.				
10	Assist physician to draw up the anesthesia by holding the vial while the physician withdraws the appropriate amount of anesthesia.				
11	Support patient as needed.				
Give Postoperative Care					
12	Apply sterile gloves.				
13	Clean area around the wound. Gently pat dry.				
14	Dress and bandage the wound as directed.				
15	Dispose of items according to OSHA guidelines. Remove gloves.				
16	Wash hands.				
17	Check the patient's vital signs.				
18	Explain wound care and provide written instruction, including symptoms of infection.				
19	Assist the patient with questions or concerns.				
20	Arrange for follow-up appointment and medication as ordered.				
21	If sending specimen to laboratory, apply gloves and eye/mouth protection. Pour aspirated fluid into a sterile container and cover tightly.				

No.	Skill	Check #1 20 pts ea	Check #2 10 pts ea	Check #3 5 pts ea	Notes
22	Label container; place into specimen transport bag. Seal. Complete laboratory requisition. Place into outside pocket of transport bag. Send to the pathology laboratory.				
23	Document the procedure, including whether a sample was sent to the laboratory.				
Student's Total Points					
Points Possible		460	230	115	
Final Score (Student's Total Points / Possible Points)					

	Notes
Start time:	
End time:	
Total time: (20 min goal)	

COMPETENCY ASSESSMENT

Procedure 31-13 Hemorrhoid Thrombectomy

Performance Objectives: To incise inflamed hemorrhoids and remove thrombus. To remove hemorrhoids with laser, electrosurgery, cryosurgery, or banding. Perform this procedure within 20 minutes with a minimum score of 100 points.

Supplies/Equipment: *On surgical field:* syringe/needle for anesthesia, mosquito hemostat (curved), sterile basin, gauze sponges, rubber bands (optional), fenestrated drape. *On side counter:* skin prep supplies, gloves (sterile in package and nonsterile), personal protective equipment (PPE), anesthesia as directed, biohazard waste container, extra gauze sponges, soft absorbent pad (similar to sanitary napkin), T-bandage (to hold pad in place).

Charting/Documentation: Enter appropriate documentation/charting in the box.

Instructor's/Evaluator's Comments and Suggestions:

SKILLS CHECKLIST Procedure 31-13: Hemorrhoid Thrombectomy

Name ______________________________

Date ______________________________

No.	Skill	Check #1 20 pts ea	Check #2 10 pts ea	Check #3 5 pts ea	Notes
1	Wash hands.				
2	Identify patient and explain the procedure.				
3	Reassure and comfort the patient as needed.				
4	Determine any known allergies and last tetanus booster.				
5	Check for signed consent form.				
6	Identify any health concerns to avoid complications.				
7	Position the patient comfortably, lying down, usually on their side or prone.				
8	Assist with adequate patient draping for comfort.				
9	Put on PPE, as necessary.				
10	Perform skin preparation.				
11	Assist physician to draw up the anesthesia by holding the vial while the physician withdraws the appropriate amount.				
12	Support patient as needed.				
Give Postoperative Care					
13	Assist the physician in placing the absorbent pad. It may be held in place with the T-bandage or the patient's underwear.				
14	Dispose of used items according to OSHA guidelines. Remove gloves and wash hands.				
15	Assist the patient as needed.				
16	Check the patient's vital signs.				
17	Explain wound care and provide written instruction, including signs of complications such as excessive bleeding and pain.				
18	Assist the patient with questions or concerns.				

No.	Skill	Check #1 20 pts ea	Check #2 10 pts ea	Check #3 5 pts ea	Notes
19	Arrange for follow-up appointment and medication as ordered.				
20	Document the procedure and the patient instructions.				
Student's Total Points					
Points Possible		400	200	100	
Final Score (Student's Total Points / Possible Points)					
		Notes			
Start time:					
End time:					
Total time: (20 min goal)					

COMPETENCY ASSESSMENT

Procedure 31-14 Suture/Staple Removal

Performance Objectives: To remove sutures or staples from a healed surgical wound. Perform this procedure within 15 minutes with a minimum score of 85 points.

Supplies/Equipment: *To remove bandage:* bandage scissors, gloves. *To remove sutures/staples:* sterile gloves, suture/staple removal kit (suture scissors and thumb dressing forceps, or staple remover, and 4 × 4 pads) *To redress:* antibiotic cream if ordered, cotton-tipped applicators, gauze sponges, and tape or adhesive strip. *Clean up:* sharps container for staples, biohazard waste container.

Charting/Documentation: Enter appropriate documentation/charting in the box.

____

____

____

____

Instructor's/Evaluator's Comments and Suggestions:

____

____

____

____

____

____

SKILLS CHECKLIST 31-14: Suture/Staple Removal

Name ______________________

Date ______________________

No.	Skill	Check #1 20 pts ea	Check #2 10 pts ea	Check #3 5 pts ea	Notes
1	Identify patient.				
2	Wash hands. Glove and remove bandage (using bandage scissors) if needed. Dispose of bandage. Remove gloves. Wash hands.				
3	Open suture or staple removal kit.				
4	Apply sterile gloves.				
If removing sutures:					
5	Using thumb forceps, gently pick up one knot of a suture. Gently pull upward toward suture line.				
6	Using suture removal scissors, cut one side of the suture as close to skin as possible. Pull up and toward the wound to remove.				
If removing staples:					
5	Using staple remover, gently apply instrument to staple.				
6	Gently squeeze the handle of the staple remover until the staple is pinched outward and upward. Pull up.				
7	Remove all sutures/staples in the same manner, noting the number of sutures or staples removed. Dispose of the sutures on a sterile gauze sponge and the staples into sharps container.				
8	Examine the wound to be certain all sutures or staples have been removed.				
9	Apply antibiotic cream as ordered, using cotton-tipped applicators.				
10	Apply dry, sterile dressing or adhesive strip if indicated.				
11	Remove gloves.				
12	Dispose of used items per OSHA guidelines.				
13	Wash hands.				
14	Check patient's vital signs if indicated.				
15	Explain wound care and provide written instructions.				

No.	Skill	Check #1 20 pts ea	Check #2 10 pts ea	Check #3 5 pts ea	Notes
16	Arrange follow-up appointment if necessary.				
17	Document the procedure, including a description of the wound.				
Student's Total Points					
Points Possible		340	170	85	
Final Score (Student's Total Points / Possible Points)					
		Notes			
Start time:					
End time:					
Total time: (15 min goal)					

COMPETENCY ASSESSMENT

Procedure 31-15 Application of Sterile Adhesive Skin Closure Strips

Performance Objectives: To approximate the edges of a wound after the removal of sutures. Sometimes used in lieu of sutures or to give additional support together with sutures. Perform this procedure within 15 minutes with a minimum score of 120 points.

Supplies/Equipment: *On sterile field:* suture removal instruments and supplies (as indicated), sterile adhesive skin closure strips, iris scissors (straight), Adson dressing forceps, tincture of benzoin (optional), sterile cotton-tipped applicators (for tincture of benzoin). *On side area:* sterile gloves in package, dressings, bandages, tape.

Charting/Documentation: Enter appropriate documentation/charting in the box.

Instructor's/Evaluator's Comments and Suggestions:

SKILLS CHECKLIST Procedure 31-15: Application of Sterile Adhesive Skin Closure Strips

Name ______________________

Date ______________________

No.	Skill	Check #1 20 pts ea	Check #2 10 pts ea	Check #3 5 pts ea	Notes
1	Identify patient and explain the procedure.				
2	Position patient comfortably.				
3	Wash hands and apply gloves.				
4	Remove bandages and dressings.				
5	Clean and dry wound.				
6	Assess the need to skin closure strips and alert the physician as indicated.				
7	Remove and dispose of gloves.				
8	Wash hands.				
9	If tincture of benzoin is ordered, open the bottle and the cotton-tipped applicators.				
10	Apply sterile gloves.				
11	Apply tincture of benzoin to edges of wound with the cotton-tipped applicators, taking care not to get any into the wound.				
12	Open package of skin adhesive strips. Cut to size if needed. Using Adson forceps, apply one end of a strip to one side of the wound. Start the first strip at the center of the wound.				
13	Secure the end to the skin by pressing firmly with the forceps.				
14	Stretch the strip across the edge of the wound and firmly secure on the other side, creating tension across the wound to hold the edges together.				
15	Apply the next two closure strips at halfway points between the middle and each end of the wound.				
16	Continue in this manner until the edges are approximated. Keep wound edges in alignment.				
17	Dress and bandage if necessary.				
18	Dispose of used items.				
19	Remove gloves and wash hands.				
20	Check the patient's vital signs as needed.				

No.	Skill	Check #1 20 pts ea	Check #2 10 pts ea	Check #3 5 pts ea	Notes
21	Explain wound care and provide written instructions.				
22	Assist the patient with questions or concerns.				
23	Arrange for follow-up appointment and medication.				
24	Document the procedure.				
Student's Total Points					
Points Possible		480	240	120	
Final Score (Student's Total Points / Possible Points)					
		Notes			
Start time:					
End time:					
Total time: (15 min goal)					

EVALUATION OF CHAPTER KNOWLEDGE

Skills	Student Self-Evaluation Good	Average	Poor
I can define surgical asepsis and differentiate between surgical asepsis and medical asepsis.	____	____	____
I can list basic rules to follow to protect sterile areas.	____	____	____
I can explain the sizing standards of suture material and the criteria used to select the most appropriate type and size.	____	____	____
I am able to identify and describe the intended use of a wide variety of surgical instruments.	____	____	____
I can demonstrate the ability to select the most appropriate types of dressings for a given situation.	____	____	____
I can state advantages and disadvantages of Betadine®, Hibeclens®, isopropyl alcohol, and hydrogen peroxide when each is used as a skin antiseptic.	____	____	____
I can define anesthesia and explain the advantages and disadvantages of epinephrine as an additive to injectable anesthetics.	____	____	____
I can recall preoperative issues to be addressed in patient preparation and education.	____	____	____
I can identify postoperative concerns to be addressed with the patient and the caregiver.	____	____	____
I can demonstrate the procedure for applying sterile gloves.	____	____	____
I can demonstrate the ability to set up a surgical tray, including laying the field, supplies, and instruments; pouring a sterile solution; using transfer forceps; and covering the sterile tray.	____	____	____
I can explain what is meant by alternative surgical methods.	____	____	____
I can document accurately.	____	____	____
I can attend to the patient's emotional needs.	____	____	____

CHAPTER 32

Diagnostic Imaging

CHAPTER PRE-TEST

Perform this test without looking at the book. This is just to see how well you have understood and can recall the information in this chapter after you have read it, but before you have completed the workbook exercises. You will not be graded on this portion (other than the grade you give yourself). Justify any "false" answers.

1. Medical assistants and other health care professionals may perform limited radiograph procedures in all states. (T or F)
2. X-rays for fractures require no special patient preparation. (T or F)
3. Radiopaque means that "x-rays" cannot penetrate it. (T or F)
4. Ultrasound uses no x-rays and can view organs while they are in motion. (T or F)
5. MRI stands for:
   a. magnetic realistic imaging
   b. magnetic resonance imaging
   c. magnetic ray imaging
   d. machine for radiologic imagining
6. Radiation for cancerous tumors uses x-rays to kill cancer cells. (T or F)

INTRODUCTION

Radiology is the use of x-rays, radioactive substances, and ultraviolet rays. Radiology can be classified into three distinct specialties: diagnostic radiology, radiation therapy, and nuclear medicine. In the medical office, the medical assistant may be expected to be familiar with the use of radiologic procedures. Most of the x-rays taken are not taken in an office setting, but rather are taken in a radiology department of a hospital or free-standing service. Medical assisting students can use this chapter to gain a basic understanding of radiology and radiology safety to properly instruct patients who will be undergoing x-ray procedures.

PERFORMANCE OBJECTIVES

After successful completion of this chapter you will be familiar with the terminology related to diagnostic imaging. You will understand the dangers and some precautions to take while working with radiation. You will be able to explain what x-rays, fluoroscopy, ultrasound, positron emissions, tomography, computed tomography (CT), magnetic resonance imaging (MRI), and flat plates are and what the differences are among radiology, radiation therapy, and nuclear medicine. You will know the proper handling and storage of radiographs and will be able to recall four possible side effects of radiation. *The following statements are related to your learning objectives for this chapter. Fill in the blanks in the following paragraph with the appropriate term(s).*

(1) ______________________ is the branch of medicine concerned with radioactive substances, including x-rays, (2) ______________________, and (3) ______________________. There are (4) ______________________ specialties into which radiology can be classified: (5) ______________________ radiology, (6) ______________________ therapy, and (7) ______________________ medicine. X-rays were named after the German physicist who discovered them in (8) ______________________. His name was (9) ______________________, and he was awarded the first (10) ______________________ in physics for his discovery. The x in x-rays stands for (11) ______________________. Some states (about 35) allow for medical assistants to have a (12) ______________________ license to perform "skeletal films" of the (13) ______________________, (14) ______________________, and so forth. This is a useful credential to have, although it does require additional (15) ______________________. When working within an x-ray area, a (16)______________________ must be worn to measure the amount of x-rays to which a person is exposed. Bones are especially dense, and therefore can absorb more (17) ______________________. Because soft tissues, such as organs, are less dense than bone, a (18) ______________________ media must be used to obtain the image. Sometimes the contrast media is (19) ______________________ to take images of the upper gastrointestinal (GI) tract or given as an (20) ______________________ to view the lower GI tract. Examples of radiographic procedures that require patient preparation include: (21) ______________________, (22) ______________________, (23) ______________________, (24) ______________________, (25) ______________________,

(26) ________________________________, (27) ________________________________, (28) ________________________________, (29) ________________________________, and (30) ________________________________. In the language of radiology, AP means (31) ____________________________, PA means (32) ____________________________, RL means (33) ____________________________, and LL means (34) ________________. The term that means "viewed at an angle" is (35) ____________________________. Fluoroscopy is the process of using a (36) ________________________ to view internal (37) ____________________________ and structures of the body so they can be seen in (38) ______________________ by the radiologist. Ultrasound, CT, and MRI allow for greater imaging (39) _________ than (40) ________________________ radiographs. Ultrasound can be used to help (41) ___________________ problems in the (42) ________________________ organs, the (43) ________________, and (44) ______________________________. It cannot be used for (45) ________________________ structures or the (46) ______________. An (47) ______________________________, or ultrasound of the heart, can view it and determine the (48) ___________________, (49) ________________, and position, as well as the motion made by the (50) ______________ opening and closing. During ultrasound, a (51) _________________ is used with a coupling agent, and (52) ______________________ are emitted from the head of the transducer. PET stands for (53) ____________________ ______________________. It is a radiologic procedure using a (54) __________________ and a (55) __________________________________ substance, which is injected into the patient's body. CT stands for (56) ______________________________________ and uses a small amount of radiation. The (57) ___________________ penetrate body (58) __________________ to produce a series of (59) _________________ sectional (60) ________________________ of the body part being examined. MRI stands for (61) ______________________________. These images are of exceptionally high quality. No (62) _________________ radiation is used, and it is (63) __________________________, safe, and (64) _________________. Flat plates are known as (65) _______________ films because they require no special technique or the use of contrast medium. Radiation therapy is generally used to treat (66) _____________________ that cannot be (67) ______________________ removed. Mammography is perhaps of the highest resolution of any x-ray, which calls for an increase in (68) _______________________ to radiation. (69) ____________________________ is the branch of medicine involved with the use of radioactive substances for (70) ___________________, (71) ____________________, and (72) ______________________.

VOCABULARY BUILDER

Find the words in Column A that are misspelled; circle them, and then correctly spell them in the spaces provided. Then match the following correct vocabulary terms listed in Column A with their corresponding definitions listed in Column B.

Column A

A. dosimeter

B. flouroscopy

C. noninvasive

D. radialpaque

E. radiolucent

F. transducer

G. PET

H. CT

I. MRI

J. flat plate

____

____

Column B

_____ 1. Use of fluorescent screen that shows the images of objects inserted between the tube and the screen

_____ 2. Sound waves are emitted from its head during ultrasound

_____ 3. Magnetic resonance imaging, a noninvasive procedure where the patient lies inside a cylinder-shaped machine in which there is an electromagnet

_____ 4. Computerized tomography, a noninvasive procedure that uses a small amount of radiation and beams that produce a series of cross-sectional images

_____ 5. Positron emission tomography, a radiographic procedure using a computer and radioactive substance

_____ 6. Term a structure is called if x-rays do not penetrate it easily

_____ 7. "Plain" films

_____ 8. Small, badgelike device worn above the waist and measures the amount of x-ray a person is exposed to

_____ 9. Not entering the body

_____ 10. Term a structure is called if x-rays penetrate it easily

LEARNING REVIEW

1. Describe the positions used during x-rays and include the direction of the x-rays, if applicable.

Position	Description	Direction of X-rays
Anteroposterior view (AP)		
Posteroanterior view (PA)		
Lateral view		
Right lateral view (RL)		
Left lateral view (LL)		
Oblique view		
Supine view		
Prone view		

2. For each radiologic test listed below, explain the purpose of the test and the patient preparation needed for the test.

Test	Purpose	Patient Preparation
Angiography		
Barium swallow (upper GI series)		
Barium enema (lower GI series)		
Cholangiography		
Cholecystography		
Cystography		
Hysterosalpingography		
Intravenous pyelography (IVP)		
Mammography		
Retrograde pyelography		

3. What part of the X-ray machine produces X-rays?
   a. the control panel
   b. the tube
   c. the table
   d. the particle beam

4. Why is exposure to radiation dangerous?
   a. radiation can damage eyes, bone marrow, and skin
   b. radiation is harmful to developing embryos
   c. radiation can destroy tissue
   d. all of the above

5. If X-rays do not penetrate a structure easily, it is termed:
   a. radiolucent
   b. radiopaque
   c. translucent
   d. none of the above

6. What test is performed to study the colon for disease?
   a. barium enema
   b. barium swallow
   c. cholangiography
   d. angiography

7. Diagnostic imaging:
   a. is accessible to all offices and hospitals
   b. is an inexpensive form of testing
   c. is easy to read
   d. is a noninvasive procedure

CERTIFICATION REVIEW

These questions are designed to mimic the certification examinations. You can use these questions like a small "Certification Examination Study Guide," but this is not meant to take the place of the more extensive study guides. Use this portion to determine in what areas to concentrate your efforts when studying for the certification examination.

1. If a patient needs to be NPO before a radiologic procedure and the patient drinks a glass of water 3 hours before the appointment, what must you do?
   a. Water is allowed but nothing else.
   b. The procedure will need to be rescheduled.
   c. The patient needs a clearer explanation of what NPO means.
   d. Three hours is long enough for the water to be through the patient's system.
   e. b and c

2. Limited license in radiology means the assistant may:
   a. take only simple skeletal films of the arms and legs
   b. take only films of bones, including sinuses, cranial films, arms and legs, and vertebral
   c. only assist a radiologist in the taking of x-rays
   d. work in the radiology department setting up patients and preparing them for radiologic procedures, but may not actually take x-rays
   e. perform any radiologic procedure that does not involve an intravenous injection

3. Possible side effects of radiation include:
   a. hair loss, weight loss, nausea, and diarrhea
   b. hair loss, nausea, dizziness, and diarrhea
   c. nausea and vomiting, inflammation of the mouth, and hair loss
   d. all of the above

4. Palliative means:
   a. relieving symptoms, as well as curing
   b. curing but not offering much relief of symptoms
   c. placebo, or an agent that does nothing but the patient thinks it helps
   d. an agent that relieves or alleviates uncomfortable symptoms but does not cure the condition

5. When storing and safeguarding radiographs:
   a. they must be protected from light, heat, and moisture
   b. the environment is of little concern; they are basically plastic and can be wiped clean
   c. they must be kept in a cool, dry place
   d. a and c

CASE STUDY

You begin working in an office where x-ray procedures are done. The physician has informed you that he will teach you the procedure for taking x-rays. In your state, special education and licensing are needed for a medical assistant to perform x-ray procedures. You also notice that no one in the office wears a dosimeter, although all are near the x-ray room during the day. Lead aprons are also not used on patients during x-ray procedures. How will you handle this situation?

SELF-ASSESSMENT

As a clinical medical assistant, if you are taking x-rays or assisting with x-ray procedures, what protective measures would you take? Would the patient take the same precautions? Why would you need more precautions than the patient?

CHAPTER POST-TEST

This is similar to the Pre-Test. Perform this test without looking at the book. This is just to see how well you have understood and can recall the information presented in this chapter after you have studied it and completed the workbook exercises. You will not be graded on this portion (other than the grade you give yourself), but this is an excellent preparation for your instructor's test. You may use this Post-Test to determine what areas you need to study more. Justify any "false" answers.

1. Medical assistants and other health care professionals may perform limited x-ray procedures in most states. (T or F)
2. X-rays for fractures require special patient preparation. (T or F)
3. Radiopaque means that "x-rays" can penetrate it. (T or F)
4. Ultrasound uses x-rays and can view organs while they are in motion. (T or F)
5. MRI stands for:
   a. magnetic realistic imaging
   b. machine for radiologic imagining
   c. magnetic resonance imaging
   d. magnetic ray imaging
6. Radiation for cancerous tumors is using x-rays and chemicals to kill cancer cells. (T or F)

CERTIFICATION CRITERIA CHECKLIST

As you go through your education and training, keep in mind the national certification examination that you will take when you graduate. Each chapter of the textbook and workbook covers a different section of the examination criteria. To keep track of your preparation for the certification examination, turn to the back of this workbook and highlight the following CMA, RMA, or CMAS certification examination criteria (if you have already highlighted them from a previous chapter, put a check mark by the criteria):

CMA

S. Treatment Area
   5. Safety precautions

T. Patient Preparation and Assisting the Physician
   3. Examinations

V. Collecting and Processing Specimens; Diagnostic Testing
   8. Medical imaging

RMA

I. General Medical Assisting Knowledge
   F. Patient Education

III. Clinical Medical Assisting
   E. Physical Examinations

CMAS

2. Basic Clinical Medical Office Assisting
   - Examination preparation

EVALUATION OF CHAPTER KNOWLEDGE

Skills	Student Self-Evaluation Good	Average	Poor
I can describe safety precautions for personnel and patients as they relate to x-rays.	_____	_____	_____
I can describe the various positions used during x-ray procedures.	_____	_____	_____
I can discuss the uses for ultrasonography, positron emission tomography, computerized tomography, magnetic resonance imaging, and flat plates.	_____	_____	_____
I can describe the proper procedures for storing x-rays.	_____	_____	_____
I can describe four radiologic procedures that require patient preparation.	_____	_____	_____
I can discuss state regulations regarding the medical assistant performing x-ray procedures.	_____	_____	_____

CHAPTER 33

Rehabilitation and Therapeutic Modalities

CHAPTER PRE-TEST

Perform this test without looking at the book. This is just to see how well you have understood and can recall the information in this chapter after you have read it, but before you have completed the workbook exercises. You will not be graded on this portion (other than the grade you give yourself). Justify any "false" answers.

1. To adduct is to go away from the midline. (T or F)
2. Range of motion is measured in inches. (T or F)
3. When lifting heavy objects, always bend from the waist and keep the object close to your body. (T or F)
4. It helps to have patients put their arms around your neck when lifting them. (T or F)
5. If a patient falls, you should protect his or her head, but otherwise, let him or her fall. (T or F)
6. Medical assistants often perform range of motion exercise on patients in the office. (T or F)

INTRODUCTION

Rehabilitation medicine is a field of medicine that specializes in both preventing disease or injury and restoring patients' physical function, using a combination of physical and mechanical agents to aid in diagnosis and treatment. The goal of rehabilitation medicine is to help restore the functions that have been affected by a patient's condition. The role of the medical assistant is to assist the physician or rehabilitation therapist in enabling a patient to regain normal or near-normal function after an illness or injury. A medical assistant might assist a patient in learning to safely ambulate after a period of sedentary recuperation; in learning the correct use of assistive devices, such as crutches, a cane, or a walker; or in performing therapeutic exercises. In addition to therapeutic exercise, a variety of therapeutic modalities such as heat, cold, light, electricity, and water can be used as part of the patient's rehabilitation program, and the medical assistant should be familiar with how these modalities act on the body and understand the safety precautions associated with each. It is important for the medical assistant to understand the goals and objectives of the rehabilitation program designed by the physician or therapist. A medical assistant's duties in the field of rehabilitation medicine often involve physical strength and coordination, such as when performing wheelchair transfers. It is important to follow proper procedures at all times to protect both the patient and the medical assistant from injury. Therapeutic communication between the medical assistant and rehabilitation patient is essential to providing encouragement and support for patients who face difficult, uncomfortable, or frustrating physical challenges.

PERFORMANCE OBJECTIVES

After successful completion of this chapter you will be able to discuss, using medical terms, rehabilitative medicine and therapeutic modalities. You will know the importance of correct body posture and body mechanics and will be able to demonstrate proper techniques to lift heavy objects, transfer patients, care for a falling patient, push a wheelchair, and help patients ambulate. You will be familiar with assistive devices and how to use them properly for your own safety and for the safety of your patients. You will have the skills and abilities to properly measure patients for crutches, walkers, and canes and to teach them how to properly use each device. You will be able to use heat and cold modalities and explain the body's physiologic reactions to both. *The following statements are related to your learning objectives for this chapter. Fill in the blanks in the following paragraph with the appropriate term(s).*

Physical disability affects (1) ____________________ of people in the United States. Some people recover (2) ____________________, and others recover to their fullest (3) ____________________ and live the rest of their lives with some type of disability. Still others suffer from (4) ____________________ conditions such as (5) ____________________ or severe (6) ____________________ that incapacitates them to the extent they cannot work or completely (7) ____________________. Rehabilitative medicine involves using (8) ____________________ and (9) ____________________ agents to aid in the (10) ____________________, (11) ____________________, and (12) ____________________ of diseases or bodily injury. Medical assistants in the field of rehabilitative medicine will generally be working in (13) ____________________ medicine, an (14) ____________________ practice, or in the (15) ____________________ or (16) ____________________ therapy department of a large hospital or other outpatient clinic or medical office. Wherever you work with rehabilitative medicine, you will most likely be a (17) ____________________ of a large team, with the (18) ____________________ in charge of prescribing the treatments. (19) ____________________ is the practice of using certain key muscle groups together with good body (20) ____________________ and proper body (21) ____________________ to reduce the risk for (22) ____________________ to both the patient and the caregiver. Always be conscious of using proper (23) ____________________ whenever moving, (24) ____________________, (25) ____________________, or (26) ____________________ heavy or (27) ____________________ objects. Use assistive devices, some of which provide (28) ____________________ and (29) ____________________, whereas some require more (30) ____________________. ROM, or (31) ____________________

______________________________ is the amount of (32) ____________________ each joint has. The instrument used to measure ROM is a (33) ____________________. ROM is always expressed in (34) ________________________. The electrical activity of a muscle can be (35) ____________________ on a graph or (36) ________________ to help determine how well the muscle (37) ______________. The instrument used to test the electrical activity of a muscle is an (38) ______________________________. Electric current can also be used to help stimulate muscles. This is called (39) ______________________________ of muscles. Heat and cold are two (40) __________________________ or physical agents, which are used in rehabilitative medicine. Heat, or (41) ______________________________, causes (42) ________________, or the dilation of the blood vessels, which increases circulation to the area. Cold application, or (43) ________________________________, is used to (44) ____________________ blood vessels and slow or stop the flow of blood to an area. Only a (45) ________________________ can order therapeutic modalities as medical treatment, and the medical assistant needs to be cautious of recommending any therapeutics without the order of his or her physician–employer. Some modalities, though, are simple enough for patients to do at home.

VOCABULARY BUILDER

A. Rehabilitation Medicine Terminology

Find the words below that are misspelled; circle them, and then correctly spell them in the spaces provided. Then match each of the following correct vocabulary terms to the example below that best describes it.

A. vasoconstriction	H. goniometry	O. modality
B. thermaltherapy	I. ambulation	P. criotherapy
C. muscle testing	J. gait	Q. gait belt
D. contractures	K. ultrasound	R. vasodialation
E. goniometer	L. activities of daily living (ADL)	S. assistive devices
F. body mechanics	M. hemaplegia	
G. atrophy	N. range of motion (ROM)	________________
________________	________________________	________________

______ 1. Patient Lenore McDonell, confined to a wheelchair since early childhood, receives continuing physical therapy to minimize the effects of any decrease of mobility or atrophy in her legs caused by inactivity.

______ 2. When examining a new patient, a physical therapist must determine which of the physical agents, such as heat, cold, light, water, and electricity, will be most beneficial in treating the patient's condition.

______ 3. As Margaret Thomas, diagnosed with Parkinson's disease, began to experience balance problems and difficulties in walking, her physical therapist prescribed the use of high-frequency sound waves to generate heat in the deep tissue of her right leg, producing a therapeutic effect.

______ 4. Cold applications are used to constrict blood vessels and slow or stop the flow of blood to an area.

______ 5. Lenny Taylor, suffering the early stages of dementia from Alzheimer's disease, works with an occupational therapist to practice methods of making everyday tasks easier to perform.

______ 6. Heat is a modality that creates a therapeutic effect by causing blood vessels to dilate, thereby increasing circulation to an area and speeding up the healing process.

______ 7. When construction worker Jaime Carrera suffers a shoulder injury on the job, Dr. James Whitney performs this process for assessing the motion, strength, and task potential of the muscle group, tendons, and associated tissues.

______ 8. Joe Guerrero, CMA, instructs patient Martin Gordon on the correct method of ambulating while using a three-point gait and axillary crutches.

______ 9. Dr. Winston Lewis recommends this heat modality to help relieve Herb Fowler's chronic lower back pain, which is caused by strain on the back muscles created by the patient's overweight condition.

______ 10. When patient Dottie Tate comes to Inner City Health Care describing a sore back and several recent falls, Dr. Whitney asks clinical medical assistant Bruce Goldman to secure a gait belt around Dottie's waist and have her walk across the room. With Bruce staying a step behind her and slightly to the side, Dr. Whitney carefully observes Dottie's progress when performing this task.

______ 11. As a muscle atrophies, shrinking and losing its strength, joints become stiff and experience development of these deformities. Without constant exercise, the musculoskeletal system deteriorates.

______ 12. Dr. Susan Rice recommends that patient Dottie Tate begin to use a walker at home to prevent further falls. Bruce Goldman, CMA, secures this safety device around Dottie's waist and positions her inside the walker as he gives her verbal instructions to begin the procedure of learning to ambulate with a walker.

______ 13. Older adult patient Abigail Johnson is afraid that because she has diabetes mellitus she is at increased risk for stroke. "I don't want to end up a vegetable and a burden to my family," she tells Dr. Elizabeth King, "all paralyzed on one side like that."

______ 14. Clinical medical assistant Joe Guerrero applies this practice of using certain key muscle groups together with correct body alignment to avoid injury when assisting patient Lenore McDonell in performing a transfer from her wheelchair to the examination table.

______ 15. Margaret Thomas's neurologist uses this instrument to measure the angle of her shoulder joint's ROM during a follow-up examination for Parkinson's disease.

______ 16. Dr. Mark Woo chooses this cold modality to treat the sprained wrist of an emergency patient, reducing inflammation.

______ 17. Canes, walkers, and crutches are examples of walking aids.

______ 18. When lying flat with arms at the sides, the average person should be able to move from a 20-degree hyperextension of the elbow joint to a 150-degree flexion.

______ 19. A physical therapist uses the measurement of joint motion to help evaluate a patient's ROM.

B. Joint Movement Terminology

Match each of the vocabulary terms listed below to its proper definition.

A. extension
B. circumduction
C. plantar flexion
D. dorsiflexion
E. eversion
F. adduction
G. hyperextension
H. flexion
I. inversion
J. pronation
K. supination
L. rotation
M. abduction

_____ 1. Moving the arm so the palm is up
_____ 2. Moving a body part outward
_____ 3. Straightening of a body part
_____ 4. Motion toward the midline of the body
_____ 5. Moving a body part inward
_____ 6. Turning a body part around its axis
_____ 7. A position of maximum extension, or extending a body part beyond its normal limits
_____ 8. Motion away from the midline of the body
_____ 9. Circular motion of a body part
_____ 10. Moving the arm so the palm is down
_____ 11. Moving the foot downward at the ankle
_____ 12. Moving the foot upward at the ankle joint
_____ 13. Bending of a body part

LEARNING REVIEW

1. Some patients require assistive devices to ambulate. Three broad types of assistive devices are listed below. For each assistive device, name the various styles available and one identifying feature of each style. Also, name the physical conditions each style is best suited to be used with as part of a physician's treatment plan.

Canes

(1) ____

____

(2) ____

____

(3) ____

____

Walkers

(1) ____

____

(2) ____

____

(3) ____

____

Crutches

(1) ____

____

(2) ____

____

(3) ____

2. Therapeutic exercise helps patients restore their bodies, protect their bodies from further damage, and prevent against the development of respiratory and circulatory complications caused by inactivity. Medical assistants need to understand the goals and objectives of therapeutic exercise programs. Patients will need support and encouragement to stick to their programs.

   Name four types of exercise programs that are used for therapeutic or preventative purposes. Then match each one to the example below that best describes it.

   ____ 1. ____

   ____ 2. ____

   ____ 3. ____

   ____ 4. ____

   A. Patient Jim Marshall, who is suffering a sports injury to the muscles surrounding the knee, performs exercises in a therapy pool.

   B. Lourdes Austen performs self-directed exercises at home to improve the ROM and increase strength in her left arm, after lumpectomy and axillary lymph node dissection.

   C. Lenore McDonell, who is confined to a wheelchair and unable to move her legs voluntarily, works regularly with a physical therapist to avoid atrophy and contractures in the legs and to improve overall circulation.

   D. Jaime Carrera, who is recovering from a shoulder injury, rebuilds upper body strength with a daily regimen of push-ups, first against the wall and then on the floor.

3. For each illustration, identify the range of motion being performed.

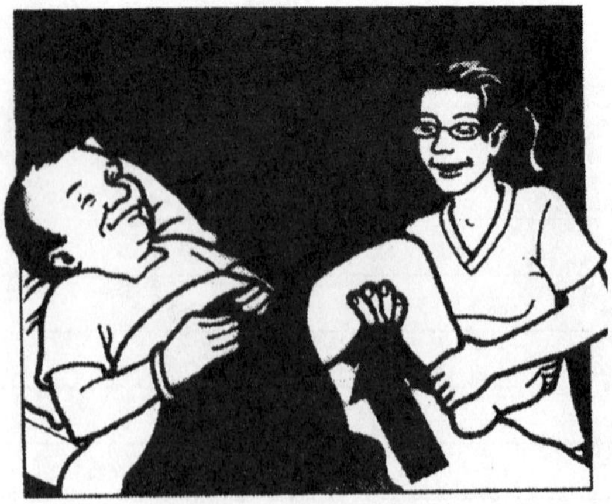

1. ______________________________

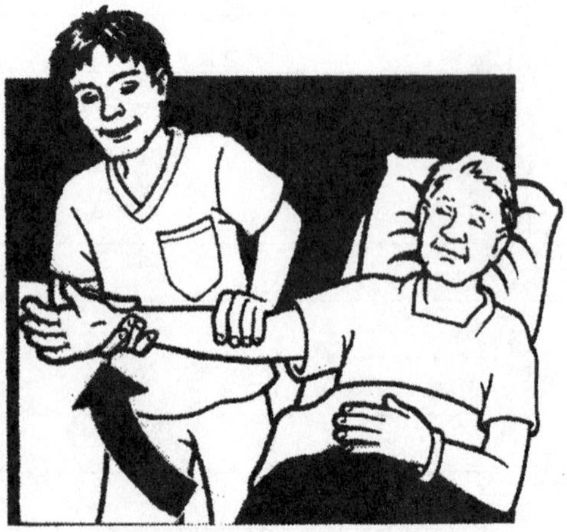

2. ______________________________

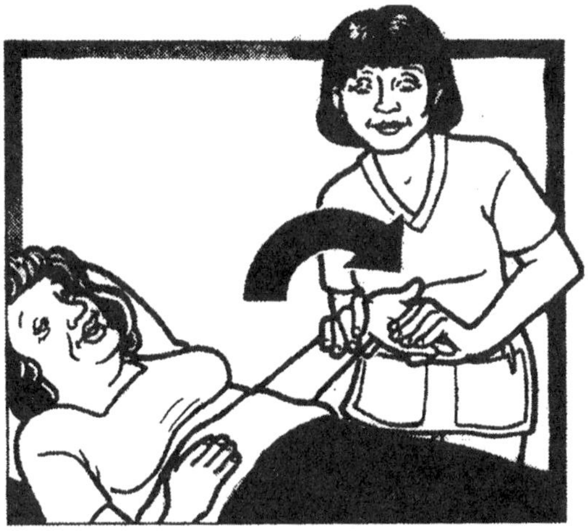

3. ______________________________

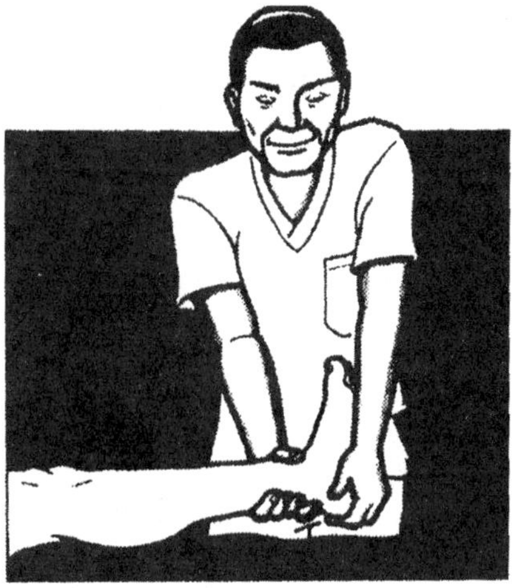

4. ______________________________

4. Therapeutic exercise is not the only way to treat painful joints or tissues. Many patients respond well to the therapeutic modalities of heat and cold, thermotherapy and cryotherapy. List six precautions that medical assistants must take when applying heat or cold modalities.

(1) ____

____

(2) ____

____

(3) ____

____

(4) ____

____

(5) ____

____

(6) ____

____

5. Identify each modality listed below as either a dry heat therapy (DHT), a moist heat therapy (MHT), a moist cold therapy (MCT), or a dry cold therapy (DCT) by placing the proper letters in the space provided. Then identify whether the modality can be performed at home by the patient, with or without caregiver assistance, or whether the modality must be performed in a clinical setting under the supervision of a health care professional. List any special precautions or concerns.

_________ A. Ice pack ____

____

_________ B. Paraffin wax bath ____

____

_________ C. Cold compress ____

____

_________ D. Hot water bottle ____

____

_________ E. Hot compress ____

____

_________ F. Whirlpool bath ____

____

_________ G. Heating pad ____

____

_________ H. Hot soak of one extremity ____

____

_________ I. Hot pack ____

____

_________ J. Total body immersion in a Hubbard tank ____________________________

____

6. For each of the following, identify the proper temperature and correct amount of time the modality should be administered to the patient.
   A. Aquamatic K-Pad for an older adult patient ____________________________
   B. Paraffin wax bath for a patient with rheumatoid arthritis ____________________
   C. An ice pack for a patient with an ankle sprain ____________________________
   D. Hot water bottle for an adult patient ____________________________
   E. A hot compress to drain pus from a patient's skin infection ____________________
   F. Hot soak of the arm and hand for a patient with osteoarthritis ________________

7. How do ultrasound waves best travel? What are the special concerns of ultrasound treatment, how long can ultrasound be administered, and who is authorized to perform ultrasound procedures on patients?

____

____

____

____

CERTIFICATION REVIEW

These questions are designed to mimic the certification examinations. You can use these questions like a small "Certification Examination Study Guide," but this is not meant to take the place of the more extensive study guides. Use this portion to determine in what areas to concentrate your efforts when studying for the certification examination.

1. When lifting or carrying heavy objects, you should rely on the following muscle groups:
   a. abdominal
   b. thoracic
   c. legs and arms
   d. back

2. The type of assistive device that does not require as much upper body strength but is not recommended for older adults is the:
   a. walker
   b. cane
   c. crutches
   d. wheelchair

3. When a patient is standing with hands on the grip of a walker, the elbow should be bent at a _____ -degree angle:
   a. 90
   b. 45
   c. 15
   d. 30

4. The type of crutch that may be used temporarily while a lower extremity heals is:
   a. axillary
   b. forearm
   c. platform
   d. Lofstrand

5. A quad cane is:
   a. two-legged
   b. four-legged
   c. one-legged
   d. three-legged

CASE STUDIES

Medical assistants must practice good body mechanics to protect themselves and their patients from injury. Often called on to lift heavy objects, perform patient transfers, and assist patients in ambulation, medical assistants need to know how to execute their duties safely and efficiently.

For each situation below, discuss the following:

1. What is the best action of the medical assistant?
2. What is the best therapeutic response of the medical assistant?
3. Could the situation have been avoided? If so, how? If not, why not?

Case 1

Ellen Armstrong, CMA, performs the annual task of assembling and moving inactive patient files into a storage filing area for safekeeping. It is the end of the day and Ellen is tired and eager to finish the job; this task has never been one of Ellen's favorites. When she gets to filling the last of three cartons of files, Ellen moves the carton to a shelf, about shoulder high, in the storage room. She returns and decides to take both of the remaining cartons in one trip. Fatigued, she bends at the waist to pick them up.

Case 2

After explaining the procedure to the patient and her son, Wanda Slawson, CMA, performs the transfer of Mary Craig, an older adult blind patient with diabetes mellitus who is suffering from atrophy of the legs, from a car to a wheelchair in the parking lot of Inner City Health Care. Unfortunately, because of Mary's position in the car, the patient must be transferred with her weaker side closest to the wheelchair. The patient panics during the transfer and throws her arms around Wanda's neck as she is lifting and pivoting Mary to the right to position her in the wheelchair. The patient's son John rushes forward to grab on to his mother.

Case 3

Dr. Susan Rice asks Bruce Goldman, CMA, to instruct patient Dottie Tate in the use of a walker to prevent further falls at home. Dottie is silent as Dr. Rice leaves the examination room and Bruce proceeds to set the walker correctly. However, when Dottie sees that Bruce must once again put Dottie in a gait belt for her protection—the belt was used earlier in the examination to assess Dottie's ability to ambulate—the patient gets feisty. She is visibly tired and ready to go home. "I'll learn to use the walker if I have to, but I won't wear that infernal contraption. It makes me feel like a baby. And it's such a bother. Who wants to go through all that? We just don't need it."

SELF-ASSESSMENT

1. Have you ever considered the field of physical or occupational therapy as a career?
2. What makes you think you would do well or not do well in those fields?
3. What do you think you would not care for in working with rehabilitative medicine? What would you like the most?

4. What are some of the skills, talents, interests, and abilities a person would need to have to do well in rehabilitative medicine? List a dozen or more, and then consider and circle all of those that you possess. Which on the list could you learn in a rehabilitative medicine program (insert an *S* for school), and which would be a natural part of your makeup (insert an *N* for natural)? Is there a direct relation between the skills, talents, interests, and abilities you possess and those that you marked with an *N*? Discuss your results with a small group of fellow students. What conclusion(s) did you reach?

POST-TEST

This is similar to the Pre-Test. Perform this test without looking at the book. This is just to see how well you have understood and can recall the information presented in this chapter after you have studied it and completed the workbook exercises. You will not be graded on this portion (other than the grade you give yourself), but this is an excellent preparation for your instructor's test. You may use this Post-Test to determine what areas you need to study more. Justify any "false" answers.

1. To abduct is to go away from the midline. (T or F)
2. ROM is measured in degrees. (T or F)
3. When lifting heavy objects, always bend from the waist and keep the object close to your body. (T or F)
4. It helps to have patients put their arms on your shoulders when helping them to ambulate. (T or F)
5. If a patient falls, you should gently ease him or her to the floor. (T or F)
6. Medical assistants must be familiar with ROM exercises that will be performed on patients by other members of the health care team. (T or F)

CERTIFICATION CRITERIA CHECKLIST

As you go through your education and training, keep in mind the national certification examination that you will take when you graduate. Each chapter of the textbook and workbook covers a different section of the examination criteria. To keep track of your preparation for the certification examination, turn to the back of this workbook and highlight the following CMA, RMA, or CMAS certification examination criteria (if you have already highlighted them from a previous chapter, put a check mark by the criteria):

CMA

E. Communication
    3. Patient instruction
P. Office Policies and Procedures
    2. Patient education
S. Treatment Areas
    2. Principles of operations (equipment)

RMA

I. General Medical Assisting Knowledge
   F. Patient Education
III. Clinical Medical Assisting
   H. Therapeutic Modalities

CMAS

3. Medical Office Clerical Assisting
   - Communication

COMPETENCY ASSESSMENT

Procedure 33-1 Transferring Patient from Wheelchair to Examination Table

Performance Objectives: To safely transfer a patient from a wheelchair to an examination table using a one-person transfer technique, and then using a two-person transfer technique. Perform each of these objectives within 15 minutes (30 minutes total) with a minimum score of 105 points.

Supplies/Equipment: Wheelchair, examination table, gait belt, step stool with rubber trips and a handle for gripping

Charting/Documentation: Enter appropriate documentation/charting in the box.

Instructor's/Evaluator's Comments and Suggestions:

SKILLS CHECKLIST Procedure 33-1: Transferring Patient from Wheelchair to Examination Table

Name ______________________________

Date ______________________________

No.	Skill	Check #1 20 pts ea	Check #2 10 pts ea	Check #3 5 pts ea	Notes
1	Wash hands.				
2	Identify patient, introduce yourself, and explain the procedure.				
3	Place the wheelchair next to the examination table and lock the brakes.				
4	Place the gait belt securely around the patient's waist. Tuck excess under belt.				
5	Move the wheelchair footrests up and out of the way or remove them. Have patient place feet firmly on floor.				
6	Position the stool in front of the examination table as close to the wheelchair as possible.				
7	Instruct the patient to move to the edge of the wheelchair.				
8	Stand directly in front of the patient with your legs slightly apart. Bend at the hips and knees, grasp the gait belt, and instruct the patient to place both hands on the armrest of the wheelchair, so he or she can push off when you give the signal. If the patient does not have the strength to push off, have him or her rest his or her arms in front of him or her.				
9	Give a signal and lift the gait belt upward, pushing with the knees. If patient has strength in his or her legs, ask patient to push up with legs and arms.				
10	Still grasping the gait belt, have the patient step onto the stool with the foot closest to the examination table and pivot so his back is to the examination table. Make sure his or her buttocks are slightly higher than the bed. Support patient's weaker leg with your leg farthest from the examination table.				

No.	Skill	Check #1 20 pts ea	Check #2 10 pts ea	Check #3 5 pts ea	Notes
11	Have the patient grasp the stool handle and place his or her other hand on examination table.				
12	Gently ease the patient to a seated position on examination table.				
13	Place the patient in proper examination position on the table.				
14	Move the wheelchair and stool out of the way.				
Modification—Two-Person Transfer					
1	Place the gait belt snugly around the patient's waist and tuck in the excess.				
2	Have one person stand in front of the patient and the other to the side, next to the examination table.				
3	Both hands should grasp the belt from underneath. Have the patient place his or her hands on the armrests (or relaxed in front).				
4	On one assistant's signal, both assistants should pull the patient straight up. The patient should push off with his or her arms if possible.				
5	The assistant nearest the examination table moves the wheelchair out of the way, whereas the other assistant pivots the patient and has the patient place his or her legs (if possible) onto the step stool. If the patient has strength, he or she can grasp the handles of the step stool.				
6	On one assistant's signal, both assistants lift the patient onto the examination table.				
7	Position the patient on the examination table as necessary.				
Student's Total Points					
Points Possible (21 total steps)		420	210	105	
Final Score (Student's Total Points / Possible Points)					

	Notes
Start time:	
End time:	
Total time: (15 min goal for each—30 min total)	

COMPETENCY ASSESSMENT

Procedure 33-2 Transferring Patient from Examination Table to Wheelchair

Performance Objectives: To safely transfer a patient from the examination table to a wheelchair. Perform this objective within 15 minutes with a minimum score of 65 points.

Supplies/Equipment: Wheelchair, examination table, gait belt, step stool with rubber tips and a handle for gripping

Charting/Documentation: Enter appropriate documentation/charting in the box.

Instructor's/Evaluator's Comments and Suggestions:

SKILLS CHECKLIST Procedure 33-2: Transferring Patient from Examination Table to Wheelchair

Name ______________________

Date ______________________

No.	Skill	Check #1 20 pts ea	Check #2 10 pts ea	Check #3 5 pts ea	Notes
1	Wash hands.				
2	Identify patient, introduce yourself, and explain the procedure.				
3	Place the wheelchair next to the examination table and lock the brakes.				
4	Position the step stool next to the wheelchair.				
5	Assist the patient to rise to a seated position; place the gait belt snugly around the patient's waist and tuck in the excess.				
6	Place your arm under the patient's arm and around the patient's shoulders. Place the other arm under the patient's knees. Pivot the patient so the legs are dangling over the side of the examination table.				
7	Keeping a hand on the patient, move directly in front of the patient.				
8	Grasp the patient by placing hand under gait belt. Plant feet shoulder's width apart and bend knees.				
9	Give signal and pull the patient slightly forward so the patient's feet come down onto the stool. Instruct the patient to push off examination table and grasp the stool handle.				
10	Still grasping gait belt, instruct the patient to step to the floor with the strong leg, pivoting at the same time so his or her back is to the wheelchair.				
11	Have the patient grasp the armrests of the wheelchair.				

No.	Skill	Check #1 20 pts ea	Check #2 10 pts ea	Check #3 5 pts ea	Notes
12	Bend from knees and hips and lower the patient into the wheelchair, making sure the patient is seated comfortably.				
13	Lower footrests and place the patient's feet on them.				
Student's Total Points					
Points Possible		260	130	65	
Final Score (Student's Total Points / Possible Points)					

	Notes
Start time:	
End time:	
Total time: (15 min goal)	

COMPETENCY ASSESSMENT

Procedure 33-3 Assisting the Patient to Stand and Walk

Performance Objectives: To help a patient ambulate safely. Perform this objective within 5 minutes with a minimum score of 55 points.

Supplies/Equipment: Gait belt, chair or wheelchair

Charting/Documentation: Enter appropriate documentation/charting in the box.

Instructor's/Evaluator's Comments and Suggestions:

SKILLS CHECKLIST Procedure 33-3: Assisting the Patient to Stand and Walk

Name ______________________________

Date ______________________________

No.	Skill	Check #1 20 pts ea	Check #2 10 pts ea	Check #3 5 pts ea	Notes
1	Wash hands.				
2	Identify patient, introduce yourself, and explain the procedure.				
3	Lock the brakes on the wheelchair if the patient is using one; place the patient's feet on the floor and move the foot plates out of the way.				
4	Instruct the patient to slide forward in the chair.				
5	Place the gait belt around the patient's waist and tuck excess under the belt.				
6	Stand directly in front of the patient, grasp the gait belt from underneath and assist the patient to stand on signal, and instruct the patient to push up on the armrests of the wheelchair.				
7	Steady the patient and watch for balance, strength, and skin color. Take pulse, if necessary.				
8	If the patient is steady and has balance, strength, and good skin color, proceed by standing slightly behind and to the side of his or her weaker side.				
9	Grasp the gait belt with one hand and place the other on the patient's bent arm for support.				
10	Start with the same foot as the patient and keep in step with him or her.				
11	Document the procedure including the date, time, duration of ambulation, response of patient, and instructions given.				
Student's Total Points					
Points Possible		220	110	55	
Final Score (Student's Total Points / Possible Points)					

	Notes
Start time:	
End time:	
Total time: (5 min goal)	

COMPETENCY ASSESSMENT

Procedure 33-4 Care of the Falling Patient

Performance Objectives: To help a patient fall safely to avoid injury. Perform this objective within 5 minutes with a minimum score of 30 points.

Supplies/Equipment: Gait belt may already be on the patient

Charting/Documentation: Enter appropriate documentation/charting in the box.

Instructor's/Evaluator's Comments and Suggestions:

SKILLS CHECKLIST Procedure 33-4: Care of the Falling Patient

Name ________________________

Date ________________________

No.	Skill	Check #1 20 pts ea	Check #2 10 pts ea	Check #3 5 pts ea	Notes
1	Keep a firm hand on the gait belt.				
2	If the patient falls backward, widen your stance to become a more stable base of support for him or her to fall against. Gently slide him or her to the floor, call for assistance, and take the patient's pulse.				
3	If the patient falls to either side, steady him or her back onto his or her feet, by moving your foot in the direction he or she is falling. Verify that the patient is well enough to continue ambulation. If necessary, call for assistance. Check for injury and check the patient's blood pressure and pulse.				
4	Should the patient fall forward, support him or her around the waist. Step forward with your outer leg and gently lower the patient to the floor, making sure to protect him or her from injury.				
5	Have the patient examined by a physician before moving him or her again.				
6	Document the fall in an incident report.				
Student's Total Points					
Points Possible		120	60	30	
Final Score (Student's Total Points / Possible Points)					

	Notes
Start time:	
End time:	
Total time: (5 min goal)	

COMPETENCY ASSESSMENT

Procedure 33-5 Assisting a Patient to Ambulate with a Walker

Performance Objectives: To help a patient to ambulate safely and independently with a walker. Perform this objective within 15 to 25 minutes with a minimum score of 65 points.

Supplies/Equipment: Gait belt, walker

Charting/Documentation: Enter appropriate documentation/charting in the box.

Instructor's/Evaluator's Comments and Suggestions:

SKILLS CHECKLIST Procedure 33-5: Assisting a Patient to Ambulate with a Walker

Name ______________________

Date ______________________

No.	Skill	Check #1 20 pts ea	Check #2 10 pts ea	Check #3 5 pts ea	Notes
1	Wash hands.				
2	Identify patient, introduce yourself, and explain the procedure.				
3	Apply the gait belt snugly around the patient's waist and tuck in excess.				
4	Check the walker to be sure the rubber section tips are secure on all legs; check the handrests for rough or damaged edges. Tighten all adjustments.				
5	Check to make sure the patient is wearing good walking shoes with a rubber (nonskid) sole.				
6	Check the height of the walker and adjust if necessary.				
7	Position the patient inside the walker and instruct the patient to hold on to the handles while keeping the walker in front of him or her.				
8	Stand behind and slightly to the side of the patient.				
9	Instruct the patient to lift the walker and place all four legs of the walker out in front so the back legs are even with the patient's toes.				
10	Instruct the patient to lean forward and transfer weight so that the patient steps into the walker, first with his or her strongest leg, then with the weaker leg. Make sure the patient brings the strong leg past the weaker leg.				
11	Monitor the patient carefully, staying alert to signs of fatigue. Stand ready to catch the patient if needed.				

No.	Skill	Check #1 20 pts ea	Check #2 10 pts ea	Check #3 5 pts ea	Notes
12	If the walker has rollers, the patient will roll the walker ahead a comfortable distance from his or her body, then walk into it. The patient can also walk normally with a rolling walker by rolling it in front and leaning into the gait, using the walker for support.				
13	Document the date, time, duration of ambulation, response of the patient, and instructions given.				
Student's Total Points					
Points Possible		260	130	65	
Final Score (Student's Total Points / Possible Points)					

	Notes
Start time:	
End time:	
Total time: (15–25 min goal)	

COMPETENCY ASSESSMENT

Procedure 33-6 Teaching the Patient to Ambulate with Crutches

Performance Objectives: To help a patient to ambulate safely using crutches. Perform this objective within 10 minutes with a minimum score of 50 points.

Supplies/Equipment: Gait belt, crutches

Charting/Documentation: Enter appropriate documentation/charting in the box.

Instructor's/Evaluator's Comments and Suggestions:

SKILLS CHECKLIST Procedure 33-6: Teaching the Patient to Ambulate with Crutches

Name ______________________

Date ______________________

No.	Skill	Check #1 20 pts ea	Check #2 10 pts ea	Check #3 5 pts ea	Notes
1	Wash hands.				
2	Identify patient, introduce yourself, and explain the procedure.				
3	Assemble the crutches and make sure they are in good working order; that is, the rubber tips are in place and not torn, the axillary bars and handrests are covered with padding and not cracked or worn, and the wing nuts are tight.				
4	Check the measurement of the crutches. Pediatric crutches must be used for pediatric patients.				
5	Apply the gait belt; assist the patient to stand and place the crutches under the patient's armpits.				
6	Instruct the patient to carry weight completely on the hands and not on the armpits.				
7	Instruct the patient to put all his or her weight on the good leg and to bend the weak leg slightly so it will not drag.				
8	Assist the patient with the required gait.				
9	Wash hands.				
10	Document the date, time, duration of ambulation, and instructions given.				
Student's Total Points					
Points Possible		200	100	50	
Final Score (Student's Total Points / Possible Points)					

	Notes
Start time:	
End time:	
Total time: (10 min goal)	

COMPETENCY ASSESSMENT

Procedure 33-7 Assisting a Patient to Ambulate with a Cane

Performance Objectives: To help a patient to ambulate safely with a cane. Perform this objective within 15 minutes with a minimum score of 65 points.

Supplies/Equipment: Gait belt, appropriate cane for patient

Charting/Documentation: Enter appropriate documentation/charting in the box.

Instructor's/Evaluator's Comments and Suggestions:

SKILLS CHECKLIST Procedure 33-7: Assisting a Patient to Ambulate with a Cane

Name ______________________

Date ______________________

No.	Skill	Check #1 20 pts ea	Check #2 10 pts ea	Check #3 5 pts ea	Notes
1	Wash hands.				
2	Ascertain what type of cane the patient will be using and assemble equipment.				
3	Identify the patient and explain the procedure.				
4	Check the cane to be sure the bottom has a rubber suction tip. If a quad or walkcane is being used, check all the tips.				
5	Apply the gait belt snugly around patient's waist and assist the patient to a standing position.				
6	Place the cane close to the body to the side of the foot of the strong leg. Adjust the cane so the handle is at the level of the patient's hip joint.				
7	During weight bearing, ascertain that the patient's elbow is to be flexed 20 to 30 degrees.				
8	Instruct the patient to move the cane and the involved leg simultaneously, depending on patient's ability.				
9	Instruct the patient to move the weak leg forward while transferring body weight to the cane.				
10	Instruct the patient to move the strong leg forward past the cane.				
11	Follow behind and to the side of the patient's weak side.				
12	Wash hands.				
13	Document the date, time, duration of ambulation, response of patient, and instructions given. Initial report.				
Student's Total Points					
Points Possible		260	130	65	
Final Score (Student's Total Points / Possible Points)					

	Notes
Start time:	
End time:	
Total time: (15 min goal)	

EVALUATION OF CHAPTER KNOWLEDGE

Skills	Student Self-Evaluation Good	 Average	 Poor
I know the definition of rehabilitation medicine and its importance in patient care.	_____	_____	_____
I understand the importance of correct posture and body mechanics and how to safely transfer patients and lift or move large objects using correct body mechanics.	_____	_____	_____
I know how to care for the falling patient.	_____	_____	_____
I know how to help a patient safely stand and walk.	_____	_____	_____
I know three types of assistive devices and how to teach patients to ambulate using each.	_____	_____	_____
I understand how to measure patients for axillary crutches.	_____	_____	_____
I can describe the ambulation gaits used with crutches.	_____	_____	_____
I understand the function of joint range of motion and how to measure joint movement.	_____	_____	_____
I understand how therapeutic exercise is used in rehabilitation medicine and know the types of therapeutic exercises.	_____	_____	_____
I know the definitions of the body movements used in range of motion exercises.	_____	_____	_____
I know the types of therapeutic modalities, can explain how the body reacts to each, and can describe the situation in which each modality would be used.	_____	_____	_____
I understand how ultrasound works.	_____	_____	_____

CHAPTER 34

Nutrition in Health and Disease

CHAPTER PRE-TEST

Perform this test without looking at the book. This is just to see how well you have understood and can recall the information in this chapter after you have read it, but before you have completed the workbook exercises. You will not be graded on this portion (other than the grade you give yourself). Justify any "false" answers.

1. Homeostasis depends on proper nutrients being made available for the body to use. (T or F)
2. Some nutrients provide energy, whereas others help with bodily processes. (T or F)
3. Fats, carbohydrates, and proteins provide energy. (T or F)
4. Fat-soluble vitamins are those vitamins that need oil to be used and stored. (T or F)
5. Water-soluble vitamins are readily depleted, and therefore must be taken in daily. (T or F)
6. Antioxidants are those substances that help the body cells recover from the damaging effects of day-to-day living. (T or F)
7. Fiber is primarily a carbohydrate and comes only from plant sources. (T or F)

INTRODUCTION

Nutrition is the study of the intake of nutrients into the body and how the body uses these nutrients. A proper balance of nutrients is required for optimum health. As individuals progress through each stage of the life span, their diets must be modified to adapt to the body's changing needs. Particular disease states may also require a change from a normal diet to control the progress of the disease and help return the patient to good health. Medical assistants who recognize the type and quantity of nutrients required to maintain good health and who understand how the diet should be changed in response to various disease states or to changes in physical development can use their knowledge of nutritional principles to encourage patients to adopt healthy, nutritional habits. Addressing the patient's eating habits and concerns also helps ensure that the patient will comply with the physician's treatment plan regarding diet and nutrition. Medical assisting students can use this chapter to learn about the vital importance of good nutrition in promoting and maintaining health.

PERFORMANCE OBJECTIVES

After successful completion of this chapter you will be able to discuss, using medical terms, the effects of nutrition on health and disease. You will know the seven basic nutrient types and will be able to explain the relation and balance among the three energy sources for the body. You will be able to recognize the differences between fat and water-soluble vitamins and what each provides. You will be able to discuss various therapeutic diets common to disease states and changes in life cycles. You will be more familiar with herbal supplements, and you will be able to intelligently read a food label to determine the nutritional facts and ingredients. *The following statements are related to your learning objectives for this chapter. Fill in the blanks in the following paragraph with the appropriate term(s).*

Nutrition includes the (1) ____________________, (2) ____________________, (3) ____________________, and (4) ____________________ of food. Nutrition serves many (5) ____________________ in the body. Some (6) ____________________ can provide energy, whereas others provide (7) ____________________ so that proteins can be made within the body or they act as (8) ____________________ to help processes such as the (9) ____________________ mechanism. Energy nutrients are (10) ____________________, (11) ____________________, and (12) ____________________. Other nutrients include (13) ____________________, (14) ____________________, (15) ____________________, and (16) ____________________. It is important to read food (17) ____________________ to help your patients learn more about nutrients. Herbal supplements are herbs from medicinal plants and are also known as (18) ____________________ or (19) ____________________. Many patients use herbs for the treatment of (20) ____________________ and (21) ____________________, and to maintain (22) ____________________. It is part of the movement toward inclusion of (23) ____________________ or (24) ____________________ therapy. Some supplements are (25) ____________________, whereas others are (26) ____________________. Medical assistants must be sure to ask patients about all (27) ____________________ and (28) ____________________ they may be using, including (29) ____________________, (30) ____________________, (31) ____________________, and (32) ____________________. Nutritional needs vary according to individual needs. Women who are (33) ____________________ or (34) ____________________ will have different nutritional needs than infants, adolescents, and older adults. Therapeutic diets are used when the body is in a state of (35) ____________________ or imbalance. In the cases of (36) ____________________, (37) ____________________, (38) ____________________, or cancers, food intake can be adjusted to counteract the disease process and help the body get back to a healthy state. Different (39) ____________________ have different diets, and the combinations of foods or the foods themselves may be (40) ________________ to the medical assistant. The medical assistant who has a good working (41) __________________________ of ethnic foods can help (42) _______________ patients that the dietary changes they need to make are within the parameters of their own (43) _________________________.

VOCABULARY BUILDER

A. Vitamins are a class of nutrients in which each specific vitamin has a function entirely of its own. These complex molecules are required by the body in minute quantities. What are the two functions of vitamins in the body?

(1) ____

(2) ____

B. *Identify the correct chemical name for each vitamin listed. Then describe what each vitamin does in the body to promote good health.*

_________________________ A. One of the B-complex vitamins, also called nicotinic acid

____

_________________________ B. Vitamin B_1

____

_________________________ C. Vitamin E

____

_________________________ D. Vitamin D

____

_________________________ E. One of the B-complex vitamins, also called folacin

____

_________________________ F. Vitamin A

____

_________________________ G. Vitamin B_{12}

____

_________________________ H. Vitamin C

____

_________________________ I. Vitamin B_2

____

_________________________ J. Vitamin B_6

____

C. *Find the words below that are misspelled; circle them, and then correctly spell them in the spaces provided. Then fill in the blanks below with the correct vocabulary term from the following list.*

absorbtion	diaretics	metabolism
amino acids	electrolytes	nutrients
antioxident	elimination	nutrition
basal metabolic rate (BMR)	extracellular	oxidation
calories	fat-soluble	preservatives
catalist	glycogen	processed foods
cellulose	homostasis	saturated fats
coenzyme	ingestion	trace minerals
digestion	major minerals	water soluable
______________	______________	______________
______________	______________	______________

1. Artificial flavors, colors, and ________________________, chemicals that keep food fresh longer, are nonnutritive substances commonly added to processed foods.
2. ________________________ is the study of the intake of nutrients into the body and how the body processes and uses these nutrients.
3. Toxicity is most likely to occur with ________________________ vitamins because they are stored in tissues composed of lipids and in the liver and are not carried easily into the bloodstream.
4. The best source of complete proteins are meats and animal products such as milk and eggs; complete proteins contain all eight of the essential ________________________.
5. Beverages that contain caffeine and alcohol, which are ________________________, will cause the body to increase urinary output and lose water. These substances should be avoided when performing activities, such as a good physical workout, and entering environments, such as an airplane passenger cabin, that promote dehydration.
6. A ________________________ is a nonprotein substance that acts with a catalyst to facilitate chemical reactions in the body.
7. ________________________ is the process of the digestive system involving the transfer of nutrients from the gastrointestinal tract into the bloodstream.
8. Chlorine (Cl) is a mineral with an important ________________________ function, one that takes place outside the cells of body tissues in the spaces between layers or groups of cells.
9. The total of all changes, or energy, chemical and physical, that takes place in the body is called ________________________.
10. Some minerals are considered ________________________ in that they become ionized and carry a positive or negative charge; these minerals must be carefully balanced in the body.

11. ________________________ begins at the mouth with chewing and progresses through the gastrointestinal tract to the small intestine.
12. ________________________ are ingested substances that help the body maintain a state of homeostasis.
13. The process of ________________________ maintains a constant internal environment of the human body, including such functions as heartbeat, blood pressure, respiration, and body temperature.
14. A ________________________ facilitates chemical reactions by speeding up the reaction time without the need for a high-energy output.
15. It is always important to analyze the nutritional labels on ________________________ purchased in the supermarket.
16. Lard is one example of ________________________, which have been found to increase the level of fats and cholesterol in the blood and are hydrogenated, or contain hydrogen.
17. The ability to reduce ________________________ is a characteristic of vitamin E that has led some researchers to suggest that vitamin E may slow the aging process, although its true effectiveness has not yet been demonstrated.
18. The excretion of waste through the anus is called ________________________, the final step of the digestive process.
19. The amount of energy a substance is able to supply is measured in large ______________.
20. Potassium is one of the seven ________________________ found in the body.
21. Vitamins that are ________________________ must be constantly ingested to maintain proper blood levels, because these vitamins are not easily stored in the body.
22. Vitamin E is a fat-soluble vitamin that belongs to a group of compounds called ________________________, which counteract the damaging effects of oxidation. Beta-carotene is another substance in this group.
23. Despite their name, ________________________ are vital to body functioning and include molybdenum and fluorine.
24. ______________________ begins the digestive process when we put food in our mouths to eat.
25. Children, pregnant women, and people with a lean body mass will have a higher ________________________ because it takes more energy to fuel the muscles than it does to store fat.
26. A type of carbohydrate, ________________________, is derived from a plant source and supplies fiber in the human diet.
27. Ingested only in small quantities, ________________________ is an important carbohydrate form for storage of glucose in the body.

LEARNING REVIEW

1. Identify each organ of the digestive system. Describe the healthy functioning of each organ in the space provided. Then, using a medical dictionary or encyclopedia, look up each organ and list one common disorder that would adversely affect the digestive process.

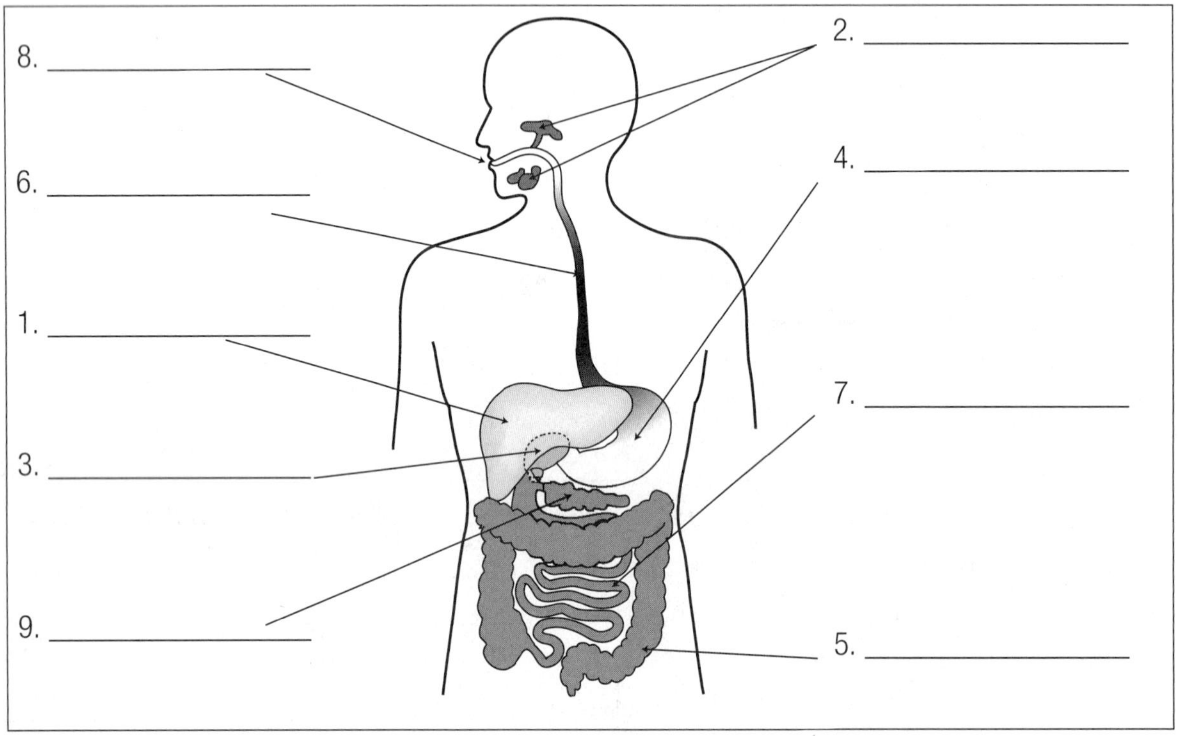

(1) Healthy function: ______________________________
______________________ Common disorder: ______________

(2) Healthy function: ______________________________
______________________ Common disorder: ______________

(3) Healthy function: ______________________________
______________________ Common disorder: ______________

(4) Healthy function: ______________________________
______________________ Common disorder: ______________

(5) Healthy function: ______________________________
______________________ Common disorder: ______________

(6) Healthy function: ______________________________
______________________ Common disorder: ______________

(7) Healthy function: ______________________________
______________________ Common disorder: ______________

(8) Healthy function: ______________________________
______________________ Common disorder: ______________

(9) Healthy function: ______________________________

______________________________ Common disorder: ______________

2. A. Nutrients are divided into two groups: those that provide energy and those that do not.

Identify the nutrients listed below as providing energy or not providing energy by checking the appropriate box.

Energy	No Energy	
☐	☐	(1) Vitamins
☐	☐	(2) Carbohydrates
☐	☐	(3) Fiber
☐	☐	(4) Minerals
☐	☐	(5) Lipids (fats)
☐	☐	(6) Proteins
☐	☐	(7) Water

B. What three chemical elements do carbohydrates, fats, and proteins all contain?

(1) ______________ (2) ______________ (3) ______________

C. Name the most important dietary complex carbohydrate. ______________

D. Name the only true essential fatty acid in the human diet. ______________

E. What additional chemical element does protein alone contain? ______________

F. What happens when the body does not have enough carbohydrates or fats in supply as an energy source? What effect does this have on the body? ______________

____

G. PEM stands for Protein Energy Malnutrition. What usually occurs with this deficiency?

____

____

H. Name two diseases/conditions associated with deficiencies in protein.

(1) ______________ (2) ______________

3. A. List two distinct ways in which minerals differ from vitamins.

(1) ______________________________

(2) ______________________________

B. For each food source, list the mineral or minerals that each provides.

(1) Eggs ______________________________

(2) Milk ______________________________

(3) Cheese ______________________________

(4) Salmon ______________________________

(5) Bananas ______________________________

(6) Green vegetables ______________________________

4. For each of the following, identify the substance as a water-soluble vitamin (WSV), fat-soluble vitamin (FSV), a major mineral (MM), or a trace mineral (TM). Then match the substance to the response below that best fits its character or properties.

____ 1. sulfur	____ 6. pyridoxine
____ 2. vitamin B_{12}	____ 7. iodine
____ 3. iron	____ 8. biotin
____ 4. vitamin K	____ 9. retinol
____ 5. sodium	____ 10. vitamin D

____ A. This substance works with potassium to maintain proper water balance and proper pH balance; the two also are involved in nervous muscular conduction and excitability.

____ B. This substance is part of the pigment rhodopsin found in the eye and is responsible in part for vision, especially night vision.

____ C. This substance is vital to life because of its role in the heme molecule, which carries oxygen to every cell in the body.

____ D. Rickets and osteomalacia are diseases caused by deficiencies in this substance; when deficiencies occur, usually in childhood, malformation of the skeleton is seen.

____ E. This member of the B-complex, together with pantothenic acid, is generally responsible for energy metabolism.

____ F. Because this substance is found only in foods from animal sources, such as liver, kidney, and dairy products, pernicious anemia, the result of deficiencies, may be a problem for some vegetarians.

____ G. This substance, found in rice, beans, and yeast, is important to protein metabolism.

____ H. This substance is a component of one of the amino acids and is found in protein; it is also involved in energy metabolism.

____ I. About half of the body's requirement for this substance is fulfilled through synthesis by intestinal bacteria; bile is required for its absorption into the bloodstream.

____ J. This substance is only found in the thyroid hormones; without it, the thyroid gland would be unable to regulate the overall metabolism of the body.

5. A. List six types of fiber that are carbohydrates.

(1) ____________________	(4) ____________________
(2) ____________________	(5) ____________________
(3) ____________________	(6) ____________________

B. What important fiber is not a carbohydrate? (1) ____________________

Americans generally do not consume enough fiber. How much fiber should be consumed each day? (2) ____________________ Why does brown rice contain more fiber than white rice? (3) ____________________

6. A. What happens when the body takes in more calories than will be expended by the body as energy? (1) ______________________________

   What happens when the body uses more energy than the calories it takes in will produce? (2) ______________________________

   What is the ideal percentage of total calories that should be consumed as carbohydrates, fats, and proteins? Carbohydrates: (3) __________ Fats: (4) __________ Proteins: (5) __________

   B. An 8-fluid-ounce serving of 1% fat soy milk contains 110 calories with 2 grams of total fat, 20 grams of total carbohydrates, and 4 grams of total protein. Calculate the total number of calories from each energy nutrient; show your calculations in the space provided below.

   Number of calories from fat: (1) __________ Number of calories from carbohydrates: (2) __________ Number of calories from protein: (3) __________

   C. Now calculate the percentage of total calories due to each energy nutrient.

   Percentage of calories from fat: (1) __________ Percentage of calories from carbohydrates: (2) __________ Percentage of calories from protein: (3) __________

   D. Compare the percentages of total calories due to fat, carbohydrates, and protein found in soy milk with the percentages you calculated for one serving of peanut butter in the textbook's Critical Thinking box on page 870.

Percentage of Total Calories	Peanut Butter	Soy Milk
Fat		
Carbohydrates		
Protein		

   How do the percentages relate to the ideal percentages for optimum energy balance in the body? ______________________________

   ____

   ____

7. Dr. Elizabeth King has confirmed that patient Mary O'Keefe is pregnant with her third child.

   A. Name two minerals that Mary must increase the intake of in her diet.

   (1) ______________________________ (2) ______________________________

   B. Name three reasons why a woman needs to increase her intake of nutrients and calories when she is pregnant.

   (1) ____

   (2) ____

   (3) ____

   C. What dietary supplement usually needs to be added to a baby's diet? ________________

8. When helping patients modify their diets, medical assistants need to be knowledgeable about the nutrients in the food we eat. The nutritional analysis label on the back or side of a food package is helpful when figuring out the levels of fat, cholesterol, sodium, carbohydrates, protein, and vitamins contained in a particular food.

   A. The percentage of daily values listed on a label report the amount of a nutrient obtained by eating how many servings of a product? (1) ________________ The percentages are based on a (2) ____________________ calorie diet. The listing for total carbohydrates is broken down into what two additional listings? (3) ____________________ (4) ____________________ Which type of carbohydrate is more beneficial and why? (5) ____

   ____

   A patient should look for a food product in which the sodium content is relatively low. What is the greatest number of milligrams of sodium a person should eat each day? (6) ____________ What is the total amount of cholesterol a person should eat each day? (7) ________________ Why is a high-fiber diet important? (8) ____________________

   ____

   ____

B. Compare the nutrition food label from a box of muesli with fruit, nuts, and seeds, with the label from a package of pretzel snacks. Which is more nutritious and why? Note that one serving of the muesli, a half cup or 55 grams, is roughly equivalent to 2 servings of pretzels, 14 pretzels or 60 grams.

____

____

____

____

____

____

____

____

____

____

____

____

____

____

____

____

____

____

____

____

____

____

____

Muesli

Nutrition Facts

Serving Size: 1/2 cup (55g)

Servings Per Container: about 8

Amount Per Serving	Cereal	Cereal + 125 mL Vitamin A & D fortified skim milk
Calories	210	250
Calories from Fat	30	35
	% Daily Value**	
Total Fat 3g*	5%	5%
Saturated Fat 0.5g	3%	3%
Cholesterol 0mg	0%	0%
Sodium 30mg	1%	4%
Total Carbohydrate 40g	13%	15%
Dietary Fiber 5g	21%	21%
Sugars 13g		
Protein 6g		
Vitamin A	0%	8%
Vitamin C	8%	8%
Calcium	4%	20%
Iron	35%	35%
Vitamin D	0%	10%
Thiamine	35%	40%
Riboflavin	25%	35%
Niacin	2%	2%
Vitamin B_6	15%	20%
Folate	10%	10%
Pantothenic Acid	4%	10%

*Amount in Cereal. One half cup skim milk contributes an additional 40 calories, 65 mg sodium, 6g total carbohydrate (6g sugars), and 4g protein.

**Percent Daily Values are based on a 2,000 calorie diet. Your daily values may be higher or lower depending on your calorie needs.

	Calories	2,000	2,500
Total Fat	Less than	65g	80g
Sat Fat	Less than	20g	25g
Cholesterol	Less than	300mg	300mg
Sodium	Less than	2,400mg	2,400mg
Total Carbohydrate		300g	375g
Dietary Fiber		25g	30g

Calories per gram:

Fat 9 • Carbohydrate 4 • Protein 4

Pretzels

Nutrition Facts

Serving Size: 7 Pretzels (30g)

Servings Per Container: 9.4

Amount Per Serving	
Calories 120	
Calories from Fat 10	
	% Daily Value*
Total Fat 1g	2%
Saturated Fat 0g	0%
Cholesterol 0g	0%
Sodium 360mg	15%
Total Carbohydrate 24g	8%
Dietary Fiber 1g	4%
Sugars 1g	
Protein 3g	

Vitamin A 0% Σ Vitamin C 0%

Calcium 0% Σ Iron 2%

*Percent Daily Values are based on a 2,000 calorie diet. Your daily values may be higher or lower depending on your calorie needs:

		Calories 2,000	2,500
Total Fat	Less than	65g	80g
Sat Fat	Less than	20g	25g
Cholesterol	Less than	300mg	300mg
Sodium	Less than	2,400mg	2,400mg
Total Carbohydrate		300g	375g
Dietary Fiber		25g	30g

Calories per gram:

Fat 9 Σ Carbohydrate 4 Σ Protein 4

Ingredients: Unbleached Wheat Flour, Water, Corn Syrup, Partially Hydrogenated Vegetable Oil (Soybean), Yeast Salt, Bicarbonates and Carbonates of Sodium.

9. Compare the advantages and disadvantages of the following diets: U.S. southern, Jewish, and Japanese.

____

____

____

____

____

____

CERTIFICATION REVIEW

These questions are designed to mimic the certification examinations. You can use these questions like a small "Certification Examination Study Guide," but this is not meant to take the place of the more extensive study guides. Use this portion to determine in what areas to concentrate your efforts when studying for the certification examination.

1. Carbohydrates, fats, and proteins have one thing in common. What is it?
   a. high calcium content
   b. their ability to convert into energy
   c. low sodium content
   d. all of the above
2. Examples of monosaccharides are:
   a. fructose
   b. sucrose
   c. a and d
   d. glucose
3. The compounds composed of carbon, hydrogen, and oxygen that exist as triglycerides in the body are:
   a. fats
   b. fiber
   c. vitamins
   d. minerals
4. The basic structural unit of a protein is:
   a. simple sugar
   b. complex sugar
   c. lipids
   d. amino acids
5. Herbal supplements are also known as:
   a. phytomedicines
   b. antioxidants
   c. amino acids
   d. trans acids

CASE STUDY

Lourdes Austen, a breast cancer survivor, regularly attends a support group for breast cancer patients and survivors held once a month. Lourdes finds the group a great source of encouragement, information, and support—a safe place to discuss her feelings and concerns about breast cancer. The group is planning a session to talk about nutrition issues, and Lourdes asks clinical medical assistant Audrey Jones if she would like to attend the meeting with her to contribute to the group's discussion. With permission from office manager Marilyn Johnson and Lourdes's physician Dr. Elizabeth King, Audrey attends the meeting. The group members are enthusiastic and ask Audrey many questions, including the following: "Why is good nutrition important for cancer patients?" "I don't have much of an appetite anymore and get nauseous all the time. What can I do?" "I keep hearing about those macrobiotic diets? Are they any good? Should I try them?"

Discuss the following:

1. What information can Audrey give in answer to the question regarding the importance of good nutrition for cancer patients?
2. What suggestion can Audrey offer to patients who have no appetite and have nausea or vomiting?
3. What can Audrey tell the group about macrobiotic diets?
4. What is the role of the medical assistant in attending the breast cancer support group meeting?

SELF-ASSESSMENT

1. Keep track of your diet for a couple of days. Track everything you eat and drink and the amounts of each item.

2. Either use the Internet to research the nutritional value of each item or look in a good dietary resource for the information. Figure the number of calories you ate each day, the amount of fiber, the amount and types of fats, how much protein, how many carbohydrates and sugars, and which vitamins and minerals you consumed. Hint: There are specific Web sites that can help you with this project. One example is: http://www.calorie-count.com. This Web site allows you to search through hundreds of different foods and drinks to find the "labels" for them. It is free! You can even create your own personal profile.

3. Now figure in any vitamins and supplements you ingested.

4. Is there any particular part of a nutritious diet that you are lacking?

5. Are there any components that you ate too much of?

POST-TEST

This is similar to the Pre-Test. Perform this test without looking at the book. This is just to see how well you have understood and can recall the information presented in this chapter after you have studied it and completed the workbook exercises. You will not be graded on this portion (other than the grade you give yourself), but this is an excellent preparation for your instructor's test. You may use this Post-Test to determine what areas you need to study more. Justify any "false" answers.

1. Homeostasis occurs properly and does not depend on proper nutrients being made available for the body to use. (T or F)
2. Nutrients provide energy. (T or F)
3. Fats and carbohydrates provide energy, whereas proteins do not. (T or F)
4. Fat-soluble vitamins are those vitamins that are stored in the fat of the body. (T or F)
5. Water-soluble vitamins are not easily depleted, and therefore can build up to dangerous levels. (T or F)
6. Antioxidants are those substances that help the body's cells overcome the damages of free radicals. (T or F)
7. Fiber is primarily a carbohydrate and comes only from plant sources. (T or F)

CERTIFICATION CRITERIA CHECKLIST

As you go through your education and training, keep in mind the national certification examination that you will take when you graduate. Each chapter of the textbook and workbook covers a different section of the examination criteria. To keep track of your preparation for the certification examination, turn to the back of this workbook and highlight the following CMA, RMA, or CMAS certification examination criteria (if you have already highlighted them from a previous chapter, put a check mark by the criteria):

CMA
C. Psychology
    2. Developmental stages of the life cycle
E. Communication
    3. Patient instruction
Z. Nutrition
    1. Basic principles
    2. Special needs

RMA
I. General Medical Assisting Knowledge
    A. Anatomy and Physiology
        2. Disorders and diseases
    F. Patient Education

CMAS
3. Medical Office Clerical Assisting
    • Communication

EVALUATION OF CHAPTER KNOWLEDGE

Skills	Student Self-Evaluation Good	Average	Poor
I understand the role of the digestive system and the processes that take place in the digestive system.	_____	_____	_____
I know the seven basic nutrient types and how each contributes to a healthy diet.	_____	_____	_____
I understand the relationship and balance among the three energy nutrients.	_____	_____	_____
I understand the difference between water- and fat-soluble vitamins and how vitamins contribute to a healthy diet.	_____	_____	_____
I can identify major and trace minerals.	_____	_____	_____
I can interpret the information on the nutrition labels of processed foods.	_____	_____	_____
I understand the need for diets to be modified in response to life cycle changes and disease states.	_____	_____	_____

CHAPTER 35

Basic Pharmacology

CHAPTER PRE-TEST

Perform this test without looking at the book. This is just to see how well you have understood and can recall the information in this chapter after you have read it, but before you have completed the workbook exercises. You will not be graded on this portion (other than the grade you give yourself). Justify any "false" answers.

1. Only licensed physicians may dispense drugs. (T or F)
2. All prescription drugs are considered to be controlled substances. (T or F)
3. Most drugs are called by their chemical names now. (T or F)
4. The *Physician's Desk Reference (PDR)* is a small, handy, easy-to-use reference for drug information. (T or F)
5. An allergic reaction to a drug is considered a side effect. (T or F)
6. Controlled substances should be flushed down the toilet when they become out of date. (T or F)
7. Parenteral means to administer a drug by injection. (T or F)

INTRODUCTION

A comprehensive understanding of pharmacology and the study of drugs is essential to medical assistants in the ambulatory care setting. Medical assistants must have a working knowledge of basic pharmacology, including uses, sources, forms, and delivery routes of drugs, and an understanding of governmental laws that oversee the distribution and administration of medications. Medical assistants should also demonstrate the ability to recognize drug classifications and identify actions that will allow them to caution patients in the use of both prescription and nonprescription medications. Medical assistants must also be able to access medical resources and reference books for information pertaining to pharmaceutical products, including drug classifications, routes, forms of storage, and side effects and contraindications. It is essential that medical assistants also have the skills to recognize the signs of drug abuse and misuse and to effectively follow the procedures delegated to instances of suspected patient mishandling of drugs. It is important to remember, however, that only a licensed physician may prescribe medications.

PERFORMANCE OBJECTIVES

After successful completion of this chapter you will be able to discuss, using medical terminology, pharmacology. You will be able to recall five medical uses for drugs, five sources of drugs, and three types of drug names and will be able to give examples. You will be familiar with drug references including the *PDR*. You will understand the law regarding controlled substances and how to store them, dispose of them, and keep records of them. You will know about administering, prescribing, and dispensing drugs and the routes of drug administrations. You will know where to look for the principle actions, contraindications, warnings, common dosages, and other information about drugs, both prescription and over the counter (OTC). You will also know about drug abuse and which drugs are most likely to be abused. You will understand and will be able to explain the medical assistant's legal role and responsibilities regarding drugs. *The following statements are related to your learning objectives for this chapter. Fill in the blanks in the following paragraph with the appropriate term(s).*

(1) ______________________________ is the study of drugs, the science that is concerned with the (2) _______________, (3) _______________, (4) ____________________, (5) ______________________________, and chemical properties; the (6) _______________; and effects of (7) _____________ on living organisms. There are basically five medical uses for drugs. They are (8) __________________, used in radiology to help diagnose; (9) _______________, used to kill or remove the cause of the disease; (10) __________________, used to treat a condition and relieve symptoms; (11) _________________________, which replaces substances; and (12) ____________________________________, which prevents or decreases the severity of a disease. Drug names are of three types: the (13) ______________________________ name, which is the drug's molecular structure; the (14) ________________________ name, which is registered by the U.S. Patent and Trademark Office; and the (15) ______________ name, which is the drug's official name. Drugs come from many sources, including (16) __________________, (17) ________________________________, (18) ________________________________, (19) ____, and (20) ______________________. All drugs available for legal use are controlled by the (21) ________________________________ ______________________________. The federal law that regulates controlled substances, or those substances with potential for (22) ________________________________, is called the (23) ____. Controlled substances are categorized into (24) ____________ schedules according to their use and potential for abuse. Controlled substances must be stored in (25) ________________________ cabinets. To give a drug is to (26) ___________________ it, to give a written order for a drug is to (27) ____________________ it, and to (28) _________________________ a drug means to hand it to the patient to take at another time. Probably the most well-known resource for drug information is the *PDR*, which stands for (29) ____. It is divided into several sections, which are color coded, making it easier to use. Drugs are often classified in drug resources

in groups according to their (30) ______________________________. For example, a drug that acts to relieve pain is classified as an (31) ______________________, whereas a drug that relieves depression is classified as a (32) ______________________________, and a drug that reduces fever is classified as a (33) ______________________________. Drugs often will have undesirable actions. Some of those actions limit the usefulness of the drug and are called (34) ______________________ effects. Some cause an unfavorable or harmful unintended action, called (35) __________________________ reactions. Drugs come in three basic types of compounds—(36) ____________________, (37) ____________________________, (38) ______________________________—and may be administered through many routes. The (39) ____________________________ route is generally by injection, but it means any route that does not involve the digestive tract. Medications may be given by mouth, called (40) ______________ route; under the tongue, called (41) ________________; applied as a cream, ointment, or lotion, called (42) ____________________; as a spray or aerosol called (43) __________________ as liquid drops to the eyes/ears called (44) __________________; or as either vaginal or rectal (45) ____________________. Patches applied to the skin are referred to as the (46) __________________________ system of delivery.

VOCABULARY BUILDER

A. *Find the words in Column A that are misspelled; circle them, and then correctly spell them in the spaces provided. Then match the following key vocabulary terms listed in Column A with their corresponding definitions listed in Column B.*

Column A

A. abuse
B. administer
C. anaphalaxis
D. contradication
E. dispense
F. pharmocology
G. perscribe

____

____

____

____

Column B

_____ 1. Term used to describe when a licensed practitioner gives a written order to be taken to a pharmacist to be filled

_____ 2. An allergic hypersensitivity reaction of the body to a foreign protein or drug

_____ 3. To give the medication to the patient to be used at another time

_____ 4. The study of drugs; the science dealing with the history, origin, sources, physical and chemical properties, uses, and effects on living organisms

_____ 5. To give a medication to a patient by mouth, injection, or any other method of delivery

_____ 6. Any symptom or circumstance for which an otherwise approved form of treatment is inadvisable

_____ 7. The misuse of legal and illegal drugs

B. *Find the words in the list below that are misspelled; circle them, and then correctly spell them in the spaces provided. Then insert the proper terms into the spaces provided in the following text, which discusses medical uses of drugs, name of drugs, and sources of drugs.*

animal	generic	replacement
chemical	genetic engineering	synthetic
curative	mineral	therapuetic
diagnostic	plant	trade or brand
gene splicing	preventive or prophalactic	

_______________ _______________

A drug is a medicinal substance that may be used to vary or modify the functions of a living being. Of the five basic medical uses for drugs, antibiotics are an example of (1) _______________ drugs, agents used for the killing or removal of the causative agent of a disease. An immunizing agent is an example of a (2) _______________ drug, one used to stave off or abate the severity of a disease. Another medical use for drugs is used in the treatment of a condition to provide symptomatic relief; this is known as (3) _______________. Insulin and hormones are examples of this medical use of drugs, known as (4) _______________. A fifth basic medical use of drugs is used in conjunction with radiology and allows physicians to pinpoint the location of diseases' manifestations. This usage is known as (5) _______________.

As essential to the medical assistant as the knowledge of basic uses for drugs is the knowledge of the names of drugs. The majority of drugs have three types of names. The (6) _______________ name is the drug's official name assigned by the U.S. Adopted Names Council. Aspirin is an example of this type of name. The drug's (7) _______________ name describes its molecular structure and identification of its chemical structure. Acetylsalicylic acid is an example of this type of name. Ecotrin is an example of a (8) _______________ name, which is registered by the U.S. Patent Office and approved for usage by the U.S. Food and Drug Administration.

Medical assistants must also have a comprehensive understanding of the five basic sources of drugs. The source of digitalis, the dried leaf of a foxglove plant, is an example of a (9) _______________ source. Insulin, a hormone derived from the pancreas of cows and hogs, is an example of a drug derived from an (10) _______________ source. Drugs that are artificially prepared in pharmaceutical laboratories are known as (11) _______________ drugs. Synthetically prepared sulfur, used in pharmaceutical products (such as certain bacteriostatic drugs), is an example of a drug derived from a (12) _______________ source. One of the latest sources for drugs has been provided by (13) _______________. Using a technique called (14) _______________, scientists are able to create hybrid forms of life that can treat certain diseases; interferon for cancer treatment is an example of this process.

LEARNING REVIEW

1. All drugs available for legal use are controlled by the:
   a. Federal Food, Drug, and Cosmetic Act
   b. the Council on Pharmacy of the American Medical Association
   c. Controlled Substance Act of 1970

2. Federal law requires that at the end of the workday, controlled substances that are used on the premises:
   a. must be locked in a physician's office by a physician
   b. must be removed from the building and stored in a government-appointed storage space
   c. must be counted, verified by two individuals, and recorded on an audit sheet

3. An inventory record of Schedule II drugs must be submitted to the Drug Enforcement Agency (DEA) every:
   a. week
   b. year
   c. 2 years

4. An example of a drug requiring a prescription is:
   a. the antibiotic penicillin
   b. the antihistamine Benadryl®
   c. the analgesic acetaminophen

5. An example of an OTC drug is:
   a. the analgesic ibuprofen
   b. the vasodilator nitroglycerin
   c. the antitussive codeine

6. When a drug acts on the area to which it is administered it has what is known as a:
   a. systemic action
   b. remote action
   c. local action

7. The four principal factors that affect drug action are absorption, distribution, biotransformation, and:
   a. elimination
   b. interaction
   c. contraindication

8. By law, outdated and expired controlled substances must be:
   a. handed over to your local law enforcement agency
   b. thrown away
   c. returned to the pharmacy

9. Patients need to realize that OTC drugs can:
   a. interact with other drugs and cause undesirable or adverse reactions or complications
   b. mask symptoms and exacerbate an existing condition
   c. a and b

10. The most frequently used routes of administering medication are:
    a. inhalation and sublingual
    b. parenteral and inhalation
    c. oral and parenteral

11. Under federal law, physicians who prescribe, administer, or dispense controlled substances must register with the DEA and renew their registration as required by state law. Describe the five schedules of classification for controlled substances and give an example for each.

    Schedule I ______________________________

    ______________________ Example: ______________________

    Schedule II ______________________________

    ______________________ Example: ______________________

    Schedule III ______________________________

    ______________________ Example: ______________________

    Schedule IV ______________________________

    ______________________ Example: ______________________

    Schedule V ______________________________

    ______________________ Example: ______________________

12. For each of the following, identify whether the drug involved is an OTC medication or a prescribed medication (PM). What patient guidelines for proper use are illustrated in each example?

    _____ A. Nora Fowler insists that Dr. Winston Lewis cannot help her rheumatoid arthritis and that simple ibuprofen is all she needs. Nora buys bulk generic bottles of ibuprofen at the drugstore for her rheumatoid arthritis and takes as many as she needs to help ease the painful inflammation in her joints and tissues.

    ____

    ____

_____ B. When Jim Marshall experiences extreme stress while finishing the architectural designs for a new office building in the community, his girlfriend offers him a tablet or two of lorazepam, a benzodiazepine drug used to treat anxiety and insomnia. "Here, Dr. King gave me these, and they work great," she says. "You can't drive when you take this stuff, though. Oh, and these pills are about 2 years old, but I'm sure they'll still work fine."

____

____

_____ C. At the slightest sniffle or sneeze, Lenore McDonell takes the strongest multisymptom cold medication she can find. Her philosophy is: "I might as well knock it out of my system."

____

____

_____ D. Abigail Johnson hates taking so many medications. So every now and then, when she feels especially good, Abigail just decides to stop taking the antihypertensive drug that is part of Dr. Elizabeth King's treatment plan to control Abigail's high blood pressure. On a bad day, she'll take an extra pill.

____

____

_____ E. Wayne Elder is susceptible to recurrent colds and ear infections. Wayne's symptoms are hard to control because he will almost always stop taking the antibiotics when he starts to feel better and he does not finish the entire regimen recommended by Dr. Lewis.

____

____

13. Proper disposal of drugs is important because expired drugs can be harmful. Identify the proper manner of disposing of each of the following forms of drugs.

    A. Liquids and ointments ______________________________

    B. Powdered drugs must be ______________________________

    C. Pills and capsules must be ______________________________

    D. Vials and ampules must be ______________________________

    E. Outdated and expired controlled substances must be ______________________________

    F. What happens if a medication is removed from its container but not used? For example, a patient refuses novocaine before a minor dental procedure. ______________________________

    ____

14. A. What factor in determining the route selection for administering a medication is illustrated by each example below and why?

    (1) A patient diagnosed with insulin-dependent diabetes mellitus performs three self-injections of insulin daily, according to the physician's treatment plan.

    ____

    (2) Chemotherapeutic drugs are used to attack cancer cells that may be traveling throughout a patient's body, and usually they are administered intravenously.

    ____

    (3) A patient in a nursing home who is in the end stages of Parkinson's disease is bedridden, has trouble swallowing, and suffers from dementia. The patient, who is also suffering from angina as a result of poor blood circulation, is prescribed a nitroglycerin transdermal system instead of a sublingual dosage, to be held under the tongue, or a time-released capsule to swallow.

    ____

    B. The most frequently used routes of administering medication are oral and parenteral. List seven additional routes of administration.

    (1) ______________ (5) ______________

    (2) ______________ (6) ______________

    (3) ______________ (7) ______________

    (4) ______________

    C. Name three recently developed systems of drug delivery. Describe each and note their specific advantages.

    (1) ______________________________

    ____

    (2) ______________________________

    ____

    (3) ______________________________

    ____

15. A. List four examples of the ways in which drugs may be classified, or arranged, in groups.

    (1) ______________________________

    (2) ______________________________

    (3) ______________________________

    (4) ______________________________

B. For each drug action, identify the correct drug classification. Then list one example of a drug contained in each class.

Action	Drug Classification	Example
(1) Controls or stops bleeding		
(2) Prevents or relieves nausea and vomiting		
(3) Neutralizes acid		
(4) Decreases blood pressure		
(5) Reduces fever		
(6) Loosens and promotes normal bowel elimination		
(7) Prevents conception		
(8) Kills or destroys malignant cells		
(9) Prevents or relieves diarrhea		
(10) Produces a calming effect without causing sleep		

16. The *PDR* is an invaluable resource and one of the most widely used publications in the medical industry. The annually updated publication is usually available in most clinics and medical offices. It provides medical professionals with practical information about thousands of medications and includes other useful data, such as lists of drugs new to the market and those that have been discontinued. It is essential that medical assistants become familiar with the publication and learn how to access the wealth of information stored within.
Use the PDR to locate the pertinent information for each of the following scenarios. Then identify the drug's source or method of production.

A. Herb Fowler, Dr. Winston Lewis's patient, calls to report he is experiencing nausea, a symptom he believes may be a negative reaction to the Chronulac Syrup Dr. Lewis recently prescribed for Herb's chronic constipation. Using the *PDR*, locate the following information:

Chronulac Syrup's generic name: ______________________________

The sugar Chronulac Syrup contains: ______________________________

Identify the drug's source or method of production: ______________________

B. Another patient of Dr. Lewis's, Michael Zamboni, has recently been diagnosed with insulin-dependent type II diabetes. Dr. Lewis prescribes Humulin®. Using the *PDR*, find the following information:

Humulin®'s generic name: ______________________________

The animal source from which Humulin® is derived: ____________________

Identify the drug's source or method of production: ______________________

C. Susan Marshall, a new patient of Dr. Elizabeth King's, acquired a high-pressure job about 1 month ago. Recently, she has been reporting an upset stomach, which has been attributed to her stressful job and poor eating habits. Dr. King orders prescription-strength Pepcid® for Susan. Using the *PDR*, locate the following information:

Pepcid®'s generic name: ______________________________

Pepcid®'s active ingredient: ______________________________

Identify the drug's source or method of production: ______________________________

D. Camille Saunders, another patient of Dr. King's, has been taking Ortho-Tri-Cyclen®, an oral contraceptive, for 6 months. It has just been discovered that Camille has epilepsy. Using the *PDR*, locate the following information:

Does Ortho-Tri-Cyclen® have any known contraindications to any drugs used in the treatment of epilepsy, and if so, which drugs?

____

____

Identify the drug's source or method of production: ______________________________

CERTIFICATION REVIEW

These questions are designed to mimic the certification examinations. You can use these questions like a small "Certification Examination Study Guide," but this is not meant to take the place of the more extensive study guides. Use this portion to determine in what areas to concentrate your efforts when studying for the certification examination.

1. Hybrid forms of life have been created that benefit human beings by providing an alternative source of drugs; an example is:
   a. ibuprofen
   b. interferon
   c. digitalis
   d. epinephrine

2. If the symbol ® follows a drug name, no other manufacturer can make or sell the drug for:
   a. 7 years
   b. 10 years
   c. 20 years
   d. 17 years

3. One compound extracted from the adrenal gland of animals and used therapeutically is:
   a. cortisone
   b. acetaminophen
   c. insulin
   d. piroxician

4. Those drugs with a potential for abuse and dependency are monitored by the:
   a. FDA
   b. AAMA
   c. DEA
   d. CDC

5. An inventory record of Schedule II drugs must be submitted to appropriate authorities every:
   a. 2 years
   b. year
   c. 5 years
   d. 7 years

CASE STUDY

While Anna Preciado, a clinical medical assistant newly hired at the offices of Drs. Lewis and King, is performing her shift duties, she notices a fellow employee exhibiting strange behavior. Audrey Jones, CMA, is usually the model of efficiency. Since Anna began working at the Northborough Family Medical Group, she has always known Audrey to be alert, friendly, and able to handle difficult clinical situations with grace under pressure. Lately, however, when Anna asks Audrey questions, Audrey seems irritable and easily confused. Anna also notices Audrey exhibiting a sloppy technique during routine clinical procedures. Anna is disturbed by Audrey's erratic behavior but does not mention anything to anyone. After all, Anna is new to the job. But while counting the contents of the controlled substance cabinet in preparation for the end of her shift, Anna notices that a bottle of phenobarbital is missing. Anna knows that office manager Marilyn Johnson will arrive shortly to verify and record the inventory count. Anna is now worried that perhaps Audrey is to blame for the missing drugs but is afraid of jumping to conclusions and of angering Audrey. Anna knows Audrey is in the staff lounge preparing to leave for a dinner break.

Discuss the following:

1. What is Anna's first action under the circumstances? Should she confront Audrey?
2. What special responsibilities do health care professionals, including medical assistants, have regarding the misuse or abuse of legal or illegal drugs?

SELF-ASSESSMENT

Organize your medicine cabinet. Or, with permission, organize the medicine cabinet of a close family member.

1. First, determine which drugs are out of date and destroy them properly.

2. Next, determine which drugs are no longer being prescribed, but rather are basically "left over" from a previous illness.

3. Make a decision. Should those leftover drugs be disposed of, or was it the intention of the physician for those medications to be available to you (or your family member) in the future? If they are not to be used in the future, dispose of them properly.

4. Separate the OTC drugs from the prescription drugs. Organize the OTC medications into categories of actions (the analgesics together, cough and cold medicines together, etc.).

5. If you (or your family member) are on a long-term drug therapy, make up a medicine card to be carried with you (or your family member) at all times. On the card, list the drug, strength, and dosage. Place this card in your wallet or purse (or that of your family member), so the medicine list is available at all times.

POST-TEST

This is similar to the Pre-Test. Perform this test without looking at the book. This is just to see how well you have understood and can recall the information presented in this chapter after you have studied it and completed the workbook exercises. You will not be graded on this portion (other than the grade you give yourself), but this is an excellent preparation for your instructor's test. You may use this Post-Test to determine what areas you need to study more. Justify any "false" answers.

1. Only licensed physicians may prescribe drugs. (T or F)
2. Only drugs that have the potential for abuse are considered to be controlled substances. (T or F)
3. Most drugs are now called by their generic names. (T or F)
4. *PDR* stands for the *Physician's Drug Reference*. (T or F)
5. An allergic reaction to a drug is considered a contraindication. (T or F)
6. Outdated drugs that are not controlled substances should be flushed down the toilet. (T or F)
7. Parenteral usually means to administer a drug by injection. (T or F)

CERTIFICATION CRITERIA CHECKLIST

As you go through your education and training, keep in mind the national certification examination that you will take when you graduate. Each chapter of the textbook and workbook covers a different section of the examination criteria. To keep track of your preparation for the certification examination, turn to the back of this workbook and highlight the following CMA, RMA, or CMAS certification examination criteria (if you have already highlighted them from a previous chapter, put a check mark by the criteria):

CMA

F. Medicolegal Guidelines & Requirements
    2. Legislation

W. Preparing (and Administering) Medications
    1. Pharmacology

RMA

III. Clinical Medical Assisting
   F. Clinical Pharmacology

CMAS

2. Basic Clinical Medical Assisting
   - Basic pharmacology

EVALUATION OF CHAPTER KNOWLEDGE

Evaluate your comprehension of basic pharmacology, including uses, sources, forms, and the delivery routes of drugs; the intent of the law regarding controlled substances and other medications; and your knowledge of the classifications and actions of drugs.

	Student Self-Evaluation		
Skills	Good	Average	Poor
I have a working knowledge of basic pharmacology, including knowing five basic uses and five basic sources for drugs, and have the ability to recall three types of drug names and give examples of each.	____	____	____
I am able to prepare and administer medications as directed by a physician.	____	____	____
I am able to maintain medication records in relation to the prescription, administration, and dispensation of drugs.	____	____	____
I can document medications accurately.	____	____	____
I understand what the Federal Food, Drug, and Cosmetic Act and Controlled Substance Act of 1970 entails.	____	____	____
I am able to handle, store, and dispose of controlled substances in compliance with governmental regulations.	____	____	____
I can define the law in terms of administering, prescribing, and dispensing drugs.	____	____	____
I am able to name the seven major sections (including the four most commonly used) of the *PDR.*	____	____	____
I am able to describe principal actions of drugs and at least three undesirable reactions.	____	____	____
I am able to list emergency drugs and supplies.	____	____	____
I am able to list commonly abused drugs and recognize their effects.	____	____	____

CHAPTER 36

Calculation of Medication Dosage and Medication Administration

CHAPTER PRE-TEST

Perform this test without looking at the book. This is just to see how well you have understood and can recall the information in this chapter after you have read it, but before you have completed the workbook exercises. You will not be graded on this portion (other than the grade you give yourself). Justify any "false" answers.

1. A prescription is a written legal document. (T or F)
2. Prescriptions for controlled substances have different requirements than prescriptions for other drugs. (T or F)
3. Dosage and dose mean the same thing. (T or F)
4. Dosages are determined by considering patient age, weight, sex, and other factors. (T or F)
5. We are required by the "Needlestick Safety Act" to use the safest needles available. (T or F)
6. The gluteus medius is the muscle of choice for a deep intramuscular (IM) injection. (T or F)
7. The deltoid muscle is the easiest and most accessible IM site. (T or F)
8. The ventrogluteal muscle is the muscle of choice for an infant IM injection. (T or F)

INTRODUCTION

To safely administer medications to patients, medical assistants must possess a fundamental knowledge of pharmacology, have the ability to calculate doses of medication, and be competent in various methods of medication administration, including oral and parenteral forms. Medical assistants must also be aware of the legal and ethical aspects of medication administration. It is the responsibility of all health care professionals to provide care only within the scope of practice of their training and knowledge, and within legal and ethical boundaries. Only a physician has the legal authority to prescribe medications for patients. Medical assistants prepare and administer medications as directed by the physician, accurately documenting and reporting according to the facility's established policies and procedures. All Standard Precautions and Occupational Safety and Health Act (OSHA) guidelines are observed to protect health care professionals, patients, and visitors from the transmission of pathogens.

PERFORMANCE OBJECTIVES

After successful completion of this chapter you will be able to discuss, using medical terminology, the legal and ethical implications of medication administration. You will know what makes up the medication order and the parts of a prescription, and you will be able to state what information is found on a medication label. You will be able to correctly calculate adult and children's dosages using metric and household systems of measurements. You will be able to list the guidelines to follow when preparing and administering medications and correctly select the proper sites to administer injections. You will know how to dispose of needles, syringes, and excess medications properly and safely. You will also be able to discuss intravenous (IV) therapy. *The following statements are related to your learning objectives for this chapter. Fill in the blanks in the following paragraph with the appropriate term(s).*

Despite that most ambulatory care centers, clinics, and physician's offices use (1) ______________________ type of medication preparation, the medical assistant still needs to know how to (2) ______________________ dosages. Members of the health care team who prepare and administer medications are (3) ______________________ and (4) ______________________ responsible for their own actions. Under law, these individuals, medical assistants included, are required to be (5) ______________________, (6) ______________________, or otherwise (7) ______________________ by a physician. Each state has laws governing the practice of (8) ______________________, (9) ______________________, and (10) ______________________. Because these laws vary from state to state, it is essential that (11) ______________________ know the law in the state where they are (12) ______________________ before (13) ______________________ any (14) ______________________. Under all the state laws, those who are administering the drugs are expected to be (15) ______________________ about the drugs they are administering and the (16) ______________________ the drugs may have on the patient. The prescription gives directions for (17) ______________________, (18) ______________________, and (19) ______________________ a medication to a patient. Federal law divides medicines into two main classes: (20) ______________________ and (21) ______________________ medicines. The medication label includes information such as the (22) ______________________ name and the (23) ______________________ name, the (24) ______________________ numbers, the (25) ______________________ in a given amount of medication, the usual (26) ______________________ and (27) ______________________ of administration, the (28) ______________________ of administration, (29) ______________________ and (30) ______________________, and the (31) ______________________ date for the medication, as well as other information for storage and mixing directions. There are many rules surrounding medications, some for patients' safety and some for the medical assistant who is administering the drug. The "Six Rights" of proper drug administration are rules that were established to help eliminate drug (32) ________________________. The first right is to be sure you are giving the right (33)________________. Then, be sure you have figured the right (34) _____________. The right (35) ______________ is important, too, because most drugs are designed to be given a certain way. The fourth right is the right (36) ______________________. This is more commonly used in hospital and inpatient settings when patients are there round the clock. The next right to be aware of is the right (37) ______________. Always check the order and identify the patient carefully. Lastly, because medical records are legal documents, be sure to (38) ___________________ exactly what you gave, how much, what route, the site, how you gave it, and whether the patient had any reactions.

VOCABULARY BUILDER

Find the words below that are misspelled; circle them, and then correctly spell them in the spaces provided. Then supply a brief definition for each vocabulary term.

1. Apnea____
2. BSA ____
3. Hypoxemia____
4. Meniscus ____
5. Nomogram____
6. Parentral____
7. Precipitate ____
8. Taut ____
9. Unit dose ____
10. Weal____

LEARNING REVIEW

1. The prescription is a written legal document that gives directions for compounding, dispensing, and administering to a patient. Refer to the prescriptions on the next page. In the spaces below, "decode" the prescriptions into layperson's terms and answer the questions that follow.

   ____

   ____

   ____

A. Dr. King prescribes an adult dosage for epilepsy.

L&K LEWIS & KING, MD
2501 CENTER STREET
NORTHBOROUGH, OH 12345

Name Lourdes Austin
Address 821 Spring Lane, Apt. 12 Date 3/1/XX

℞

Dilantin 100 mg tab
#90
Sig 100 mg p.o. tid

Generic Substitution Allowed Susan Rice M.D.
Dispense As Written M.D.
REPETATUR 0 1 2 3 p.r.n.
☑ LABEL

1. How many grains are in each dose?______ __ teaspoons

2. How many days of medication are dispensed? ______________________

B. Dr. Lewis prescribes a child's dosage for an ear infection.

L&K LEWIS & KING, MD
2501 CENTER STREET
NORTHBOROUGH, OH 12345

Name Felicia Lawrence
Address 362 Owen's View Way Date 3/1/XX

℞

Amoxicillin 250 mg/5 cc.
#150cc
Sig 500 mg p.o. tid

Generic Substitution Allowed Winston Lewis M.D.
Dispense As Written M.D.
REPETATUR 0 1 2 3 p.r.n.
☑ LABEL

1. Perform the conversion: 5 cc = ________

2. How many doses are included in the amount dispensed? ______________

2. A. Identify the following measures as weight (W) or volume (V). Then name the measure each abbreviation stands for and what system of measurement it belongs to.

Weight	Volume	Abbreviation	Measure	System
☐	☐	Gm		
☐	☐	Tbsp		
☐	☐	ml		
☐	☐	qt		
☐	☐	gtt		
☐	☐	μg		

B. Perform the following conversions:

(1) 4 tsp = ________ ml

(2) 3.5 in. = _______ cm

(3) 1,200 mg = _________Gm

(4) 30 mg =________ gr

(5) 8 ml = ________ gtt

C. What are proportions? How are proportions useful in calculating dosages of medication?

____

____

3. A. Identify the type of syringe typically used for each of the following; list the size and calibration as well.

(1) Venipuncture: ________________________________

(2) Insulin administration: _________________________

(3) Allergy testing: ______________________________

B. For each syringe-needle combination below, identify the most likely parenteral route: subcutaneous injection (SC), intramuscular injection (IM), or intradermal injection (ID). Also identify the proper angle of injection.

		Angle of injection
_____	1. 3-ml syringe/22G, 1 1/2-inch needle	____________
_____	2. 1-ml syringe/25G, 5/8-inch needle	____________
_____	3. U-100 (1 ml)/26G, 1/2-inch needle	____________
_____	4. 3-ml syringe/25G, 5/8-inch needle	____________

CERTIFICATION REVIEW

These questions are designed to mimic the certification examinations. You can use these questions like a small "Certification Examination Study Guide," but this is not meant to take the place of the more extensive study guides. Use this portion to determine in what areas to concentrate your efforts when studying for the certification examination.

1. The hard copy of a prescription is filed and kept for a minimum of:
   a. 10 years
   b. 7 years
   c. 5 years
   d. indefinitely

2. The portion of the prescription that gives directions to the patient is called the:
   a. superscription
   b. inscription
   c. subscription
   d. signature

3. The metric prefix that refers to 1,000 units is:
   a. kilo-
   b. milli-
   c. micro-
   d. deca-

4. Dosage of insulin is always measured in:
   a. cubic centimeters
   b. milliliters
   c. units
   d. milliequivalents

5. The hollow core of a needle is called the:
   a. bevel
   b. gauge
   c. lumen
   d. hilt

CASE STUDY

Louise Kipperley comes to the urgent care center at Inner City Health Care when she experiences the third severe migraine headache in only one month. The headache has lasted two days, and Louise has experienced symptoms of nausea and vomiting. Dr. Rice gives written orders to administer Imitrex® 25 mg IM stat, together with a prescription for the patient to fill and use at home. Liz Corbin, CMA, makes a medicine card from the physician's order sheet of Louise's medical record and prepares the stat dosage for Louise according to the correct procedure for administering oral medications. Liz is about to transport the medication to Louise in examination room 3 when she reads the physician's written order for Louise, which calls for 25 mg IM stat. The written prescription is for Imitrex® every four hours as needed. Liz discards the dosage she has prepared for the patient, and instead gives Louise Dr. Rice's prescription and tells her to have it filled immediately.

Discuss the following:

1. What medication error has Liz made? What effect will the error likely have on the patient?
2. What should Liz have done? What standard procedures should be followed when a medication error occurs?

SELF-ASSESSMENT

Have you ever been given a shot? Do you remember how you felt just before the injection? Most people are more afraid of the pain of the injection than anything having to do with the medication. Do you think there are ways you can behave that will help your fearful patients feel less afraid? What could you do or say to alleviate their fears? Do you think it is just children who are afraid of needles? Write down a couple of things you will do and say to help your patients. Discuss your ideas with a few classmates and listen to their ideas.

POST-TEST

This is similar to the Pre-Test. Perform this test without looking at the book. This is just to see how well you have understood and can recall the information presented in this chapter after you have studied it and completed the workbook exercises. You will not be graded on this portion (other than the grade you give yourself), but this is an excellent preparation for your instructor's test. You may use this Post-Test to determine what areas you need to study more. Justify any "false" answers.

1. A prescription is a legal document only if its written. (T or F)
2. Prescriptions for controlled substances have the same requirements as prescriptions for other drugs. (T or F)
3. Dosage and dose have different meanings. (T or F)
4. Doses are determined by considering patient age, weight, sex, and other factors. (T or F)
5. We are required to use the safest needles available by OSHA. (T or F)
6. The gluteus maximus is the muscle of choice for a deep IM injection. (T or F)
7. The bicep muscle is the easiest and most accessible IM site. (T or F)
8. The vastus lateralis muscle is the muscle of choice for an infant IM injection. (T or F)

CERTIFICATION CRITERIA CHECKLIST

As you go through your education and training, keep in mind the national certification examination that you will take when you graduate. Each chapter of the textbook and workbook covers a different section of the examination criteria. To keep track of your preparation for the certification examination, turn to the back of this workbook and highlight the following CMA, RMA, or CMAS certification examination criteria (if you have already highlighted them from a previous chapter, put a check mark by the criteria):

CMA

R. Principles of Infection Control
    3. Disposal of biohazardous material
    4. Practice of Standard Precautions

W. Preparing (and Administering) Medications

RMA

III. Clinical Medical Assisting
    F. Clinical Pharmacology

CMAS

2. Basic Clinical Medical Assisting
    - Basic pharmacology

COMPETENCY ASSESSMENT

Procedure 36-1 Administration of Oral Medications

Performance Objectives: To correctly administer an oral medication after receiving a physician's order. Perform this objective within 5 minutes with a minimum score of 105 points.

Supplies/Equipment: Medication order by physician, medication, medicine note, medicine tray, medicine cup, water

Charting/Documentation: Enter appropriate documentation/charting in the box.

Instructor's/Evaluator's Comments and Suggestions:

SKILLS CHECKLIST Procedure 36-1: Administration of Oral Medications

Name ______________________

Date ______________________

No.	Skill	Check #1 20 pts ea	Check #2 10 pts ea	Check #3 5 pts ea	Notes
1	Verify the physician's order.				
2	Follow the "Six Rights."				
3	Wash hands.				
4	Work in a well-lit, quiet, clean area.				
5	Assemble equipment and supplies.				
6	Obtain the correct medication using the medication note.				
7	Compare the medication label with the medication note (first check).				
8	Check the expiration date.				
9	Calculate dosage, if necessary.				
10	Correctly prepare: • solid medication from multi-dose bottle • unit dose medication • liquid medication from multi-dose bottle				
11	Compare medicine label with medication note (second check).				
12	Properly transport the dose of medicine to the patient. Also bring the original container.				
13	Identify the patient and explain the procedure.				
14	Assess patient. Take vital signs if indicated.				
15	Assist patient to a comfortable position.				
16	Check the medication order the third time. Provide water.				
17	Administer the medication. Make sure the patient takes the medicine.				
18	Provide for the patient's safety by observing the patient for any adverse reactions.				
19	Clean medication tray if used, dispose of medication cup according to OSHA guidelines.				

No.	Skill	Check #1 20 pts ea	Check #2 10 pts ea	Check #3 5 pts ea	Notes
20	Document the medication administration in the patient's chart using the medication note. Destroy the medication note.				
21	Return the medication container to the proper storage area/shelf.				
Student's Total Points					
Points Possible		420	210	105	
Final Score (Student's Total Points / Possible Points)					

	Notes
Start time:	
End time:	
Total time: (5 min goal)	

COMPETENCY ASSESSMENT

Procedure 36-2 Withdrawing Medication from a Vial

Performance Objectives: To correctly withdraw medication from a vial with 100% accuracy. Perform this objective within 5 minutes with a minimum score of 90 points.

Supplies/Equipment: Medication order by physician, vial of medication, medication note, appropriately sized safety syringe and needle, alcohol wipes, gloves, sharps container

Charting/Documentation: Enter appropriate documentation/charting in the box.

Instructor's/Evaluator's Comments and Suggestions:

SKILLS CHECKLIST Procedure 36-2: Withdrawing Medication from a Vial

Name ______________________________

Date ______________________________

No.	Skill	Check #1 20 pts ea	Check #2 10 pts ea	Check #3 5 pts ea	Notes
1	Read the medication order and assemble equipment. Read the vial label by holding it next to the medication card (first check).				
2	Wash hands, then apply gloves.				
3	Select the proper size safety needle and syringe for the medication and the route. If necessary, attach the needle to the syringe.				
4	Check the vial label against the medication note (second check). Check expiration date.				
5	Remove the metal or plastic cap from the vial. If the vial has been opened previously, clean the rubber stopper by applying a disinfectant (alcohol) wipe in a firm, circular motion.				
6	Remove the needle cover, pulling it straight off in a decisive move.				
7	Inject air into the vial equal to the amount of medication to be withdrawn.				
8	Invert the vial. Hold the vial and syringe steady in one hand. Pull back on plunger to withdraw the measured dose. Measure accurately. Keep the tip of the needle in the liquid to prevent air from entering syringe. Keep syringe at eye level.				
9	Check the syringe for air bubbles. Remove air bubbles by tapping sharply on the syringe (while the needle is still in the vial). Push the air bubbles back into the vial and withdraw more medication if necessary. Double-check the syringe for accuracy.				
10	Remove the needle from the vial. Replace the sterile needlecover using the scoop method. Be extremely careful to safeguard the sterility of the needle.				
11	Check the vial label and the withdrawn amount against the medication card (third check).				

No.	Skill	Check #1 20 pts ea	Check #2 10 pts ea	Check #3 5 pts ea	Notes
12	Place the filled syringe on a medicine tray with an antiseptic wipe and the medication note.				
13	Change needles if the medication is an irritant.				
14	Immediately after use, activate the safety mechanism and discard used syringe-needle unit into a sharps container (located within reach).				
15	Properly dispose of used equipment and supplies. Disinfect medicine tray. Remove gloves.				
16	Wash hands.				
17	Document the procedure.				
18	Return the multi-dose vial to the proper storage area (cabinet or refrigerator). Destroy the medication note. Dispose of unused medication in a single-dose vial according to facility procedures.				
Student's Total Points					
Points Possible		360	180	90	
Final Score (Student's Total Points / Possible Points)					
		Notes			
Start time:					
End time:					
Total time: (5 min goal)					

COMPETENCY ASSESSMENT

Procedure 36-3 Withdrawing Medication from an Ampule

Performance Objectives: To properly withdraw medication from an ampule with 100% accuracy. Perform this objective within 5 minutes with a minimum score of 75 points.

Supplies/Equipment: Medicine tray, medication order by physician, ampule of medication, medication note, appropriately sized safety syringe and filter needle, antiseptic wipes (alcohol), gloves, sharps container

Charting/Documentation: Enter appropriate documentation/charting in the box.

Instructor's/Evaluator's Comments and Suggestions:

SKILLS CHECKLIST Procedure 36-3: Withdrawing Medication from an Ampule

Name ______________________

Date ______________________

No.	Skill	Check #1 20 pts ea	Check #2 10 pts ea	Check #3 5 pts ea	Notes
1	Check the physician's order. Write out medication card.				
2	Wash hands and gather equipment. Apply gloves.				
3	Select ampule of medication. Read label and check medication note for correct medication and dose (first check). Check medication expiration date.				
4	Flick ampule using a sharp flick of the wrist to dislodge medication from top.				
5	Thoroughly disinfect the neck with an alcohol swab. Check label (second check).				
6	Wipe dry the neck of the ampule or let air dry. Completely surround the ampule with the gauze and forcefully snap off the top of the ampule by pulling the top toward the body. Discard top into sharps container.				
7	Place ampule on medication tray. Check label (third time).				
8	With prepared safety syringe and filter needle unit, aspirate the required dose (usually all the medication) into syringe. Cover needle with sheath using sterile scoop method and transport on a medicine tray to the patient.				
9	Change needles				
10	Identify the patient.				
11	Administer the medication.				
12	Discard the syringe-needle unit into sharps container. Discard alcohol wipes and cotton balls into biohazard waste container.				
13	Remove gloves and dispose into biohazard waste. Dispose of ampule into sharps container.				

No.	Skill	Check #1 20 pts ea	Check #2 10 pts ea	Check #3 5 pts ea	Notes
14	Wash hands.				
15	Correctly document the procedure. Destroy medication note.				
Student's Total Points					
Points Possible		300	150	75	
Final Score (Student's Total Points / Possible Points)					

	Notes
Start time:	
End time:	
Total time: (5 min goal)	

COMPETENCY ASSESSMENT

Procedure 36-4 Administration of Subcutaneous, Intramuscular, and Intradermal Injections

Performance Objectives: To correctly administer subcutaneous, intramuscular, and intradermal injections with 100% accuracy. Perform this objective within 5 minutes with a minimum score of 135 points.

Supplies/Equipment: Medication order by physician, medication vial, medication note, appropriately sized safety needle-syringe unit, antiseptic (alcohol) wipes, gloves, cotton balls, adhesive strip, sharps container

Charting/Documentation: Enter appropriate documentation/charting in the box.

Instructor's/Evaluator's Comments and Suggestions:

SKILLS CHECKLIST Procedure 36-4: Administration of Subcutaneous, Intramuscular, and Intradermal Injections

Name ______________________________

Date ______________________________

No.	Skill	Check #1 20 pts ea	Check #2 10 pts ea	Check #3 5 pts ea	Notes
1	Verify the physician's order. Make out medication note taking information from physician's order sheet in the patient record.				
2	Follow the "Six Rights."				
3	Wash hands.				
4	Work in a well-lit, quiet, clean area.				
5	Select the appropriate safety syringe-needle unit and an alcohol wipe.				
6	Select the correct medication.				
7	Compare the medication label with the medication note (first check).				
8	Check the expiration date.				
9	Calculate dosage, if necessary.				
10	Prepare safety syringe-needle unit for use.				
11	Withdraw medication from vial.				
12	Compare medicine label with medication note (second check).				
13	Place filled safety syringe-needle unit on the medicine tray with medication note and the vial. Check medication order against the vial and the syringe for a third time.				
14	Carefully transport the medicine to the patient.				
15	Identify the patient and explain the procedure.				
16	Apply gloves.				
17	Prepare the patient for the injection (drape, position, and allay patient apprehension).				
18	Select an appropriate injection site. Follow a rotating schedule, if appropriate.				
19	Cleanse the injection site with a sterile antiseptic wipe. Use a circular motion, working from the center out to about 2 inches beyond the planned injection site.				

No.	Skill	Check #1 20 pts ea	Check #2 10 pts ea	Check #3 5 pts ea	Notes
20	Allow the skin to dry.				
21	Administer the injection. Aspirate first to be certain the needle is not in a blood vessel (except for intradermal injections), then administer the injection. Immediately after withdrawing the needle, activate the safety mechanism, and then dispose of syringe-needle unit into a sharps container.				
22	Massage injection site with cotton ball unless contraindicated.				
23	Observe the patient for signs of difficulty.				
24	Inspect the injection site for bleeding, then apply adhesive strip if necessary.				
25	Properly dispose of used equipment and supplies. Remove gloves.				
26	Wash hands.				
27	Correctly document the procedure including the medication, dosage and strength, route, site, and any patient reactions. Return the vial to storage and destroy the medication note.				
Student's Total Points					
Points Possible		540	270	135	
Final Score (Student's Total Points / Possible Points)					

	Notes
Start time:	
End time:	
Total time: (5 min goal)	

COMPETENCY ASSESSMENT

Procedure 36-5 Administering a Subcutaneous Injection

Performance Objectives: To correctly administer a subcutaneous injections with 100% accuracy. Perform this objective within 5 minutes with a minimum score of 150 points.

Supplies/Equipment: Medication order by physician, medication note, appropriately sized safety needle-syringe unit, antiseptic (alcohol) wipes, gloves, cotton balls, adhesive strip, sharps container

Charting/Documentation: Enter appropriate documentation/charting in the box.

Instructor's/Evaluator's Comments and Suggestions:

SKILLS CHECKLIST Procedure 36-5: Administering a Subcutaneous Injection

Name ______________________________

Date ______________________________

No.	Skill	Check #1 20 pts ea	Check #2 10 pts ea	Check #3 5 pts ea	Notes
1	Verify the physician's order. Make out medication note.				
2	Follow the "Six Rights."				
3	Wash hands. Adhere to OSHA guidelines.				
4	Work in a well-lit, quiet, clean area.				
5	Select the appropriate safety syringe-needle unit and other supplies.				
6	Select the correct medication.				
7	Compare the medication label with the medication note (first check).				
8	Check the expiration date of the medicine.				
9	Calculate dosage, if necessary.				
10	Correctly prepare the injection.				
11	Compare medicine label with medication note (second check).				
12	Carefully transport the medicine to the patient on the medicine tray with the vial and other supplies.				
13	Identify the patient and explain the procedure.				
14	Apply gloves.				
15	Prepare the patient for the injection (drape, position, and allay patient apprehension).				
16	Check medication order against the vial and the syringe for a third time.				
17	Select an appropriate injection site.				
18	Cleanse the injection site with a sterile antiseptic wipe. Use a circular motion, working from the center out to about 2 inches beyond the planned injection site. Allow the skin to dry.				
19	Remove the needle cover using a quick, decisive motion.				
20	Grasp skin to form a 1-inch fold.				

No.	Skill	Check #1 20 pts ea	Check #2 10 pts ea	Check #3 5 pts ea	Notes
21	Insert the needle quickly at a 45-degree angle.				
22	Aspirate first to be certain the needle is not in a blood vessel.				
23	Inject the medicine.				
24	Quickly remove the needle and immediately activate the safety mechanism. Release the skin.				
25	Immediately dispose of syringe-needle unit into a sharps container.				
26	Cover the site and massage with a cotton ball (except insulin, interferon, and heparin). Apply adhesive strip if needed.				
27	Provide for patient safety. Check for any reaction to the injection.				
28	Properly dispose of used equipment and supplies. Remove gloves and wash hands.				
29	Document the procedure including the medication, dosage and strength, route, site, and any patient reactions. Destroy the medication note.				
30	Return the vial to the storage area.				
Student's Total Points					
Points Possible		600	300	150	
Final Score (Student's Total Points / Possible Points)					

	Notes
Start time:	
End time:	
Total time: (5 min goal)	

COMPETENCY ASSESSMENT

Procedure 36-6 Administering an Intramuscular Injection

Performance Objectives: To correctly administer an intramuscular injection with 100% accuracy. Perform this objective within 5 minutes with a minimum score of 165 points.

Supplies/Equipment: Medication ordered by physician, medication note, appropriately sized safety needle-syringe unit, antiseptic (alcohol) wipes, gloves, cotton balls, adhesive strip, sharps container

Charting/Documentation: Enter appropriate documentation/charting in the box.

Instructor's/Evaluator's Comments and Suggestions:

SKILLS CHECKLIST Procedure 36-6: Administering an Intramuscular Injection

Name ______________________

Date ______________________

No.	Skill	Check #1 20 pts ea	Check #2 10 pts ea	Check #3 5 pts ea	Notes
1	Verify the physician's order. Make out medication note.				
2	Follow the "Six Rights."				
3	Wash hands. Adhere to OSHA guidelines.				
4	Work in a well-lit, quiet, clean area.				
5	Select the appropriate safety syringe-needle unit and other supplies.				
6	Select the correct medication.				
7	Compare the medication label with the medication note (first check).				
8	Check the expiration date of the medicine.				
9	Calculate dosage, if necessary.				
10	Correctly prepare the injection.				
11	Compare medicine label with medication note (second check).				
12	Carefully transport the medicine to the patient on the medicine tray with the vial and other supplies.				
13	Identify the patient and explain the procedure.				
14	Apply gloves.				
15	Prepare the patient for the injection (drape, position, and allay patient apprehension).				
16	Check medication order against the vial and the syringe for a third time.				
17	Select an appropriate injection site.				
18	Cleanse the injection site with a sterile antiseptic wipe. Use a circular motion, working from the center out to about 2 inches beyond the planned injection site. Allow the skin to dry.				
19	Remove the needle cover using a quick, decisive motion.				
20	Stretch the skin taut.				

No.	Skill	Check #1 20 pts ea	Check #2 10 pts ea	Check #3 5 pts ea	Notes
21	Using a dartlike motion, insert the needle to the hub at a 90-degree angle.				
22	Release the skin.				
23	Aspirate to be certain the needle is not in a blood vessel.				
24	Inject the medicine.				
25	Quickly remove the needle and immediately activate the safety mechanism.				
26	Immediately dispose of syringe-needle unit into a sharps container.				
27	Cover the site and massage with a cotton ball. Apply adhesive strip if needed.				
28	Properly dispose of used equipment and supplies. Remove gloves.				
29	Wash hands.				
30	Observe the patient for signs of difficulty.				
31	Provide for patient safety. Check for any reaction to the injection.				
32	Document the procedure including the medication, dosage and strength, route, site, and any patient reactions. Destroy the medication note.				
33	Return the vial to the storage area.				
Student's Total Points					
Points Possible		660	330	165	
Final Score (Student's Total Points / Possible Points)					
		Notes			
Start time:					
End time:					
Total time: (5 min goal)					

COMPETENCY ASSESSMENT

Procedure 36-7 Administering an Intradermal Injection of Purified Protein Derivative (PPD)

Performance Objectives: To correctly administer an intradermal injection of purified protein derivative (PPD) with 100% accuracy. Perform this objective within 5 minutes with a minimum score of 160 points.

Supplies/Equipment: Medication ordered by physician, medication note, appropriately sized safety needle-syringe unit, antiseptic (alcohol) wipes, gloves, sharps container

Charting/Documentation: Enter appropriate documentation/charting in the box.

____

____

____

____

Instructor's/Evaluator's Comments and Suggestions:

____

____

____

____

____

____

SKILLS CHECKLIST Procedure 36-7: Administering an Intradermal Injection of Purified Protein Derivative (PPD)

Name ______________________

Date ______________________

No.	Skill	Check #1 20 pts ea	Check #2 10 pts ea	Check #3 5 pts ea	Notes
1	Verify the physician's order. Make out medication note.				
2	Follow the "Six Rights."				
3	Wash hands. Adhere to OSHA guidelines.				
4	Work in a well-lit, quiet, clean area.				
5	Select the appropriate safety syringe-needle unit and other supplies.				
6	Select the correct medication—PPD.				
7	Compare the medication label with the medication note (first check).				
8	Check the expiration date of the medicine.				
9	Calculate dosage, if necessary.				
10	Correctly prepare the injection.				
11	Compare medicine label with medication note (second check).				
12	Carefully transport the medicine to the patient on the medicine tray with the vial and other supplies.				
13	Identify the patient and explain the procedure.				
14	Assess the patient. Apply gloves.				
15	Prepare the patient for the injection (drape, position, and allay patient apprehension).				
16	Check medication order against the vial and the syringe for a third time.				
17	Select an appropriate injection site, usually the anterior forearm.				
18	Cleanse the injection site with a sterile antiseptic wipe. Using a circular motion, work from the center out to about 2 inches beyond the planned injection site. Allow the skin to dry.				
19	Remove the needle cover using a quick, decisive motion.				
20	Stretch the skin taut.				

No.	Skill	Check #1 20 pts ea	Check #2 10 pts ea	Check #3 5 pts ea	Notes
21	Carefully insert the needle, bevel up, at a 5- to 10-degree angle to about 1/8 inch. Do not aspirate. Release the skin.				
22	Steadily inject the PPD to form a wheal.				
23	Carefully remove the needle after a brief delay.				
24	Immediately activate the safety mechanism.				
25	Immediately dispose of syringe-needle unit into a sharps container.				
26	Gently blot the site of blood if needed. Do not massage! Warn patient not to rub or press on the site. Dispose of supplies into biohazard waste container. Disinfect medicine tray. Remove gloves.				
27	Wash hands.				
28	Observe the patient for signs of difficulty.				
29	Provide for patient safety. Check for any reaction to the injection.				
30	Caution the patient not to press on the wheal.				
31	Document the procedure including the medication dosage and strength, route, site, and any patient reactions. Destroy the medication note and return the vial to the storage area.				
32	The injected area will be read in 48 to 72 hours for the amount of induration or reaction to the PPD. Measure the induration. If the area is hardened 10 mm or greater, alert the physician to the positive reaction.				
Student's Total Points					
Points Possible		640	320	160	
Final Score (Student's Total Points / Possible Points)					

	Notes
Start time:	
End time:	
Total time: (5 min goal)	

COMPETENCY ASSESSMENT

Procedure 36-8 Reconstituting a Powder Medication for Administration

Performance Objectives: To correctly reconstitute a powder medication and calculate correct dosage with 100% accuracy. Perform this objective within 5 minutes with a minimum score of 55 points.

Supplies/Equipment: Medication order by physician, vial of medication, vial of diluent, medication note, two appropriately sized safety syringes and needles, alcohol wipes, gloves, sharps container

Charting/Documentation: Enter appropriate documentation/charting in the box.

Instructor's/Evaluator's Comments and Suggestions:

SKILLS CHECKLIST Procedure 36-8: Reconstituting a Powder Medication for Administration

Name ______________________________

Date ______________________________

No.	Skill	Check #1 20 pts ea	Check #2 10 pts ea	Check #3 5 pts ea	Notes
1	Prepare the needle syringe unit.				
2	Remove top of both the diluent and the powder medication. Wipe with alcohol.				
3	Draw air into the syringe equal to the amount of diluent you will need. Insert the needle of a syringe needle unit through the center of the rubber stopper on the vial of diluent.				
4	Withdraw the appropriate amount of diluent to be added to the powder medication.				
5	Inject the diluent into the powder medication vial.				
6	Remove the needle from the vial and discard into sharps container.				
7	Roll the vial between the palms of the hands to completely mix the powder with the diluent. Label the multi-dose vial with the dilution or strength of the medication you have just prepared. Add the date, time, expiration date, and your initials.				
8	Using the second needle and syringe, inject an equal amount of air and withdraw the desired amount of medication according to the physician's order and your calculations.				
9	Flick away any air bubbles from the syringe. Push the air bubbles back into the vial. Adjust medication withdrawal as needed.				
10	The medicine tray with reconstituted medication is ready for transport to the patient.				
11	Proceed with injection type and route as indicated.				
Student's Total Points					
Points Possible		220	110	55	
Final Score (Student's Total Points / Possible Points)					

	Notes
Start time:	
End time:	
Total time: (5 min goal)	

COMPETENCY ASSESSMENT

Procedure 36-9 Z-Track Intramuscular Injection Technique

Performance Objectives: To correctly administer a Z-track intramuscular injection with 100% accuracy. Perform this objective within 5 minutes with a minimum score of 165 points.

Supplies/Equipment: Medication order by physician, medication note, medication vial, appropriately sized safety needle-syringe unit, antiseptic (alcohol) wipes, gloves, cotton balls, adhesive strip, sharps container

Charting/Documentation: Enter appropriate documentation/charting in the box.

Instructor's/Evaluator's Comments and Suggestions:

SKILLS CHECKLIST Procedure 36-9: Z-Track Intramuscular Injection Technique

Name ______________________

Date ______________________

No.	Skill	Check #1 20 pts ea	Check #2 10 pts ea	Check #3 5 pts ea	Notes
1	Verify the physician's order. Make out medication note.				
2	Follow the "Six Rights."				
3	Wash hands. Adhere to OSHA guidelines.				
4	Work in a well-lit, quiet, clean area.				
5	Organize the appropriate supplies.				
6	Select the correct medication.				
7	Compare the medication label with the medication note (first check).				
8	Check the expiration date of the medicine.				
9	Calculate dosage, if necessary.				
10	Correctly prepare the injection.				
11	Compare medicine label with medication note (second check).				
12	Carefully transport the medicine to the patient on the medicine tray with the vial and other supplies.				
13	Identify the patient and explain the procedure.				
14	Assess the patient. Apply gloves.				
15	Prepare the patient for the injection (drape, position, and allay patient apprehension).				
16	Check medication order against the vial and the syringe for a third time.				
17	Select an appropriate injection site.				
18	Cleanse the injection site with a sterile antiseptic wipe. Using a circular motion, work from the center out to about 6 inches beyond the planned injection site. Allow the skin to dry.				
19	Remove the needle cover using a quick, decisive motion.				
20	Pull the skin laterally 1.5 inches away from the injection site (keep eye on exact injection site before pulling skin).				

No.	Skill	Check #1 20 pts ea	Check #2 10 pts ea	Check #3 5 pts ea	Notes
21	Using a dartlike motion, insert the needle to the hub at a 90-degree angle. Maintain the pull on the skin.				
22	Aspirate to be certain the needle is not in a blood vessel.				
23	Inject the medicine.				
24	Wait 10 seconds before removing needle.				
25	Quickly remove the needle at the same angle as insertion.				
26	Immediately, as the needle is withdrawn, release the traction on the skin. This will seal off the medication.				
27	Immediately activate the safety mechanism and dispose of syringe-needle unit into a sharps container.				
28	Cover the site. Do not massage. Apply adhesive strip if needed.				
29	Properly dispose of used equipment and supplies. Remove gloves and wash hands.				
30	Observe the patient for signs of difficulty.				
31	Provide for patient safety. Check for any reaction to the injection.				
32	Return the vial to the storage area.				
33	Document the procedure including the medication, dosage and strength, route, site, and any patient reactions. Destroy the medication note.				
Student's Total Points					
Points Possible		660	330	165	
Final Score (Student's Total Points / Possible Points)					

	Notes
Start time:	
End time:	
Total time: (5 min goal)	

EVALUATION OF CHAPTER KNOWLEDGE

Skills	Student Self-Evaluation		
	Good	Average	Poor
I can discuss legal and ethical implications of medication administration.	____	____	____
I can describe the medication order.	____	____	____
I can describe the parts of a prescription.	____	____	____
I can state information contained on a medication label and can discuss the significance of the information.	____	____	____
I understand ratios and proportions.	____	____	____
I am able to use metric and household systems of measurement and convert between the two.	____	____	____
I understand units of medication dosage.	____	____	____
I can correctly calculate adult and child dosages.	____	____	____
I can list guidelines to follow when preparing and administering medications.	____	____	____
I know to only use safety needles and syringes.			
I can describe safe disposal of syringes, needles, and biohazardous materials.	____	____	____
I can describe site selection for administration of injections.	____	____	____
I understand allergenic extracts.	____	____	____
I can describe inhalation medications and how to administer them.	____	____	____
I can exhibit therapeutic communication skills in administering medications to patients and attend to patients' emotional needs.	____	____	____
I document accurately.	____	____	____
I can comply with governmental regulations in the administration and disposal of controlled substances.	____	____	____
I possess the ability to competently prepare and administer oral and parenteral medications as directed by a physician.	____	____	____

CHAPTER 37

Electrocardiography

CHAPTER PRE-TEST

Perform this test without looking at the book. This is just to see how well you have understood and can recall the information in this chapter after you have read it, but before you have completed the workbook exercises. You will not be graded on this portion (other than the grade you give yourself). Justify any "false" answers.

1. The skin is a great conductor of electricity. (T or F)
2. Electrolytes provide moisture, and electrodes provide metal to the conduction process. (T or F)
3. The heart is like a two-sided pump that routes blood where it needs to go. (T or F)
4. Only certain cells in the heart are able to conduct electricity. (T or F)
5. Artifacts are electrical nuisances. (T or F)
6. The heart beats approximately 60 times a minute only resting in between beats. (T or F)

INTRODUCTION

Electrocardiography is a noninvasive, safe, and painless procedure many physicians include as part of a complete physical examination. An electrocardiogram (ECG or EKG) measures the amount of electrical activity produced by the heart and the time it takes for the electrical impulses to travel through the heart during each heartbeat. The ECG is used in conjunction with other laboratory and diagnostic tests to assess total cardiac health. During an ECG, the medical assistant is responsible for patient preparation; patient education; operation of the electrocardiograph; elimination of artifacts; mounting, labeling, and placing the ECG reading in the patient's medical record; and proper maintenance and care of the equipment. It is important that the medical assistant perform ECGs skillfully and accurately.

PERFORMANCE OBJECTIVES

After successful completion of this chapter, you will be familiar with the terminology related to electrocardiography; the basic structure, function, and physiology of the heart; the electrical circuitry through the heart; and some of the pathology related to the heart conduction system. You will become familiar with the machines, equipment, and supplies associated with electrocardiography and other cardiac monitoring systems. You will know how to reassure patients, prepare them for a variety of cardiac diagnostic procedures, and answer their questions. You will be able to perform an ECG, apply a Holter monitor, and schedule many other tests and procedures. *The following statements are related to your learning objectives for this chapter. Fill in the blanks in the following paragraph with the appropriate term(s).*

The heart has (1) ____________ chambers, two upper chambers known as (2) ____________ and two lower chambers known as (3) ____________________. The (4) ____________________ blood enters the (5) ________________ atrium from the body and passes to the right ventricle, and then to the (6) ______________________, where it receives (7)__________________________. From the lungs, the blood goes through the (8) ____________________ side of the heart in much the same route before it goes back out to the (9) ______________________. The electrical conduction system of the heart begins with the body's natural pacemaker, called the (10) __________________________ node, or (11) ______ for short. The pacemaker sends its electrical message to the (12) ____________________________ node, which is abbreviated (13) ________. The electrical current travels through the septum of the heart in an area called the bundle of (14) _______, which has two branches, the right and left bundle branches. From there the charge goes to the (15) __________________________ fibers, which surround the ventricles, causing those cells to contract. This entire route is called the (16) _________________ cycle. On paper, the cycle presents itself with a series of (17) _______________ that are designated letters for identification purposes. We are able to amplify the electricity of the heart and record it on paper using a machine called an (18) ________________________________. The medical assistant needs to be sure to get a true tracing of the heart's electrical activity without any interference called (19) ____________________. The ECG can give the physician quite a bit of information about the conduction and excitability of the heart muscle, especially any irregularities in rhythm known as (20) ___________________________. Occasionally, a portable monitor, called a (21) ___________________________, will be a useful diagnostic tool. If the physician wants to see what the patient's heart is doing while exercising, he might order a (22) ______________________________ or (23) ______________________________________. Ultrasound and (24) _______________________________ are noninvasive diagnostic tests that also can be performed.

VOCABULARY BUILDER

Crossword Puzzle

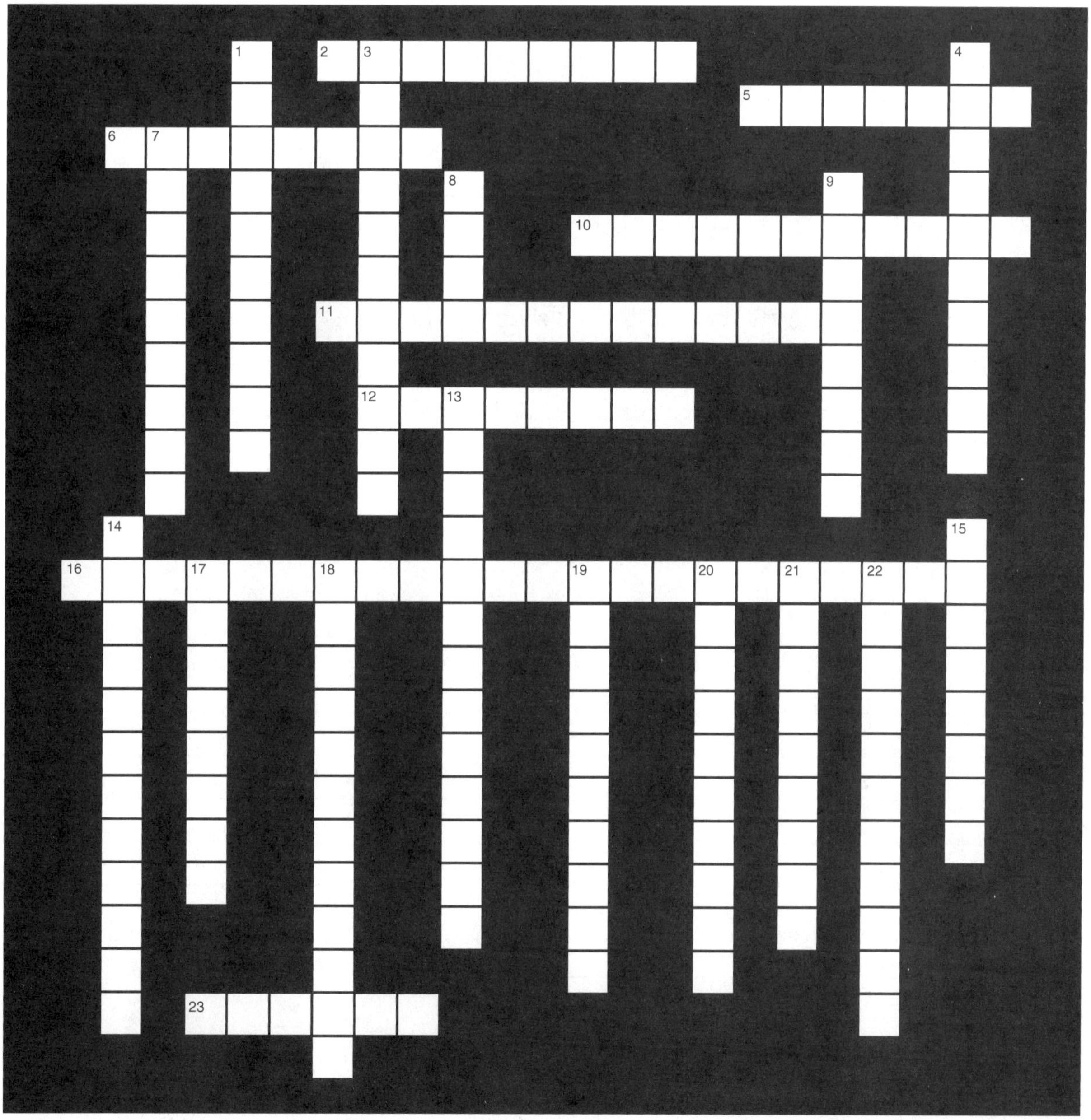

Across

2. A series of x-rays of a blood vessel(s) after injection of a radiopaque substance
5. The part of the heart cycle in which the heart is in contraction
6. The flat, horizontal line that separates the various waves of the ECG cycle
10. Chemical substance that enhances the conduction of electrical activity
11. Conversion of a pathologic cardiac rhythm (arrhythmia) to normal sinus rhythm
12. Local and temporary lack of blood to an organ or a part because of obstruction of circulation
16. Procedure used to obtain cardiac blood samples, detect abnormalities, and determine intracardiac pressure
23. Heated slender wire of the electrocardiograph that melts the wax off the ECG paper during the recording

Down

1. Pertaining to the area on the anterior surface of the body overlying the heart
3. Procedures that do not require entering the body or puncturing the skin
4. Sensors used to conduct electricity from the body to the electrocardiograph
7. To add or increase
8. The machine has several __________ wires
9. Process of applying in sequence a portion of each of the 12 leads of the ECG recording onto a document placed in the patient's chart
13. Applications of electric current to the heart, directly or indirectly, to alter a disturbance in cardiac rhythm
14. Mechanism in the electrocardiograph that changes the voltage into a mechanical motion for recording purposes
15. Having or pertaining to a one-pole process
17. The normal period in the cardiac cycle during which the myocardial fibers lengthen, the heart dilates, and the cavities fill with blood
18. One complete heartbeat
19. During an ultrasound procedure, this device picks up echoes and converts them to electrical energy
20. An area of tissue in an organ or a part that becomes necrotic after cessation of blood supply
21. Amount, extent, size, abundance, or fullness
22. Having equal electrical potentials; represented on the ECG as the baseline

LEARNING REVIEW

1. List five reasons why electrocardiography is performed.

   (1) ______________________________

   (2) ______________________________

   (3) ______________________________

   (4) ______________________________

   (5) ______________________________

2. A. The first three leads recorded on a standard ECG are Lead I, Lead II, and Lead III. These are ______________________________ leads because each of them uses two-limb electrodes that record simultaneously.

   For each lead, what electrical activity of the heart is recorded? Draw it on each figure.

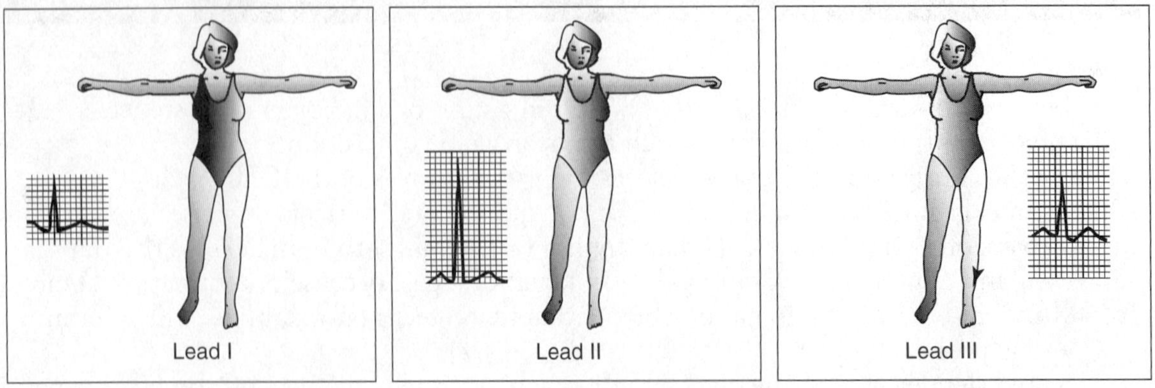

(a) **(b)** **(c)**

Lead I records electrical activity between the ________________ and ________________.

Lead II records electrical activity between the ________________ and ________________.

Lead III records electrical activity between the ________________ and ________________.

B. The next group of leads recorded on a standard ECG are augmented leads, designated, aVR, aVL, and aVF. These are ______________________________ leads.

For each lead, what electrical activity of the heart is recorded? Draw it on each figure.

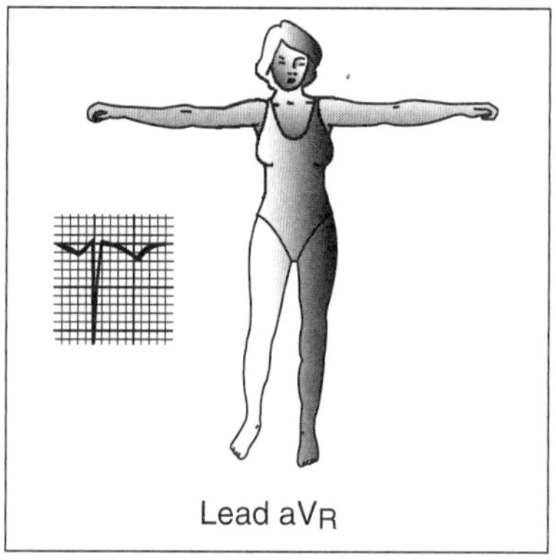

(d)

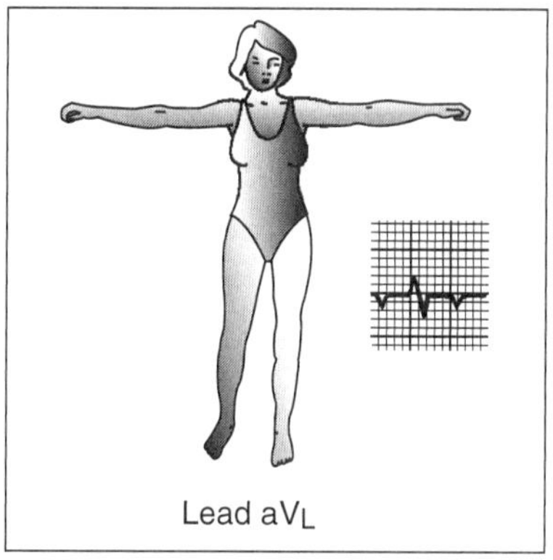

(e)

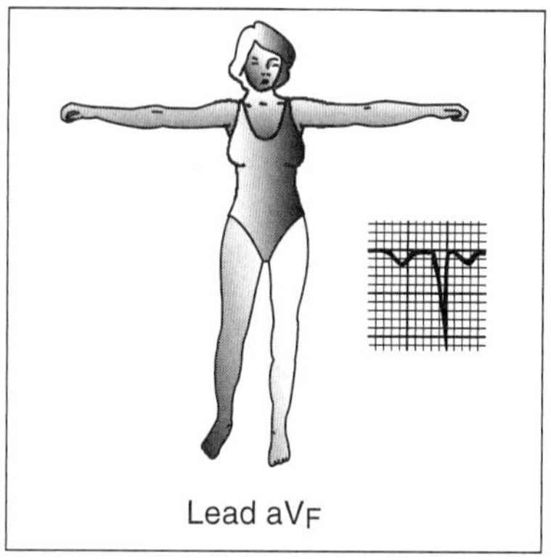

(f)

Lead aVR records electrical activity from ______________________________.

Lead aVL records electrical activity from ______________________________.

Lead aVF records electrical activity from ______________________________.

C. The remaining 6 leads of the standard 12-lead ECG are the chest leads or ________________ leads. These leads are unipolar/bipolar (select one).

Where are the leads placed on the body?

V_1 ______________________________

V_2 ______________________________

V_3 ______________________________

V_4 ______________________________

V_5 ______________________________

V_6 ______________________________

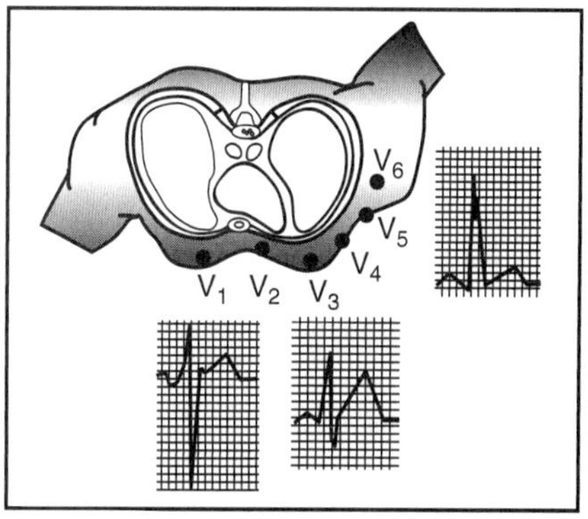

3. Artifacts are unusual and unwanted activity in the ECG tracing not caused by the electrical activity of the heart. Match each circumstance below to the artifact ECG tracing it would produce and identify the type of artifact in the space provided.

A. A broken patient cable or lead wire has become detached from an electrode.

B. The patient sings to himself or herself during the ECG procedure.

C. The patient uses body lotion.

D. The lead wires are crossed and do not follow the patient's body contour.

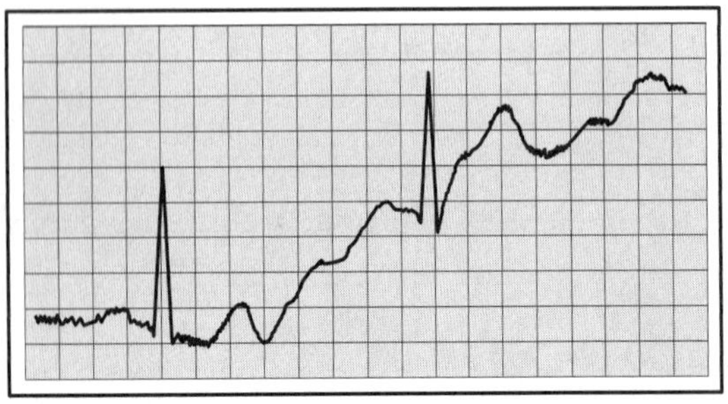

(a)

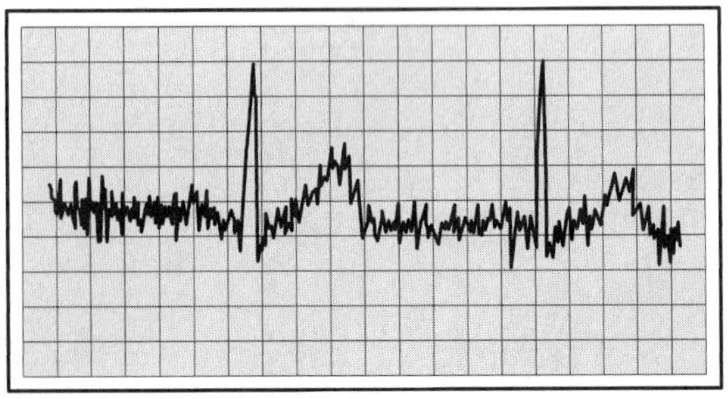

(b)

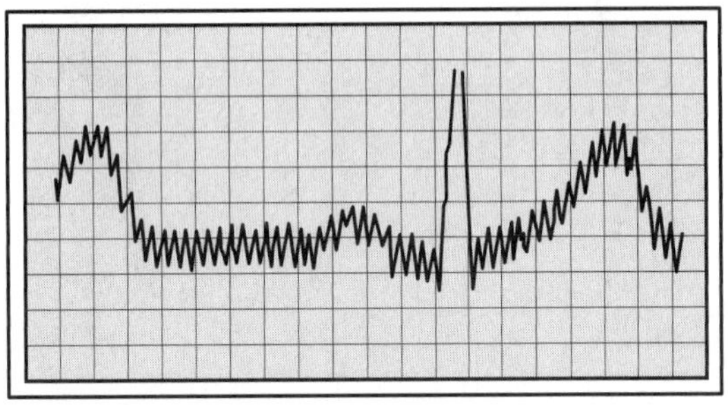

(c)

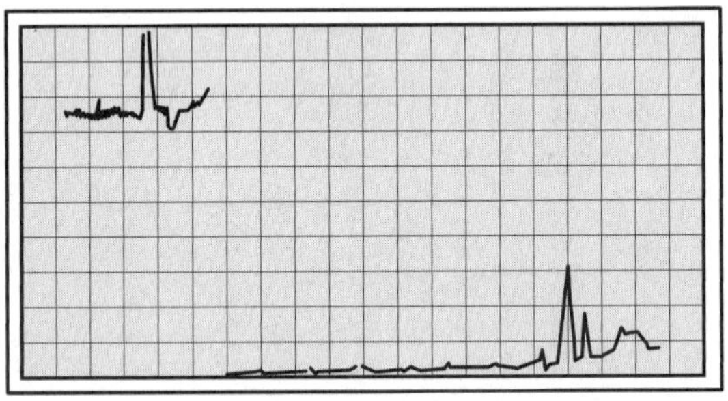

(d)

CERTIFICATION REVIEW

These questions are designed to mimic the certification examinations. You can use these questions like a small "Certification Examination Study Guide," but this is not meant to take the place of the more extensive study guides. Use this portion to determine in what areas to concentrate your efforts when studying for the certification examination.

1. Repolarization takes place while the heart muscle:
   a. contracts
   b. stops
   c. skips a beat
   d. relaxes

2. A type of chest electrode that consists of a disposable adhesive sensor is known as:
   a. precordial
   b. limb
   c. augmented
   d. bipolar

3. Augmented leads are also called:
   a. unipolar
   b. bipolar

c. precordial

d. standard

4. One millivolt of cardiac electrical activity will deflect the stylus exactly:
   a. 5 mm high
   b. 10 mm high
   c. 25 mm high
   d. 40 mm high

5. A wandering baseline may be caused by:
   a. lotions, creams, or oils on the patient's skin
   b. electrical interference
   c. crossed lead wires
   d. improper grounding

CASE STUDY

Jim Marshall, a prominent local architect in his late 30s, stays in good physical condition, works out regularly at the gym, and maintains a low-fat, low-cholesterol, low-sodium diet. Aggressive and ambitious, Jim enjoys pushing his mind and body to the limit. His favorite sports are skiing and sailing. At work, Jim is a perfectionist who puts in long hours and demands the same of his employees. Lately, though, Jim is more aware of the high-stress lifestyle he is leading and is worried about his family history of heart failure and diabetes. During periods of high physical exertion, Jim experiences mild chest pain and palpitations. Dr. Lewis prescribes an exercise tolerance test for Jim.

Discuss the following:

1. What is an exercise tolerance test? How is it performed?
2. Under what conditions would the test be discontinued?
3. At the conclusion of the test, what patient care is given? What special instructions for home care should the patient observe?
4. What is the proper insurance coding for the patient's exercise tolerance test or cardiovascular stress test? Is the code a diagnosis or procedures code?

SELF-ASSESSMENT

Keep a strict diary of everything you eat and drink for the next three days (a week is better).

1. Count up the total fats you have eaten each day.
2. Separate the types of fats and total each type for each day.
3. Go online and using search words such as "saturated fats" or "trans fats" to learn more about the different fats.
4. Find out about omega-3 fatty acids. Are you eating enough? How could you take in more?
5. What else should you be doing to stay "heart healthy"?

CHAPTER POST-TEST

This is similar to the Pre-Test. Perform this test without looking at the book. This is just to see how well you have understood and can recall the information presented in this chapter after you have studied it and completed the workbook exercises. You will not be graded on this portion (other than the grade you give yourself), but this is an excellent preparation for your instructor's test. You may use this Post-Test to determine what areas you need to study more. Justify any "false" answers.

1. The skin is a poor conductor of electricity. (T or F)
2. Electrodes provide moisture and electrolytes provide metal to the conduction process. (T or F)
3. The heart is like a four-sided pump that routes blood where it needs to go. (T or F)
4. All cardiac cells are able to conduct electricity. (T or F)
5. Artifacts are part of the heart's electrical circuitry. (T or F)
6. The heart beats approximately 24 times a minute resting only in between beats. (T or F)

CERTIFICATION CRITERIA CHECKLIST

As you go through your education and training, keep in mind the national certification examination that you will take when you graduate. Each chapter of the textbook and workbook covers a different section of the examination criteria. To keep track of your preparation for the certification examination, turn to the back of this workbook and highlight the following CMA, RMA, or CMAS certification examination criteria (if you have already highlighted them from a previous chapter, put a check mark by the criteria):

CMA

B. Anatomy and Physiology
  2. Systems, including structure, function, related conditions and diseases

S. Treatment Area
  1. Equipment preparation and operation
  2. Principles of operation (equipment)

V. (Collecting and Processing Specimens;) Diagnostic Testing
  3. Quality control
  4. Performing selected tests

RMA

III. Clinical Medical Assisting
  J. Electrocardiography

COMPETENCY ASSESSMENT

Procedure 37-1 Perform Single-Channel or Multichannel Electrocardiogram

Performance Objectives: To perform a standard 12-lead electrocardiogram (ECG). Perform this objective within 15 minutes with a minimum score of 95 points.

Supplies/Equipment: Electrocardiograph machine, lead wires with end clips, tabbed adhesive electrodes, tracing paper, patient gown, small pillow, blanket/sheet, alcohol, razor (optional), mounting card/paper

Charting/Documentation: Enter appropriate documentation/charting in the box.

Instructor's/Evaluator's Comments and Suggestions:

SKILLS CHECKLIST Procedure 37-1: Perform Single-Channel or Multichannel Electrocardiogram

Name ______________________

Date ______________________

No.	Skill	Check #1 20 pts ea	Check #2 10 pts ea	Check #3 5 pts ea	Notes
1	Perform tracing in a quiet, warm, and comfortable room away from electrical interference.				
2	Wash hands, gather equipment, identify the patient, introduce yourself, and explain the procedure.				
3	Have the patient remove clothing from the waist up and uncover lower legs. Nylon stockings must be removed, but socks can be worn. Provide a sheet or blanket for comfort if needed. Place the patient in supine position with arms and legs supported.				
4	Explain that the procedure is painless and why it is necessary to not talk or move during the procedure.				
5	Place the electrocardiograph with the power cord pointing away from the patient. Do not allow the cable to go underneath the examination table.				
6	Apply the limb electrodes first. Lead connectors of the electrodes should be positioned so the wires will not be pulling off the electrodes. If the electrodes do not adhere well, wipe with alcohol, let dry, and apply a fresh electrode. Shave site of excess hair if necessary.				
7	Place the chest leads according to standard protocol. The electrode tabs should be positioned downward.				
8	Connect all the lead wires. Make certain that the proper wires are connected to the right sites. (Some machines have six chest lead wires, and others have only one. If your machine has only one, you will need to turn off the amp between running each V lead to reposition the lead wire onto the next electrode.				

No.	Skill	Check #1 20 pts ea	Check #2 10 pts ea	Check #3 5 pts ea	Notes
9	Position the main cable centrally, usually on the patient abdomen, so the wires do not pull off the electrodes.				
10	Turn on the machine.				
11	Enter information into machine's database (patient name, birth date, age, height, weight, sex, blood pressure, identification number, and any cardiac medications the patient is taking). For manual machines, this information is entered onto the mounting card.				
12	Remind the patient not to talk and to try not to move. If he or she has a neuromuscular condition such as Parkinson's disease and cannot remain still, have the patient slide his or her hands under his or her buttocks, then relax his or her muscles.				
13	Press "auto" and the machine will run the strip. For manual machines, standardize if needed. Turn the lead selector switch to STD. Center the stylus. Position the Run speed to 25 mm/sec. Standardize manually to 10 mm and adjust if necessary.				
14	Run through all 12 leads. Manually recording four to five complexes of each before turning to the next lead. Single-channel machines print on a strip while multichannel (three) machines will print out the full size paper.				
15	Check the quality of the tracing and eliminate any artifact before repeating the ECG. For manual machines, place another standardization at the end of the tracing. Run the paper through and turn off the machine. Remove the tracing from the machine and label with the patient's name, the date, and time of day. Initial.				
16	If patient has symptoms, show tracing to the physician immediately. If doing a routine (well physical) ECG, unplug the power cord, disconnect the lead wires, and remove the electrodes from the patient.				
17	Assist the patient as needed.				

No.	Skill	Check #1 20 pts ea	Check #2 10 pts ea	Check #3 5 pts ea	Notes
18	Be certain all the patient information is with the tracing and give the uncut tracing to the physician with the mounting card. When physician is done with it, cut and mount the tracing. Label appropriately and place in patient's record.				
19	Clean and return the machine to the central area. Dispose of waste according to OSHA guidelines. Wash hands. Document procedure.				
Student's Total Points					
Points Possible		380	190	95	
Final Score (Student's Total Points / Possible Points)					
		Notes			
Start time:					
End time:					
Total time: (15 min goal)					

COMPETENCY ASSESSMENT

Procedure 37-2 Perform Holter Monitor Application

Performance Objectives: To apply a Holter monitor and teach the patient how to wear the monitor, record the incidents, keep the activity log/diary, and when to return. Perform this objective within 20 minutes with a minimum score of 90 points

Supplies/Equipment: Holter monitor, patient activity diary/log, blank magnetic tape cassette, disposable electrodes, alcohol, razor, gauze, carrying case, belt or shoulder strap

Charting/Documentation: Enter appropriate documentation/charting in the box.

Instructor's/Evaluator's Comments and Suggestions:

SKILLS CHECKLIST Procedure 37-2: Perform Holter Monitor Application

Name ______________________

Date ______________________

No.	Skill	Check #1 20 pts ea	Check #2 10 pts ea	Check #3 5 pts ea	Notes
1	Wash hands. Assemble equipment.				
2	Prepare the equipment by removing used battery from the monitor and replacing it with a fresh battery. Insert a blank magnetic tape cassette into the monitor.				
3	Wash hands.				
4	Identify the patient, introduce yourself, and explain the procedure.				
5	Have the patient remove clothing from the waist up.				
6	Have the patient sit on the examination table or chair.				
7	Locate the correct electrode placement sites. Prepare the skin by shaving if needed, rub the site with alcohol, let dry, and abrade the skin slightly with gauze.				
8	Remove the electrodes from the package and check that they are moist.				
9	Apply the adhesive-backed electrodes to the appropriate sites. Apply pressure at the center of the electrode first, then move outward until the electrode is well adhered to the site. Run your fingers along the outer rim to ensure firm attachment. Avoid pressing from one side to the other, which can cause uneven electrolyte coverage.				
10	Attach the lead wires to the electrodes, then connect them to the patient cable.				
11	Plug the monitor into an electrocardiograph machine with the test cable; run a baseline tracing (this step is optional with some monitors).				
12	Place the electrode cable so that it extends from between the buttons of the patient's shirt or from the bottom of the shirt.				

No.	Skill	Check #1 20 pts ea	Check #2 10 pts ea	Check #3 5 pts ea	Notes
13	Place the recorder into its carrying case and either attach it to the patient's belt or over the patient's shoulder. Be certain there is no pulling on the lead wires.				
14	Plug the electrode cable into the monitor. Record the starting time in the patient activity log/diary.				
15	Give the activity log to the patient and explain how to keep track of activities.				
16	Schedule the patient's return time the following day for removal and follow-up. Remind the patient to bring the activity log.				
17	Wash hands.				
18	Document the procedure in the patient's record.				
Student's Total Points					
Points Possible		360	180	90	
Final Score (Student's Total Points / Possible Points)					

	Notes
Start time:	
End time:	
Total time: (20 min goal)	

EVALUATION OF CHAPTER KNOWLEDGE

Skills	Student Self-Evaluation Good	Average	Poor
I can follow the circulation of blood through the heart, starting at the vena cavae.	_____	_____	_____
I can describe the electrical conduction system of the heart and trace its pathway.	_____	_____	_____
I can identify reasons a patient requires an ECG.	_____	_____	_____
I can identify the various positive and negative deflections and describe what each represents in the cardiac cycle.	_____	_____	_____
I can explain the purpose of standardization of the electrocardiograph.	_____	_____	_____
I can identify the 12 leads of an ECG and describe what area of the heart each lead represents.	_____	_____	_____
I can state the function of ECG graph paper, electrodes (sensors), and electrolyte.	_____	_____	_____
I can describe various types of ECGs and their capabilities.	_____	_____	_____
I can explain each type of artifact and how each can be eliminated.	_____	_____	_____
I can name and describe the purposes of the various cardiac diagnostic tests.	_____	_____	_____
I can identify the placement of Holter monitor electrodes.	_____	_____	_____
I can describe the reason for a patient activity diary during ambulatory cardiography.	_____	_____	_____
I can identify common arrhythmias and explain the causes of each.	_____	_____	_____
I can explain how to calculate heart rates from an ECG tracing.	_____	_____	_____
I can identify a common coding system used to code each lead on an ECG tracing.	_____	_____	_____
I can describe the procedure for mounting an ECG tracing.	_____	_____	_____
I document accurately.	_____	_____	_____
I can prepare a patient for a procedure and attend to his or her emotional needs.	_____	_____	_____

CHAPTER 38

Safety and Regulatory Guidelines in the Medical Laboratory

CHAPTER PRE-TEST

Perform this test without looking at the book. This is just to see how well you have understood and can recall the information in this chapter after you have read it, but before you have completed the workbook exercises. You will not be graded on this portion (other than the grade you give yourself). Justify any "false" answers.

1. Clinical Laboratory Improvement Amendments (CLIA) is a federal mandate that protects the laboratory worker. (T or F)

2. Aegis means:
   a. sponsorship or protection
   b. the part of the laboratory sample that is discarded
   c. a reagent or chemical used in laboratory tests
   d. a region or area of concern

3. Quality control is a way of:
   a. ensuring that the chemicals or reagents used are of good quality
   b. ensuring the test is run correctly
   c. ensuring that the patient sample is stored correctly
   d. all of the above

4. MSDS stands for:
   a. Material Safety Data Sheets
   b. Manual for Safety Documents/Sheets
   c. Mandated Standards for Documentation and Safety
   d. Manual of Supplies and Data for Safety

5. MSDS information must be:
   a. read by all employees
   b. indexed and alphabetized in a notebook or manual
   c. made readily available to all employees
   d. all of the above

INTRODUCTION

While treating patients in the medical facility, health care professionals, including medical assistants, come into contact with many specimens and hazardous fluids that may be highly infectious and dangerous. To protect patients and health care providers from the many hazards, medical asepsis and infection control measures are practiced to prevent or limit dangers that can be encountered in the laboratory. State and federal agencies such as the Centers for Disease Control and Prevention (CDC), the Clinical Laboratory Improvement Amendments of 1988 (CLIA '88), and the Occupational Safety and Health Administration (OSHA) establish guidelines and regulations for health care providers and employers to follow to reduce the risk for exposure and possible transmission of infectious diseases. Medical assistants must understand the regulations set forth by these government agencies and implement them in the ambulatory care setting for the health and safety of patients and health care professionals. Medical assistants must be aware of CLIA regulations regarding testing in the office and must adhere to safe practices according to OSHA regulations.

PERFORMANCE OBJECTIVES

After successful completion of this chapter, you will be familiar with the terminology related to safety and regulation guidelines in the medical laboratory. You will be familiar with various government agencies, mandates, regulations, forms, and guidelines having to do with safety in medical laboratories. You will understand the role of the medical assistant in the medical laboratory and know what tests you will be authorized to perform and under what conditions those tests will be performed for quality control. You will be knowledgeable about chemicals and reagents used in laboratory testing and how to handle them, store them, and dispose of them safely. *The following statements are related to your learning objectives for this chapter. Fill in the blanks in the following paragraph with the appropriate term(s).*

The purpose of (1) ________ is to safeguard the public by (2) ____________________ all testing of specimens taken from the (3) ______________________________. OSHA, in contrast, works to ensure (4) ____________________________________ safety in the laboratory. CLIA has (5) ____________________ categories of testing. They are (6) ________________________ tests, (7) ____________________________________ tests, which includes (8) ________, and (9) _______________________________ tests. Waived tests are simple, unvarying, and require a minimum of (10) ________________________ and (11) ___________________________. Test errors carry a minimum or (12) _______________ to the patient. PPM, which stands for (13) ____________________________________, are moderately complex and require the expertise of the provider or physician. The criteria used to determine CLIA categories include the degree of (14) ____________________________________ needed, the necessary

(15) ____________________ and (16) ____________________ the operator possesses, and the degree of (17) ____________________ and (18) ____________________ needed to perform the tests. Medical assistants may perform the tests within the (19) ____________________ category only, unless they possess advanced education and training. The PPM most often performed in the physician's office laboratory (POL) or (20) ____________________ is the microscopic examination of urine. The medical assistant may perform the physical and chemical examinations of urine, but not the PPM part. Because students are not (21) ____________________, they do not fall under the aegis of OSHA. Nevertheless, schools should follow all OSHA requirements for the (22) ____________________ of all; also, medical assisting students need to learn safe practices and how to use safety equipment for their careers.

VOCABULARY BUILDER

A. *Find the words in Column A that are misspelled; circle them, and then correctly spell them in the spaces provided. Then match the following correct vocabulary terms listed in Column A with their corresponding definitions listed in Column B.*

Column A

A. spill kit
B. standard
C. proficiency testing
D. waved
E. fume hood
F. federal register
G. calabration
H. requisition
I. mandate
J. quality control

____

____

Column B

_____ 1. Rules set up and established to measure quality, weight, extent, or value

_____ 2. The determination of the accuracy of an instrument by comparing the information provided with an accepted standard known to be accurate

_____ 3. Used to describe a category of clinical laboratory tests that are simple, unvarying, and require a minimum of judgment and interpretation

_____ 4. Measures used to monitor the processing of laboratory specimens

_____ 5. Commercially packaged materials containing supplies and equipment needed to clean a spill of biohazardous substances

_____ 6. Formal order to obey certain rules and regulations

_____ 7. A written request for laboratory analysis to be performed on a specimen

_____ 8. A barrier used in the laboratory to capture chemical vapors

_____ 9. Federal agency from which written CLIA '88 documents may be obtained

_____ 10. Sample tests performed in a clinical laboratory to determine that a specific degree of accuracy is achieved

B. *To test your spelling skills, unscramble the correct vocabulary terms that follow; then define each term in the space provided.*

1. TANOECE ______________________________
2. PATMIRHEEHCUTEOC TANGES ______________________________
3. TELHY LOCOLAH ______________________________
4. SEGAI ______________________________
5. DOYEFAMEDLRH ______________________________

LEARNING REVIEW

1. The three categories of laboratory testing are waived, moderate complexity (which include physician-performed microscopy), and high complexity. All laboratories are required to register with CLIA '88 and receive certification to perform specific categories of tests within strict boundaries of compliance. Waived tests deliver simple unvarying results and require a minimum of judgment and interpretation. Name 10 waived tests.

   (1) ____________________ (6) ____________________
   (2) ____________________ (7) ____________________
   (3) ____________________ (8) ____________________
   (4) ____________________ (9) ____________________
   (5) ____________________ (10) ____________________

2. CLIA '88 requires every facility that tests human specimens for diagnosis, treatment, and prevention of disease to meet specific federal requirements. Name five specific duties a medical assistant may perform that will make an impact on the medical facility's compliance with CLIA '88 regulations.

   (1) ______________________________
   (2) ______________________________
   (3) ______________________________
   (4) ______________________________
   (5) ______________________________

3. A written chemical hygiene plan (CHP) is required of all medical facilities to comply with safety standards outlined by OSHA. To comply with OSHA regulations, chemicals must be labeled using the National Fire Protection Association's (NFPA's) color and number methods.

   A. Match the colors below to the type of hazard each signifies.

   ______ blue — 1. fire
   ______ white — 2. reactivity
   ______ yellow — 3. use of personal protective equipment (PPE)
   ______ red — 4. health

B. For each configuration listed, use the NFPA color and number method to describe the hazardous properties of each chemical.

(1) CHEMICAL X: Red/2; Blue/3; Yellow/3; White/F

____

(2) CHEMICAL Y: Red/0; Blue/1; Yellow/0; White/X

____

(3) CHEMICAL Z: Red/1; Blue/2; Yellow/1; White/E

____

CERTIFICATION REVIEW

These questions are designed to mimic the certification examinations. You can use these questions like a small "Certification Examination Study Guide," but this is not meant to take the place of the more extensive study guides. Use this portion to determine in what areas to concentrate your efforts when studying for the certification examination.

1. CLIA was passed in an effort to:
   a. teach staff how to read test results accurately
   b. establish standards to ensure test results are kept confidential
   c. establish standards to ensure accurate test results
   d. all of the above
2. CLIA was passed in what year?
   a. 1902
   b. 1975
   c. 1988
   d. 1999
3. Which of the following procedures is a requirement of qualifying protocol for automated hematology instruments?
   a. control samples
   b. proficiency testing
   c. calibration
   d. all of the above
4. Material Safety Data Sheets (MSDSs) do *not* contain:
   a. product/chemical information
   b. emergency response procedures
   c. manufacturer information
   d. training information for using the product/chemical
5. When skin comes into contact with chemicals, it is best to:
   a. wash the area with water immediately
   b. apply a neutralizing agent to the site
   c. consult the MSDS before treatment
   d. rinse area with vinegar

SELF-ASSESSMENT

1. Choose a chemical you have at home or in the basement, garage, or storage area.
2. Look at the label.
   a. Does it have any precautionary statements or warnings?
   b. Does it have any fire hazard information?
3. Complete the following form.
   a. Name of chemical (brand name) ______________________________
   b. What chemicals are included in the active ingredients?

      ____

   c. What precautions are listed?

      ____

   d. What instructions are listed for contamination of eyes or skin, ingestion, and so forth?

      ____

   e. What is the number in your area for Poison Control?

      ____

CHAPTER POST-TEST

This is similar to the Pre-Test. Perform this test without looking at the book. This is just to see how well you have understood and can recall the information presented in this chapter after you have studied it and completed the workbook exercises. You will not be graded on this portion (other than the grade you give yourself), but this is an excellent preparation for your instructor's test. You may use this Post-Test to determine what areas you need to study more. Justify any "false" answers.

1. CLIA is a federal mandate that protects the patient. (T or F)
2. Aegis means:
   a. a reagent or chemical used in laboratory tests
   b. the part of the laboratory sample that is discarded
   c. sponsorship or protection
   d. a region or area of concern
3. Quality control is a way of:
   a. ensuring the test is run correctly
   b. ensuring that the chemicals or reagents used are of good quality
   c. ensuring that the patient sample is stored correctly
   d. all of the above

4. MSDS stands for:
   a. Material Safety Data Sheets
   b. Mandated Standards for Documentation and Safety
   c. Manual for Safety Documents/Sheets
   d. Manual of Supplies and Data for Safety

5. MSDS information must be:
   a. readily available to all employees
   b. organized in a notebook or manual
   c. indexed and alphabetized
   d. all of the above

CERTIFICATION CRITERIA CHECKLIST

As you go through your education and training, keep in mind the national certification examination that you will take when you graduate. Each chapter of the textbook and workbook covers a different section of the examination criteria. To keep track of your preparation for the certification examination, turn to the back of this workbook and highlight the following CMA, RMA, or CMAS certification examination criteria (if you have already highlighted them from a previous chapter, put a check mark by the criteria):

CMA
F. Medicolegal Guidelines & Requirements
R. Principles of Infection Control
V. Collecting and Processing Specimens; Diagnostic Testing
    3. Quality control
X. Emergencies
    1. Preplanned actions

RMA
I. General Medical Assisting Knowledge
    C. Medical Law
III. Clinical Medical Assisting
    A. Asepsis
    I. Laboratory procedures
        1. Safety
        4. Laboratory equipment

CMAS
1. Medical Assisting Foundation
    • Legal (and ethical) considerations
2. Basic Clinical Medical Office Assisting
    • Asepsis in the medical office
    • Medical office emergencies
8. Medical Office Management
    • Safety
    • Supplies and equipment

EVALUATION OF CHAPTER KNOWLEDGE

	Student Self-Evaluation		
Skills	Good	Average	Poor
I can identify government regulatory agencies responsible for setting standards.	_____	_____	_____
I know categories of testing and understand CLIA '88 requirements.	_____	_____	_____
I understand the purpose of the MSDS manual and can apply the NFPA system of chemical hazard labeling.	_____	_____	_____
I can identify situations of potential risk for exposure to hazards in the ambulatory setting.	_____	_____	_____
I can identify items to be covered in the safety training program regarding OSHA laws and exposure to chemicals, blood, body fluids, or other potentially infectious materials.	_____	_____	_____

CHAPTER 39

Introduction to the Medical Laboratory

CHAPTER PRE-TEST

Perform this test without looking at the book. This is just to see how well you have understood and can recall the information in this chapter after you have read it, but before you have completed the workbook exercises. You will not be graded on this portion (other than the grade you give yourself). Justify any "false" answers.

1. Cytology is the study of cells. (T or F)
2. A urine culture would be performed in which department of a regional laboratory?
   a. bacteriology department
   b. urinalysis department
   c. culture department
   d. cytology department
3. Which of the following is a description of a profile?
   a. many tests all billed together at one time
   b. all the tests for one patient during one calendar year
   c. all the tests a doctor orders consistently throughout her or his practice
   d. a related set of tests about an organ, system, or function
4. Proficiency tests are required by the Occupational Safety and Health Administration (OSHA). (T or F)
5. Fasting means that the patient may have water but nothing else by mouth for 12 hours. (T or F)

INTRODUCTION

Together with clinical laboratory personnel, medical assistants perform a key role in laboratory testing. Medical assistants may be responsible for patient preparation and instruction, obtaining specimens, and testing or sending specimens to the laboratory. It is important that medical assistants have a knowledge of laboratory procedures, perform quality controls, and observe standard precautions for infection control to ensure accurate testing and to safeguard the health of patients and health care personnel. When collecting, processing, or analyzing specimens, medical assistants are aiding in the physician's diagnosis and treatment of conditions and illnesses. Attention to detail and accuracy are essential skills for the medical assistant to possess in performing duties in the medical laboratory.

PERFORMANCE OBJECTIVES

After successful completion of this chapter you will be able to explain the terminology related to laboratory procedures, the main purposes of laboratory testing, as well as the similarities and differences when comparing regional laboratories to physician's office laboratories (POLs). You will be able to cite the main departments within laboratories, the usual tests performed within each department, and the common categories of laboratory tests. You will also know the purpose of the tests included in the most common laboratory profiles, at least which body system, organ, or function the doctor is testing. In any laboratory, there are quality-control and quality-assurance measures in place. You will be able to explain why those are important and even name a few examples. *The following statements are related to your learning objectives for this chapter. Fill in the blanks in the following paragraph with the appropriate term(s).*

Physicians and other health care providers depend on medical laboratory tests to aid in determining the patient's state of health and (1) ________________. You might use laboratory tests to record an individual's (2) ______________________________. You might take tests to satisfy (3) ____________________, (4) ____________________, or (5) ____________________ requirements. You might need to gain (6) ________________________ for research and clinical trials, or to detect (7) __________________________ conditions or diseases that the patient might not be aware that they have. You might be able to diagnose the condition, but need to (8) ________________ that diagnosis, or you might be trying to (9) ____________________ between two or more similar diagnoses. Sometimes a laboratory test is performed to actually put a name to or (10) ____________________a condition that has vague symptoms. Sometimes that physician is already treating a disease, or the patient has changed his or her lifestyle and you will want to run some laboratory tests to determine the (11) ________________ of treatments, and then you might need to keep the disease from getting worse by testing. When you need to protect an unborn child or society or family members from a disease, you might run a laboratory test to (12) ________________ them from getting the disease. Laboratories can be small enough to be in a small room of a doctor's office, called a (13) __________________________, or huge enough to take up entire buildings and blocks, such as the large campus of a (14) ____________ ________________ laboratory. If a laboratory is large and can offer many services, it will probably have many departments and personnel. Some of the departments within the larger laboratories include the (15) ______________________ department, in which cells are microscopically examined, the (16) ________________________ department, in which tissues are examined, the (17) ______________________________ department, where blood tests are performed, and the chemistry within our bodies is tested in the (18) ________________________ department. There are other departments such as the (19) ________________________, (20) __________________________, and (21) ____________________________ departments, and many more, depending on how the laboratory is organized. As medical assistants working in ambulatory care, you will combine services of your own with services from independent regional laboratories. The current health care environment offers numerous options in the methods used to process laboratory tests. You might refer the (22) ________________________ to an outside laboratory for the entire test, you might perform the entire test in your (23) __________________, or you might (24) _____________________ the specimen in your laboratory and send it to an independent laboratory for testing. However you are involved in laboratory testing, you need to be aware of the importance of ensuring accuracy through (25) ______________________________________ measures, safety within the laboratory, and accuracy in recordkeeping. The request for a laboratory test is called a (26) _______________________, and the results are sent back to the physician on a (27) ________________________. There are specific types of information that need to be included on each of those documents. The properly completed requisition contains the following data: the physician's (28) ______________________, account number, address, and telephone number; the patient's (29) __________________, address and telephone numbers, their (30) ____________________________ information, (31) _____________________, and identification number; any unique patient identifier; the patient's (32) _______________, date of birth, and sex. The (33) ______________ of the specimen, the (34) ___________________ and (35) _________________ the specimen was collected, the (36) ________________ requested, any (37) __________________________ the patient is taking, the clinical (38) _________________________, the urgency of the results, any special collection or patient (39) _________________, and whether the results are to be sent to a (40) ____________________________. Reports generated by the laboratory are to include the (41) ____________________________ name, address, and telephone numbers, the (42) _____________________ physician's information, the (43) ______________________ information, the date the specimen was (44) ___________________ by the laboratory, the date and time it was (45) ____________________________, and the date the laboratory (46) _____________________ the results. Of course, also included is the test name, the (47) ______________, and the (48) ______________________ reference ranges, if applicable. How you handle the results when they are received in the office is up to individual office's protocol; but all results, whether normal or abnormal, should be (49) ___________________ by the physician before being filed. If the specimen is obtained in the POL, the guidelines need to be followed. You should check the (50) ______________________________ and identify the patient; refer to the laboratory (51) ____________________ manual or call for specific instructions; instruct the patient in any needed (52) __________________________ restrictions; instruct the patient to (53) ________________ any special food or take other substances if required, select and provide for the patient appropriate (54) ____________________ with the proper (55) ____________________________________ in them, if required; label the specimen properly, according to protocol; obtain the specimen or instruct the patient to provide the specimen according to the laboratory's instructions; and follow applicable (56) ____ guidelines when packaging the specimen for transport.

VOCABULARY BUILDER

A. *Find the words below that are misspelled; circle them, and then correctly spell them in the spaces provided. Then insert the proper correct vocabulary terms into the sentences below. Each sentence describes a situation you might find in a POL or in a reference laboratory.*

assay	diagnosis	objective
asymptomatic	diaphram	profile
baseline	differential diagnosis	qualitative tests
biopsy	electrolytes	quantative tests
clinical diagnosis	glucose	reagents
condensor	invasive	requisition
control test	normal flora	serum
________________	________________	________________

1. Wanda Slawson, CMA, is examining a specimen in the laboratory using a compound microscope. The ______________________ is the lens system closest to the specimen she is viewing.
2. Dr. Mark Woo orders laboratory tests for a female emergency patient experiencing severe abdominal cramps to make a ________________________ that will distinguish between a diagnoses of appendicitis or an ovarian cyst.
3. Ralph Samson receives a job offer from a construction company that requires all employees to be tested for misuse or abuse of legal or illegal drugs before they can work on the site. Bruce Goldman, CMA, performs Ralph's blood test under the direction of Dr. Whitney; his test comes back clean. The results of Ralph's test can be used in the future as a ________________________ measurement, a record of healthy normal results.
4. Dr. King needs a red blood cell (RBC) count, a white blood cell (WBC) count, and a platelet count for Maria Jover. Joe Guerrero, CMA, performs a venipuncture on Maria and sends a tube of her blood to the laboratory, together with a written ________________________ containing specific information and instructions about what tests to perform on the specimens.

5. Bruce Goldman, CMA, is examining a specimen under a compound microscope. Because he is having difficulty seeing clearly, Bruce opens the microscope's ________________ to increase the amount of light on the specimen.
6. Dr. Lewis asks Audrey Jones, CMA, to send a tube of Herb Fowler's blood to the laboratory for analysis. Dr. Lewis wants to determine the constituents and relative proportion of each of the enzymes in Herb's serum; this type of analysis is called an ________________.
7. Jim Marshall comes to see Dr. Lewis reporting that he has been constantly tired for the past two or three months. Because Jim's symptoms are so vague, Dr. Lewis orders a blood __________________________ to help narrow the diagnosis possibilities.
8. Bruce Goldman, CMA, always follows Standard Precautions and washes his hands before touching a patient. Although everyone's body contains many natural microorganisms, called __________________________, aseptic handwashing reduces the potential for exposure to or transmission of pathogens.
9. Hematology laboratories count the WBCs or RBCs in a sample of a patient's blood. In general, these type of counting tests are known as __________________________.
10. As a method of quality control, a __________________________ sample is tested together with a patient's sample as a method of ensuring the accuracy of test results.
11. Joe Guerrero, CMA, asks Abigail Johnson, who he knows is diagnosed with diabetes mellitus, whether she regularly tests her blood at home to measure her ________________ level.
12. The hematology laboratory performs tests that measure characteristics of blood such as size, shape, and maturity of cells. These types of tests are known in general as ________________.
13. Histology is the study of tissue samples to determine disease. In most cases, a frozen tissue sample or ______________ is sliced, stained, and microscopically examined for anomalies.
14. Urinalysis performed on a urine specimen from patient Annette Samuels shows that she has a mild bladder infection. Annette is surprised at this diagnosis; she does not feel sick. Dr. Esposito explains that it is possible to be __________________________ and still have an infection.
15. Most of the patient samples that Audrey Jones, CMA, prepares to send to the laboratory are samples of __________________________, the liquid portion of blood obtained after blood has been allowed to clot or has been separated.
16. If a control sample shows inaccurate results after testing, one possible explanation is that the __________________________ are faulty or have expired.
17. In microscopic analysis of specimens, the light, or image, is reflected by the __________ onto the specimen to the ocular lenses for visualization.

18. Fine-needle aspiration is an ________________________ procedure used in a preliminary diagnosis of breast cancer; the test involves inserting a needle into the suspicious breast lump and extracting cells for analysis under a microscope. Because this test is not always reliable, often a mammogram is also performed.
19. A ______________________ of Lyme disease can be confirmed by performing laboratory tests on patient blood specimens.
20. Dr. Rice makes a ________________________ of asthma for patient Rhea Epstein, based on subjective and objective information gathered after obtaining an in-depth patient history and performing a complete physical examination.
21. ________________________ are substances that split into electrically charged particles, or ions, when dissolved or melted. These electricity conductors are important in maintaining fluid and acid-base homeostasis in the body.

B. *Match each laboratory facility or department to the statement below that best describes it, then fill in the additional blanks.*

A. reference laboratories
B clinical chemistry
C. cytology
D. hematology
E. histology
F. immunology/immunohematology
G. hospital-based laboratories
H. parasitology
I. microbiology
J. mycology
K. physician's office laboratories
L. procurement stations
M. urinalysis

____ 1. This laboratory department performs blood typing procedures, cross-matching, and the separation and storage of blood components for transfusion, as well as antibody–antigen reactions.

____ 2. This subdivision of the microbiology department detects the presence of disease–producing human parasites or ova present in patient specimens such as feces and blood. Name three diseases caused by parasites.

(1) ________________ (2) ________________ (3) ________________

____ 3. Independent laboratories often have smaller satellite or ________________ located near isolated medical facilities or in areas convenient to patients.

____ 4. This laboratory department performs qualitative and quantitative tests on blood and blood components. Identify each test named below.

Hgb ________________________ ESR ________________________

Diff ________________________ Hct ________________________

____ 5. This subdivision of the microbiology department is where fungi are grown and identified.

____ 6. ____________________________ are independent, regionally located laboratories used by hospitals and physicians for complex, expensive, or specialized tests.

____ 7. Some procedures performed by this department include assays of enzymes in the serum, serum glucose, or electrolyte levels. Name three electrolytes.

(1) ________________ (2) ________________ (3) ________________

____ 8. This laboratory department analyzes patient specimens for the presence of disease-producing microorganisms. Name three infectious diseases.

(1) ________________ (2) ________________ (3) ________________

____ 9. ____________________________ perform medical laboratory tests easily and inexpensively in the office by the medical assistant.

____ 10. ______________________________ perform most of the tests required for inpatient clinics and hospitals.

____ 11. ____________________ is the microscopic study of the form and structure of the various tissues making up living organisms. Tissue analysis and biopsy studies are performed in this area of the laboratory.

____ 12. This laboratory department performs microscopic examinations of cells to detect irregularities in growth and development. Name two types of tests performed.

(1) ________________________ (2) ________________________

____ 13. ______________________ involves the physical, chemical, and microscopic examination of urine as a diagnostic tool for physicians.

LEARNING REVIEW

1. Physicians depend on medical laboratories to help them ascertain a patient's state of health or state of disease. There are eight main reasons why a physician might need a laboratory test performed. Identify the proper reason laboratory testing is required for each example given.

A. After feeling the abdomen for bladder distention and performing a rectal examination, Charles Williams's symptoms suggest to Dr. Lewis that Charles may be suffering from an enlarged prostate. Dr. Lewis orders blood tests and a urinalysis to confirm his diagnosis.

____

B. Patient Janet Renquiz, a retired homemaker, complies with the treatment plan for her diagnosed case of chronic lymphocytic leukemia by submitting to a regular testing of her blood for the presence of leukemic cells, which monitors the progress of the disease.

____

C. Anna Ortiz, who is pregnant, has had genital herpes for several years. In the week before her child is to be born, Dr. King takes a culture of Anna's cervical and vaginal mucosa to determine whether her baby is at risk for contracting herpes in the birth canal.

____

D. Dr. Mark Woo has been treating Edith Leonard, who describes having poor vision and fainting spells. Because Edith's symptoms are vague and he cannot make a firm diagnosis, Dr. Woo orders a complete blood profile to give him additional information about Edith's case.

____

E. Louise Kipperly comes to Inner City Health Care for her yearly medical checkup. Dr. Esposito orders a series of blood tests to make sure that Louise's cholesterol level is within a normal, healthy range.

____

F. Fifteen-year-old Corey Boyer comes to Inner City Health Care with what seems to be a severe sore throat. A physical examination demonstrates the presence of fever, headache, difficulty swallowing, and inflamed tonsils. Dr. Whitney orders a complete blood cell count (CBC) and a heterophil antibodies test to confirm a diagnosis of either tonsillitis or infectious mononucleosis. When the results of Corey's blood tests come back from the laboratory, however, atypical lymphocytes in the blood indicate the early onset of infectious mononucleosis.

____

G. When Jaime Carrera's laboratory tests come back positive for herpesvirus hominis, his girlfriend Eleanor is instructed to come into Inner City Health Care for testing. Eleanor, who has no symptoms, is tested for herpes simplex and nonspecific urethritis.

____

H. Maria Jover, who was diagnosed with HIV, takes protease inhibitors to help her immune system fight the disease. Dr. King orders blood tests to determine how Maria is responding to the treatment.

____

2. A. Name five tests commonly performed in a POL.

(1) ____

(2) ____

(3) ____

(4) ____

(5) ____

B. Name three reasons point-of-care testing might be used to obtain laboratory results.

(1) ____________ (2) ____________ (3) ____________

3. Identify each entry that follows as a way an infectious agent leaves the body of a sick person (L), the way an organism may be transmitted (T), or the way an organism enters the body (E).

____ A. discharges from infected eyes

____ B. contaminated needles and syringes

____ C. milk from an infected cow

____ D. directly onto mucous membrane

____ E. breast milk

____ F. towels

____ G. health care workers exposed to blood

____ H. transplacentally to fetus

____ I. contact with blood and body fluids

____ J. discharges from respiratory tract

____ K. feces and urine

____ L. flies

____ M. excreta from intestinal tract

____ N. directly on the conjunctiva

4. The accuracy of any laboratory test result depends on the performance of quality controls by all health care workers who handle a specimen. Medical assistants must have a thorough knowledge of quality controls and standards.

   A. List five factors that can compromise the accuracy of laboratory test results.

      (1) ______________________________

      (2) ______________________________

      (3) ______________________________

      (4) ______________________________

      (5) ______________________________

   B. What is the reason for using a control test sample? Explain in detail.

      ____

      ____

      ____

5. Knowing how to perform tasks safely is critical when working in a medical laboratory. Medical assistants must understand the different types of hazards present in a medical laboratory and know how to protect themselves and other health care professionals from possible harm.

   A. It is important to avoid ingestion or exposure to chemicals and pathogens. Name four ways this can be avoided.

      (1) ______________ (3) ______________

      (2) ______________ (4) ______________

   B. What is the first action to take when a surface becomes contaminated?

      ____

   C. Explain why it is important to avoid wearing loose clothing or accessories in the laboratory.

      ____

      ____

   D. In terms of safety issues, why is it important to properly maintain laboratory equipment?

      ____

      ____

6. For each method of exposure, list one circumstance in which pathogens may be transmitted in the ambulatory care setting and Standard Precautions that are effective in reducing or preventing the transmission of pathogens under each circumstance.

   A. **Direct contact**

      Pathogens may be transmitted ______________________________

      Standard precautions: ______________________________

   B. **Ingestion**

      Pathogens may be transmitted ______________________________

      Standard precautions: ______________________________

C. **Mucous membranes**

Pathogens may be transmitted ____________________

Standard precautions: ____________________

7. A. What is the purpose of a microscope?

B. Name the five parts of a microscope.

(1) ____________________

(2) ____________________

(3) ____________________

(4) ____________________

(5) ____________________

C. The ____________________ microscope is the most commonly used microscope in a medical laboratory.

D. Name three other types of microscopes and explain what each is designed for viewing.

(1) ____________________

(2) ____________________

(3) ____________________

E. Name the two adjustments found on a microscope and explain the purpose of each.

(1) ____________________

(2) ____________________

F. Name six practices that should always be followed to properly care for a microscope.

(1) ____________________

(2) ____________________

(3) ____________________

(4) ____________________

(5) ____________________

(6) ____________________

CERTIFICATION REVIEW

These questions are designed to mimic the certification examinations. You can use these questions like a small "Certification Examination Study Guide," but this is not meant to take the place of the more extensive study guides. Use this portion to determine in what areas to concentrate your efforts when studying for the certification examination.

1. Choosing to perform the simplest and least invasive procedure to rule out a particular disease before requiring more extensive testing is known as a:
   a. clinical diagnosis
   b. cumulative diagnosis
   c. developmental diagnosis
   d. differential diagnosis

2. ______________________ involve actual number counts such as done in WBC counts, RBC counts, and platelet levels.
   a. Qualitative tests
   b. Quantitative tests
   c. CLIA waived tests
   d. Functional tests

3. The area of the clinical laboratory where organisms such as bacteria and fungi are grown and identified is called the:
   a. cytology department
   b. chemistry department
   c. microbiology department
   d. histology department

4. A hepatic function panel will include a:
   a. creatinine level
   b. rheumatoid factor
   c. cholesterol level
   d. bilirubin level

5. Serum separator tubes used in hematology may not be used when collecting blood for a:
   a. lipid profile
   b. thyroid profile
   c. cardiac profile
   d. toxicologic study

CASE STUDY

At Abigail Johnson's annual physical examination on June 5, 20XX, at 2 PM, Dr. Elizabeth King orders several laboratory tests to monitor Abigail's diagnosed conditions of hypertension, diabetes mellitus, and moderate angina pectoris. Dr. Frank Jones, Abigail's cardiologist, will also receive a copy of the final laboratory report. Ellen Armstrong, CMA, prepares the laboratory requisition form. Complete Ellen's laboratory requisition form for Abigail's laboratory work.

Patient:

Abigail Johnson
225 River Street
Northborough, OH 12336
Phone: 389-2631
Date of Birth: March 1, 1920
Social Security Number: 011-11-1231
Medicare #: 021-45-6712-D

Physicians:

Dr. Elizabeth King
Northborough Family Medical Group
2501 Center Street
Northborough, OH 12345
Phone: 651-8000
Dr. Frank Jones
815 Heart Health Blvd.
Northborough, OH 12339
Phone: 655-7000

Physician's Order for Laboratory Testing: Blood profile to include BUN, Chloride, Cholesterol, Creatinine, Glucose, LDH, Potassium, SGOT, SGPT, Sodium, Triglycerides.

NORTHBOROUGH REFERENCE LABORATORIES
128 Analysis Way
Northborough, OH 12468

[redacted] ❑ GROUP ACCOUNT ❑ PATIENT

LAST NAME	FIRST NAME	MI	SEX	DATE OF BIRTH
ADDRESS	CITY		STATE	ZIP
PHONE # Home Work	SOC. SEC #			

Ordering Physician Signature

PRIMARY CARE PHYSICIAN __________

SPECIMEN INFORMATION
❑ **STAT**
Date of Collection __________
Time of Collection __________
❑ Serum ❑ Plasma
❑ Urine (Volume) __________
Hours __________
❑ Other __________
CALL RESULTS TO: __________
Phone #:( ) __________
Copy Results to: __________

COMPLETE SHADED BOX BELOW FOR PATIENT AND THIRD PARTY BILL ONLY

RESPONSIBLE PARTY LAST NAME	FIRST NAME	MI	MEDICARE ❑ AMERICAID ❑ \#	
ADDRESS CITY	STATE	ZIP	PHONE #	
INSURED NAME	INSURANCE CO. NAME/ADDRESS			
INSURED'S EMPLOYER	RELATIONSHIP TO PATIENT ❑ Self ❑ Spouse ❑ Dependent		CONTRACT #	GROUP #

REASON FOR TEST (A DIAGNOSIS IS NECESSARY FOR ALL INSURANCE CLAIMS) *SEE REVERSE FOR CODES*

SPECIMEN CODES: G - GEL, L - LAVENDER, R - RED, B - BLUE, BK - BLACK, U - URINE

PROFILES

❑ BIOCHEM BASIC	1G	❑ BIOCHEM PROFILE III	2G, 1L	❑ LIPID 12-16 HOUR FAST REQUIRED	1G	❑ THYROID	1G
❑ BIOCHEM PROFILE I	1G, 1L	❑ ARTHRITIS	2G,1BK	❑ LIVER	1G	❑ HYPERTHYROID	1G
❑ BIOCHEM PROFILE II	1G, 1L	❑ HEPATITIS	1G	❑ PRENATAL	1G, 1L, 1R	❑ HYPOTHYROID	1G
						❑ TORCH PROFILE	1G

INDIVIDUAL TESTS

❑ ALBUMIN	G	❑ FSH	G	❑ PROSTATE SPECIFIC ANTIGEN	G
❑ ALK. PHOSPHATASE	G	❑ GC CULTURE, SOURCE _____		❑ PT W/INR	B
❑ AMYLASE	G	❑ GLUCOSE	G	❑ PTT	B
❑ ANA SCREEN	G	❑ GLYCATED HEMOGLOBIN	L	❑ RHEUMATOID FACTOR	G
❑ BILIRUBIN, TOTAL	G	❑ hCG, BETA SUBUNIT QUANT.	G	❑ RPR	G
❑ BILIRUBIN, TOTAL + DIRECT	G	❑ HDL	G	❑ RUBELLA IgG ANTIBODY	G
❑ BILIRUBIN, NEONATAL	G	❑ HEPATITIS B SURF. ANTIBODY	G	❑ SEDIMENTATION RATE	BK
❑ BUN	G	❑ HEPATITIS B SURF. ANTIGEN	G	❑ SGOT	G
❑ CALCIUM, TOTAL	G	❑ HEPATITIS C ANTIBODY	G	❑ SGPT	G
❑ CBC W/AUTOMATED DIFF	L	❑ HIV ANTIBODY (SIGNED CONSENT REQUIRED)	G	❑ SPUTUM CULTURE	
❑ CBC W/MANUAL DIFF	L	❑ LACTIC DEHYDROGENASE	G	❑ STOOL CULTURE	
❑ CHLAMYDIA SCREEN, SOURCE _____		❑ LEAD, PEDIATRIC	L	❑ THROAT, GROUP A STREP CULTURE	
❑ CHOLESTEROL	G	❑ LH	G	❑ TOTAL PROTEIN	G
❑ CREATININE	G	❑ LIPASE	G	❑ TSH	G
❑ CULTURE, SOURCE _____		❑ LITHIUM	G	❑ URIC ACID	G
❑ ELECTROLYTES	G	❑ OVA & PARASITE PREP.		❑ URINALYSIS	U
❑ ESTRADIOL	G	❑ PHOSPHORUS	G	❑ URINE CULTURE	U
❑ FERRITIN	G	❑ PREGNANCY TEST, BLOOD	G	❑ VITAMIN B12	G
❑ FOLIC ACID	G	❑ PROGESTERONE	G		
❑ FREE T4	G	❑ PROLACTIN	G		

ICD-9-CM DIAGNOSIS CODES

- ☐ 648.80 ABN GLUC TOL/PREG OR PP
- ☐ 682.9 ABSCESS
- ☐ 042 AIDS
- ☐ 477.9 ALLERGIC RHINITIS
- ☐ 626.0 AMENORRHEA
- ☐ 285.9 ANEMIA
- ☐ 413.9 ANGINA
- ☐ 716.90 ARTHRITIS
- ☐ 414.00 ASHD
- ☐ 493.90 ASTHMA
- ☐ 600 BENIGN PROSTATIC HYPERTROPHY
- ☐ 466.0 BRONCHITIS
- ☐ 199.1 CA SPECIFY SITE:______________
- ☐ 428.0 CHF
- ☐ 496 COPD
- ☐ 436 CVA
- ☐ E934.9 COUMADIN THERAPY
- ☐ 250.00 DIABETES
- ☐ 558.9 DIARRHEA
- ☐ 562.11 DIVERTICULITIS
- ☐ 780.4 DIZZINESS
- ☐ 276.9 ELECTROLYTE IMBALANCE
- ☐ 259.9 ENDOCRINE DISORDERS
- ☐ 530.10 ESOPHAGITIS
- ☐ 780.6 FEVER
- ☐ 558.9 GASTROENTERITIS
- ☐ 784.0 HEADACHE
- ☐ 599.7 HEMATURIA
- ☐ 573.3 HEPATITIS
- ☐ 070.9 HEPATITIS, VIRAL
- ☐ 272.4 HYPERLIPIDEMIA
- ☐ 401.9 HYPERTENSION
- ☐ 244.9 HYPOTHYROID
- ☐ 628.9 INFERTILITY, FEMALE
- ☐ 487.1 INFLUENZA
- ☐ 774.6 JAUNDICE OF NEWBORN
- ☐ 782.4 JAUNDICE NOT NEWBORN
- ☐ V72.6 LAB EXAMINATION
- ☐ 709.8 LESION, SKIN
- ☐ 573.9 LIVER DISEASE
- ☐ 785.6 LYMPHADENOPATHY
- ☐ 780.7 MALAISE & FATIGUE
- ☐ 382.9 OTITIS MEDIA
- ☐ 789.0 PAIN, ABDOMEN
- ☐ 724.5 PAIN, BACK
- ☐ 723.1 PAIN, CERVICAL NECK
- ☐ 786.50 PAIN, CHEST
- ☐ 719.40 PAIN, JOINT
- ☐ V76.2 PAP SMEAR
- ☐ 614.9 PID
- ☐ 462 PHARYNGITIS
- ☐ 486 PNEUMONIA
- ☐ V22.2 PREGNANCY, NORMAL
- ☐ 593.9 RENAL DISEASE
- ☐ 461.9 SINUSITIS
- ☐ 462 SORE THROAT
- ☐ V67.0 SURGICAL FOLLOW UP
- ☐ 780.2 SYNCOPE
- ☐ 465.9 URI
- ☐ 599.0 UTI
- ☐ 616.10 VAGINITIS
- ☐ 079.9 VIRAL SYNDROME
- ☐ 998.5 WOUND INFECTION
- ☐ OTHER: ______________
- ☐ ______________
- ☐ ______________
- ☐ ______________

PROFILES / CPT CODES

BIOCHEM BASIC / 80019

Albumin
Alkaline Phosphatase
Anion Gap
Bicarbonate
Bilirubin, Total
BUN
Calcium
Chloride
Cholesterol
Creatinine
GGTP
Glucose
LDH
Phosphorus
Potassium
Protein, Total
SGOT (AST)
SGPT (ALT)
Sodium
Triglycerides
Uric Acid

BIOCHEM PROFILE I / 80019, 85025, 85029

Biochem Basic
CBC w/Automated Diff

BIOCHEM PROFILE II / 80019, 85025, 85029, 83718

Biochem Basic
CBC w/Automated Diff
Lipid Profile

BIOCHEM PROFILE III / 80019, 85025, 85029 83718, 80091

Biochem Basic
CBC w/Automated Diff
Lipid Profile
Thyroid Profile

ARTHRITIS PROFILE / 80072

ANA
Rheumatoid Factor
Sed Rate
Uric Acid

HEPATITIS PROFILE / 80059

Hepatitis A Ab (HAAB)
Hepatitis B Core Ab (HBCAB)
Hepatitis B Surf Ab (HBSAB)
Hepatitis B Surf Ag (HBSAG)
Hepatitis C Ab (HCAB)

LIPID PROFILE / 80061
12-16 Hour Fast Required

Cholesterol
HDL
LDL
Triglycerides

LIVER PROFILE / 80058

Albumin
Alkaline Phosphatase
Bilirubin, Total
SGOT (AST)
SGPT (ALT)

PRENATAL PROFILE / 80055

ABO/Rh type
Antibody Screen
CBC w/Automated Diff
Hepatitis B Surf Antigen
Rubella IgG Antibody
RPR

THYROID PROFILE / 80091

Free Thyroxine Index
T_3 Uptake
T_4

HYPERTHYROID PROFILE / 80091, 84480

Thyroid Profile
T_3 Total

HYPOTHYROID PROFILE / 80092

Thyroid Profile
TSH

TORCH PROFILE / 80090

CMV IgG Ab
Herpes I and II Ab
Rubella IgG Antibody
Toxoplasma IgG Ab

SELF-ASSESSMENT

Working in a medical laboratory requires spending large amounts of time performing extremely detail-oriented procedures, such as observing specimens through a microscope for signs of disease. Laboratory analysis also involves maintaining high-quality controls and safety standards to ensure the accuracy and reliability of results. The way you deal with details in your everyday life can reveal much about your predisposition for detail-oriented analytic tasks. For each statement, circle the response that best describes you.

1. When walking along a city street, I:
   a. notice each person who passes me, remember details from storefronts, and even recognize the make and model of cars as they drive by
   b. like to listen to other people's conversations and enjoy interacting with friends who are accompanying me
   c. usually spend my time daydreaming
2. If I think about the way a pine tree looks, I:
   a. visualize the rough texture of its bark and see its long, thin leaves perfectly in my head
   b. think about the great Christmas trees my family always had when I was a kid
   c. see two blobs of color, green and brown
3. I prefer working in an atmosphere:
   a. that is structured and involves analytic thinking
   b. where the decision-making process is cut-and-dry and the options are well-defined
   c. where I do not have to make decisions or interpret anything
4. When preparing a meal or recipe, I:
   a. am very careful to make sure I read the recipe over twice before I start and have each of the ingredients on hand
   b. read the recipe quickly just to make sure I understand the basics
   c. just wing it; I cook by intuition
5. When preparing for a trip or vacation, I:
   a. know exactly where my passport and other important papers are located, make a list of all essential items to bring and check off the list as each is packed, and leave detailed written instructions for the housesitter
   b. know pretty much what I need and where I can find it; but I wait until the day before to get it all together
   c. let someone else do all the packing and handle all the arrangements; too many details for me
6. After a conversation with someone I have just met, I:
   a. remember the exact color of his or her eyes
   b. would be able to make a pretty good guess about what color his or her eyes are
   c. have no idea what color his or her eyes are

7. When giving people driving directions to a destination, I:
   a. make sure to give detailed instructions, using at least two different routes, noting landmarks and the location of gas stations along the way
   b. say basically what area of town they need to head toward and the street address; I know they can figure out the rest on their own
   c. usually give people the wrong directions, so I tell them to ask someone else

8. In regard to friends' birthdays, I:
   a. have them all written down in my calendar, and I send cards out four days before the date
   b. know what month they fall in, and make sure to wish them a happy birthday somewhere around the middle of the month
   c. I am usually embarrassed when I find out a friend's birthday has passed; I can never remember dates

Scoring: If most of your answers were *A*s, you are an extremely detail-oriented and observant person. You are well-suited to the tasks performed in the medical laboratory. If your answers were mostly *B*s, you can be observant, but you do not always pay close attention to details. If your answers were mostly *C*s, you will need to work on your observation skills.

POST-TEST

This is similar to the Pre-Test. Perform this test without looking at the book. This is just to see how well you have understood and can recall the information presented in this chapter after you have studied it and completed the workbook exercises. You will not be graded on this portion (other than the grade you give yourself), but this is an excellent preparation for your instructor's test. You may use this Post-Test to determine what areas you need to study more. Justify any "false" answers.

1. Histology is the study of cells. (T or F)

2. A urine culture would be performed in which department of a regional laboratory?
   a. urinalysis department
   b. bacteriology department
   c. culture department
   d. cytology department

3. NPO means that the patient may have water but nothing else by mouth for 12 hours. (T or F)

4. Which of the following is a description of a profile:
   a. all the tests for one patient during one calendar year
   b. all the tests a doctor orders consistently throughout his or her practice
   c. many tests all billed together at one time
   d. a related set of tests about an organ, system, or function

5. Proficiency tests are required by CLIA. (T or F)

CERTIFICATION CRITERIA CHECKLIST

As you go through your education and training, keep in mind the national certification examination that you will take when you graduate. Each chapter of the textbook and workbook covers a different section of the examination criteria. To keep track of your preparation for the certification examination, turn to the back of this workbook and highlight the following CMA, RMA, or CMAS certification examination criteria (if you have already highlighted them from a previous chapter, put a check mark by the criteria):

CMA

F. Medicolegal Guidelines & Requirements
R. Principles of Infection Control
S. Treatment Area
    2. Principles of operation
V. Collecting and Processing Specimens; Diagnostic Testing
    3. Quality control

RMA

I. General Medical Assisting Knowledge
    C. Medical Law
III. Clinical Medical Assisting
    I. Laboratory Procedures

CMAS

1. Medical Assisting Foundation
    - Legal and ethical considerations
2. Basic Clinical Medical Office Assisting
    - Asepsis in the medical office
8. Medical Office Management
    - Supplies and equipment

COMPETENCY ASSESSMENT

Procedure 39-1 Using the Microscope

Performance Objectives: To properly use a microscope to view organisms using the coarse and fine adjustments, as well as the low- and high-power and oil-immersion objectives. Perform this procedure within 20 minutes with a minimum score of 190 points.

Supplies/Equipment: Microscope, lens paper, lens cleaner, prepared slides, immersion oil, disinfectant

Charting/Documentation: Enter appropriate documentation/charting in the box.

Instructor's/Evaluator's Comments and Suggestions:

SKILLS CHECKLIST Procedure 39-1: Using the Microscope

Name ______________________

Date ______________________

No.	Skill	Check #1 20 pts ea	Check #2 10 pts ea	Check #3 5 pts ea	Notes
1	Wash hands.				
2	Assemble equipment and supplies.				
3	Clean the oculars and objectives with lens paper.				
4	Use the coarse adjustments to raise the eyepiece or lens unit.				
5	Rotate the low power (10×) objective into position.				
6	Turn on the light.				
7	Open the diaphragm until maximum light comes up through the condenser.				
8	Place the slide on the stage.				
9	Locate the coarse adjustment.				
10	Look directly at the stage and 10x objective and turn the coarse adjustment until the slide is as close to the objective as it will go.				
11	Look into the oculars and slowly turn the coarse adjustment so the stage lowers, until the object comes into view.				
12	Locate the fine adjustment.				
13	Turn the fine adjustment to sharpen the image.				
	a. For binocular microscopes, adjust the distance between the oculars until one image is seen.				
	b. Use the adjustments to bring the image into focus.				
	c. Close the right eye, and with the left eye, bring the image into sharp focus using the left ocular collar.				
	d. Look into the oculars with both eyes to see if the image is in clear focus. If it is not, repeat from step a.				
14	Scan the slide by either method:				
	a. Use the stage knobs to move the slide while looking through the oculars.				
	b. Move the slide with fingers while looking through the oculars.				
15	Rotate the high-power (40×) objective into position while looking directly at the objective and slide so the slide does not touch the objective.				

No.	Skill	Check #1 20 pts ea	Check #2 10 pts ea	Check #3 5 pts ea	Notes
16	Look through the oculars to view the slide.				
17	Locate the fine adjustment.				
18	Look through the oculars and fine focus the slide.				
19	Adjust the light.				
20	Scan the slide as in step 14, keeping the slide in focus.				
21	Rotate the oil-immersion objective to the side slightly so no objective is in position.				
22	Place one drop of immersion oil on the portion of the slide that is directly over the condenser.				
23	Rotate the oil immersion objective into position.				
24	Look to see that the oil immersion objective is touching the drop of oil.				
25	Look through the oculars and slowly turn the fine adjustment until slide is in focus.				
26	Adjust the light.				
27	Scan the slide.				
28	Rotate the 10× objective into position.				
29	Remove the slide from the stage and clean.				
30	Clean the 10× and 40× objectives with lens cleaner and lens paper.				
31	Clean the 100× objective with lens cleaner and lens paper to remove all the oil.				
32	Clean any oil from the stage and condenser.				
33	Turn off the light and disconnect.				
34	Position the eyepiece in the lowest position using the coarse adjustment.				
35	Center the stage.				
36	Cover the microscope and return it to storage.				
37	Clean the work area and return slides to storage.				
38	Wash hands.				
Student's Total Points					
Points Possible		760	380	190	
Final Score (Student's Total Points / Possible Points)					

	Notes
Start time:	
End time:	
Total time: (20 min goal)	

EVALUATION OF CHAPTER KNOWLEDGE

	Student Self-Evaluation		
Skills	Good	Average	Poor
I can explain the purposes of laboratory testing.	_____	_____	_____
I understand the differences and similarities between independent laboratories and POLs.	_____	_____	_____
I can identify departments within the medical laboratory and list the types of testing performed within each department.	_____	_____	_____
I know nine of the most common laboratory profiles and the body system that each covers.	_____	_____	_____
I understand quality-control programs in the medical laboratory.	_____	_____	_____
I know the general safety rules within the medical laboratory.	_____	_____	_____
I know how to fill out a laboratory requisition form.	_____	_____	_____
I understand the information required on a written laboratory requisition form.	_____	_____	_____
I can explain the function of and identify the parts of a compound microscope.	_____	_____	_____
I understand how to properly use and care for a compound microscope.	_____	_____	_____
I can follow all Standard Precautions.	_____	_____	_____

CHAPTER 40

Phlebotomy: Venipuncture and Capillary Puncture

CHAPTER PRE-TEST

Perform this test without looking at the book. This is just to see how well you have understood and can recall the information in this chapter after you have read it, but before you have completed the workbook exercises. You will not be graded on this portion (other than the grade you give yourself).

1. Red blood cells (RBCs) are produced in the:
   a. liver
   b. lymph nodes
   c. spleen
   d. bone marrow

2. What type of blood is the most common for laboratory tests?
   a. arterial blood
   b. venous blood
   c. capillary blood
   d. coronary blood

3. What is a buffy coat made of?
   a. white blood cells (WBCs)
   b. RBCs
   c. platelets
   d. a and c

4. Which way should the bevel of the needle be held when performing venipuncture?
   a. up
   b. down
   c. sideways
   d. any of the above
5. Which of the following tubes contains no anticoagulants?
   a. green
   b. red
   c. gray
   d. lavender
6. What position should patients be in while they are having their blood drawn?
   a. standing
   b. lying down
   c. sitting
   d. either b or c
7. What is the maximum amount of time the tourniquet should be left on?
   a. 30 seconds
   b. 60 seconds
   c. 90 seconds
   d. 120 seconds
8. What is the most common method used to draw blood from an adult?
   a. syringe
   b. vacuum tube
   c. butterfly
   d. intravenous needle

INTRODUCTION

Venipuncture is the process of collecting patients' blood samples for the purpose of diagnostic testing. Although the health care professional responsible for performing this important task varies according to the type and needs of the ambulatory care setting, medical assistants often are required to perform venipuncture. The goal of venipuncture is to obtain blood specimens that are collected and processed in a manner that will provide accurate and reliable diagnostic test results. To achieve this goal, medical assistants will draw on a combination of clinical, social, and administrative skills. Aseptic technique and Standard Precautions for infection control, including the proper handling and disposal of sharps, must be observed when performing venipuncture.

PERFORMANCE OBJECTIVES

After successful completion of this chapter you will be able to explain the medical terms related to venous and capillary puncture. You will understand your role as a medical assistant and your responsibility toward your patients in the area of phlebotomy. You will have the skills to give your patients reassurance before and during blood draws. You will know a lot more about blood and its components, the difference between plasma and serum, the characteristics of blood when reacting to various chemicals and clot enhancers, and the tests that will be run on differently prepared specimens of blood. You will understand and be able to demonstrate the technical part of obtaining blood specimens, how to properly tie a tourniquet, how to use the various needles and the different collection methods for different patients in different situations. You will be well versed in the problem-solving processes you will need to go through during unsuccessful blood draws. You will also understand your responsibility toward safety of your patient, your colleagues, and society in general when handling needles and biohazard waste. *The following statements are related to your learning objectives for this chapter. Fill in the blanks in the following paragraph with the appropriate word(s).*

Phlebotomy is the process of (1) ______________________ for (2) ______________ purposes. A (3) ______________________________________ is a person trained to (4) ______________ blood specimens either by (5) ______________________ or (6) __________________________ puncture. Medical assistants, by the nature of their professions, are often in the position to serve patients and physician–employers by procuring blood samples within the physician's office laboratory (POL). To perform this aspect of your job better, you need to understand the (7) ________________________ and physiology of the circulatory system, especially the venous system. Arteries have (8) ______________ walls, usually contain oxygenated blood, have a pulse, and are located in deeper tissues than veins. Veins are easier and safer to access for blood specimens. The word (9) ______________________ actually means "to puncture a vein." Capillaries are close to the surface and are used when only a (10) ____________________ of blood is needed for testing. Blood is a combination of liquid and cellular components. Plasma is the fluid that provides a (11) ________________ for (12) __________________________, (13) __________________________, (14) ____________________, and (15) ____________________ to travel through our bodies via the (16) ____________________________. The most common vein used in venipuncture is the (17) __________________________, but there are many other veins available, even veins of the hand and foot. A (18) ______________________ is required to access a vein of the foot, though. The three common methods used to obtain blood samples are the (19) ______________ method, the (20) ______________________ method, and the (21) ____________________ method. You will need to become comfortable with all three methods. Whichever method is used, the sample will probably be transferred to a (22) __________________ eventually. This is because the vacuum tube contains the (23) ____________________ and (24) ___________________________ necessary for maintaining the specimen (25) ______________________ for the blood tests to be performed. The (26) ________________________ stoppers on vacuum tubes are different colors. These colors indicate the contents of the tube. Most of the vacuum tubes contain (27) __________________ of some sort, either (28) _________________________, to prevent the specimen from clotting, (29) ________________ to maintain the quality of the specimen, clot (30) _________________ to hasten the clotting process, or even (31) _______________________ separator gels to keep the cells/clot from the plasma/serum. The color/type of tube selected will depend on the test being run on the blood. Regardless of the technique used to obtain the blood sample, whether it is venipuncture or capillary puncture, the (32) ______________________ needles and syringes available must be used. This protects the (33) _________________________________ and the (34) ______________________ from accidental (35) __________________________. The skilled phlebotomist will (36) _________________________ patient reactions to blood draws and respond (37) ________________________ as quickly as possible. To prevent injury to the patient from fainting and falling, the patient should always be either sitting in a chair with arms or (38) ______________________________. If the blood sample is not obtained with the puncture, it may be necessary to (39) ________________________ the position of the needle. To do this, (40) ____________________ the needle a half turn. The (41) __________________ of the needle may be against the (42) ___________ of the vein. If the needle has not penetrated far enough, (43) ______________________ it slightly farther. If the needle has penetrated through the vein, (44) _____________________ a little. Try another (45) ___________________ before withdrawing the needle. The point is, problem solving is an important part of a successful blood draw. (46) ____________________ is never recommended. It is (47) _________________ to the patient and will almost certainly cause damage to the vessel, resulting in a (48) ________________________________. If the blood sample cannot be obtained after (49) _________ attempts, ask a colleague to perform the draw. Patients present with a variety of situations that can lead to unsuccessful (50) ______________________. There is no shame in asking for someone else to attempt the draw. The primary (51) ________________ of the medical assistant is to (52) _________________ an (53) ________________________ specimen for testing and to do it safely.

VOCABULARY BUILDER

1. *Find the words listed below that are misspelled; circle them, and then correctly spell them in the spaces provided. Then match each of the vocabulary terms listed below to its correct definition.*

aliquot	hemololysis	phlebotomy
anticoagulant	leukocytes	therapeutic
canulla	luer	torniquet
edematous	lipemia	viscosity
erythrocytes	palpitate	______________
______________	______________	______________

______________________ A. WBCs

______________________ B. A small sample of the whole

______________________ C. Swollen from abnormal fluid accumulation

______________________ D. RBCs

______________________ E. A tube used for insertion into a body cavity

______________________ F. Device that screws into an evacuated tube holder

______________________ G. The liberation of hemoglobin

______________________ H. A band to be drawn around a limb to restrict blood flow and distend the veins

______________________ I. Thickness or stickiness, resistance to flow

______________________ J. The act of feeling with the hand or fingers

______________________ K. A condition in which there are increased amounts of lipids in the blood

______________________ L. Puncture or the incision of a vein

______________________ M. Used in the treatment of disease

______________________ N. A substance used to prevent blood clotting

2. *Find the words listed below that are misspelled; circle them, and then correctly spell them in the spaces provided. Then match the vocabulary terms with the correct definitions below.*

hypoglycemia	diurnal	plasma
additive	thirotrophic gel	serum
hemotoma	hemoconcentration	thrombocytes
venipuncture	______________	______________

______________________ A. The fluid portion of blood from an anticoagulated tube

______________________ B. The state of having a lower than normal blood glucose level

______________________ C. The process of collecting blood

______________________ D. Any material placed in a tube that maintains or facilitates the integrity and function of the specimen

________________ E. The body's daily cycle; levels fluctuate during this cycle

________________ F. An accumulation of blood around the venipuncture site during or after venipuncture, caused by the leakage of blood from where the needle punctured the vein

________________ G. The fluid portion of the blood after clotting has taken place

________________ H. A gel material capable of forming an interface between the cells and fluid portion of the blood as a result of centrifugation

________________ I. Platelets

________________ J. Leaving a tourniquet on the arm longer than 1 minute, causing blood to pool at the location of the venipuncture, resulting in inaccurate blood samples

3. *Write a brief definition of the following vocabulary words.*
   A. Integrity ________________
   B. Oxygenated ________________
   C. Primary container ________________
   D. Dilate ________________
   E. Centrifuge ________________
   F. Buffy coat ________________
   G. Constrict ________________

LEARNING REVIEW

1. Identify and describe the first, second, and third choices of sites on the human body used to perform venipuncture.
   (1) ________________
   (2) ________________
   (3) ________________

2. Tourniquets play a critical role in venipuncture and must be applied and used properly to obtain a blood specimen for analysis.
   A. What is the purpose of a tourniquet? ________________
   B. Where is the tourniquet placed? ________________
   C. How long should the tourniquet remain on the arm during the procedure? ________________
   D. At what point during the procedure should the tourniquet be removed? Why is the timing of removal so important? ________________

3. Match the collection tubes containing anticoagulants with their corresponding color stoppers: green, gray, blue, and lavender.
   A. Coagulation "citrate" tube: ______________________
   B. EDTA tube: ______________________
   C. Oxalate/fluoride tube: ______________________
   D. Heparin tube: ______________________

4. Discuss how the five factors listed below might have an effect on blood test results.
   (1) Exercise ______________________
   ____
   (2) Tourniquet ______________________
   ____
   (3) Volume of blood drawn ______________________
   ____
   (4) Heparin ______________________
   ____
   (5) Temperature of specimen ______________________
   ____

5. Vein stimulation refers to techniques used when initial attempts to obtain a blood sample are not successful. What are five techniques used to stimulate veins?
   (1) ______________________
   (2) ______________________
   (3) ______________________
   (4) ______________________
   (5) ______________________

6. What is the purpose of additives? How do they differ from anticoagulants? Give examples of each.
   ____
   ____
   ____
   ____

7. A. How can medical assistants be sure they have found a vein and not an artery or a tendon when preparing to draw blood from a patient? Describe the characteristics of each.
   ____
   ____
   ____

B. Arteries and veins are crucial elements of the circulatory system. Indicate which of the following are functions or characteristics of arteries (A) and which are functions of veins (V).

_____ 1. Normally brighter in color

_____ 2. No pulse

_____ 3. Carry blood to heart; carry deoxygenated blood (except pulmonary)

_____ 4. Thin wall and less elastic

_____ 5. Carry blood from heart, carry oxygenated blood (except pulmonary)

_____ 6. No valves

8. Identify the recommended venipuncture method for each of the situations listed below.

_________________________ A. When drawing blood from a 75-year-old patient with thin veins.

_________________________ B. For collecting a blood specimen from children, who have small veins and a tendency to move during the venipuncture procedure.

_________________________ C. When elimination of any risk for needlestick accident is desired.

_________________________ D. When multiple blood samples must be obtained from one venipuncture procedure.

CERTIFICATION REVIEW

These questions are designed to mimic the certification examinations. You can use these questions like a small "Certification Examination Study Guide," but this is not meant to take the place of the more extensive study guides. Use this portion to determine in what areas to concentrate your efforts when studying for the certification examination.

1. To speed removal of serum from a tube of blood, an instrument called a _______________ is used.
   a. autoclave
   b. centrifuge
   c. calibrator
   d. incubator

2. Plasma contains:
   a. fibrinogen
   b. a buffy coat
   c. RBCs
   d. a clot

3. Needle insertion for venipuncture should be at an angle of:
   a. 90 degrees
   b. 30 degrees
   c. 45 degrees
   d. 15 degrees

4. The first step in a successful venipuncture is to:
   a. select the site
   b. put the patient at ease
   c. tie the tourniquet appropriately
   d. apply gloves

5. Syncope refers to:
   a. fasting
   b. relaxation
   c. fainting
   d. reclining

CASE STUDY

Wanda Slawson, CMA, performs a successful venipuncture on Jaime Carrera using the evacuated tube system and a 21-gauge needle. Wanda is now preparing to label the tubes for laboratory analysis. She is careful to label all tubes at the patient's side before leaving the examination room.

Discuss the following:

1. What information must be included on the specimen labels for the specimen to be accepted for analysis?
2. What guidelines must Wanda follow during the venipuncture procedure to ensure that anticoagulated blood specimens are acceptable for analysis?
3. Once Wanda has followed all procedures for the correct labeling and processing of the blood specimens, what Standard Precautions must she perform?

SELF-ASSESSMENT

1. Make your own flashcards using the examples provided in this chapter. Tear out the page of flashcards and copy them double-sided onto a cardstock or heavy-weight paper. Cut them apart. Color in the "0" with the same color as the vacuum tube tops (brick red, lavender, green, blue, etc.) and fill in the information. Use the cards to drill yourself and your classmates.

2. During your career as a medical assistant, you will probably run into a patient who refuses to have his or her blood drawn.
   a. How will you calm the patient?
   b. What measures will you take that might be different from typical blood draws?
   c. What would make you decide not to continue with a blood draw?

d. How would you chart each situation? In the first situation, you are able to convince the patient and end up with a successful blood draw. In the other situation, you decide to stop the procedures without obtaining a blood draw. On the lines below, chart both situations.

(1) ____

____

(2) ____

____

POST-TEST

This is similar to the Pre-Test. Perform this test without looking at the book. This is just to see how well you have understood and can recall the information presented in this chapter after you have studied it and completed the workbook exercises. You will not be graded on this portion (other than the grade you give yourself), but this is an excellent preparation for your instructor's test. You may use this Post-Test to determine what areas you need to study more.

1. Blood cells are produced in the:
   a. liver
   b. lymph nodes
   c. spleen
   d. bone marrow

2. The most common type of blood for laboratory tests is:
   a. capillary blood
   b. venous blood
   c. arterial blood
   d. coronary blood

3. A buffy coat is a combination of:
   a. RBCs
   b. WBCs
   c. platelets
   d. b and c

4. The bevel of the needle should be held in which of the following positions when performing venipuncture?
   a. down
   b. up
   c. sideways
   d. any of the above

5. Which tube color contains no anticoagulants?
   a. red top
   b. gray top
   c. green top
   d. lavender top

6. Which of the following position(s) should patients be in while they are having their blood drawn?
   a. lying down
   b. standing
   c. sitting
   d. either a or c

7. What is the maximum amount of time the tourniquet should be left on?
   a. 30 seconds
   b. 60 seconds
   c. 90 seconds
   d. 120 seconds

8. The most common method used to draw blood from an adult is:
   a. syringe
   b. butterfly
   c. vacuum tube
   d. intravenous needle

CERTIFICATION CRITERIA CHECKLIST

As you go through your education and training, keep in mind the national certification examination that you will take when you graduate. Each chapter of the textbook and workbook covers a different section of the examination criteria. To keep track of your preparation for the certification examination, turn to the back of this workbook and highlight the following CMA, RMA, or CMAS certification examination criteria (if you have already highlighted them from a previous chapter, put a check mark by the criteria):

CMA

B. Anatomy and Physiology
   2. Systems, including structure, function, related conditions and diseases

D. Professionalism
   4. Maintaining confidentiality

J. Records Management

R. Principles of Infection Control

S. Treatment Area
   2. Equipment preparation and operation
   5. Safety precautions

V Collecting and Processing Specimens; Diagnostic Testing
   3. Quality control

RMA

I. General Medical Assisting Knowledge
    A. Anatomy and Physiology
    E. Human Relations
III. Clinical Medical Assisting
    A. Asepsis
    I. Laboratory Procedures

CMAS

1. Medical Assisting Foundation
    - Anatomy and physiology
    - Professionalism
2. Basic Clinical Medical Office Assisting
    - Asepsis in the medical office
3. Medical Office Clerical
    - Communication

O	Color: Additive: Specimen type: Tests:
O	Color: Additive: Specimen type: Tests:
O	Color: Additive: Specimen type: Tests:
O	Color: Additive: Specimen type: Tests:
O	Color: Additive: Specimen type: Tests:
O	Color: Additive: Specimen type: Tests:
O	Color: Additive: Specimen type: Tests:
O	Color: Additive: Specimen type: Tests:

COMPETENCY ASSESSMENT

Procedure 40-1 Palpating a Vein for Venipuncture

Performance Objectives: To palpate for an appropriate vein for venipuncture using a tourniquet. Perform this objective within 10 minutes with a minimum score of 40 points.

Supplies/Equipment: Gloves, goggles and mask, alcohol swab, tourniquet

Charting/Documentation: Enter appropriate documentation/charting in the box.

Instructor's/Evaluator's Comments and Suggestions:

SKILLS CHECKLIST Procedure 40-1: Palpating a Vein for Venipuncture

Name ______________________________

Date ______________________________

No.	Skill	Check #1 20 pts ea	Check #2 10 pts ea	Check #3 5 pts ea	Notes
1	Identify the patient. Ask the patient's name and verify it with the computer label or identification number. If a fasting specimen is required, verify that the patient has not had anything to eat or drink except water.				
2	Wash hands. Put on gloves, safety glasses, and mask.				
3	Apply tourniquet 3 to 4 inches above the venipunture site. Apply tightly enough to slow blood flow but not so tight that blood flow in the arteries is stopped.				
4	Have the patient close the hand, and place the patient's arm in a downward position.				
5	Palpate the antecubital space of the arm, feeling for the basalic or cephalic vein with the tip of your index finger.				
6	Feel for a soft bounce and a roundness to the vein. Follow the direction of the vein.				
7	After locating an acceptable vein, mentally map the location. Visualize the puncture site.				
8	If a vein cannot be found in the antecubital space of the arm, then the hand veins must be checked following the same procedure. Venipuncture of the hand is more successful when a butterfly is used.				
Student's Total Points					
Points Possible		160	80	40	
Final Score (Student's Total Points / Possible Points)					

	Notes
Start time:	
End time:	
Total time: (10 min goal)	

COMPETENCY ASSESSMENT

Procedure 40-2 Venipuncture by Syringe

Performance Objectives: Using a syringe to obtain venous blood acceptable for laboratory testing as required by a physician. Perform this objective within 15 minutes with a minimum score of 125 points.

Supplies/Equipment: Gloves, goggles and mask, 10-ml syringe, 21-gauge safety needle, vacuum tube(s) or special collection tube(s), vacuum tube safety holder, tourniquet, 70% isopropyl alcohol swab, cotton balls, gauze, adhesive bandage or tape, sharps container, test tube rack

Charting/Documentation: Enter appropriate documentation/charting in the box.

Instructor's/Evaluator's Comments and Suggestions:

SKILLS CHECKLIST Procedure 40-2: Venipuncture by Syringe

Name ______________________

Date ______________________

No.	Skill	Check #1 20 pts ea	Check #2 10 pts ea	Check #3 5 pts ea	Notes
1	Position and identify the patient. Ask the patient's name and verify it with the computer label or identification number. If a fasting specimen is required, verify that the patient has not had anything to eat or drink except water.				
2	Wash hands. Put on gloves, safety glasses, and mask.				
3	Open the sterile needle and sterile syringe packages and assemble if necessary. Pull the plunger halfway out and push it all the way in again.				
4	Select the proper vacuum tubes for later transfer of the specimen, tap all tubes containing anticoagulants, and check the expiration dates. Arrange them in a holding rack.				
5	Select a site and apply the tourniquet.				
6	Ask the patient to close the hand. The patient must not pump the hand. Place the hand in a downward position.				
7	Select a vein, noting the location and direction of the vein.				
8	Clean the site with an alcohol swab with one firm swipe.				
9	Avoid touching the site after cleansing.				
10	Draw the skin taut with your thumb by placing it 1 to 2 inches below the puncture site.				
11	With the bevel up, line up the needle with the direction of the vein and perform the puncture. The point of the needle should enter the skin about 0.25 inch below where the vein was palpated. Once the vein has been entered, do not move the needle.				

No.	Skill	Check #1 20 pts ea	Check #2 10 pts ea	Check #3 5 pts ea	Notes
12	Let go of the skin and use that hand to pull back on the plunger. Pull gently and only as fast as the syringe fills. If the vein collapses, stop pulling on the plunger and let the vein refill.				
13	When the syringe is full, have the patient open the hand. Remove the tourniquet.				
14	Lightly place a cotton ball above the puncture site and remove the needle in the same direction as inserted.				
15	Apply pressure to the site for 2 to 3 minutes. Let the patient assist by holding the pressure if desired. The patient may elevate the arm but should be instructed not to bend the elbow.				
16	Aliquot blood into the appropriate tubes in the rack in the proper order. Refer to the "Order of Draw" instructions in Chapter 40 of the textbook. During transfer, you may hold each tube at the base only.				
17	Puncture the vacuum tube through the rubber stopped with the syringe needle and allow the blood to enter the tube until the flow stops. Never push on the plunger or force blood into the tube.				
18	Implement safety mechanisms or devices on the needle immediately.				
19	Mix any anticoagulant tubes immediately.				
20	Discard the syringe and needle into a sharps container and the contaminated cotton ball and other waste into a red bag.				
21	Label all tubes before leaving the room. If any special treatment is required for the specimens, institute the handling protocol right away.				
22	Check the patient. Observe him or her for signs of stress.				

No.	Skill	Check #1 20 pts ea	Check #2 10 pts ea	Check #3 5 pts ea	Notes
23	When sufficient pressure has been applied to stop the bleeding, apply a small pressure bandage by pulling a cotton ball in half, applying it to the puncture site, and placing an adhesive bandage or tape over it. Instruct the patient to remove the bandage in 20 minutes. If the patient is sensitive or allergic to latex, be sure to use nonlatex paper tape. If the bleeding has not stopped after 2 to 3 minutes, have the patient continue to hold direct pressure on the site for another 5 minutes with the arm elevated above the heart. The patient can do this by lying down with his or her arm on a pillow.				
24	Disinfect tray and supplies and dispose of all contaminated items properly. Remove gloves using the proper technique.				
25	Wash hands, record the procedure, and complete the laboratory requisition.				
Student's Total Points					
Points Possible		500	250	125	
Final Score (Student's Total Points / Possible Points)					

	Notes
Start time:	
End time:	
Total time: (15 min goal)	

COMPETENCY ASSESSMENT

Procedure 40-3 Venipuncture by Vacuum Tube System

Performance Objectives: Using the vacuum tube system to obtain venous blood acceptable for laboratory testing as required by a physician. Perform this objective within 15 minutes with a minimum score of 130 points.

Supplies/Equipment: Gloves, goggles and mask, vacuum tube adapter/holder, 21-gauge multidraw needle, vacuum tube(s) or special collection tube(s), tourniquet, 70% isopropyl alcohol swab, cotton balls, adhesive bandage or tape, sharps container

Charting/Documentation: Enter appropriate documentation/charting in the box.

Instructor's/Evaluator's Comments and Suggestions:

SKILLS CHECKLIST Procedure 40-3: Venipuncture by Vacuum Tube System

Name ____________________

Date ____________________

No.	Skill	Check #1 20 pts ea	Check #2 10 pts ea	Check #3 5 pts ea	Notes
1	Position and identify the patient. Ask the patient's name and verify it with the computer label or identification number. If a fasting specimen is required, verify that the patient has not had anything to eat or drink except water.				
2	Wash hands. Put on gloves, safety glasses, and mask.				
3	Break the seal on the shorter needle; thread the shorter needle into the holder/adapter.				
4	Tap all tubes containing anti-coagulants and check the expiration dates.				
5	Insert the first tube in the holder/adapter without penetrating the stopper. Reference the "Order of Draw" chart in Chapter 40 of the textbook to select the tube in the proper order.				
6	Select a site and apply the tourniquet.				
7	Ask the patient to close the hand. The patient must not pump the hand. Place the hand in a downward position, which further enlarges the vein allowing for easier venipuncture.				
8	Select a vein, noting the location and direction of the vein.				
9	Cleanse the site with alcohol with one firm swipe.				
10	Avoid touching the site after cleansing.				
11	Draw the skin taut with your thumb by placing it 1 to 2 inches below the puncture site.				
12	With the bevel line up, line up the needle with the direction of the vein and perform the puncture. The point of the needle should enter the skin about 0.25 inch below where the vein was palpated. Once the vein has been entered, do not move the needle.				

No.	Skill	Check #1 20 pts ea	Check #2 10 pts ea	Check #3 5 pts ea	Notes
13	Let go of the skin and use that hand to grasp the vacuum tube holder. Using the flange, push the tube forward until the shorter needle has completely entered the tube. Do not change hands while performing venipuncture. One hand is securely holding the adapter/holder, and the other hand is free for tube insertion and removal.				
14	Rotate tube so the label is down for better viewing. Fill the tube until the vacuum is exhausted and the blood flow stops.				
15	When the blood ceases, gently remove the vacuum tube from the needle and holder without moving the needle in the patient's arm.				
16	Immediately mix the blood in the anticoagulant tubes by gently inverting them several times.				
17	Insert the second tube onto the needle by using the same motion as with the first tube. Let it fill; then remove it with the same motion as the first tube. Invert it several times if it contains anticoagulants.				
18	When the last tube has filled, remove it from the needle. Ask the patient to open his or her hand. Release the tourniquet.				
19	Lightly place the cotton ball above the puncture site and smoothly remove the needle from the arm in the same direction as insertion. Apply pressure on the site.				
20	Implement safety mechanisms or devices on the needle immediately.				
21	Continue the pressure on the site for 2 to 3 minutes. Let the patient assist by holding the pressure. Ask the patient not to bend his or her arm, but he or she may elevate the arm while applying pressure.				
22	Dispose of the needle into a sharps container and the contaminated cotton ball and other waste into a biohazard red bag.				

No.	Skill	Check #1 20 pts ea	Check #2 10 pts ea	Check #3 5 pts ea	Notes
23	Label all tubes before leaving the patient. If any special treatment is required for the specimens, institute the handling/storage protocol right away.				
24	Check the patient. Observe him or her for signs of stress. The patient should stop bleeding within 2 to 3 minutes. If the bleeding has stopped, apply a small pressure bandage by pulling a cotton ball in half, applying it to the puncture site, and placing an adhesive bandage or tape over it. Instruct the patient to remove the bandage in 20 minutes. If the patient is sensitive or allergic to latex, be sure to use nonlatex paper tape. If the bleeding has not stopped after 2 to 3 minutes, have the patient continue to hold direct pressure on the site for another 5 minutes with his or her arm elevated above the heart. He or she can do this by lying down with the arm on a pillow.				
25	Disinfect tray and supplies and dispose of all contaminated items properly. Remove gloves using the proper technique.				
26	Wash hands, record the procedure, and complete the laboratory requisition.				
Student's Total Points					
Points Possible		520	260	130	
Final Score (Student's Total Points / Possible Points)					

	Notes
Start time:	
End time:	
Total time: (15 min goal)	

COMPETENCY ASSESSMENT

Procedure 40-4 Venipuncture by Butterfly Needle System

Performance Objectives: Using a butterfly needle system to obtain venous blood acceptable for laboratory testing as required by a physician. Perform this objective within 15 minutes with a minimum score of 150 points.

Supplies/Equipment: Gloves, goggles and mask, vacuum tube adapter/holder (if using a vacuum tube connection), a 10- to 15-ml syringe (if using a syringe connection), butterfly needle system with 21-gauge needle (use a multisample needle system with a luer adapter for attaching to the vacuum tube and a hypodermic needle for syringe attachment), vacuum tube rack (syringe collection), vacuum tubes, tourniquet, 70% isopropyl alcohol swab, gauze or cotton balls, adhesive bandage or tape, sharps container

Charting/Documentation: Enter appropriate documentation/charting in the box.

Instructor's/Evaluator's Comments and Suggestions:

SKILLS CHECKLIST Procedure 40-4: Venipuncture by Butterfly Needle System

Name ______________________

Date ______________________

No.	Skill	Check #1 20 pts ea	Check #2 10 pts ea	Check #3 5 pts ea	Notes
1	Position and identify the patient. Ask the patient's name and verify it with the computer label or identification number.				
2	If a fasting specimen is required, verify that the patient has not had anything to eat or drink except water.				
3	Wash hands.				
4	Put on gloves, as well as safety glasses and mask.				
5	Assemble equipment.				
6	Open the package of butterfly needle system. If using the multi-sample needle, connect the needle to the vacuum tube holder/adapter. If using the hypodermic needle and syringe, connect the needle to the syringe. If using a syringe, set the vacuum tubes in a rack for later use.				
7	Tap the vacuum tubes to be sure any additive is dislodged from the stopper and sides of the tube. Check the expiration dates.				
8	Apply the tourniquet.				
9	Ask the patient to close his or her hand. The patient should not pump his or her hand. If possible, place the arm in a downward position.				
10	Select a vein, noting the location and direction of the vein.				
11	Clean the site with an alcohol swab using one swift firm swipe and allow to dry.				
12	Avoid touching the site after cleansing.				
13	Draw the skin taut by placing your thumb 1 to 2 inches below the site and pulling down firmly.				
14	Hold the wings of the butterfly together with the bevel up; line up the needle with the vein and smoothly insert it into the vein at about a 5- to 10-degree angle.				

No.	Skill	Check #1 20 pts ea	Check #2 10 pts ea	Check #3 5 pts ea	Notes
15	Remove your hand from holding the skin taut.				
16	If you are connected to a vacuum tube holder, grasp the flange of the vacuum tube holder and push the tube forward until the needle has completely entered the tube.				
17	If you are connected to a syringe, pull gently on the syringe.				
18	Do not change hands while performing the venipuncture. The hand performing the venipuncture is holding the needle steady. The other hand is for inserting and removing the vacuum tubes or manipulating the syringe.				
19	If you are collecting directly into vacuum tubes, remove and replace the vacuum tubes as explained in Procedure 40-3, until you have drawn the necessary amounts. If you are drawing into a syringe, you will be limited to the size of the syringe being used.				
20	When the syringe is filled, ask the patient to open his or her hand and release the tourniquet.				
21	Lightly place a cotton ball above the puncture site and smoothly remove the needle from the arm in the same direction as insertion. Apply pressure immediately.				
22	Activate the safety device of the butterfly needle immediately.				
23	Continue to apply pressure on the site. Let the patient assist by holding the pressure. Ask the patient not to bend the arm. They may elevate the arm while applying pressure, though.				
24	If using a syringe, aliquot blood into the appropriate tubes as outlined in Procedure 40-2.				
25	Dispose of the butterfly needle and tubing into a sharps container.				
26	Label all the tubes.				
27	Check the patient. Observe him or her for signs of stress.				

No.	Skill	Check #1 20 pts ea	Check #2 10 pts ea	Check #3 5 pts ea	Notes
28	The patient should stop bleeding within 2 to 3 minutes. If the bleeding has stopped, apply a small pressure bandage. The patient should be instructed to remove the bandage in about 20 minutes. If the bleeding has not stopped, have the patient continue to hold pressure another 5 minutes with the arm elevated above his or her heart, then recheck.				
29	Clean up tray and supplies; dispose of contaminated cotton ball. Remove gloves using the proper technique. Discard gloves into biohazard container and disinfect goggles.				
30	Wash hands, record the procedure, and complete the laboratory requisition.				
Student's Total Points					
Points Possible		600	300	150	
Final Score (Student's Total Points / Possible Points)					

	Notes
Start time:	
End time:	
Total time: (15 min goal)	

COMPETENCY ASSESSMENT

Procedure 40-5 Capillary Puncture

Performance Objectives: To obtain capillary blood acceptable for laboratory testing as required by a physician. Perform this objective within 10 minutes with a minimum score of 65 points.

Supplies/Equipment: Gloves, goggles and mask (optional), alcohol swab, microcollection tubes, capillary tubes or specific test kit, safety lancet, gauze, cotton balls, adhesive bandage or tape, sharps container

Charting/Documentation: Enter appropriate documentation/charting in the box.

Instructor's/Evaluator's Comments and Suggestions:

SKILLS CHECKLIST Procedure 40-5: Capillary Puncture

Name ______________________________

Date ______________________________

No.	Skill	Check #1 20 pts ea	Check #2 10 pts ea	Check #3 5 pts ea	Notes
1	Assemble the supplies.				
2	Identify the patient, introduce yourself, and explain the procedure. Recheck the physician's orders.				
3	Wash hands and apply gloves.				
4	Organize the equipment and supplies.				
5	Select the puncture site on the fleshy part of the ring or middle finger, avoiding the tip and the sides.				
6	Have the patient wash their hands in warm water. If necessary, apply a warming pack to the fingertip, encourage the patient to relax, and provide a comfortable, professional atmosphere.				
7	Clean the selected puncture site with alcohol and allow it to air dry or dry it with a gauze pad.				
8	Holding the distal phalange firmly, perform the puncture across the lines of the fingerprint rather than along the lines.				
9	Using a gauze pad, wipe away the first drop.				
10	Collect the specimen according to the test being performed				
11	Check the patient. He or she should hold direct pressure on the site for at least 2 minutes (120 seconds). If the bleeding has stopped, apply an adhesive bandage. If the bleeding has not stopped, have the patient hold direct pressure for 5 minutes, and then recheck.				

No.	Skill	Check #1 20 pts ea	Check #2 10 pts ea	Check #3 5 pts ea	Notes
12	Discard the gloves into a biohazard container and either discard or disinfect the goggles. Wash hands.				
13	Record the procedure and complete the laboratory requisition or test.				
Student's Total Points					
Points Possible		260	130	65	
Final Score (Student's Total Points / Possible Points)					
		Notes			
Start time:					
End time:					
Total time: (10 min goal)					

COMPETENCY ASSESSMENT

Procedure 40-6 Obtaining a Capillary Specimen for Transport Using a Microtainer Transport Unit

Performance Objectives: To obtain a specimen of capillary blood for transport to a laboratory for testing, using a Microtainer transport unit. Perform this objective within 20 minutes with a minimum score of 90 points.

Supplies/Equipment: Capillary puncture supplies (gloves, alcohol pad, safety lancet, cotton ball, adhesive bandage), Microtainer transport unit, laboratory requisition, small sturdy container with a tightly fitting lid (such as a urine specimen cup), pen, biohazard specimen transport bag

Charting/Documentation: Enter appropriate documentation/charting in the box.

Instructor's/Evaluator's Comments and Suggestions:

SKILLS CHECKLIST Procedure 40-6: Obtaining a Capillary Specimen for Transport Using a Microtainer Transport Unit

Name ______________________

Date ______________________

No.	Skill	Check #1 20 pts ea	Check #2 10 pts ea	Check #3 5 pts ea	Notes
1	Determine the appropriateness of submitting a capillary specimen for the specific test you are performing.				
2	Assemble the supplies.				
3	Identify the patient, introduce yourself and explain the procedure.				
4	Perform the capillary puncture with the safety lancet.				
5	Discard the first drop of blood by wiping it away with the gauze.				
6	Allow another drop to form.				
7	Scoop the drop into the Microtainer tube.				
8	Tip the Microtainer tube, allowing the blood drop to slide into the tube.				
9	Gently agitate the tube to mix the additive.				
10	Continue collection of blood until the tube is filled.				
11	Provide the patient with a cotton ball and ask him or her to hold pressure on the puncture wound.				
12	Remove the scoop from the Microtainer unit and discard the scoop into a sharps container.				
13	Remove the colored cap from the back of the Microtainer tube and place it securely onto the opening.				
14	Place the capped Microtainer tube into a small sturdy container (such as a sterile urine specimen cup) and tightly apply the lid.				
15	Label the container.				
16	Fill out the laboratory requisition while the patient is there. Place container into biohazard specimen transport bag. Place the requisition into the outer pocket of the transport bag.				

No.	Skill	Check #1 20 pts ea	Check #2 10 pts ea	Check #3 5 pts ea	Notes
17	Check the patient. If the bleeding has stopped, apply an adhesive strip; answer any questions; and release the patient.				
18	Document the procedure in the patient's chart/medical record.				
Student's Total Points					
Points Possible		360	180	90	
Final Score (Student's Total Points / Possible Points)					
		Notes			
Start time:					
End time:					
Total time: (20 min goal)					

EVALUATION OF CHAPTER KNOWLEDGE

	Student Self-Evaluation		
Skills	Good	Average	Poor
I understand the principles and usage of venipuncture procedures.	_____	_____	_____
I can identify and describe venipuncture equipment and techniques.	_____	_____	_____
I can demonstrate an understanding of the physiology of the circulatory system.	_____	_____	_____
I can differentiate between serum and plasma.	_____	_____	_____
I can describe the purposes of additives and anticoagulants.	_____	_____	_____
I can demonstrate the ability to respond correctly to adverse patient reactions to venipuncture.	_____	_____	_____
I recall vein stimulation techniques.	_____	_____	_____
I can identify correct color-coded tubes used with specific anticoagulants.	_____	_____	_____
I can identify the correct order of draw for blood collection.	_____	_____	_____
I can facilitate therapeutic communication with patients, putting them at ease during venipuncture.	_____	_____	_____
I can demonstrate aseptic techniques and Sandard Precautions for infection control, including proper disposal of sharps.	_____	_____	_____
I understand variables that can affect laboratory test results.	_____	_____	_____
I possess the ability to handle and process acceptable specimens for accurate analysis in the laboratory.	_____	_____	_____

CHAPTER 41

Hematology

CHAPTER PRE-TEST

Perform this test without looking at the book. This is just to see how well you have understood and can recall the information in this chapter after you have read it, but before you have completed the workbook exercises. You will not be graded on this portion (other than the grade you give yourself). Justify any "false" answers.

1. Hematology is the study of blood cells and coagulation. (T or F)
2. Hematopoiesis is the formation of blood cells. (T or F)
3. Increased neutrophils is indicative of a bacterial infection. (T or F)
4. White blood cells (WBCs) are responsible for carrying oxygen to the body's cells. (T or F)
5. Platelets assist with clotting. (T or F)
6. Red blood cells (RBCs) are the most numerous of all the body's blood cell components. (T or F)

INTRODUCTION

Hematology is the study of the blood in both normal and diseased states. As a diagnostic tool, hematologic tests are invaluable to the physician in determining illness, evaluating a patient's progress, and deciding on treatment modalities. The most common hematologic tests include hemoglobin, hematocrit, WBC count, RBC count, platelet count, differential WBC count, erythrocyte sedimentation rate (ESR), and prothrombin time. Included in the study of hematology is the study of hematopoiesis, the formation of blood cells. It is important for the clinical medical assistant to understand the process of normal blood values and how to perform various blood collection and testing procedures. Following safety and quality-control guidelines will protect medical assistants and others and contribute to the accuracy of test results.

PERFORMANCE OBJECTIVES

After successful completion of this chapter you will be able to explain the medical terms related to blood and its components and characteristics. A lot about the body can be determined by looking at the characteristics of blood. You will be able to describe how blood cells are formed, the identifying characteristics of each, what purpose each component serves, the normal values of each component, and what changes occur during diseased states. You will be able to describe how the WBC differentiation and the RBC indices are used in diagnoses. You will know what a hematocrit, hemoglobin, and ESR is, and what information they give us. You will, of course, also become familiar with the equipment, supplies, and procedures associated with blood tests, especially Clinical Laboratory Improvement Act (CLIA) waived categories of blood tests. *The following statements are related to your learning objectives for this chapter. Fill in the blanks in the following paragraph with the appropriate term(s).*

(1) ____________________ is the study of blood cells and coagulation in both normal and (2) ________________ states. It does not include the (3) ____________________ of blood. The two main components of blood are the (4) ____________________ portion and the (5) ____________________. The RBCs are called (6) ____________________ and are responsible for carrying (7) ________________________ to the body's cells and (8) ______________________________________ away from the cells. WBCs are called (9) __________________________ and are responsible for fighting diseases. The platelets are called (10) ______________________________, and they assist with blood clotting. There are (11) ________________ different types of WBCs, and each serves a different purpose in fighting diseases. The part of the complete blood cell count (CBC) that counts and indexes the various white cells is called the WBC (12) ________________________. The part of the CBC that indexes and counts the red cells is called the RBC (13) ____________________. Hemoglobin, abbreviated (14) ___________, and hematocrit, abbreviated (15) ___________, are two tests that help to determine the oxygen-carrying efficiency of the red cells. The erythrocyte sedimentation rate, abbreviated (16) ________________ and sometimes called (17) __________________________ for short, is a test to determine the speed at which the (18) __________________ fall in a column of blood within (19) ______ hour. During disease conditions in the body, the (20) ____________________ membrane of the RBCs is (21) _____________, and this affects the (22) _____________ at which the RBCs fall. The ESR rate is (23) ______________________ in infections and inflammatory diseases and other conditions.

VOCABULARY BUILDER

Find the words listed below that are misspelled; circle them, and then correctly spell them in the spaces provided. Then match each of the vocabulary terms listed below to its correct definition.

_______ 1. complete blood count
_______ 2. erythrocysts
_______ 3. esinophil
_______ 4. microcytic
_______ 5. luekocytes
_______ 6. hematacrit
_______ 7. hemaglobin
_______ 8. basophil
_______ 9. thrombocytes
_______ 10. lymphocytes
_______ 11. monocytes
_______ 12. macrocytic
_______ 13. hypochromic
_______ 14. erythropoitin

____
____
____
____
____
____

A. A hormone triggered by the kidneys that helps produce RBCs
B. Having less color than normal
C. A larger than normal cell
D. A WBC without cytoplasmic granules that has a large, convoluted, nonsegmented nucleus
E. A smaller cell than normal
F. WBCs, one of the formed elements of blood
G. WBC with a dense, nonsegmented nucleus that lacks granules in the cytoplasm
H. Platelets
I. Granulocytic WBC with dark purple cytoplasmic granules
J. Molecule of the RBC that transports oxygen
K. Percentage of RBCs within a specimen of anticoagulated whole blood
L. A granulocytic WBC with red-stained granules in the cytoplasm that is increased with allergies
M. RBCs, one of the formed elements of blood
N. A hematologic test consisting of a Hct, Hgb, RBC and WBC counts, differential WBC count, and the erythrocyte indices

LEARNING REVIEW

1. When Dr. Winston Lewis orders CBCs on his patients, what are the six general parameters the physician will study to help him make a diagnosis?

(a) ______________________ (d) ______________________
(b) ______________________ (e) ______________________
(c) ______________________ (f) ______________________

2. While Dr. Elizabeth King is reviewing bloodwork drawn on one of her patients, she notes the hematocrit is normal, yet the hemoglobin is low. This is an indication of which of the following diseases?

a. sickle cell anemia
b. Rouleau
c. leukemia
d. iron deficiency anemia
e. malaria

3. Match the appropriate adult parameters with the following blood tests.

______ 1. 36–55%	A. hemoglobin
______ 2. 80–100 fl	B. WBC count
______ 3. 4,500–11,000/mm^3	C. mean corpuscular volume
______ 4. 3236 g/dl	D. hematocrit
______ 5. 4.0–6.0 million/mm^3	E. mean corpuscular hemoglobin concentration
______ 6. 12–18 g/dl	F. RBC count
______ 7. 27–33 pg	G. mean corpuscular hemoglobin

4. What two WBC features on a stained differential slide are studied to assist in the identification of the cell?

   (1) ______________________ (2) ______________________

5. Identify the following erythrocyte indices and list the correct formula for determining each one.

   MCH ____

   MCV ____

   MCHC ____

6. A. In Dr. Lewis's office, Audrey Jones, CMA, performs an ESR using the Wintrobe method, whereas at Inner City Health Care, Walter Seals, CMA, uses the Westergren method. Describe the difference between the two procedures.

   ____

   ____

   B. Sedimentation rate results vary with different states of health. Name two factors that influence the sedimentation rate. Why is the ESR a more accurate tool in diagnosing the onset of a disease than in checking on the progress of treatment?

   ____

   ____

   ____

7. A. At Inner City Health Care, Karen Ritter, CMA, uses automated hematology instruments. Automated hematology procedures have many advantages over the manual methods. List five of these advantages.

   (1) ______________________ (4) ______________________

   (2) ______________________ (5) ______________________

   (3) ______________________

   B. Name three procedures required by CLIA '88 regulations for automated hematology instruments.

   (1) ____

   (2) ____

   (3) ____

CERTIFICATION REVIEW

These questions are designed to mimic the certification examinations. You can use these questions like a small "Certification Examination Study Guide," but this is not meant to take the place of the more extensive study guides. Use this portion to determine in what areas to concentrate your efforts when studying for the certification examination.

1. When a physician collects a bone marrow sample in the adult, the site chosen is the iliac crest or the:
   a. femur
   b. sternum
   c. tibia
   d. scapula
2. The central ion of each heme group is:
   a. magnesium
   b. calcium
   c. potassium
   d. iron
3. A buffy coat contains WBCs and:
   a. RBCs
   b. plasma
   c. platelets
   d. serum
4. When a patient has iron deficiency anemia, the erythrocytes will appear:
   a. hyperchromic
   b. hypochromic
   c. polychromic
   d. bichromic
5. Increased eosinophils may indicate:
   a. hay fever or other allergic conditions
   b. leukemia
   c. appendicitis
   d. tuberculosis

CASE STUDIES

Case 1

Wayne Elder is a regular patient at Inner City Health Care. Two days ago, he began to feel fatigued, experiencing development of a cough, fever, and chills. Dr. Ray Reynolds has examined Mr. Elder and, based on the presented symptoms, makes a clinical diagnosis of influenza.

Discuss the following:

1. What type of blood test will Dr. Reynolds order to confirm his diagnosis?
2. What type of results are to be expected based on a diagnosis confirming clinical data?

Case 2

Maria Jover is describing a constant rundown feeling. After examining her, Dr. Elizabeth King has ordered a hemoglobin determination. Also, because of a past history of blood transfusion, she has also ordered an HIV test to be done at an outside reference laboratory. Dr. King asks Ellen Armstrong, CMA, to perform the venipuncture procedure on Maria to obtain the blood specimens for analysis.

Discuss the following:

1. What tube will Ellen use to collect the blood sample to be used for the hemoglobin determination test?
2. What is Dr. King hoping to learn from the hemoglobin determination results?
3. With the fact that HIV infection cannot yet be ruled out, what Standard Precautions should Ellen follow in performing the venipuncture and the automated hemoglobin determination test?

SELF-ASSESSMENT

What are your personal feelings about performing venipuncture and testing the blood of individuals who may be infected with HIV?

1. Do you think you will be more cautious?
2. Do you think you should be notified if the blood you are drawing or testing is known to be HIV positive?
3. Do you have the same concerns with hepatitis infections?

POST-TEST

This is similar to the Pre-Test. Perform this test without looking at the book. This is just to see how well you have understood and can recall the information presented in this chapter after you have studied it and completed the workbook exercises. You will not be graded on this portion (other than the grade you give yourself), but this is an excellent preparation for your instructor's test. You may use this Post-Test to determine what areas you need to study more. Justify any "false" answers.

1. Hematology is the study of blood cells, coagulation, and chemistry. (T or F)
2. Hematosis is the formation of blood cells. (T or F)
3. Increased lymphocytes is indicative of a bacterial infection. (T or F)
4. RBCs are responsible for carrying oxygen to the body's cells. (T or F)
5. Thrombocytes assist with clotting. (T or F)
6. RBCs are the least numerous of all the body's blood cell components. (T or F)

CERTIFICATION CRITERIA CHECKLIST

As you go through your education and training, keep in mind the national certification examination that you will take when you graduate. Each chapter of the textbook and workbook covers a different section of the examination criteria. To keep track of your preparation for the certification examination, turn to the back of this workbook and highlight the following CMA, RMA, or CMAS certification examination criteria (if you have already highlighted them from a previous chapter, put a check mark by the criteria):

CMA

R. Principles of Infection Control

V. Collecting and Processing Specimens; Diagnostic Testing
  2. Processing specimens
  3. Quality control
  4. Performing selected tests

RMA

III. Clinical Medical Assisting
  A. Asepsis
  I. Laboratory Procedures

CMAS

2. Basic Clinical Medical Office Assisting
  - Asepsis in the medical office

COMPETENCY ASSESSMENT

Procedure 41-1 Hemoglobin Determination (HemoCue®)

Performance Objectives: To properly and safely perform an automated hemoglobin determination to evaluate the oxygen capacity of the blood. Perform this objective within 15 minutes with a minimum score of 65 points.

Supplies/Equipment: Gloves, disinfectant, capillary puncture equipment or blood samples collected in EDTA, HemoCue® system or other hemoglobin analyzer with supplies appropriate for the analyzer, biohazard red bag, biohazard sharps container

Charting/Documentation: Enter appropriate documentation/charting in the box.

____

____

____

____

Instructor's/Evaluator's Comments and Suggestions:

____

____

____

____

____

____

SKILLS CHECKLIST Procedure 41-1: Hemoglobin Determination (HemoCue®)

Name ______________________

Date ______________________

No.	Skill	Check #1 20 pts ea	Check #2 10 pts ea	Check #3 5 pts ea	Notes
1	Wash hands and put on gloves.				
2	Assemble equipment and materials.				
3	Turn on instrument to warm it up. Calibrate or standardize the instrument according to the manufacturer's directions.				
4	Perform a capillary puncture observing the Bloodborne Pathogen Standards. Wipe away the first drop of blood.				
5	Collect blood from the puncture using a capillary tube or cuvette appropriate for the analyzer to be used. Avoid trapping air bubbles in the collection device.				
6	Wipe excess blood from the outside of the collection device (if appropriate), being careful not to touch the open end of the device.				
7	Insert the filled cuvette into the HemoCue® photometer within 10 minutes of filling the cuvette. Read the hemoglobin value from the display and record.				
8	Discard all contaminated materials into biohazard containers.				
9	Return all equipment to proper storage.				
10	Wipe counters with surface disinfectant.				
11	Remove and discard gloves into biohazard container.				
12	Wash hands.				
13	Document the results.				
Student's Total Points					
Points Possible		260	130	65	
Final Score (Student's Total Points / Possible Points)					

	Notes
Start time:	
End time:	
Total time: (15 min goal)	

COMPETENCY ASSESSMENT

Procedure 41-2 Microhematocrit

Performance Objectives: To properly and safely perform the microhematocrit procedure using a few microliters of blood in a capillary tube to separate the cellular elements of the blood from the plasma by centrifugation. Perform this objective within 15 minutes with a minimum score of 115 points.

Supplies/Equipment: Gloves, capillary tubes (heparinized), sealing clay, microhematocrit centrifuge and reader, alcohol swabs, gauze and cotton balls, safety lancets, adhesive strip, disinfectant, biohazard red bag, sharps container. OPTIONAL: If obtaining blood from a vacuum tube: vacuum tube of anticoagulated blood, safety shield for cap removal, face shield

Charting/Documentation: Enter appropriate documentation/charting in the box.

Instructor's/Evaluator's Comments and Suggestions:

SKILLS CHECKLIST Procedure 41-2: Microhematocrit

Name ______________________

Date ______________________

No.	Skill	Check #1 20 pts ea	Check #2 10 pts ea	Check #3 5 pts ea	Notes
1	Wash hands and put on gloves.				
2	Assemble equipment and materials for capillary puncture and microhematocrit procedure.				
3	Fill two to three capillary tubes from a capillary puncture:				
	a. Perform a capillary puncture (see Procedure 40-5).				
	b. Wipe away the first drop of blood, then dispose of gauze into biohazard waste.				
	c. Touch one end of heparinized capillary tube to the second drop.				
	d. Allow the tube to fill three-fourths full by capillary action. Hold tube level so air does not enter the tube.				
	e. Fill second tube in the same manner.				
	f. Wipe the outside of the filled capillary tube with gauze to remove excess blood.				
	g. Seal the capillary tube by placing it into the sealing clay.				
4	*or* Fill two capillary tubes using a tube of EDTA anticoagulated blood:				
	a. Mix the tube of blood thoroughly by gently rocking for 2 minutes.				
	b. Remove the cap from the tube using a safety shield.				
	c. Tilt the tube so the blood is near the top of the tube.				
	d. Insert the tip of a plain capillary tube into the blood and fill three-fourths full. Wipe the outside of the capillary tube with gauze to remove excess blood.				
	e. Seal the tube by placing the end into the sealing clay.				
	f. Fill the second tube in the same manner.				
5	Check to see if the interior sealing clay edge appears level in the tubes.				

No.	Skill	Check #1 20 pts ea	Check #2 10 pts ea	Check #3 5 pts ea	Notes
6	Place tubes into the microhematocrit centrifuge with sealed ends securely against the rubber gasket. Balance the centrifuge by placing tubes opposite each other. Make a note of which patients' sample are in which slots.				
7	Fasten lid(s) securely.				
8	Set the timer and adjust the speed if necessary.				
9	Centrifuge for the prescribed time.				
10	Allow the centrifuge to come to a complete stop before unlocking the lid(s).				
11	Determine the microhematocrit values using the scale on the reader.				
12	Average the values from the two tubes and record the microhematocrit as a percentage.				
13	Discard the capillary tubes into the sharps container.				
14	Clean and return equipment to proper storage.				
15	Clean the work area with disinfectant.				
16	Remove and discard gloves into biohazard container and wash hands.				
17	Document the results.				
Student's Total Points					
Points Possible (23 total steps)		460	230	115	
Final Score (Student's Total Points / Possible Points)					

	Notes
Start time:	
End time:	
Total time: (15 min goal)	

COMPETENCY ASSESSMENT

Procedure 41-3 Erythrocyte Sedimentation Rate

Performance Objectives: To properly and safely perform an erythrocyte sedimentation rate (ESR). Perform this objective within 1 hour and 15 minutes with a minimum score of 80 points.

Supplies/Equipment: Gloves, sample of venous blood collected in EDTA, Sediplast® or other ESR kit (sedival and sedirack, Sediplast® autozeroing pipette, pipette capable of delivering up to 1.0 ml), Wintrobe method (Wintrobe sedimentation tube, Wintrobe sedimentation rack, long-stem Pasteur-type pipette with rubber bulb), timer, 10% chlorine bleach solution/disinfectant, face shield or goggles and mask, biohazard red bag waste, sharps container

Charting/Documentation: Enter appropriate documentation/charting in the box.

Instructor's/Evaluator's Comments and Suggestions:

SKILLS CHECKLIST Procedure 41-3: Erythrocyte Sedimentation Rate

Name ______________________________

Date ______________________________

No.	Skill	Check #1 20 pts ea	Check #2 10 pts ea	Check #3 5 pts ea	Notes
1	Wash hands and put on gloves.				
2	Assemble equipment and material.				
3	Gently mix blood sample for 2 minutes.				
4	Perform either Sediplast® ESR or Wintrobe method.				
Sediplast Method					
	a. Remove stopper on sedivial and fill to mark with 0.8 ml anticoagulated blood. Replace stopper and invert several times to mix.				
	b. Place sedivial in Sediplast rack on a level surface.				
	c. Gently insert the Sediplast pipette through the pierceable stopper with a twisting motion and push down until the pipette rests on the bottom of the vial. The pipette will autozero the blood, and any excess will flow into the sealed reservoir compartment.				
	d. Set timer for 1 hour.				
	e. Return blood sample to proper storage.				
	f. Let the pipette stand undisturbed for exactly 1 hour, then read the results according to the scale on the tube.				
	g. Record the sedimentation rate: ESR (Westergren, 1 hour) = ___ mm.				
	h. Dispose of tube and vial in sharps container; dispose of other supplies into red bag.				
Wintrobe Method					
	a. Place tube into Wintrobe sedimentation rack.				
	b. Check the leveling bubble to ensure the rack is level.				

No.	Skill	Check #1 20 pts ea	Check #2 10 pts ea	Check #3 5 pts ea	Notes
	c. Fill the Wintrobe tube to the zero mark with well-mixed blood using the Pasteur pipette and take care not to overfill and avoid getting bubbles in the tube by filling from the bottom.				
	d. Set timer for 1 hour. Be certain the tube is level and undisturbed for the entire hour.				
	e. Return rest of blood sample to proper storage.				
	f. After exactly 1 hour, measure the distance the RBCs have fallen in millimeters using the scale on the side of the tube.				
	g. Record the sedimentation rate: ESR (Wintrobe, 1 hour) = _____ mm				
	h. Disinfect and clean the equipment and return to storage.				
5	Clean work area with disinfectant.				
6	Remove gloves and discard into biohazard container.				
7	Wash hands.				
8	Document the results.				
Student's Total Points					
Points Possible (16 total steps)		320	160	80	
Final Score (Student's Total Points / Possible Points)					

	Notes
Start time:	
End time:	
Total time: (1 hour and 15 min goal)	

COMPETENCY ASSESSMENT

Procedure 41-4 Obtaining Blood for Blood Culture

Performance Objectives: While performing venipuncture from two separate sites, prepare two culture bottles of blood from each site for culture (four total). Perform this objective within 20 minutes with a minimum score of 80 points.

Supplies/Equipment: Nonsterile glove for use with povidone-iodine solution, sterile gloves, laboratory requisition, blood cultures, anaerobic and aerobic (usually four: two bottles each for two sets of cultures), 70% isopropyl alcohol, povidone-iodine solution swabs or towelettes, venipuncture supplies (according to method used) for two separate sites, biohazard red bag, biohazard sharps container, labeling pen

Charting/Documentation: Enter appropriate documentation/charting in the box.

____

____

____

____

Instructor's/Evaluator's Comments and Suggestions:

____

____

____

____

____

____

SKILLS CHECKLIST Procedure 41-4: Obtaining Blood for Blood Culture

Name ______________________________

Date ______________________________

No.	Skill	Check #1 20 pts ea	Check #2 10 pts ea	Check #3 5 pts ea	Notes
1	Identify the patient, introduce yourself, and explain the procedure.				
2	Ensure that the patient has not initiated antimicrobial therapy.				
3	Wash hands and put on gloves.				
4	Assemble equipment and supplies according to the venipuncture procedure being used and the laboratory requirements.				
5	Place the culture bottles on a flat surface within reach during the procedure. Mark the correct fill line on both bottles at 10 ml per bottle (1–2 ml per bottle for pediatric patients).				
6	Prepare the venipuncture site with isopropyl alcohol and allow to dry, then apply povidone-iodine in progressively larger concentric circles from the inside outward. The iodine must remain on the skin for one full minute and be allowed to dry naturally. The venipuncture site should not be touched after the skin is disinfected.				
7	Cleanse the bottle tops with alcohol and povidone-iodine solution just as the skin was.				
8	Remove the preparation glove and apply the sterile gloves using sterile procedure.				
9	Perform venipuncture according to method used. Insert the aerobic culture bottle onto the needle. Fill to the appropriate line, usually 10 ml per bottle (1–3 for pediatric patients). Remove the first bottle, invert 8 to 10 times, and apply the second (anaerobic) bottle. Fill. Remove the second bottle and invert 8 to 10 times.				
10	Complete the venipuncture procedure as determined by the method used. Remove the remaining iodine from the skin with isopropyl alcohol.				

No.	Skill	Check #1 20 pts ea	Check #2 10 pts ea	Check #3 5 pts ea	Notes
11	Perform venipuncture at the second site, repeating the process as stated above. The second and subsequent culture bottles must be collected within 30 minutes of the first.				
12	The culture bottles should be stored at room temperature, not refrigerated.				
13	Label the bottles with the patient's name, date, time, and other required information.				
14	Dispose of all contaminated supplies, disinfect all surfaces, remove gloves, and wash hands.				
15	Complete the laboratory requisition including the date and time of each specimen collected, any antibiotic therapy the patient is receiving, the name and strength of the antibiotic, the dosage, duration, and the last dose taken. Include the clinical diagnosis and any special organisms suspected or to rule out. The laboratory requisition must indicate if the culture is for *brucella* or *francisella*. The information on the laboratory requisition should exactly match the information given on the bottles.				
16	Document the procedure in the laboratory section of the patient's chart/medical record.				
Student's Total Points					
Points Possible		320	160	80	
Final Score (Student's Total Points / Possible Points)					

	Notes
Start time:	
End time:	
Total time: (20 min goal)	

EVALUATION OF CHAPTER KNOWLEDGE

Skills	Student Self-Evaluation		
	Good	Average	Poor
I can discuss the role and importance of hematologic studies as a diagnostic tool.	____	____	____
I can discuss the clinical science of hematology.	____	____	____
I can compare normal and abnormal values of CBC parameters and understand how the CBC is used in diagnosis and treatment of disease.	____	____	____
I can maintain aseptic technique and follow Standard Precautions throughout all procedures.	____	____	____
I understand the importance of following all quality-control guidelines.	____	____	____
I display the appropriate techniques in collecting and processing specimens.	____	____	____
I perform tests with the competent skills necessary for entry-level employment.	____	____	____
I can document all procedures according to laboratory policy.	____	____	____
I can describe physiologic reasons for different variations of test results in different states of health and disease.	____	____	____
I can operate and maintain facility supplies and equipment safely.	____	____	____
I can exhibit empathy for patients and attend to patient's emotional needs during the collection of blood samples.	____	____	____

CHAPTER 42

Urinalysis

CHAPTER PRE-TEST

Perform this test without looking at the book. This is just to see how well you have understood and can recall the information in this chapter after you have read it, but before you have completed the workbook exercises. You will not be graded on this portion (other than the grade you give yourself). Justify any "false" answers.

1. Which part of the urinalysis is to be performed by the physician?
   a. the chemical examination
   b. the physical examination
   c. the specific gravity
   d. the microscopic examination
2. Ketones in urine indicate:
   a. diabetes
   b. glomerulonephritis
   c. cystitis
   d. fat hemolysis
3. If the patient brings a urine sample in a household container from home, you would:
   a. accept it this time, but after this, you will give them a proper container
   b. provide the patient with an appropriate container and ask for a fresh sample
   c. accept it if it is a first morning void and the container is clean
   d. b and c

4. The most common collection of urine in the physician's office laboratory (POL) is the:
   a. random collection
   b. timed specimen
   c. clean-catch, midstream specimen
   d. a and c

5. The written patient instructions for a midstream, clean catch should be:
   a. posted in the restroom behind the toilet
   b. posted in the restroom beside the toilet
   c. posted in the restroom behind the door
   d. both a and b

6. The minimum amount of urine needed for a complete urinalysis is 10 ml. (T or F)

7. Pyridium, a bladder analgesic, can:
   a. increase urine flow
   b. turn the urine a bright orange to red and may stain clothes
   c. quiet down bladder irritation
   d. both b and c

INTRODUCTION

Urinalysis refers to the examination of urine as an aid in patient diagnosis or to follow the course of a disease. Urinalysis is a routine procedure in most physical examinations. Physicians often order a variety of tests on urine to make accurate patient diagnoses. It is essential that medical assistants understand both the importance of urinalysis and their own role in assisting in patient diagnosis and treatment. In this chapter, medical assisting students learn the basics of urinalysis; examination of urine specimens; including proper collection techniques for urine specimens, safety guidelines involved in collecting and handling specimens; and measures to ensure a consistent quality-control program. Students learn to properly perform urinalysis testing and become aware of factors that may intervene with urinalysis accuracy. Observing Standard Precautions is mandatory in urinalysis procedures.

PERFORMANCE OBJECTIVES

After successful completion of this chapter you will be able to explain the medical terms related to urinalysis. You will be able to explain the anatomy, physiology, and common pathology of the urinary tract. You will know the normal and abnormal constituents of urine, what their significance is in urine, and how to test for them and report them. You will be competent in teaching patients, both male and female patients, how to perform a midstream, clean-catch urine collection. You will know the procedures of performing urinalysis and confirmatory testing of urine, as well as a sterile collection of urine for culture and sensitivity. You will also know how the physician will probably treat a given condition or disease and when further testing might be indicated. You will be able to give your patient the proper instructions in preparation for further testing. *The following statements are related to your learning objectives for this chapter. Fill in the blanks in the following paragraph with the appropriate term(s).*

Urine is formed in the (1) ____________________, transported to the bladder via the (2) ____________________, and transported to the outside of the body through the (3) ____________________. The actual filtering of the blood takes place in the (4) ____________________, which is located in the nephron, where most of the work of the kidney takes place. By examining (5) ____________________, we can determine many functions of many systems of the body. According to CLIA, the health care professional performing urine testing must have (6) ____________________ training, an (7) ____________________ of quality-control (QC) procedures, (8) ____________________ in the use of instrumentation, (9) ____________________ of the stability and proper storage of (10) ____________________, (11) ____________________ of the factors that will influence test results, and knowledge of how to (12) ____________________ the results. Urine is examined for amount, color, clarity, and specific gravity, which are parts of the (13) ____________________ examination of urine. The (14) ____________________ examination of urine consists of using a reagent test strip that is dipped into the urine. The (15) ____________________ examination of urine consists of spinning a test tube of urine in a (16) ____________________ machine, then placing a drop of the (17) ____________________ onto a slide for viewing under the microscope. The presence of blood, bacteria, and (18) ____________________ esterace in the urine is indicative of a UTI or (19) ____________________. The presence of (20) ____________________ in the urine indicates a need for further testing for diabetes. The presence of epithelial cells in the urine indicates that the specimen was probably not a (21) ____________________.

VOCABULARY BUILDER

A. *Find the words listed below that are misspelled; circle them, and then correctly spell them in the spaces provided. Then match the following terms listed in Column A with corresponding definitions listed in Column B.*

Column A

_______ 1. Clinitest

_______ 2. ketone

_______ 3. pH

_______ 4. urochrome

_______ 5. sedament

_______ 6. amorphus

_______ 7. Ictotest

_______ 8. cultures

Column B

A. Urine testing that includes physical, chemical, and microscopic testing of a urine sample

B. Crystalline material found in urine sediment; shapeless; possessing no definite form

C. Tiny structures usually formed by deposits of protein (or other substances) on the walls of renal tubes

D. Reagent table test that confirms the presence of reducing sugars in the urine

_______ 9. casts
_______ 10. urinalysis
_______ 11. Acetest
_______ 12. quality control (QC)
_______ 13. specific gravity
_______ 14. hyaline
_______ 15. crystals
_______ 16. midstream collection
_______ 17. panic values
_______ 18. reagent test strip
_______ 19. urea
_______ 20. meniscus
_______ 21. turbid
_______ 22. screening
_______ 23. acid–base balance

____

____

E. Found in normal urine sediment, these structures generally have no particular significance; the presence of a few should be noted because they may indicate disease states.

F. Microorganisms cultivated in a nutrient medium

G. Transparent, clear casts that are often hard to see in urine; these casts should be examined under subdued lighting

H. Confirmatory test for bilirubin

I. Chemical compound produced during increased metabolism of fat; tested on a reagent strip

J. Curvature appearing in a liquid's upper surface when the liquid is placed in a container

K. Urine sample collected in the middle of the flow of urine

L. Test results that indicate a potentially life-threatening or greatly debilitating situation that must be reported to a physician immediately

M. Scale that indicates the relative alkalinity or acidity of a solution; measurement of hydrogen ion concentration

N. Program that ensures accurate and dependable test results

O. Narrow strip of plastic on which pads containing reagents are attached; used in urinalysis to detect a variety of substances and values

P. Insoluble matter that settles to the bottom of a liquid; material examined in the urinalysis microscopic examination

Q. Ratio of weight of a given volume of a substance to the weight of the same volume of distilled water at the same temperature; test often performed during the urinalysis physical examination (can also appear on the reagent strip)

R. Opaque; lack of clarity

S. Product used to test for the presence of abnormal amounts of acetone in the urine

T. Principal end product of protein metabolism

U. Yellow pigment that provides color to urine

V. Condition that occurs when the net rate at which the body produces acids or bases is equal to the net rate at which acids or bases are excreted

W. Preliminary examination used to detect the most characteristic signs of a disorder that may entail further investigation

B. *Fill in the proper terms relating to urinalysis.*

1. ______________________________ Orange–yellow pigment that forms from the breakdown of hemoglobin in red blood cells. It usually travels in the bloodstream to the liver, where it is converted to a water-soluble form and excreted into the bile.

2. ______________________________ Abnormal presence of blood in urine, symptomatic of many disorders of the genitourinary system and renal diseases.

3. ______________________________ Simple sugar that is a major source of energy in the human body; monitoring of its levels in the urine and blood is a vital diagnostic test in diabetes and other disorders; a test on a reagent strip.

4. ______________________________ Test on a reagent strip that indicates the presence of white blood cells in the urinary tract.

5. ______________________________ Colorless compound produced in the intestine after the breakdown by bacteria of bilirubin.

6. ______________________________ Chemical substances that detect or synthesize other substances in a chemical reaction and are used in laboratory analyses because they are known to react in a specific way.

7. ______________________________ Accumulation of ketones in the body, occurring primarily as a compilation of diabetes mellitus; if left untreated, it could cause coma.

8. ______________________________ Pattern based on 24-hour cycle that emphasizes the repetition of certain physiologic phenomena such as eating and sleeping.

9. ______________________________ Waste product formed in muscle that is excreted by the kidneys; increased in blood and urine when kidney function is abnormal.

10. ______________________________ Instrument that measures the refractive index of a substance or solution; used in the urinalysis chemical examination to measure the urine specimen's specific gravity.

11. ______________________________ Device used to measure specific gravity; consists of a float with a calibrated stem.

12. ______________________________ Urine that appears to be above the sediment when centrifuged; poured off before sediment is examined in the urinalysis microscopic examination.

13. ______________________________ Mucoprotein excreted by the epithelial cells of the renal tubules.

LEARNING REVIEW

1. *Fill in the blanks in the following paragraphs with the appropriate term(s).*

A.

electrolytes	metabolism	tubule
excess fluid	milliliters	urea
filtration	nephron	urine
glomerulus	salts	waste products
homeostasis	soluble	

The formation and excretion of ________________ is the principal method by which the body excretes water and the ________________ waste products of ________________. The kidneys control this process and also regulate the fluid outside the cells of the body, carefully maintaining the body's balance of fluids eliminated or retained, or ________________ of body fluids. The kidneys are responsible for the ______________ of ______________, ______________, and ________________ from the blood. Substances filtered out of the body can include water, ammonia, ______________, glucose, amino acids, creatinine, and ________________. These wastes leave the body through the eliminated urine. The filtering unit of the kidney is called the ________________. The ________________ is the part of the kidney that concentrates the filtered material. Together, these elements of the kidney form the ________________________. Each minute, more than 1,000 ________________ of blood flows through the kidney to be cleansed.

B.

amino acids	creatinine	protein
blood	glucose	threshold
concentration	kidney	

While passing through the ______________________________, some substances, such as ______________________________ and ______________________________, need to be reabsorbed into the ______________________________. These substances are reabsorbed in relation to their ______________________________ in the blood and are known as ______________________________. Some of these substances need only be partially reabsorbed, such as ______________________________ and ______________________________.

C.

ammonium	hydrogen	sodium
blood	kidney	urine
drugs	secreted	

Toward the end of the ________________'s sojourn through the ________________, other substances that have not already been filtered are secreted into the ______________. For instance, substances such as ________________ and ________________ ions may be __________ in the urine in exchange for __________________. In addition, certain __________________ in the blood at this point may also be secreted into the urine.

2. A. After passing through a healthy kidney, urine composition is approximately ____ percent water and _____ percent dissolved substances, which generally come from dietary intake or metabolic waste products.

   B. Identify each substance below as a normal (N) or an abnormal (AB) substance found in urine.

____ (1) Urobilinogen	____ (4) Multiple leukocytes	____ (7) Erythrocytes
____ (2) Potassium	____ (5) Lipids	____ (8) Creatinine
____ (3) Uric acid	____ (6) 1+ Protein	____ (9) Chloride

   C. When certain disease processes occur in the human body, changes in urine production can occur. List six possible changes.

   (1) ______________________________ (4) ______________________________
   (2) ______________________________ (5) ______________________________
   (3) ______________________________ (6) ______________________________

3. When handling urine specimens, Standard Precautions must be followed to ensure that proper infection control standards are observed. In the spaces provided below, list five precautions used when handling urine specimens.

   (1) ____
   (2) ____
   (3) ____
   (4) ____
   (5) ____

Circle the correct response for each multiple choice question below.

4. QC programs:
   a. provide a random spot-check of accuracy
   b. ensure accurate and reliable results for the patient
   c. provide comparisons with patient specimens necessary to interpret urinalysis test results

5. Equipment and instruments used for urine testing:
   a. must be disposed of properly in biohazard containers after each procedure
   b. are self-calibrating and require no adjustment
   c. should be checked daily for proper calibration

6. QC procedures should be performed:
   a. exactly as procedures are performed on patient specimens
   b. on every other urine specimen tested
   c. only by a licensed health care professional trained to interpret the results

7. Urine control samples:
   a. have no special storage requirements
   b. are purchased commercially from manufacturers
   c. are used to obtain baseline urinalysis results from healthy patients

8. Documentation of QC testing:
   a. must be recorded in a daily urinalysis QC log and kept for at least 3 years
   b. is not necessary unless the equipment is malfunctioning
   c. should be recorded in the patient's medical record

9. List six Clinical Laboratory Improvement Amendments (CLIA) regulations that apply to the clinical medical assistant performing urine testing.
   (1) ______________________________
   (2) ______________________________
   (3) ______________________________
   (4) ______________________________
   (5) ______________________________
   (6) ______________________________

10. A. One of the most important steps in the collection of urine specimens is to correctly identify the specimen through proper labeling. Make up your own identification (ID), use Dr. Mark Woo as your physician and write out complete labeling information for a specimen of your own urine below.

    Correct urine specimen label: ______________________________

    ____

    B. What is the proper procedure for testing an unlabeled or incorrectly labeled specimen?

    ____

    C. Name the four types of urine specimens frequently ordered by physicians.
    (1) ______________ (3) ______________
    (2) ______________ (4) ______________

    D. Name the four methods of urine collected ordered by physicians.
    (1) ______________ (3) ______________
    (2) ______________ (4) ______________

11. A. What are the four steps in a physical examination of a urine specimen?
    (1) ______________________________
    (2) ______________________________
    (3) ______________________________
    (4) ______________________________

B. What does the specific gravity of urine indicate? ______________________

C. Name three methods of measuring the specific gravity of a urine specimen and state the advantages or disadvantages of each. Place a C by the method that is available in conjunction with chemical testing.

(1) ______________________

(2) ______________________

(3) ______________________

12. Reagent test strips, or dipsticks, are used to test urine for many metabolic processes, including kidney and liver functions, urinary tract infection, and pH balance.

A. *Match each test below to the information that best describes it.*

______ 1. glucose	______ 5. nitrites	______ 8. ketones
______ 2. pH	______ 6. leukocyte	______ 9. protein
______ 3. urobilinogen	______ 7. specific gravity	______ 10. bilirubin
______ 4. blood		

A. These occur during prolonged fasting. They appear when excessive amounts of fatty acids are broken down into simpler compounds and when glucose availability is limited.

B. Increased levels of this substance suggest liver disease or bleeding disorders. It is a degradation product of bilirubin formed by intestinal bacteria.

C. This substance in a urine sample indicates infection, urinary tract trauma, kidney bleeding, and menses.

D. This substance can increase during a high fever and also indicates injury to the kidney, specifically to the glomerular membrane.

E. This test indicates white blood cells in the urinary tract, presumably attracted by invading bacteria.

F. This test detects unsuspected diabetes or is used to check the efficiency of insulin therapy in patients with diabetes.

G. This test changes color, depending on the ion concentration in urine. The highest reading available on the test is 1.030.

H. This test has a range of 4.6 to 8.0 and measures the acidity or alkalinity of the urine. A reading less than 7.0 indicates increased acidity; greater than 7.0 indicates increased alkalinity.

I. The presence of this substance indicates a urinary tract infection, because it is normally absent from urine. It is formed from the conversion of nitrates by certain species of bacteria.

J. This substance, a product of the breakdown of hemoglobin, breaks down in the light; a urine sample should be protected from light during testing.

B. How should reagent test strips be handled and stored?

____

____

____

13. The results of reagent strips are screening results; some positive results must be confirmed by further testing. For each substance below, identify the confirming test used. Then match each entry to the information that best fits each test.

_________________________________ (1) Reducing sugars

_________________________________ (2) Protein

_________________________________ (3) Ketones

_________________________________ (4) Bilirubin

______ A. This test includes a tablet and an absorbent mat. A purple color will develop when a urine drop is placed on a moist mat if the substance is present.

______ B. This test is used to detect lactose and galactose and is performed when the glucose test is positive on the reagent test strip.

______ C. In this test, a 2+ result is cloudy and granular.

______ D. A drop of urine added to a tablet will produce a purple color when this substance, produced during an increased metabolism of fat, is present.

14. Microscopic examination of urine sediment is also a valuable diagnostic tool for physicians.

A. *Match each type of sediment listed to the statement that best describes it.*

A. white blood cells	D. renal epithelial cells	G. red blood cells
B. yeast	E. bacteria	H. protozoa
C. squamous epithelial cells	F. artifacts	I. sperm

______ 1. Hair, fiber, air bubbles, and oil are common examples

______ 2. These skin cells are not medically significant and are sloughed off continuously in urine

______ 3. *Trichomonas vaginalis* is the most common example

______ 4. Cocci, bacilli, and spirilla

______ 5. These cells appear as pale, light-refractive disks; they are counted in a microscopic field and reported as cells per high-power field (HPF)

______ 6. These cells are larger than erythrocytes, have a visible nucleus, and may appear granular; they are reported as cells per HPF

______ 7. These are reported only when seen in male urine, unless specifically requested by the physician

______ 8. *Candida albicans* is the most common example

______ 9. These cells can indicate kidney disease if present in large numbers and are easily confused with leukocytes and other skin cells. If suspected, the slide should be reviewed by the physician. They are reported as cells per HPF.

B. *In the circles below, draw an example of the sediment as seen under a microscope.*

1. Fiber, hair, air bubble artifact 2. Yeast 3. Squamous epithelial cells 4. Bacteria

15. Crystals are the most insignificant part of urinary sediment and are not usually an important element of microscopic analysis, though many laboratories do report them. However, a few crystals may indicate disease states; name three.

    (1) ____________________ (2) ____________________ (3) ____________________

16. Casts are formed when protein accumulates and precipitates in the kidney tubules and are then washed into the urine. Identify each cast below and draw an example in the circle provided.

A. **B.** **C.**

______________________________ A. These casts contain remnants of disintegrated cells that have a fine or coarse appearance.

______________________________ B. These casts contain leukocytes, erythrocytes, or skin cells.

______________________________ C. These casts are difficult to see under the microscope without some light adjustment because of their near transparency.

CERTIFICATION REVIEW

These questions are designed to mimic the certification examinations. You can use these questions like a small "Certification Examination Study Guide," but this is not meant to take the place of the more extensive study guides. Use this portion to determine in what areas to concentrate your efforts when studying for the certification examination.

1. The filtering unit of the kidney is called the:
   a. meatus
   b. glomerulus
   c. ureter
   d. urethra

2. A common medication used to treat bladder infections and that turns the urine bright orange is:
   a. Pyridium®
   b. Zestoretic®
   c. propranolol
   d. Neurontin

3. The urine of a diabetic patient with ketoacidosis may smell:
   a. musty
   b. sour
   c. putrid
   d. sweet

4. The curvature that appears in a liquid's upper surface when placed in a container is the:
   a. specific gravity
   b. urobilinogen
   c. meniscus
   d. buffy coat

5. The most common type of cast seen in urine sediment is:
   a. hyaline
   b. granular
   c. waxy
   d. cellular

CASE STUDIES

Case 1

At Inner City Health Care, Wanda Slawson, CMA, gives patient Wendy Janus written directions for a 24-hour urine collection to be performed at home, but Wendy misplaces them. Wanda must give directions to Wendy over the telephone.

1. What directions should be given to the patient to correctly perform the urine collection?
2. What communication techniques should Wendy use to make sure the patient understands the collection procedures? What other potential alternatives for communicating the information, besides the telephone, are available?

Case 2

Wanda Slawson, CMA, is asked to give a male adolescent patient the proper procedure for a clean catch specimen. The 15-year-old boy is visibly embarrassed and will not hold eye contact with Wanda as she relates the instructions for collection to him.

1. What instructions are relevant for a clean-catch specimen for this patient?
2. What communication techniques should Wanda use in working with this patient?

SELF-ASSESSMENT

1. Have you ever had a urinalysis test performed?
2. Were you ever given proper instructions? If not, why do you think you were not instructed properly. If you were, did you understand clearly what you were to do?
3. Were instructions clearly written and posted in the restroom at a location that was readable during the collection?
4. Do you think good patient preparation and instructions influence the result of the test performed? In what way?
5. Now that you know the importance of proper patient teaching, how will your experience and training influence your work as a medical assistant in other areas of patient education?

POST-TEST

This is similar to the Pre-Test. Perform this test without looking at the book. This is just to see how well you have understood and can recall the information presented in this chapter after you have studied it and completed the workbook exercises. You will not be graded on this portion (other than the grade you give yourself), but this is an excellent preparation for your instructor's test. You may use this Post-Test to determine what areas you need to study more. Justify any "false" answers.

1. Which part of the urinalysis is to be performed by the medical assistant?
   a. the chemical examination
   b. the physical examination
   c. the specific gravity
   d. all of the above
2. Fat hemolysis is indicated by what in the urine?
   a. sugar
   b. bacteria
   c. protein
   d. ketones
3. If the patient brought a urine sample in a mayonnaise jar from home, you would:
   a. provide the patient with an appropriate container and ask for a fresh sample
   b. politely accept it this time, but after this, you will give the patient a proper container
   c. accept it if it is a first morning void and the container is clean
   d. a and c
4. The most common collection of urine in the POL is the:
   a. clean-catch, midstream specimen collection
   b. random collection
   c. timed specimen
   d. a and b

5. The written patient instructions for a midstream, clean catch should be:
   a. posted in the restroom beside the toilet
   b. posted in the restroom above the sink
   c. posted in the restroom behind the door
   d. handed to the patient as he or she enters
6. The minimum amount of urine needed for a complete urinalysis is 20 ml. (T or F)
7. Pyridium, a bladder analgesic, can:
   a. turn the urine a bright orange to red and may stain clothes
   b. decrease urine flow
   c. quiet down bladder irritation
   d. a and c

CERTIFICATION CRITERIA CHECKLIST

As you go through your education and training, keep in mind the national certification examination that you will take when you graduate. Each chapter of the textbook and workbook covers a different section of the examination criteria. To keep track of your preparation for the certification examination, turn to the back of this workbook and highlight the following CMA, RMA, or CMAS certification examination criteria (if you have already highlighted them from a previous chapter, put a check mark by the criteria):

CMA
B. Anatomy and Physiology
    2. Systems, including structure, function related conditions and diseases
F. Medicolegal Guidelines & Requirements
    2. Legislation
R. Principles of Infection Control
T. Patient Preparation and Assisting the Physician
    5. Explanation and instructions
V. Collecting and Processing Specimens; Diagnostic Testing

RMA
I. General Medical Assisting Knowledge
    A. Anatomy and Physiology
    F. Patient Education
III. Clinical Medical Assisting
    A. Asepsis
    I. Laboratory Procedures

CMAS
1. Medical Assisting Foundation
    • Anatomy and physiology
2. Basic Clinical Medical Office Assisting
    • Asepsis in the medical office
3. Medical Office Clerical
    • Communication

COMPETENCY ASSESSMENT

Procedure 42-1 Assessing Urine Volume, Color, and Clarity

Performance Objectives: Determine and document the volume, color, and clarity of a urine sample. Perform this objective within 5 minutes with a minimum score of 55 points.

Supplies/Equipment: Gloves, urine container, biohazard container, disinfectant cleaner, laboratory report form

Charting/Documentation: Enter appropriate documentation/charting in the box.

____

____

____

____

Instructor's/Evaluator's Comments and Suggestions:

____

____

____

____

____

____

SKILLS CHECKLIST Procedure 42-1: Assessing Urine Volume, Color, and Clarity

Name ______________________

Date ______________________

No.	Skill	Check #1 20 pts ea	Check #2 10 pts ea	Check #3 5 pts ea	Notes
1	Wash hands and put on gloves.				
2	Assemble equipment and supplies.				
3	Follow all safety guidelines, being careful not to splash the urine specimen. Wipe up any spills immediately with disinfectant.				
4	Examine the specimen for proper labeling. The cup should be labeled, not the lid. If the label is missing or illegible, request a new sample from the patient and notify the physician that there will be a delay.				
5	Ensure the lid is tightened, then mix thoroughly.				
6	Measure and note the amount of urine in the specimen if it is less than 10 ml. The amount of the specimen does not need to be noted if it is more than 10 ml.				
7	Assess and note the urine color against a white background with good lighting.				
8	Assess the clarity of the urine using the white background. Record any cloudiness as appropriate.				
9	Dispose of the specimen into the toilet or designated sink and dispose of all supplies into appropriate biohazard containers.				
10	Remove gloves, then wash hands.				
11	Document.				
Student's Total Points					
Points Possible		220	110	55	
Final Score (Student's Total Points / Possible Points)					

	Notes
Start time:	
End time:	
Total time: (5 min goal)	

COMPETENCY ASSESSMENT

Procedure 42-2 Using the Refractometer to Measure Specific Gravity

Performance Objectives: Measure and record the specific gravity of a urine specimen. Perform this objective within 5 minutes with a minimum score of 30 points.

Supplies/Equipment: Refractometer, gloves, urine sample, pipettes, distilled water, lint-free (lens) tissues, biohazard container, disinfectant, laboratory report form

Charting/Documentation: Enter appropriate documentation/charting in the box.

Instructor's/Evaluator's Comments and Suggestions:

SKILLS CHECKLIST Procedure 42-2: Using the Refractometer to Measure Specific Gravity

Name ______________________

Date ______________________

No.	Skill	Check #1 20 pts ea	Check #2 10 pts ea	Check #3 5 pts ea	Notes
1	Wash hands and put on gloves.				
2	Assemble equipment and supplies.				
3	Follow all safety guidelines, being careful not to splash the urine specimen. Wipe up all spills immediately with disinfectant cleanser.				
4	Perform quality control on the refractometer by checking it using distilled water:				
	a. Clean the surface of the prism and the cover with lint-free tissue and distilled water. Dry.				
	b. Depending on the type of refractometer being used, either close the cover and then apply a drop of distilled water, or apply the water and then close the cover. Either way, the water should flow over the surface of the prism.				
	c. With the instrument toward a light, view the scale. It should read exactly 1.000.				
	d. If the reading is correct, document it. If the reading is off, adjust the calibration with a small screwdriver.				
5	Test the urine sample exactly as the distilled water was tested and record the specific gravity on the urinalysis report form.				
6	Dispose of the specimen into the toilet or designated sink and all supplies into the appropriate containers. The slide, coverslip, and test tube should be put into a sharps container. Disinfect all reusable equipment and all surfaces.				
Student's Total Points					
Points Possible		120	60	30	
Final Score (Student's Total Points / Possible Points)					

	Notes
Start time:	
End time:	
Total time: (5 min goal)	

COMPETENCY ASSESSMENT

Procedure 42-3 Performing a Urinalysis Chemical Examination

Performance Objectives: Detect any abnormal chemical constituents of a urine specimen. Perform this objective within 15 minutes with a minimum score of 75 points.

Supplies/Equipment: Gloves, urine test strips, urine specimen, biohazard container, disinfectant cleaner, laboratory report form

Charting/Documentation: Enter appropriate documentation/charting in the box.

Instructor's/Evaluator's Comments and Suggestions:

SKILLS CHECKLIST Procedure 42-3: Performing a Urinalysis Chemical Examination

Name ______________________

Date ______________________

No.	Skill	Check #1 20 pts ea	Check #2 10 pts ea	Check #3 5 pts ea	Notes
1	Wash hands and put on gloves.				
2	Assemble equipment and supplies.				
3	Follow all safety guidelines, being careful not to splash the urine specimen. Wipe up all spills immediately with disinfectant cleanser.				
4	Examine the specimen for proper labeling. The cup should be labeled, not the lid. If the label is incorrect, missing, or illegible, notify the patient to submit a new sample, notify the physician of the delay, and document.				
5	Ensure the lid is securely tightened and mix the urine thoroughly.				
6	If you are planning to perform a complete urinalysis, label a urine centrifuge tube with the patient's name and pour 10 ml into the tube for the microscopic examination. Set aside in the centrifuge.				
7	Read and follow the manufacturer's instructions exactly. The following is a generic guideline.				
8	Remove a test strip from the container and replace the cap tightly.				
9	Immerse the test strip completely in the well-mixed urine and remove it immediately. While removing, tap it gently onto a paper towel to remove excess urine.				
10	Properly time the test for each test pad.				
11	Holding the test strip close to the container or chart, but not touching it, compare the color of the pads on the test strip with the color guide.				
12	Record the results on the laboratory report form.				

No.	Skill	Check #1 20 pts ea	Check #2 10 pts ea	Check #3 5 pts ea	Notes
13	Dispose of the specimen into the toilet or designated sink and all supplies into appropriate bio-hazard containers.				
14	Remove gloves and wash hands.				
15	Document in the patient's chart or medical record.				
Student's Total Points					
Points Possible		300	150	75	
Final Score (Student's Total Points / Possible Points)					

	Notes
Start time:	
End time:	
Total time: (15 min goal)	

COMPETENCY ASSESSMENT

Procedure 42-4 Preparing Slide for Microscopic Examination of Urine Sediment

Performance Objectives: Prepare a slide for a microscopic examination of urine sediment. Perform this objective within 15 minutes with a minimum score of 60 points.

Supplies/Equipment: Gloves, microscope, centrifuge, microscope slides, cover slips, disposable pipettes, centrifuge tubes and holder, urine atlas guide, disinfectant cleaner, biohazard container, sharps container, SediStain (optional)

Charting/Documentation: Enter appropriate documentation/charting in the box.

Instructor's/Evaluator's Comments and Suggestions:

SKILLS CHECKLIST Procedure 42-4: Preparing Slide for Microscopic Examination of Urine Sediment

Name ______________________

Date ______________________

No.	Skill	Check #1 20 pts ea	Check #2 10 pts ea	Check #3 5 pts ea	Notes
1	Wash hands and put on gloves.				
2	Assemble equipment and supplies.				
3	Follow all safety guidelines, being careful not to splash the urine specimen. Wipe up all spills immediately with disinfectant cleanser.				
4	Examine the specimen for proper labeling. The label should be on the cup, not the lid. If the label is incorrect, illegible, or missing, request a new sample from the patient and notify the physician of the delay.				
5	Ensure the lid is securely tightened and mix the urine thoroughly.				
6	Label a urine centrifuge tube with the patient's name and pour 10 ml into the tube. Set into the centrifuge. Balance the centrifuge, securely close and lock the lid, and spin at 1,500 rpm for 5 minutes.				
7	After centrifugation, pour off the supernatant leaving about 1 ml in the bottom of the tube. Add two drops of SediStain if desired. Remix the sediment by tapping on the counter or with your fingernail.				
8	Place a drop of the well-mixed sediment onto a clean microscope slide. Cover with a coverslip by holding the coverslip at an angle to the drop, bringing the edge close to the drop until the urine spreads along the edge of the cover slip, then gently lower the cover slip onto the drop.				
9	Place the slide on to the microscope stage but do not leave the light on.				
10	Alert the physician that the slide is ready for viewing.				

No.	Skill	Check #1 20 pts ea	Check #2 10 pts ea	Check #3 5 pts ea	Notes
11	The following steps are included, though the physician must perform the actual assessment:				
	a. When examining urine sediment, keep the light subdued by lowering the condenser and constantly varying the fine-focus adjustment.				
	b. Scan the sediment using a 100× (low-power) magnification.				
	c. View 10 to 15 fields and around the edge of the slide for casts.				
	d. Scan the slide using the 40× objective for other cells and formed elements.				
12	Dispose of the specimen into the toilet or designated sink and all supplies into appropriate biohazard containers. The slide, coverslip, and tube should go into sharps container.				
Student's Total Points					
Points Possible		240	120	60	
Final Score (Student's Total Points / Possible Points)					
		Notes			
Start time:					
End time:					
Total time: (15 min goal)					

COMPETENCY ASSESSMENT

Procedure 42-5 Performing a Complete Urinalysis

Performance Objectives: Perform a complete urinalysis, including the physical and chemical examinations, and prepare for the microscopic examination test within 30 minutes of obtaining the specimen. Perform this objective within 20 minutes with a minimum score of 70 points.

Supplies/Equipment: Gloves, urine specimen, pipettes, centrifuge tube, centrifuge, microscope, microscope slides, cover slip, permanent marker, reagent strips (dipsticks), urine atlas, refractometer, distilled water, lint-free tissues, biohazard container, sharps container, disinfectant cleaner, laboratory report form, SediStain (optional)

Charting/Documentation: Enter appropriate documentation/charting in the box.

Instructor's/Evaluator's Comments and Suggestions:

SKILLS CHECKLIST Procedure 42-5: Performing a Complete Urinalysis

Name ______________________

Date ______________________

No.	Skill	Check #1 20 pts ea	Check #2 10 pts ea	Check #3 5 pts ea	Notes
1	Wash hands and put on gloves.				
2	Assemble equipment and supplies.				
3	Follow all safety guidelines, being careful not to splash the urine specimen. Wipe up all spills immediately with disinfectant.				
4	Examine the specimen for proper labeling. The label must be on the cup, not the lid. If the label is incorrect, illegible, or missing, request a new sample from the patient and notify the physician of the delay.				
5	Ensure the lid is securely tightened and mix the urine thoroughly.				
6	Label a urine centrifuge tube with the patient's name and pour 10 ml into the tube for the microscopic examination. Set into the centrifuge. Balance the centrifuge, securely close and lock the lid, and spin at 1,500 rpm for 5 minutes.				
7	While the sample is being centrifuged, assess and record the color and clarity.				
8	Perform quality control on the refractometer. Perform the specific gravity test using a refractometer if specific gravity is not included in the chemical test strip. Record.				
9	Perform the chemical examination following the manufacturer's instructions. Record the results.				
10	After centrifugation, pour off the supernatant leaving about 1 ml in the bottom of the tube. Add two drops of SediStain if desired. Remix the sediment by tapping on the counter or with your fingernail.				
11	Place a drop of the well-mixed sediment onto a clean microscope slide. Cover with a coverslip.				

No.	Skill	Check #1 20 pts ea	Check #2 10 pts ea	Check #3 5 pts ea	Notes
12	Place the slide onto the microscope stage and alert the physician that the slide is ready for viewing. Do not leave on the light of the microscope.				
13	Dispose of the specimen into the toilet or designated sink and all supplies into appropriate biohazard containers.				
14	File the completed laboratory report form into the laboratory section of the patient's medical record/chart. Document the procedure.				
Student's Total Points					
Points Possible		280	140	70	
Final Score (Student's Total Points / Possible Points)					

	Notes
Start time:	
End time:	
Total time: (20 min goal)	

COMPETENCY ASSESSMENT

Procedure 42-6 Utilizing a Urine Transport System for C&S

Performance Objectives: Prepare a urine specimen for transport using a culture and sensitivity transport kit. Perform this objective within 10 minutes with a minimum score of 50 points.

Supplies/Equipment: Gloves, sterile urine cup and specimen, urine culture and sensitivity transport kit, laboratory requisition, paper towel

Charting/Documentation: Enter appropriate documentation/charting in the box.

Instructor's/Evaluator's Comments and Suggestions:

SKILLS CHECKLIST Procedure 42-6: Utilizing a Urine Transport System for C&S

Name ______________________

Date ______________________

No.	Skill	Check #1 20 pts ea	Check #2 10 pts ea	Check #3 5 pts ea	Notes
1	Wash hands and put on gloves.				
2	Assemble equipment and supplies (Figure 42-21A shows one system).				
3	Follow all safety guidelines, being careful not to splash the urine specimen. Wipe up all spills immediately with disinfectant cleanser.				
4	Examine the specimen for proper labeling. The label should be on the cup, not the lid. If the label is incorrect, missing, or illegible, request a new sample from the patient and notify the physician of the delay.				
5	Check the urine culture and sensitivity transport kit expiration date.				
6	Open the urine culture and sensitivity transport kit package (see Figure 42-21B). Remove the cap from the specimen cup, placing the lid upside down on the paper towel.				
7	Follow the manufacturer's instructions exactly (depending on the system being used):				
	a. Place the urine tube into the adapter (see Figure 42-21C) and the specimen straw into the urine (see Figure 42-21D).				
	b. Advance the urine tube into the adapter, pushing the tube onto the needle while keeping the specimen straw submerged in urine.				
	c. Allow the vacuum in the urine tube to draw up the urine. Fill to the exhaustion of the vacuum tube (see Figure 42-21E).				
	d. Remove the tube and the specimen straw/adapter unit and dispose of it into biohazard waste.				
	e. Gently invert the tube 8 to 10 times to mix the preservative within the tube.				

No.	Skill	Check #1 20 pts ea	Check #2 10 pts ea	Check #3 5 pts ea	Notes
8	Label the tube with patient's name, date, time, and other required information.				
9	Dispose of all contaminated supplied, disinfect all surfaces, remove gloves, and wash hands.				
10	Complete the laboratory requisition. Document the procedure in the patient's chart/medical record.				
Student's Total Points					
Points Possible		200	100	50	
Final Score (Student's Total Points / Possible Points)					

	Notes
Start time:	
End time:	
Total time: (10 min goal)	

COMPETENCY ASSESSMENT

Procedure 42-7 Instructing a Patient in the Collection of a Clean-Catch, Midstream Urine Specimen

Performance Objectives: To instruct a patient in the proper technique of collecting a urine specimen suitable for urinalysis testing. Perform this objective within 15 minutes with a minimum score of 60 points.

Supplies/Equipment: Gloves, urine cup with a secure lid, cleansing towelettes, marking pen, written instructions posted appropriately in the bathroom

Charting/Documentation: Enter appropriate documentation/charting in the box.

____

____

____

____

Instructor's/Evaluator's Comments and Suggestions:

____

____

____

____

____

____

SKILLS CHECKLIST Procedure 42-7: Instructing a Patient in the Collection of a Clean-Catch, Midstream Urine Specimen

Name ______________________

Date ______________________

No.	Skill	Check #1 20 pts ea	Check #2 10 pts ea	Check #3 5 pts ea	Notes
1	Wash hands and assemble the supplies.				
2	Identify the patient, introduce yourself, and provide for a private area with no distractions.				
3	Provide the patient with a capped urine cup labeled with his or her name, a pair of gloves, and the cleansing towelettes.				
4	Show the patient the written instructions posted in the bathroom.				
5	Explain to the patient why the urine sample should be a mid-stream clean-catch sample and what that means.				
6	Ask the patient to first wash his or her hands and apply the gloves.				
7	Explain the cleansing process for a clean-catch:				
	a. For the male patient, explain that he is to cleanse the urethral opening twice, using two separate towelettes, before he begins to urinate.				
	b. For the female patient, explain that she will need to spread her labia and cleanse from front to back first on one side, then the other, and finally in the middle. Explain that she is to hold her labia apart until the urine sample is obtained.				
8	Explain the process of obtaining the midstream specimen: For both male and female patients, they are to bring the cup into the stream and obtain about half a cup before removing the cup from the stream.				
9	Explain to the patient the he or she should then secure the cap onto the cup.				
10	The patient may rinse the outside of the capped cup if needed and dry it with a towel.				

No.	Skill	Check #1 20 pts ea	Check #2 10 pts ea	Check #3 5 pts ea	Notes
11	The patient is to then remove the gloves, dispose of them into the red bag waste recepticle, and wash her or his hands.				
12	The cup may be returned to the medical assistant or placed in the laboratory recepticle as directed.				
Student's Total Points					
Points Possible		240	120	60	
Final Score (Student's Total Points / Possible Points)					

	Notes
Start time:	
End time:	
Total time: (15 min goal)	

EVALUATION OF CHAPTER KNOWLEDGE

Evaluate your comprehension of urinalysis, including proper collection and handling techniques; safety guidelines involved; and how to properly perform a complete urinalysis, including physical, chemical, and microscopic examinations.

Skills	Student Self-Evaluation Good	Average	Poor
I understand the importance of urinalysis as a diagnostic tool.	_____	_____	_____
I understand how urine is formed and excreted in the human body.	_____	_____	_____
I can define key terms related to urinalysis found in the glossary.	_____	_____	_____
I understand the crucial role that safety procedures and quality control play in performing a urinalysis.	_____	_____	_____
I can accurately perform a physical examination of urine and explain causes of abnormal physical characteristics in urine specimens.	_____	_____	_____
I can accurately perform a chemical examination of urine and explain causes of abnormal chemical characteristics in urine specimens.	_____	_____	_____
I can explain causes of abnormal microscopic characteristics in urine specimens.	_____	_____	_____
I am able to describe confirmatory tests for ketones, glucose, protein, and bilirubin.	_____	_____	_____
I can identify the proper method of preparing urine sediment for microscopic examination.	_____	_____	_____
I am able to identify both normal and abnormal structures discovered during the microscopic examination of urine sediment.	_____	_____	_____
I am aware of and can describe factors that may interfere with the accuracy of the urinalysis.	_____	_____	_____
I can perform proper documentation of urine testing procedures.	_____	_____	_____
I can follow Standard Precautions.	_____	_____	_____

CHAPTER 43

Basic Microbiology

CHAPTER PRE-TEST

Perform this test without looking at the book. This is just to see how well you have understood and can recall the information in this chapter after you have read it, but before you have completed the workbook exercises. You will not be graded on this portion (other than the grade you give yourself). Justify any "false" answers.

1. The field of microbiology does not include the study of:
   a. mice
   b. bacteria
   c. fungi
   d. parasites
2. The presence of any bacteria in the body is harmful. (T or F)
3. Media is:
   a. the microscopic slide that is smeared with a specimen
   b. the laboratory chemical that is used in testing
   c. a nutritional mixture specific to a particular type of bacteria
   d. a sample of body secretions that contains harmful pathogens
4. Mycology is the study of viruses. (T or F)
5. A safety hood is part of the medical assistant's protective equipment. (T or F)
6. Anaerobic organisms do not grow well in the presence of oxygen. (T or F)

7. Appropriate handling of specimens includes:
   a. wearing personal protective equipment (PPE)
   b. washing hands often
   c. wearing gloves
   d. all of the above

8. Microbial waste can be thrown out with the regular waste. (T or F)

9. Which of the following is not an important quality-control measure?
   a. Monitor the refrigerator temperatures daily.
   b. Culture media should be checked for accuracy with positive and negative controls.
   c. Occupational Safety and Health Administration (OSHA) manuals have to be updated periodically.
   d. Respect the expiration date of testing materials.

10. The Rapid Strep Test is popular because it eliminates false positives, is easy to read, and gives results in minutes. (T or F)

INTRODUCTION

Microbiology is an area of enormous importance in health care and one in which medical assistants play a role. Specimens are processed in either the physician's office laboratory (POL) or a reference laboratory. The emergence of pathogens increasing in resistance to antibiotics makes this area even more significant to the health professions. Rapid and precise culturing and identification of pathogens allows for appropriate treatment of the patient. The quality of the diagnosis and treatment of an infection is rooted in the quality of the specimen obtained and processed. Although laboratories will vary in size and extent of work, one thing will remain constant. Safety precautions and quality-control procedures must be carefully followed for the protection of health care professionals and for the integrity of test results.

PERFORMANCE OBJECTIVES

After successful completion of this chapter you will be able to explain the medical terms related to microbiology. You will be able to describe bacterial cell structure, site differences between pathogenic and nonpathogenic microorganisms, explain how to safely handle microbiologic specimens, and describe how microorganisms are cultured and identified in a medical laboratory setting. You will become proficient in safely and accurately obtaining specimens and using Clinical Laboratory Improvement Amendments (CLIA)-waived tests to assist in diagnosing infections. You will be familiar with treatments that are appropriate for various infections and will be able to educate your patients in preventing infections and the spread of infections from person to person. *The following statements are related to your learning objectives for this chapter. Fill in the blanks in the following paragraph with the appropriate term(s).*

The field of (1) ________________ encompasses the study of all microorganisms. The medical assistant's role in microbiology in the POL is to (2) ____________________ the specimen, test the specimen within (3) ___________________________________ categories, and prepare the slide and (4) ____________________ for examination by the physician. Some of the equipment used by the medical assistant within the POL for microbiological tests are the (5) ____________________ used to sterilize equipment, the (6) ____________________ to examine microscopic organisms, the (7) ____________________ to protect the workers from airborne particles, and (8) ____________________ to create a warm environment for growing cultures; some (9) ____________________ equipment for those microbes that do not do well in oxygen environments, the (10) ____________________ equipment that will consist mostly of wires, loops, and needles. Also found in the microbiology laboratory is an (11) ____________________ for quick sterilization of the inoculating instruments, a variety of (12) ____________________ for the various needs of different microbes, and a small (13) ____________________ to store media and kits that require cooler temperatures. Safety is always a major concern in the medical laboratory, but especially when handling dangerous potential (14) ____________________. PPE or (15) ____________________ should always be worn. The work area should be (16) ____________________ with strong (17) ____________________ on a regular basis and whenever it becomes contaminated. Whenever specimens are brought into the POL for testing, the medical assistant should be careful the check for (18) ____________________ and contaminations on the outside of the containers; and, of course, all specimens should be handled as if they were (19) ____________________. Biohazard waste is usually placed in (20) ____________________ biohazard bags marked with the (21) ____________________ biohazard symbol. The best disinfectant for biohazard spills is a 10% solution of household (22) ____________________.

VOCABULARY BUILDER

Find the words listed below that are misspelled; circle them, and then correctly spell them in the spaces provided. Then match each of the vocabulary terms listed below with its correct definition.

_______ 1. erobic	A. The science and study of fungi
_______ 2. culture	B. The act of coughing up material from the air passages
_______ 3. genus	C. Deoxyribonucleic acid
_______ 4. imunosuppressed	D. Infection acquired in a hospital
_______ 5. anerobic	E. A microorganism or substance capable of producing disease
_______ 6. mycology	F. The study of parasites
_______ 7. dermatophyte	G. Living only in the presence of oxygen
_______ 8. mordant	H. Prevention of the activation of an immune response
_______ 9. innoculate	I. A class that includes the true roundworm or threadworm
_______ 10. nosocomial	J. Living only in the absence of oxygen
_______ 11. DNA	K. A fungal parasite that grows on the skin
_______ 12. expectorate	L. The propagation of microorganisms in a special media conducive to their growth
_______ 13. microbiology	
_______ 14. morphology	
_______ 15. nematode	

_______ 16. parasitology

_______ 17. pathogen

____

____

____

____

M. The classification between family and species

N. To inject an antigen, antiserum, or antitoxin to produce immunity

O. A substance that fixes a stain or dye

P. The scientific study of microorganisms

Q. The science of structure and form without regard to function

LEARNING REVIEW

1. Infections from parasites have increased as more people travel and public awareness of the symptoms grow.
   A. The most common parasite infections seen in the laboratory are _______________ _______________, a nematode that causes pinworm infections and _______________ _______________, a flagellate that causes a sexually transmitted disease in both men and women.
   B. Specimens collected for parasites need to be checked for _______________, _______________, and _______________.
   C. Labeling specimens sent for testing with _______________, _______________, and _______________ collected is important, as well as noting if the patient has been _______________ to a specific place and what the physician suspects.
   D. To diagnose the presence of a parasite, either the _______________ _______________ or _______________ must be located in the specimen.
   E. Obtaining the specimen to test for pinworms is performed by using a _______________ _______________ _______________ that is placed sticky side down to the skin around the anal area.
   F. _______________ _______________ _______________ should be worn when working with specimens. Assuming that all specimens are _______________ is an important element of following Standard Precautions for infection control.
   G. The practice of proper aseptic _______________ _______________ several times a day, including after glove removal, is essential and should become a _______________.

2. Specimen containers will arrive at the laboratory inside biohazard plastic transport bags to avoid danger to laboratory personnel. What precautions are taken before opening the bags?

____

____

3. A laboratory's success in finding and identifying the pathogenic organism depends on multiple factors. Name nine.

(1) _______________ (6) _______________

(2) _______________ (7) _______________

(3) _______________ (8) _______________

(4) _______________ (9) _______________

(5) _______________

4. Describe how you feel about working with patients who have an infection, which is possibly communicable. What, if anything, concerns you? What resources do you have in addressing your concerns?

____

____

____

5. The medical assistant in a physician's office will most likely frequently assist in the care and treatment of patients with sore throats.

   Why is it necessary to rapidly identify the cause? _______________

   What test would be used? _______________

   What five rules should be followed?

   (1) _______________
   (2) _______________
   (3) _______________
   (4) _______________
   (5) _______________

6. *Label the parts of the cell and check off "Some" for the parts that are sometimes present and "All" for the parts that are always present.*

Basic Bacterial Cell

	Some	All
A. _______________	☐	☐
B. _______________	☐	☐
C. _______________	☐	☐
D. _______________	☐	☐
E. _______________	☐	☐
F. _______________	☐	☐

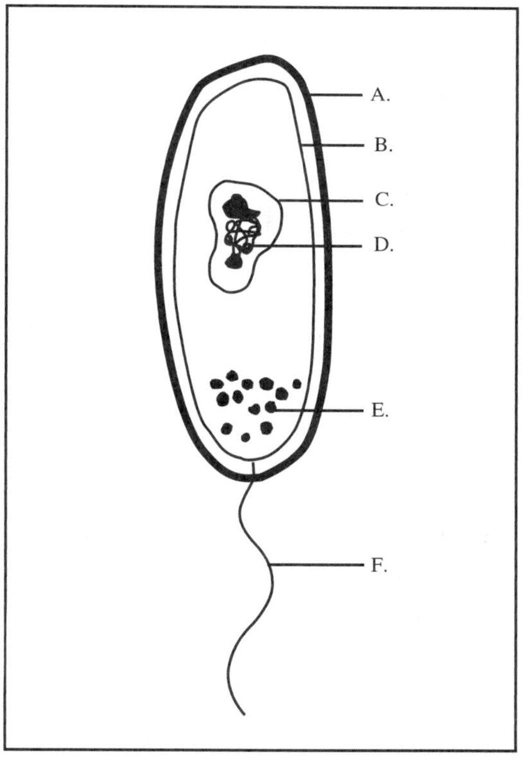

CERTIFICATION REVIEW

These questions are designed to mimic the certification examinations. You can use these questions like a small "Certification Examination Study Guide," but this is not meant to take the place of the more extensive study guides. Use this portion to determine in what areas to concentrate your efforts when studying for the certification examination.

1. Common nosocomial infections are caused by:
   a. salmonella
   b. staphylococcus
   c. shigella
   d. protista
2. Some bacteria produce __________, which are so resistant that they can live 150,000 years.
   a. flagella
   b. cell walls
   c. nuclei
   d. spores
3. Septicemia is a:
   a. blood infection
   b. throat infection
   c. urinary tract infection
   d. respiratory infection
4. Bacilli are:
   a. rod shaped
   b. round
   c. spiral shaped
   d. found in clusters
5. Gram-negative bacteria stain:
   a. purple
   b. pink
   c. red
   d. green

CASE STUDIES

Case 1

Winston Lewis, MD, has ordered a series of three sputum cultures for Herb Fowler, who has been suffering with a productive cough for several months and extreme fatigue. Audrey Jones, CMA, is assigned to obtain the cultures. When each culture is obtained from Mr. Fowler, Audrey brings it to the POL for culturing.

Discuss the following:

1. What is the procedure for obtaining a sputum specimen? Why are detailed patient instructions critical?
2. Mr. Fowler wishes to give all three specimens in one day to save on the transportation to and from the physician's office. Audrey explains that the specimens must be obtained one each day, on awakening, for three days. What is the reason for this?
3. What microorganisms might the physician suspect, and how should the specimen be treated in the POL? Under what circumstances should the specimen be sent to an outside reference laboratory for further testing?

Case 2

Mary O'Keefe calls for an emergency appointment for her 3-year-old son, Chris, because he awakened during the night with a high fever and severe pain in his right ear, which is draining. Dr. King performs the examination, assisted by Ellen Armstrong, CMA. During the examination, Dr. King takes a specimen of the fluid ear discharge for laboratory analysis, which the physician suspects will confirm a clinical diagnosis of otitis media. Dr. King asks Ellen to perform a Gram stain on a portion of the patient specimen and to send the remainder of the specimen to an outside reference laboratory for culturing.

Discuss the following:

1. What equipment will Ellen require to perform the Gram staining of the specimen?
2. What Standard Precautions must Ellen observe while performing the Gram stain procedure?
3. If a strain of *Streptococcus* or *Staphylococcus* bacteria is responsible for the infection producing the patient's condition of otitis media, what Gram staining result will Ellen receive? What will the Gram-stained specimen look like under the microscope? (Consult a medical reference or encyclopedia, if necessary)

SELF-ASSESSMENT

Make a list of all the things that are done to keep your food and environment free of pathogens. This would include water purification, food processing, homogenization, antibacterial soap and cleansers, immunizations, and any other process you can think of.

1. After each item on the list, place a check mark by those that are available only to certain populations but not to underdeveloped countries and areas.
2. Discuss with fellow students which of the things on your lists could be implemented fairly simply and inexpensively.
3. Reorganize the lists starting with the easiest to implement and going toward the most expensive/difficult.
4. List other items or processes that would need to be done to implement each item on your list.

POST-TEST

This is similar to the Pre-Test. Perform this test without looking at the book. This is just to see how well you have understood and can recall the information presented in this chapter after you have studied it and completed the workbook exercises. You will not be graded on this portion (other than the grade you give yourself), but this is an excellent preparation for your instructor's test. You may use this Post-Test to determine what areas you need to study more. Justify any "false" answers.

1. The field of microbiology includes:
   a. bacteria, fungi, vectors, and parasites
   b. mice, their parasites, and bacteria
   c. fungi, bacteria, viruses, and other microbes
   d. parasites, fungi, viruses, bacteria, and vectors
2. Many bacteria are normal in our bodies. (T or F)
3. Media is:
   a. the laboratory chemical that is used in testing
   b. the microscopic slide that is smeared with a specimen
   c. a sample of body secretions that contains harmful pathogens
   d. a nutritional mixture specific to a particular type of bacteria
4. Mycology is the study of fungi. (T or F)
5. An incubator is part of the medical assistant's protective equipment. (T or F)
6. Anaerobic organisms grow well in the presence of oxygen. (T or F)
7. Appropriate handling of specimens includes:
   a. wearing PPE
   b. wearing gloves
   c. washing hands often
   d. all of the above
8. Microbial waste should not be thrown out with the regular waste. (T or F)
9. Which of the following is not an important quality-control measure?
   a. OSHA manuals have to be updated periodically.
   b. Check the refrigerator temperatures daily.
   c. Culture media should be checked for accuracy with positive and negative controls.
   d. Respect the expiration date of testing materials.
10. The Rapid Strep Test is popular because it is easy to read and is available in minutes, but it does often result in false positives. (T or F)

CERTIFICATION CRITERIA CHECKLIST

As you go through your education and training, keep in mind the national certification examination that you will take when you graduate. Each chapter of the textbook and workbook covers a different section of the examination criteria. To keep track of your preparation for the certification examination, turn to the back of this workbook and highlight the following CMA, RMA, or CMAS certification examination criteria (if you have already highlighted them from a previous chapter, put a check mark by the criteria):

CMA

F. Medicolegal Guidelines & Requirements
R. Principles of Infection Control
S. Treatment Area
    1. Equipment preparation and operation
    2. Principles of operation (equipment)
V. Collecting and Processing Specimens; Diagnostic Testing

RMA

I. General Medical Assisting Knowledge
    C. Medical Law
III. Clinical Medical Assisting
    A. Asepsis
    I. Laboratory Procedures

CMAS

1. Medical Assisting Foundation
    - Anatomy and physiology
2. Basic Clinical Medical Office Assisting
    - Asepsis in the medical office
3. Medical Office Clerical
    - Communication

COMPETENCY ASSESSMENT

Procedure 43-1 Procedure for Obtaining a Throat Specimen for Culture

Performance Objectives: To obtain secretions from the nasopharnyx and tonsillar area as a means of identifying pathogenic microorganisms. Perform this objective within 15 minutes with a minimum score of 65 points.

Supplies/Equipment: Tongue depressor, culture tube with applicator stick or commercially prepared culture collection system (culturette), label and requisition form, gloves and face shield, good light source

Charting/Documentation: Enter appropriate documentation/charting in the box.

Instructor's/Evaluator's Comments and Suggestions:

SKILLS CHECKLIST Procedure 43-1: Procedure for Obtaining a Throat Specimen for Culture

Name ______________________

Date ______________________

No.	Skill	Check #1 20 pts ea	Check #2 10 pts ea	Check #3 5 pts ea	Notes
1	Identify yourself and explain the procedure to the patient.				
2	Have an emesis basin and tissues ready.				
3	Have the patient in a sitting position.				
4	Wash hands, gather supplies, and apply gloves and face shield.				
5	Ask the patient to open his or her mouth wide, and then adjust the light source.				
6	Remove the swab from the culturette using sterile technique.				
7	Ask the patient to say "ah." Depress the tongue with the tongue depressor and swab the back of the throat and tonsillar area. Concentrate primarily on any red, raw areas and pustules. Take care not to touch the swab on the inside of the cheeks or on the tongue.				
8	Place the swab back into the culturette using sterile technique and crush the glass capsule containing the medium. If using a different type of culturette, pierce the membrane in the tube with the swab to release the culture medium.				
9	Label the culturette according to the physician's office laboratory policy and requirements.				
10	Ensure patient comfort and answer any questions related to the testing.				
11	Discard contaminated supplies into a biohazard waste container. Disinfect all work surfaces. Properly remove gloves and face shield and discard appropriately.				

No.	Skill	Check #1 20 pts ea	Check #2 10 pts ea	Check #3 5 pts ea	Notes
12	Wash hands.				
13	Complete laboratory requisition and record the procedure in the patient's medical record/chart.				
Student's Total Points					
Points Possible		260	130	65	
Final Score (Student's Total Points / Possible Points)					
		Notes			
Start time:					
End time:					
Total time: (15 min goal)					

COMPETENCY ASSESSMENT

Procedure 43-2 Wet Mount and Hanging Drop Slide Preparations

Performance Objectives: To prepare a slide for viewing live microorganisms for motility and identifying characteristics. Perform this objective within 15 minutes with a minimum score of 40 points.

Supplies/Equipment: Gloves, glass slide and coverslip, special slide with a well, petroleum jelly, dropper

Charting/Documentation: Enter appropriate documentation/charting in the box.

Instructor's/Evaluator's Comments and Suggestions:

SKILLS CHECKLIST Procedure 43-2: Wet Mount and Hanging Drop Slide Preparations

Name ______________________________

Date ______________________________

No.	Skill	Check #1 20 pts ea	Check #2 10 pts ea	Check #3 5 pts ea	Notes
1	Wash hands and apply gloves.				
2	Assemble equipment and supplies.				
3	**For wet mount slide preparation:**				
	a. Place a drop of the bacterial suspension onto a glass slide (Figure 43-21A).				
	b. Place petroleum jelly around the edges of the coverslip and place the coverslip on top of the bacterial suspension.				
	For hanging drop slide preparation:				
	a. Place the bacterial specimen (in suspension) in the center of the coverslip with the petroleum jelly around the edges.				
	b. Invert the slide and place the concave well of the slide over the specimen drop of the coverslip.				
	c. Turn the slide right side up for the physician to perform the microscopic examination.				
Student's Total Points					
Points Possible (8 steps total for both processes)		160	80	40	
Final Score (Student's Total Points / Possible Points)					

	Notes
Start time:	
End time:	
Total time: (15 min goal)	

COMPETENCY ASSESSMENT

Procedure 43-3 Performing Strep Throat Testing

Performance Objectives: To test for streptococcus infection of the throat for diagnostic purposes. The following steps are intentionally general, so a variety of kits can be used. Perform this objective within 15 minutes with a minimum score of 40 points.

Supplies/Equipment: Gloves, commercial strep throat testing kit including controls and standards, disinfectant, tongue blade, adjustable light source, biohazard container

Charting/Documentation: Enter appropriate documentation/charting in the box.

____

____

____

____

Instructor's/Evaluator's Comments and Suggestions:

____

____

____

____

____

____

SKILLS CHECKLIST Procedure 43-3: Performing Strep Throat Testing

Name ______________________________

Date ______________________________

No.	Skill	Check #1 20 pts ea	Check #2 10 pts ea	Check #3 5 pts ea	Notes
1	Assemble all necessary equipment and materials.				
2	Introduce yourself, identify the patient, and explain the procedure.				
3	Wash hands and apply gloves.				
4	Use the tongue blade, the light source, to obtain the specimen from the throat as described in Procedure 43-1, except do not fill out the laboratory requisition form.				
5	Follow the manufacturer's instructions *exactly* to perform the strep throat test. Be sure to also run the control tests.				
6	Properly dispose of all waste in biohazard container. Disinfect the area and any equipment used.				
7	Complete the laboratory report form and notify the physician of the results.				
8	Document the procedure in the patient's medical record.				
Student's Total Points					
Points Possible		160	80	40	
Final Score (Student's Total Points / Possible Points)					

	Notes
Start time:	
End time:	
Total time: (15 min goal)	

EVALUATION OF CHAPTER KNOWLEDGE

Skills	Student Self-Evaluation Good	Average	Poor
I can identify the components of PPE and important safety procedures.	_____	_____	_____
I can identify quality-control measures and describe uses of them in the laboratory.	_____	_____	_____
I understand the importance and methods of collecting high-quality specimens.	_____	_____	_____
I can list different types of specimens.	_____	_____	_____
I can describe bacterial cell structure and can discuss identification systems for bacteria.	_____	_____	_____
I can cite a variety of parasites and fungi.	_____	_____	_____
I can describe sensitivity testing	_____	_____	_____
I can describe the difference between the presence of microorganisms as normal flora and as pathogens.	_____	_____	_____
I understand the importance of patient education in obtaining specimens.	_____	_____	_____
I understand the importance of the use of quality controls in the laboratory and with laboratory equipment.	_____	_____	_____
I can describe the need to discard media and reagents that have passed the expiration date.	_____	_____	_____
I recognize the role of the medical assistant in the laboratory.	_____	_____	_____
I can follow precisely the correct procedures in performing tests in the laboratory.	_____	_____	_____

CHAPTER 44

Specialty Laboratory Tests

CHAPTER PRE-TEST

Perform this test without looking at the book. This is just to see how well you have understood and can recall the information in this chapter after you have read it, but before you have completed the workbook exercises. You will not be graded on this portion (other than the grade you give yourself). Justify any "false" answers.

1. How many different blood types are there?
   a. 3
   b. 5
   c. 4
   d. 8
2. The phenylketonuria (PKU) test is mandatory for all infants in all states. (T or F)
3. During pregnancy, the human chorionic gonadotropin (hCG) levels peak at 8 weeks. (T or F)
4. About 15% of the general population is Rh negative. (T or F)
5. The Rh system was named for the rhesus monkeys used in the experiments that led to the discovery of an Rh factor. (T or F)
6. Insulin helps regulate glucose levels in the blood. (T or F)
7. A purified protein derivative (PPD) is administered with an intradermal injection. (T or F)

INTRODUCTION

More tests than ever before are performed in the ambulatory care setting. As a result, the medical assistant's role in laboratory testing is expanding. To meet the challenge, medical assistants must have a solid understanding of medical terminology, laboratory procedures, safety procedures, and Standard Precautions for infection control. Quality-control programs and accuracy in the collection and handling of specimens, including blood specimens obtained by venipuncture, ensure accurate and reliable test results. Therapeutic communication, which helps gain the patient's cooperation in obtaining a good specimen for analysis, is an important skill for medical assistants to develop.

PERFORMANCE OBJECTIVES

After successful completion of this chapter you will be able to explain the medical terms related to specialty laboratory tests such as those tests for PKU, infectious mononucleosis, pregnancy, and glucose levels, as well as other waived tests performed with the use of a manufactured kit. You will also become familiar with preparing patients for nonwaived tests such as semen analysis, postprandial blood glucose, blood typing, and many others. You will learn the pathology of many specialized conditions and the transmission, prevention, treatment, and prognosis. You will learn about normal and abnormal blood values for glucose, triglycerides, cholesterol, phenylalanine, and blood urea. *The following statements are related to your learning objectives for this chapter. Fill in the blanks in the following paragraph with the appropriate term(s).*

Pregnancy testing is used when (1) ________________ is suspected and before prescribing (2) _____________, (3) ____________________, (4) ______________________ or other drugs, and before (5) __________________. The home pregnancy tests differ little from the physician's office laboratory (POL) test kits except for the appropriate (6) ________________________ measures and (7) ________________________ personnel. A positive pregnancy test does not necessarily diagnose a normal pregnancy. It could indicate an abnormal condition such as (8) ____________________ pregnancy, developing (9) __________________________ of the uterus, (10) __________________, or (11) ____________________________. Infectious mononucleosis is a (12) ___________________ disease that may have vague (13) _______________ symptoms and can mimic other diseases. Blood typing and Rh-factor testing are not considered (14) _____________ waived, but it is a fun test to perform in the medical assisting laboratory classroom because it shows (15) ______________________. Semen analysis requires considerable patient education before obtaining the sample because many factors can (16) ___________ the results. PKU stands for (17) _____________________ and is an (18) ___________________ condition. With a properly (19) ___________________________ diet, patients can do well. TB or (20) _______________________ screening is a commonly performed test in the POL. It consists of injecting a small amount of (21) ________________________________, and then observing a (22) _________________ 48 to 72 hours later. Blood glucose is commonly performed at home by (23) _____________________ patients and also in the POL. Another test performed in the POL that tells of the glucose control for the past 4 to 6 weeks is the (24) __________________________________, or hemoglobin A1c for short. Screening tests for cholesterol, (25) ______________________, and (26) ________________________ are also readily available automated tests performed in the POL. The chemical within the blood may be tested in a test called a chemistry (27) ___________________________, which is performed almost routinely now in many laboratories.

VOCABULARY BUILDER

Find the words listed below that are misspelled; circle them, and then correctly spell them in the spaces provided. Then insert the following correct vocabulary terms into the sentences that follow.

ABO blood group
agglutinition
antibody
antigen
antiserum
billirubin
blood urea nitrogen
cholesterol
choriocarcinoma
Cushing's syndrome
diabetes melitis
eptopic
Epstein–Barr virus
Guthrie screening test
heterophile antibodies
high-density lipoprotein
human chorionic gonadotropin (hCG)
hydatidiform
hemolytic anemia
hyperglycemia
hypoglycemia
infectious mononucleosis
immunoessay
insulin
latex beads
low-density lipoprotein
Mantoux test
phenylketonuria (PKU)
purified protein derivative (PPD)
Rh factor
semen
tine test
triglyceride
tuberculosis

__________________ __________________ __________________

__________________ __________________ __________________

1. Although the ___________ is still used in some areas to test for ________________, most physicians, including Drs. Lewis and King, use the Mantoux test.

2. When a patient's glucose levels test high, Audrey Jones, CMA, knows it could be an indication of diabetes mellitus. She understands, however, that the high glucose levels could also be a sign of ______________ ______________, a hormonal disorder caused by an excess of corticosteroid hormones secreted by the adrenal glands, or a sign of acute stress response. A glucose tolerance test should be performed.

3. When Mary O'Keefe's enzyme ____________________ test is positive, Ellen Armstrong, CMA, suspects that this positive reaction indicates a normal pregnancy. However, detection of hCG, _____________________, can also indicate abnormal conditions such as an ____________________ pregnancy; a developing _____________________ mole of the uterus; or _______________________, a rare malignant neoplasm, usually of the uterus.

4. When Ellen Armstrong, CMA, performs a test for pregnancy using a slide test, she makes sure that after she adds hCG __________________ (___________________ to hCG) to the urine on a microscope slide; she then adds an _________________ reagent containing _________________ coated with hCG to the mixture.

5. Bruce Goldman, CMA, commonly performs tests for blood glucose levels at Inner City Health Care. The results are used to screen for carbohydrate disorders such as ___________ ______, in which a patient has a low blood glucose level.

6. Joe Guerrero, CMA, performs a slide test for pregnancy, remembering that negative ______ __________ indicates positive pregnancy.

7. When renal disease is suspected, a physician will order, as one of several tests, a BUN or ______________ ______________ ______________ test, which measures the concentration of urea in the blood.

8. Abigail Johnson has been diagnosed with ______________, which is a type of carbohydrate disorder usually characterized by a deficiency of ______________, a hormone secreted by the pancreas.

9. High levels of ____________________, the "bad" cholesterol, are associated with an increased risk for coronary artery disease. Cholesterol bound to ____________________, the "good" cholesterol, is transported to the liver where it is excreted in the form of bile.

10. To determine the severity of ____________________, the quantity of ______________ in the amniotic fluid of pregnant women is evaluated.

11. Serum ________________ concentration will increase moderately after ingesting a meal containing fat, peaking 4 to 5 hours later.

12. When a ______________ sample is required of a male patient for analysis, Wanda Slawson, CMA, instructs patients to avoid ejaculation for 3 days before collection of the sample.

13. Liz Corbin performs a ______________________ on Lenny Taylor's arm, raising a wheal where 0.1 ml PPD was administered properly with an intradermal injection.

14. Bruce Goldman, CMA, explains to Corey Boyer that his case of IM, ______________ ________________________, is a result of infection of the lymphocytes by the ________________ (EBV). Dr. Whitney confirmed the diagnosis from hematologic and clinical findings combined with the detection of ______________________ ______________________.

15. Nora Fowler was born with ____________________, an inherited condition in which the amino acid phenylalanine is not metabolized.

16. To evaluate a newborn for PKU, Audrey Jones, CMA, uses the ____________________ to evaluate the baby's blood.

17. The symptoms of ____________________ are similar to those of diabetes mellitus: excessive thirst; passing large amounts of urine; glycosuria, high levels of glucose in the urine; and ketosis, the high levels of ketones.

18. Patients exhibiting a positive or questionable ________________________ reaction should have a chest x-ray to examine for tubercules, and a sputum sample should be stained to search for acid-fast rods. The presence of tubercules and acid-fast rods confirms active tuberculosis.

19. Two categories of blood typing are for the ________________________ and the ________________________.

LEARNING REVIEW

1. A. Name three reasons for performing a semen analysis on a male patient.
   (1) ______________________________
   (2) ______________________________
   (3) ______________________________

   B. When a semen analysis is performed as part of a fertility work-up, seminal fluid is analyzed to determine what three factors?
   (1) ____________ (2) ____________ (3) ____________

2. A. Name the four blood group categories.
   (1) ________ (2) ________ (3) ________ (4) ________

   B. Fill in the missing information in the chart below.

Blood Group/Type	Antigen on RBC	Serum Antibodies
1. AB	____________	____________
2. ____________	B	____________
3. ____________	____________	No anti-D

   C. The Rh type of most North Americans is ____________. How can most cases of hemolytic disease of the newborn (HDN) be prevented? ____________________

Circle the best answer or answers to the following questions.

3. Which of the following factors can alter the results of semen analysis?
   a. eating foods containing garlic
   b. smoking cigarettes
   c. riding a bicycle on the day of the analysis
   d. drinking milk

4. To ensure an accurate reading, the following precautions should be taken when performing a pregnancy test.
   a. The patient should abstain from having sex within 2 days of the test.
   b. Refrigerated urine samples and test reagents should be allowed to come to room temperature before testing.
   c. The patient should drink at least eight glasses of water in the 6 hours preceding the test.
   d. First morning urine or urine with a specific gravity of at least 1.010 should be used.

5. The wheal produced on a patient's arm in response to a Mantoux test is positive for a past or present infection of *Mycobacterium tuberculosis* if it is:
   a. almost invisible
   b. 15 mm or more of induration
   c. 10 mm or more of induration
   d. exactly 2 mm of induration

6. *Fill in the blanks with the correct term.*

   A. Glucose is the principal carbohydrate found circulating in the ________________.

   B. In glucose analyzers based on ____________________, the glucose in the sample reacts with the reagents in the pad, causing a color to develop.

   C. Excess glucose is converted into ____________________ for short-term storage in the liver and muscle cells.

   D. The blood glucose level of ____________________ patients usually peaks 30 to 60 minutes after consumption of the glucose test solution leading to a level of 160 to 180 mg/dl, and then returns to the fasting level after 2 to 3 hours.

   E. A patient should be instructed to eat a diet high in ____________________ for 3 days before the glucose tolerance test.

   F. To determine whether diabetic patients are consistently adhering to their diets, physicians can administer the ______________________ test.

7. A. Describe the cholesterol molecule.

   ____

   ____

   B. Explain the difference between saturated, monounsaturated, and polyunsaturated fats and give an example of each.

   ____

   ____

   C. Look at Table 44-6, reference values for total blood cholesterol. What are the levels found in the U.S. population for your age and sex?______________

   D. Describe the function of cholesterol.

   ____

   ____

CERTIFICATION REVIEW

These questions are designed to mimic the certification examinations. You can use these questions like a small "Certification Examination Study Guide," but this is not meant to take the place of the more extensive study guides. Use this portion to determine in what areas to concentrate your efforts when studying for the certification examination. Justify any "false" answers.

1. Antigens present or absent on the surface of the red blood cell (RBC) are used to determine blood types. These are ______________ molecules.

   a. carbohydrate

   b. protein

   c. fat

   d. electrolyte

2. A potentially life-threatening situation during incompatible blood transfusion is called:
   a. Epstein–Barr
   b. intravascular hemolysis
   c. hydatidiform mole
   d. phenylketonuria

3. Men with oligspermia should be evaluated for which type of disorder?
   a. pancreatic
   b. liver
   c. thyroid
   d. kidney

4. A negative reaction to a Mantoux test would include an induration of:
   a. 10 mm or more
   b. 5–9 mm
   c. 12–15 mm
   d. less than 5 mm

5. Postprandial refers to:
   a. after eating
   b. after medication
   c. after sleeping
   d. after urinating

6. Insulin is secreted by which organ?
   a. liver
   b. spleen
   c. kidney
   d. pancreas

7. When performing the Mantoux test, what size needle would you choose?
   a. 25–26 gauge, 1/2 inch
   b. 26–27 gauge, 3/8 inch
   c. 27–28 gauge, 1/2 inch
   d. 29–30 gauge, 3/8 inch

8. The urine hCG test is more accurate than the blood enzyme immunoassay. (T or F)

CASE STUDY

Mary Alexander is an established patient of Dr. Esposito's at Inner City Health Care. Mary, 32 years old, is about 10 pounds overweight for her height. Mary has been diagnosed with type I insulin-dependent diabetes mellitus since childhood. Dr. Esposito's treatment plan includes administration of 30 units of U-100 NPH insulin by injection everyday. Dr. Esposito knows that Mary has trouble complying with the dietary restrictions included in her treatment plan and in observing regular mealtimes. Every now and then, the lifetime rigor of the diet wears Mary down and she begins to eat whatever she likes, whenever she feels like it. To guard against this, Mary must report her average glucose levels to Bruce Goldman, CMA, twice monthly as a safeguard.

At her next regular follow-up examination with Dr. Esposito, the physician orders a glycosated hemoglobin determination and discovers that Mary has been cheating on her diet again and has been reporting inaccurate glucose levels to the physician's office, hoping she would not get caught.

Discuss the following:

1. How is Dr. Esposito able to tell from the glycosated hemoglobin determination that Mary is not adhering to her diet and health guidelines?
2. What is glycosated hemoglobin?
3. What is the role of the medical assistant in this situation?

SELF-ASSESSMENT

1. Do you think all states should require PKU testing on all newborns? List three advantages and three disadvantages of each.

2. Do an Internet investigation to see if your state requires PKU testing on newborns.

   A. If not, why do you think it is not required? Is the test recommended? How much does it cost? What can you do to change the law?

   B. If your state does require it, Are parents allowed to refuse? Why would a parent refuse? How would you react if a parent refused?

POST-TEST

This is similar to the Pre-Test. Perform this test without looking at the book. This is just to see how well you have understood and can recall the information presented in this chapter after you have studied it and completed the workbook exercises. You will not be graded on this portion (other than the grade you give yourself), but this is an excellent preparation for your instructor's test. You may use this Post-Test to determine what areas you need to study more. Justify any "false" answers.

1. What are the different blood types?

   a. A, B, O, and AB

   b. B, O, A, and OB

   c. A, B, C, and O

   d. O, B, A, and AC

2. The PKU test is not mandatory for all infants in all states. (T or F)

3. During pregnancy, the hCG levels peak at 22 weeks. (T or F)

4. About 85% of the general population is Rh negative. (T or F)

5. The Rh system was named for the rhesus rats used in the experiments that led to the discovery of an Rh factor. (T or F)

6. Insulin helps regulate glucose levels in the urine. (T or F)

7. A PPD is administered with a subcutaneous injection. (T or F)

CERTIFICATION CRITERIA CHECKLIST

As you go through your education and training, keep in mind the national certification examination that you will take when you graduate. Each chapter of the textbook and workbook covers a different section of the examination criteria. To keep track of your preparation for the certification examination, turn to the back of this workbook and highlight the following CMA, RMA, or CMAS certification examination criteria (if you have already highlighted them from a previous chapter, put a check mark by the criteria):

CMA

F. Medicolegal Guidelines & Requirements

T. Patient Preparation and Assisting the Physician

  5. Explanation and instructions

V. Collecting and Processing Specimens; Diagnostic Testing

RMA

I. General Medical Assisting Knowledge

  C. Medical Law

III. Clinical Medical Assisting

  F. Patient Education

  I. Laboratory Procedures

CMAS

1. Medical Assisting Foundation
   - Legal and ethical considerations
3. Medical Office Clerical
   - Communication

COMPETENCY ASSESSMENT

Procedure 44-1 Pregnancy Test

Performance Objectives: To perform the enzyme immunoassay or agglutination inhibition test to detect human chorionic gonadotropin (hCG) in urine to determine positive or negative pregnancy results. Perform this objective within 15 minutes with a minimum score of 40 points.

Supplies/Equipment: Gloves, urine specimen, stopwatch, surface disinfectant, biohazard container, hCG negative and positive urine control, pregnancy test kit

Charting/Documentation: Enter appropriate documentation/charting in the box.

Instructor's/Evaluator's Comments and Suggestions:

SKILLS CHECKLIST Procedure 44-1: Pregnancy Test

Name ______________________

Date ______________________

No.	Skill	Check #1 20 pts ea	Check #2 10 pts ea	Check #3 5 pts ea	Notes
1	Wash hands and put on gloves.				
2	Assemble all equipment and supplies.				
3	Perform the test following the manufacturer's instructions. The following steps are intentionally general.				
	a. All materials must be at room temperature.				
	b. Apply urine to the test unit using dispenser provided.				
	c. Wait appropriate time interval.				
	d. Apply first reagent/antibody to test unit using dispenser provided.				
	e. Observe color development after appropriate time interval.				
	f. Stop reaction.				
	g. Consult manufacturer's package insert to interpret test results.				
4	Record the results on laboratory report form.				
5	Repeat step with positive and negative controls.				
6	Disinfect reusable equipment. Discard disposable supplies into biohazard container. Dispose of specimen according to biohazard policy. Disinfect work area.				
7	Remove gloves. Wash hands.				
8	Document the results in patient's chart.				
Student's Total Points					
Points Possible		160	80	40	
Final Score (Student's Total Points / Possible Points)					

	Notes
Start time:	
End time:	
Total time: (15 min goal)	

COMPETENCY ASSESSMENT

Procedure 44-2 Performing Infectious Mononucleosis Test

Performance Objectives: To perform an accurate test of serum or plasma to detect the presence or absence of antibodies of mononucleosis. Perform this objective within 15 minutes with a minimum score of 40 points.

Supplies/Equipment: Gloves, goggles (optional), safety lancet, alcohol swabs, cotton balls, gauze, adhesive strip, glucose analyzer, control solutions for glucose analyzer, test strips for glucose analyzer, laboratory tissue

Charting/Documentation: Enter appropriate documentation/charting in the box.

____

____

____

____

Instructor's/Evaluator's Comments and Suggestions:

____

____

____

____

____

____

SKILLS CHECKLIST Procedure 44-2: Performing Infectious Mononucleosis Test

Name ______________________

Date ______________________

No.	Skill	Check #1 20 pts ea	Check #2 10 pts ea	Check #3 5 pts ea	Notes
1	Wash hands and put on gloves.				
2	Assemble all the equipment and supplies.				
3	Perform the test according to the manufacturer's instructions exactly. These steps are intentionally general.				
4	After the test, record the results on a laboratory report form, following laboratory policy.				
5	Repeat the test procedure using the positive and negative controls.				
6	Discard contaminated materials into biohazard container. Dispose of specimen appropriately. Disinfect reusable equipment. Disinfect work area.				
7	Remove gloves, discard appropriately, and wash hands.				
8	Document results.				
Student's Total Points					
Points Possible		160	80	40	
Final Score (Student's Total Points / Possible Points)					
		Notes			
Start time:					
End time:					
Total time: (15 min goal)					

COMPETENCY ASSESSMENT

Procedure 44-3 Obtaining Blood Specimen for Phenylketonuria (PKU) Test

Performance Objectives: To obtain a blood specimen using a phenylketonuria (PKU) test card or "filter paper" to determine phenylalanine levels in newborns who are at least 3 days old. Perform this objective within 20 minutes with a minimum score of 75 points.

Supplies/Equipment: Gloves, PKU filter paper test card and mailing envelope, alcohol swabs, cotton balls or gauze pad, sterile pediatric-sized lancet, biohazard waste container

Charting/Documentation: Enter appropriate documentation/charting in the box.

Instructor's/Evaluator's Comments and Suggestions:

SKILLS CHECKLIST Procedure 44-3: Obtaining Blood Specimen for Phenylketonuria (PKU) Test

Name ______________________________

Date ______________________________

No.	Skill	Check #1 20 pts ea	Check #2 10 pts ea	Check #3 5 pts ea	Notes
1	Wash hands and put on gloves.				
2	Identify the infant. Explain the purpose of the test and the procedure to the parents. Discuss the health of the infant before to beginning the procedure.				
3	Select and clean an appropriate puncture site. Allow the alcohol to dry before the puncture.				
4	Grasp the infant's foot. Make a puncture approximately 2 to 3 mm deep in the infant's heel, making sure the infant's lateral, or side, portion of the heel pad is used.				
5	Wipe away the first drop of blood with a gauze pad.				
6	To collect blood for the test, press the back side of the filter paper test card against the infant's heel while exerting gentle pressure on the heel. The drop of blood should be large enough to completely fill and soak through the circle. Do not layer the multiple blood drops within a single circle. Completely fill all the circles on the test card.				
7	Hold a cotton ball over the puncture and apply pressure until the bleeding stops. Do not apply a bandage.				
8	Properly dispose of all waste in a biohazard container.				
9	Remove the gloves and wash hands.				
10	Allow the PKU test card to completely dry on a nonabsorbent surface at room temperature (approximately 2 hours). If performing more than one test, do not let the specimens touch each other while still wet.				
11	After the test card is dry, complete the PKU test card with all the patient and physician information.				

No.	Skill	Check #1 20 pts ea	Check #2 10 pts ea	Check #3 5 pts ea	Notes
12	Place the test card in the mailer envelope and send it to the laboratory within 2 days.				
13	Dispose of contaminated supplies into biohazard container and disinfect work area.				
14	Remove the gloves and wash hands.				
15	Document the procedure in the patient's medical record. When the test results are returned, they should be initialed by the physician and placed in the patient's medical record.				
Student's Total Points					
Points Possible		300	150	75	
Final Score (Student's Total Points / Possible Points)					
		Notes			
Start time:					
End time:					
Total time: (20 min goal)					

COMPETENCY ASSESSMENT

Procedure 44-4 Screening Test for PKU

Performance Objectives: Test a urine specimen using the diaper test or the Phenistik test to determine phenylalanine levels in infants who are at least 6 weeks old. This is a quick screening test only and *does not* take the place of the blood test. Perform this objective within 5 minutes with a minimum score of 35 points.

Supplies/Equipment: Gloves, 10% ferric chloride for the diaper test or Phenistik Method Test, biohazard waste container

Charting/Documentation: Enter appropriate documentation/charting in the box.

Instructor's/Evaluator's Comments and Suggestions:

SKILLS CHECKLIST Procedure 44-4: Screening Test for PKU

Name ______________________________

Date ______________________________

No.	Skill	Check #1 20 pts ea	Check #2 10 pts ea	Check #3 5 pts ea	Notes
1	Identify the infant. Verify that the infant is at least 6 weeks of age. Explain the purpose of the test and the procedure to the parents.				
2	Wash hands and apply gloves.				
3	Follow one of the following two procedures:				
	a. **Diaper test:** Apply several drops of 10% ferric chloride to a diaper that contains fresh urine. Development of a green color indicates a positive test.				
	b. **Phenistik test:** Dip the Phenistik test strip into fresh urine or press it against a diaper containing fresh urine. Development of a green color indicates a positive test.				
4	A positive urine test should be followed up with a blood test.				
5	Properly dispose of all waste in a biohazard waste container.				
6	Remove gloves and wash hands.				
7	Document the procedure and results in the patient's medical record.				
Student's Total Points					
Points Possible		140	70	35	
Final Score (Student's Total Points / Possible Points)					

	Notes
Start time:	
End time:	
Total time: (5 min goal)	

COMPETENCY ASSESSMENT

Procedure 44-5 Measurement of Blood Glucose Using an Automated Analyzer

Performance Objectives: To measure blood glucose at timed intervals after the patient's ingestion of a standard glucose dose. Perform this objective within 15 minutes with a minimum score of 65 points.

Supplies/Equipment: Gloves, goggles (optional), safety lancet, alcohol swabs, cotton balls, gauze, adhesive strip, glucose analyzer, control solutions for glucose analyzer, test strips for glucose analyzer, laboratory tissue

Charting/Documentation: Enter appropriate documentation/charting in the box.

Instructor's/Evaluator's Comments and Suggestions:

SKILLS CHECKLIST Procedure 44-5: Measurement of Blood Glucose Using an Automated Analyzer

Name ______________________

Date ______________________

No.	Skill	Check #1 20 pts ea	Check #2 10 pts ea	Check #3 5 pts ea	Notes
1	Review the manufacturer's manual for the specific glucose analyzer being used. Turn on the analyzer.				
2	Clean the work area and assemble all materials and supplies.				
3	Wash hands and put on gloves.				
4	Record the control ranges, control lot number, and test strip lot number.				
5	Perform the check test and the control test according to the manufacturer's instructions. If both tests are within range, proceed to the glucose test. Repeat both tests if either is out of acceptable range.				
To perform the glucose test:					
1	Remove the test strip from the bottle and replace the lid.				
2	Insert the test strip into the test chamber.				
3	Perform a capillary puncture. Wipe away the first drop with gauze.				
4	Apply a large drop of blood to the test strip. Apply cotton ball to puncture site.				
5	After the appropriate time interval has passed, read the glucose concentration.				
6	Document the results. Check site, then apply adhesive strip.				
7	Remove gloves and wash hands.				
8	Properly dispose of all waste in a biohazard waste container.				
Student's Total Points					
Points Possible (13 steps total)		260	130	65	
Final Score (Student's Total Points / Possible Points)					

	Notes
Start time:	
End time:	
Total time: (15 min goal)	

COMPETENCY ASSESSMENT

Procedure 44-6 Cholesterol Testing

Performance Objectives: To test for cholesterol, high-density lipoprotein, or triglyceride level for monitoring purposes. The following steps are intentionally general, so a variety of kits can be used. Perform this objective within 15 minutes with a minimum score of 30 points.

Supplies/Equipment: Gloves, blood collection equipment, pipettes with disposable tips, chlorine bleach, commercial kit for manual determination of cholesterol, controls and standards, marking pen, biohazard container

Charting/Documentation: Enter appropriate documentation/charting in the box.

Instructor's/Evaluator's Comments and Suggestions:

SKILLS CHECKLIST Procedure 44-6: Cholesterol Testing

Name ______________________

Date ______________________

No.	Skill	Check #1 20 pts ea	Check #2 10 pts ea	Check #3 5 pts ea	Notes
1	Assemble all necessary equipment and materials.				
2	Wash hands, then apply gloves.				
3	Obtain a blood sample from the patient, either by fingerstick or venipuncture, depending on the manufacturer's instructions.				
4	Follow the manufacturer's instructions *exactly* to perform the cholesterol test. These instructions are intentionally general. Be sure to also run the control tests.				
5	Properly dispose of all waste in biohazard container.				
6	Document results.				
Student's Total Points					
Points Possible		120	60	30	
Final Score (Student's Total Points / Possible Points)					
		Notes			
Start time:					
End time:					
Total time: (15 min goal)					

EVALUATION OF CHAPTER KNOWLEDGE

Skills	Student Self-Evaluation Good	Average	Poor
I can identify the three main precautions to be observed during the collection and testing of samples.	_____	_____	_____
I know how to collect samples and perform and interpret test results.	_____	_____	_____
I can discuss factors to be considered when evaluating test results.	_____	_____	_____
I can discuss transmission, incubation period, and symptoms of Epstein–Barr virus (infectious mononucleosis).	_____	_____	_____
I know the blood group antigens and antibodies found in each of the four ABO groups and the Rh factors.	_____	_____	_____
I can identify the cause of PKU and the symptoms caused by untreated PKU.	_____	_____	_____
I can recognize the seriousness of increased levels of phenylalanine and the dietary restrictions to be observed by PKU patients.	_____	_____	_____
I understand the cause of tuberculosis and some major characteristics of *Mycobacterium tuberculosis.*	_____	_____	_____
I recognize the role of insulin in the regulation of blood glucose levels.	_____	_____	_____
I know the differences between the testing fasting blood glucose, 2-hour postprandial glucose, and the glucose tolerance test.	_____	_____	_____
I can explain the importance of cholesterol and triglyceride testing to identify patients at high risk for coronary heart disease.	_____	_____	_____
I know the average values of cholesterol for adults, children, infants, and newborns.	_____	_____	_____
I know the acceptable level of low-density lipoprotein (LDL) in persons with or without coronary heart disease and the role of high-density lipoprotein and LDL in coronary heart disease	_____	_____	_____
I can identify the normal values of urea nitrogen for adults, children, infants, and newborns and the significance of increased blood urea levels.	_____	_____	_____
I recognize the importance of quality-control programs, including instrument maintenance, reagent shelf life, and test controls.	_____	_____	_____
I can document results accurately.	_____	_____	_____
I am respectful of the patient's emotional needs.	_____	_____	_____

CHAPTER 45

The Medical Assistant as Office Manager

CHAPTER PRE-TEST

Perform this test without looking at the book. This is just to see how well you have understood and can recall the information in this chapter after you have read it, but before you have completed the workbook exercises. You will not be graded on this portion (other than the grade you give yourself). Justify any "false" answers.

1. Teamwork results in getting more accomplished with the resources available. (T or F)
2. Office managers do not need effective communication skills. (T or F)
3. It is not necessary to update the office procedures manual. (T or F)
4. Minutes should be sent only to the team members who attended the meeting. (T or F)
5. When working with an externing student, each step should be explained together with the rationale. (T or F)
6. Office managers need to be able to accept and offer criticism constructively. (T or F)
7. The person who is the office manager is also the human resources manager. (T or F)

INTRODUCTION

In the ambulatory care setting, the office manager is an important and essential staff member involved in the daily operation of the practice. The office manager is responsible for a wide variety of duties, including supervision, time management, finances, purchasing, marketing, education, and personnel. In some cases, the same individual serves as both the office manager and the human resources manager. With more facilities turning to managed care as a way to ensure consumer use of the appropriate level of care and to facilitate cost containment, opportunities exist for medical assistants to advance to the office manager position. Use this workbook chapter to explore the role of the office manager in the ambulatory care setting.

PERFORMANCE OBJECTIVES

After successful completion of this chapter you will be able to explain the medical terms related to managing a medical office. You will become familiar with the qualities a good manager and leader should possess and cultivate; you will recognize different management styles and will be able to determine which might be more effective in a given situation. You will be more aware of effective teamwork and how to properly coordinate and run meetings. You will have tools to increase productivity and effectively manage time. You will be able to describe the concepts of marketing and recall effective marketing tools, as well as how to create patient brochures and information flyers. You will have an understanding of payroll processing, employee benefits, taxes, financial management, risk management, liability coverage, and bonding. *The following statements are related to your learning objectives for this chapter. Fill in the blanks in the following paragraph with the appropriate term(s).*

The position of office manager may include the duties of (1) ______________________________ person. Good managers are also good (2) ____________________ and possesses many qualities. They provide their coworkers with (3) ____________________, (4) ____________________, and a feeling of ownership in the process. They manage to accomplish things without (5) ____________________, usually by the power of their personal (6) ____________________. It is also important that managers (7) ____________________ convey their (8) ____________________ to their employees. A source of ill feelings is often the (9) ____________________ to let employees know what is (10) ____________________ of them. Among the specific traits a manager should possess are effective (11) ____________________ skills, (12) ____________________, (13) ____________________, (14) ____________________ skills, (15) ____________________, (16) ____________________ skills, (17) ____________________ expertise, and (18) ____________________. A good manager is continually (19) ____________________. People who succeed will take responsibility for their (20) ____________________. People who do not manage well will (21) ____________________ others for their failures. Mindsets can be changed by coming to terms with what you have to (22) ____________________, (23) ____________________ what you really want to (24) ____________________, put your goals in writing using (25) ____________________ terms, begin with small (26) ____________________ goals, (27) ____________________ poor work habits such as (28) ______________________________, and tune out (29) ____________________ thoughts while focusing on positive thoughts. Office managers must wear many hats. They will often serve as a Security Officer. The responsibilities of the (30) ____________________ include (31) ____________________ and (32) ____________________ the various impacts of (33) ____________________ on each department and assisting with (34) ____________________ issues related to Health Insurance Portability and Accountability Act (HIPAA) regulations. There are two basic management styles: (35) ______________________________ style and (36) ______________________________ style. A technique used by managers to stay informed and connected with the health of the office is called MBWA or (37) ______________________________. The office manager should (38) ______________________________ a (39) __________ management procedure that assesses the risks to which he or she and the (40) ____________________ are exposed and takes steps to develop (41) ______________________________ that (42) ____________________ those risks. Some common risks are: loss of a (43) ______________________________ employee, failure of a (44) ________________ or contractor, (45) ____________________ disclosure of (46) _______________ information through error or (47) ____________________ entry, (48) ___________ failure, (49) ________________ to a staff member or nonemployee, and a personal (50) ______________________________ change. New personnel orientation consists of (51) ________________________ and training new employees in the medical protocols and procedures (52) _______________ to that practice. If the (53) ____________________ manual is detailed and accurate, the manual becomes a (54) _____________ for the new employee. Assigning a (55) ________________ who can respond to questions is also important. Most new employees will be on (56) ______________________________ for (57) ________________________. Supervising student (58) ____________________ is another important part of medical office management, although the direct supervision can be (59) ______________________________ to another supervisor who will work more directly with the student. Performance evaluations and salary reviews should be done on a (60) ______________________ basis that is predetermined by office policy. Conflict resolution is a skill that managers need to become (61) __________________ at. There are many guidelines that are helpful in (62) ________________________ and (63) ____________________ conflict. Dismissing employees is another duty of the office manager. In this case, the written (64) ____ actually provides the format for the dismissal when necessary.

VOCABULARY BUILDER

Find the words listed below that are misspelled; circle them, and then correctly spell them in the spaces provided. Then insert the correct vocabulary terms into the sentences that follow.

agenda	"going bare"	practicum
ancilliary services	liability	procedures manual
benchmarking	malpractice	professional liability insurance
benefits	marketing	risk management
bond	minutes	teamwork
embezzle	negligance	work statement
externs	___________	___________

1. ________________________________ refers to professional occupational companies hired to complete a specific job.
2. Legal responsibility is commonly referred to as _________________.
3. ________________________________ describes the situation of a physician who does not carry professional liability insurance.
4. Making a comparison between different organizations relative to how they accomplish tasks, remunerate employees, and so on is called ______________________________.
5. ____ is designed to protect assets in the event a liability claim is filed and awarded.
6. ________________________________ are a written record of topics discussed and actions taken during meeting sessions.
7. A _________________________________ provides a concise description of the work you plan to accomplish.
8. A _______________________________ is a binding agreement with an employee ensuring recovery of financial loss should funds be stolen or embezzled.
9. A printed list of topics to be discussed during a meeting is called an _________________.
10. ________________________________ is the process by which the provider of services makes the consumer aware of the scope and quality of those services. Examples might include public relations, brochures, patient education seminars, and newsletters.
11. ________________________________ involves persons synergistically working together.
12. The failure to perform an act that a reasonable and prudent physician would or would not perform is ______________________________.
13. The student ______________________________ is a transitional stage providing an opportunity to apply theory learned in the classroom to a health care setting through practical, hands-on experience.
14. Remuneration that is in addition to the salary is a ______________________________.
15. The office manager should schedule an informational interview with the ________________ student before the practicum begins.
16. To appropriate fraudulently for one's own use is to ______________________________.
17. ________________________________ involves the identification, analysis, and treatment of risks within the medical office or facility.
18. The ____________________________________ provides detailed information relative to the performance of tasks within the job description.
19. _____________________ is the term commonly used today to describe professional liability.

LEARNING REVIEW

1. The office manager of a medical office or ambulatory care facility can have many varied responsibilities based on individual facility needs. What are five duties that are the responsibility of the office manager in a health care setting?

   (1) ____________________

   (2) ____________________

   (3) ____________________

   (4) ____________________

   (5) ____________________

2. Most marketing tools used in a medical environment provide educational and office services information to patients, potential patients, and the local community. Match the following marketing tools with their potential use in the ambulatory care facility setting.

   A. Seminars
   B. Brochures
   C. Newsletters
   D. Press releases
   E. Special events

   1. ______ These are used for announcing new equipment, new staff, expanded or remodeled office space, and so on.
   2. ______ These typically come in two types—patient education and office services—and present a professional image of the ambulatory care setting.
   3. ______ These provide an effective way to join with other community organizations to promote wellness.
   4. ______ These can educate patients and provide good will in the community. All facility staff can work as a team to organize these.
   5. ______ These can include a wide range of information from health-related topics to staff introductions to insurance updates. They may form the nucleus of a marketing program.

3. What are five attributes needed to perform as a quality manager in any office setting?

   (1) ____________________

   (2) ____________________

   (3) ____________________

   (4) ____________________

   (5) ____________________

CERTIFICATION REVIEW

These questions are designed to mimic the certification examinations. You can use these questions like a small "Certification Examination Study Guide," but this is not meant to take the place of the more extensive study guides. Use this portion to determine in what areas to concentrate your efforts when studying for the certification examination.

1. There is a direct correlation between a person's management style and his or her:
   a. technical expertise
   b. educational level
   c. personality
   d. salary
2. When managers delegate as much responsibility as possible to those they supervise, it is called:
   a. management by style
   b. management by exception
   c. management by decision model
   d. management by competitive edge
3. The person who applies the team-oriented management style is often comfortable with:
   a. teaching and coaching
   b. building, constructing, and modeling
   c. ideas, information, and data
   d. all of the above
4. A comprehensive safety program is essential to:
   a. marketing functions
   b. team building
   c. risk management
   d. equipment and supply maintenance
5. Leadership for the twenty-first century includes components of flexibility, mentoring, and:
   a. networking
   b. domination
   c. hierarchy
   d. rigidity

CASE STUDY

Office manager Shirley Brooks is responsible for the preparation and distribution of payroll checks at the offices of Drs. Lewis and King. Because the group practice is in the process of upgrading the computer system to accommodate a recent influx of new patients, Shirley is temporarily preparing the payroll using the manual write-it-once bookkeeping system. She is careful to consult payroll records for each employee, which include the employee's name, address, and telephone number; Social Security number; number of exemptions claimed on the W-4 form; gross salary; deductions withheld for all taxes, including Social Security, federal, state, local, unemployment, and disability; and date of employment.

Discuss the following:

1. As Shirley writes out the payroll check for Audrey Jones, CMA, what information should be included on the paycheck stub?
2. What must the physician's office have to process payroll?
3. What responsibility does the office manager have with regard to the confidentiality of payroll records? How might employees' rights to privacy be maintained?

SELF-ASSESSMENT

Put yourself in the place of the office manager.

1. What type of management style do you think you are the most comfortable with?
2. Carefully read about each type of style and explain why you think you are that type.
3. What skills will come naturally to you?
4. What skills will you have to work on the most?

POST-TEST

This is similar to the Pre-Test. Perform this test without looking at the book. This is just to see how well you have understood and can recall the information presented in this chapter after you have studied it and completed the workbook exercises. You will not be graded on this portion (other than the grade you give yourself), but this is an excellent preparation for your instructor's test. You may use this Post-Test to determine what areas you need to study more. Justify any "false" answers.

1. Teamwork results in getting less accomplished with the resources available. (T or F)
2. Office managers need effective communication skills. (T or F)
3. It is necessary to update the office procedures manual. (T or F)
4. Minutes should be sent all team members, not just those who attended the meeting. (T or F)
5. When working with an externing student, each step does not need to be explained together with the rationale, because they already have training. (T or F)
6. Office managers need to be able to offer criticism constructively, but they should not have to accept criticism. (T or F)
7. The person who is the office manager is never the human resources manager. (T or F)

CERTIFICATION CRITERIA CHECKLIST

As you go through your education and training, keep in mind the national certification examination that you will take when you graduate. Each chapter of the textbook and workbook covers a different section of the examination criteria. To keep track of your preparation for the certification examination, turn to the back of this workbook and highlight the following CMA, RMA, or CMAS certification examination criteria (if you have already highlighted them from a previous chapter, put a check mark by the criteria):

CMA

C. Psychology
  1. Basic principles

D. Professionalism
  5. Working as a team member to achieve goals

E Communication
  5. Evaluating and understanding communication

F. Medicolegal Guidelines & Requirements

M. Resource Information and Community Services

N. Managing Physician's Professional Schedule and Travel

O. Managing the Office

P. Office Policies and Procedures

Q. Managing Practice Finances
  5. Employee payroll

RMA

I. General Medical Assisting Knowledge
  C. Medical Law
  D. Medical Ethics
  E. Human Relations
  F. Patient Education
    2. Patient resource materials

CMAS

1. Medical Assisting Foundation
    - Legal and ethical considerations
    - Professionalism
3. Medical Office Clerical Assisting
    - Patient information and community resources
4. Medical Records Management
6. Medical Office Financial Management
8. Medical Office Management

COMPETENCY ASSESSMENT

Procedure 45-1 Preparing a Meeting Agenda

Performance Objectives: To prepare a meeting agenda with an established list of specific items to be discussed or acted on, or both. Perform this objective within 20 minutes with a minimum score of 30 points.

Supplies/Equipment: List of participants, the order of business, names of individuals giving reports, names of any guest speakers, a computer, paper to print agendas on

Charting/Documentation: Enter appropriate documentation/charting in the box.

Instructor's/Evaluator's Comments and Suggestions:

SKILLS CHECKLIST Procedure 45-1: Preparing a Meeting Agenda

Name ______________________________

Date ______________________________

No.	Skill	Check #1 20 pts ea	Check #2 10 pts ea	Check #3 5 pts ea	Notes
1	Confirm the proposed dates and place of meeting.				
2	Collect information from previous meetings' minutes for old agenda items. Check with others for report items and determine any new business.				
3	Prepare the meeting agenda and have it approved by the meeting chair.				
4	Send agenda to participants 2 weeks in advance.				
5	Reserve the meeting room.				
6	Schedule food items, equipment, and supplies that may be needed.				
Student's Total Points					
Points Possible		120	60	30	
Final Score (Student's Total Points / Possible Points)					

	Notes
Start time:	
End time:	
Total time: (20 min goal)	

COMPETENCY ASSESSMENT

Procedure 45-2 Supervising a Student Practicum

Performance Objectives: To prepare a training path for a student extern being assigned to the office, make the involved personnel aware of their responsibilities, preplan the jobs the student will perform and in what sequence they will be assigned, and try to make the externship successful by providing as much supervision and assistance as necessary. Perform this objective within 30 minutes with a minimum score of 55 points.

Supplies/Equipment: A schedule log, calendar, office procedures manual, any criteria presented by the program director

Charting/Documentation: Enter appropriate documentation/charting in the box.

Instructor's/Evaluator's Comments and Suggestions:

SKILLS CHECKLIST Procedure 45-2: Supervising a Student Practicum

Name ________________________

Date ________________________

No.	Skill	Check #1 20 pts ea	Check #2 10 pts ea	Check #3 5 pts ea	Notes
1	Determine the amount of supervision the student will require.				
2	Indentify the supervisor who will be immediately responsible for the extern.				
3	Follow Web page instructions for making arrangements.				
4	Plan which tasks the extern will be perfoming.				
5	Create a schedule outlining the time the student will be assigned to each unit/area.				
6	Begin orientation for the extern as soon as he or she arrives. Include a tour of the office and an introduction to the staff.				
7	Maintain an accurate record of the hours the extern works. Log the dates and reasons for any missed days, late arrivals, or early dismissals.				
8	Check with the extern frequently to be sure the student is receiving meaningful training from the work experience.				
9	Consult with the physicians and staff members with whom the student has worked for their opinion of the student's capabilities. Follow up with any problems that might be identified.				
10	Report the extern's progress to the medical assisting program director either during an on-site visit or via phone/e-mail.				
11	Prepare the student's evaluation report from input from all who worked with the student.				
Student's Total Points					
Points Possible		220	110	55	
Final Score (Student's Total Points / Possible Points)					

	Notes
Start time:	
End time:	
Total time: (30 min goal, including meeting with director, setting schedule, etc.)	

COMPETENCY ASSESSMENT

Procedure 45-3 Making Travel Arrangements

Performance Objectives: To make travel arrangements for the physician. Perform this objective within 20 minutes with a minimum score of 30 points.

Supplies/Equipment: A travel plan/preferences, telephone, directory, computer, and the physician's or office credit card to secure reservations

Charting/Documentation: Enter appropriate documentation/charting in the box.

Instructor's/Evaluator's Comments and Suggestions:

SKILLS CHECKLIST Procedure 45-3: Making Travel Arrangements

Name ______________________

Date ______________________

No.	Skill	Check #1 20 pts ea	Check #2 10 pts ea	Check #3 5 pts ea	Notes
1	Confirm the details of the trip: dates, times, places of departures and arrivals, preferred transportation method, number of travelers, preferred lodging type and price range, and if traveler's checks will be required.				
2	Telephone travel agent or use online ticket services.				
3	Pick up tickets, arrange for delivery, or secure confirmation of electronic tickets.				
4	Checks that arrangements are accurate and confirmed.				
5	Check that car rental and room reservations are accurate and confirmed.				
6	Make additional copies of the itinerary or create the itinerary: list dates and times of arrivals and departures, including flight numbers and seat assignments; modes of transportation; names, addresses, phone numbers, and e-mail addresses of hotels and meeting places. Maintain a copy for the office. Forward several copies to the physician.				
Student's Total Points					
Points Possible		120	60	30	
Final Score (Student's Total Points / Possible Points)					

	Notes
Start time:	
End time:	
Total time: (20 min goal)	

COMPETENCY ASSESSMENT

Procedure 45-4 Making Travel Arrangements via the Internet

Performance Objectives: To make travel arrangements for the physician using the Internet. Perform this objective within 20 minutes with a minimum score of 35 points.

Supplies/Equipment: A travel plan/preferences, computer, physician's or office credit card to secure reservations

Charting/Documentation: Enter appropriate documentation/charting in the box.

Instructor's/Evaluator's Comments and Suggestions:

SKILLS CHECKLIST Procedure 45-4: Making Travel Arrangements via the Internet

Name ______________________________

Date ______________________________

No.	Skill	Check #1 20 pts ea	Check #2 10 pts ea	Check #3 5 pts ea	Notes
1	Confirm the details of the trip: dates, times, places of departures and arrivals, preferred transportation method, number of travelers, preferred lodging type and price range, and if traveler's checks will be required.				
2	Access the Internet; select a search engine and locate Web pages under air fares with links to car rentals and hotels.				
3	Follow Web page instructions for making arrangements.				
4	Review and copy confirmations of transactions.				
5	Confirm how tickets will arrive, that is, picked up or electronic.				
6	Make additional copies of the itinerary for the office.				
7	Forward several copies to the physician.				
Student's Total Points					
Points Possible		140	70	35	
Final Score (Student's Total Points / Possible Points)					
		Notes			
Start time:					
End time:					
Total time: (20 min goal)					

COMPETENCY ASSESSMENT

Procedure 45-5 Developing and Maintaining a Procedure Manual

Performance Objectives: To develop and maintain a comprehensive, up-to-date procedures manual covering each medical, technical, and administrative procedure in the office with step-by-step directions and rationale for performing each task. Perform this objective (one procedure) within 20 minutes with a minimum score of 45 points.

Supplies/Equipment: A computer, three-ring binder, paper, procedures and criteria

Charting/Documentation: Enter appropriate documentation/charting in the box.

Instructor's/Evaluator's Comments and Suggestions:

SKILLS CHECKLIST Procedure 45-5: Developing and Maintaining a Procedure Manual

Name ______________________________

Date ______________________________

No.	Skill	Check #1 20 pts ea	Check #2 10 pts ea	Check #3 5 pts ea	Notes
1	Write detailed step-by-step procedures and rationale for each medical, technical, and administrative function. Each procedure is written by experienced employees close to the function and reviewed by a supervisor or the office manager.				
2	Include regular maintenance (cleaning, servicing, and calibrating) instructions and flow sheets for all office equipment, both in the clinical area and in the office/business areas.				
3	Include step-by-step procedures on how to accomplish each task both in the clinical area and in the office/business areas.				
4	Include local and out of the area resources for clinical staff, office/business staff, physicians/providers, and patients. Provide a listing in each area with contact information and services provided.				
5	Include basic rules and regulations, state and federal, which are related to processes performed in both clinical and office/business areas.				
6	Include the clinic procedures and flow sheets for taking inventory in each of the areas and instructions on ordering procedures.				
7	Collect the procedures into the office procedures manual.				

No.	Skill	Check #1 20 pts ea	Check #2 10 pts ea	Check #3 5 pts ea	Notes
8	Store one complete manual in a common library area. One complete copy goes to the physician–employer, to the office manager, and to each department.				
9	Review the manual annually; add any new procedures and delete and modify as needed.				
Student's Total Points					
Points Possible		180	90	45	
Final Score (Student's Total Points / Possible Points)					
		Notes			
Start time:					
End time:					
Total time: (20 min goal)					

EVALUATION OF CHAPTER KNOWLEDGE

	Student Self-Evaluation		
Skills	Good	Average	Poor
I understand payroll processing and other employee-related financial duties, including computing taxes.	_____	_____	_____
I exercise efficient time management techniques.	_____	_____	_____
I understand risk management issues.	_____	_____	_____
I understand the importance of developing and maintaining policy and procedures manuals.	_____	_____	_____
I understand methods of public relations for the ambulatory care setting.	_____	_____	_____
I can describe liability coverage and bonding.	_____	_____	_____
I can describe the qualities of an effective office manager.	_____	_____	_____
I am able to describe the process of supervising a student practicum.	_____	_____	_____
I understand the importance of teamwork and its role when supervising personnel.	_____	_____	_____

CHAPTER 46

The Medical Assistant as Human Resources Manager

CHAPTER PRE-TEST

Perform this test without looking at the book. This is just to see how well you have understood and can recall the information in this chapter after you have read it, but before you have completed the workbook exercises. You will not be graded on this portion (other than the grade you give yourself). Justify any "false" answers.

1. Which of the following is *not* a function of the human resources (HR) manager?
   a. creating and updating a policy manual
   b. recruiting and hiring office personnel
   c. orienting new personnel
   d. training new personnel
2. Wage and salary policies should be in writing. (T or F)
3. A policy manual should contain daily step-by-step instructions. (T or F)
4. Job descriptions are not always useful because they change so often. (T or F)
5. All job applicants should be interviewed. (T or F)
6. It is acceptable to ask job applicants about the last place they worked and a conflict they had there. (T or F)
7. References are usually checked upon after the first interview. (T or F)
8. The HR manager is responsible for dismissing employees. (T or F)
9. Employees have a right to review their personnel files at any time. (T or F)

INTRODUCTION

In some health care practices, particularly in that of the solo practitioner, the office manager also functions as the HR manager. In other cases, these management functions are assumed by two separate individuals. The HR manager is concerned with both group and individual employee issues. The HR manager performs such duties as formulating job descriptions, recruitment and hiring, payroll and salary review, training, benefits, advancement, grievances, dismissals, and maintaining employee personnel records. Use this workbook chapter to explore the role of the HR manager in the ambulatory care setting.

PERFORMANCE OBJECTIVES

After successful completion of this chapter you will be able to explain the medical terms related to HR management. You will be familiar with the duties of an HR manager; the functions of formal policies and the policy manual; and the methods and rules surrounding the recruitment, interviewing, and orienting of new employees. You will also know about the laws surrounding personnel issues and management. You will be aware of the reasons and purposes of exit interviews and maintaining accurate personnel records. *The following statements are related to your learning objectives for this chapter. Fill in the blanks in the following paragraph with the appropriate term(s).*

Tasks usually assigned to the HR manager include determining job (1) ______________________; scheduling, hiring, and (2) ____________________ new employees; and (3) ________________ employee personnel (4) ____________________. One difference between a procedures manual and a policy manual is that the procedures manual is a daily, step-by-step guide with instructions, whereas a policy manual is about (5) ____________________ practices and (6) _____________ of an office. The HR manager also needs to make sure (7) ________________________ are in place for every position. Included in the job description are the (8) __________________ of the ideal applicant; the necessary (9) _______________________, (10) _____________, (11) _______________________; and any special (12) __________________ or licensure that is expected. The job description should be reviewed and updated every (13) _________. A major challenge of HR managers today is that of (14) ____________________. Medical assistants are listed as the number one fastest growing occupation through 2012 by the (15) ____. The need is so great that some clinics have turned to contracting out such work as (16) _____________________ and (17) _____________________. Before interviews, it is a good idea to establish a set of (18) _____________________ for the (19) _____________________. This helps alleviate one applicant being given (20) ____________________ over another. At the close of the interview, the applicant should be told when the (21) ______________ will be made or whether a (22) _____________________ will be conducted, as well as how (23) ___________________ will be made. At the time the offer for hire is made, the candidate should understand the (24) ____________________ offered, the (25) ___________________________, the practice (26) __________________, and the (27) ________________. When the candidate accepts the position, a (28) ______________________ letter should be written with further details. Orienting the new employee is the responsibility of both the (29) ______________ and lead personnel. Training is usually the responsibility of the office manager and the staff supervisors where the new employee will be working. Important elements of orientation include (30) ______________ to other (31) ______________ members and (32) ______________ a mentor. Dismissing employees usually falls to the (33) ______________ with the HR manager involved in the exit interview. An important aspect of the HR manager is to maintain (34) ______________. This confidential employee file should include all documentation and correspondence related to each employee from (35) ______________ to (36) ______________, from (37) ______________ to (38) ______________ including the formal (39) ______________ and all demographic information. These files are kept for (40) ______________ after the employee leaves the practice. HR managers must always comply with (41) ______________ laws against (42) ______________ on the basis of race, color, religion, sex, age, or national origin.

VOCABULARY BUILDER

Find the words listed below that are misspelled; circle them, and then correctly spell them in the spaces provided. Insert the correct vocabulary terms into the following sentences.

conflict resolution	job description	overtime
educational history	letter of referance	probation
evaluation	letter of resignation	résumés
exit interveiw	menter	salary review
involuntary dismisal	networking	work history
______________	______________	______________
______________		

1. Clinical medical assistant Anna Preciado, who is approaching 1 year of employment at the offices of Drs. Lewis and King, is due to have her ______________ to assess her job performance.
2. Because of an unexpected staffing shortfall, Audrey Jones, CMA, has volunteered to work ______________ this week. She will receive 1½ times the regular rate of pay for hours above her regular 40-hour week.
3. Office manager Marilyn Johnson, acting as the HR manager, will conduct a ______________ ______________ at the beginning of the new calendar year with each employee. If necessary, she will then inform the employee of his or her revised base pay rate.
4. An ______________ has been scheduled for administrative/clinical medical assistant Liz Corbin before she leaves the clinic to continue her education. This session will give Liz an opportunity to provide her positive and negative opinions of the position and the facility.

5. Jane O'Hara, co-office manager at Inner City Health Care, has been asked by her physician–employers to use ______________________________ to solve several problems occurring between two coworkers at the facility.
6. Office manager Marilyn Johnson has received a ______________________________ from the former instructor of a current job applicant describing the applicant's performance, attitude, and qualifications.
7. In interviews for a new Certified Medical Assistant position, office manager Walter Seals asks applicants to outline their ______________________________, including employers, positions, duties, and responsibilities.
8. Office manager Walter Seals reviews ________________________ received from applicants for the new medical assisting position to ensure that the applicants interviewed meet the physician–employer's minimum qualifications for education and work experience.
9. The ______________________________ listed on each résumé reveals to the office manager the applicant's places of learning and degrees or certificates earned.
10. The violation of office policies at Inner City Health Care led to the ____________________ of one of the part-time employees.
11. Administrative medical assistant Ellen Armstrong, in her first job since leaving school, has had office manager Marilyn Johnson as her ______________________, to assist in the training, guidance, and coaching she will need in her first position.
12. Winston Lewis, MD, is active in his state medical society; the ____________________ has resulted in beneficial and long-lasting social, business, and professional relationships.
13. Liz Corbin, CMA, submitted a ______________________________ to her current employer when she decided to leave her present position to return to school to pursue an advanced degree.
14. Office manager Marilyn Johnson will inform all of the job applicants that they will be on ____________________ for their first 3 months on the job. During this period, the employee and supervisory personnel can determine if the environment and the position are satisfactory for the employee.
15. Office manager Jane O'Hara, updating the employee manual, includes a ____________________ for every position in the office that details tasks, duties, and responsibilities.

LEARNING REVIEW

1. The manual that identifies clear guidelines and directions required of all employees is known as the policy manual. What are four topics that would be included in a policy manual regardless of the size of the practice identified in this chapter.

   (1) ______________________________

   (2) ______________________________

   (3) ______________________________

   (4) ______________________________

2. Office manager Marilyn Johnson has the responsibility of dismissing an employee for a serious violation of office policies. From the list below, select key points to keep in mind when dismissal is necessary by circling the letters of the statements that apply.
   A. Have employee pack his or her belongings from desk.
   B. The dismissal should be made in private.
   C. Take no longer than 20 minutes for the dismissal.
   D. Be direct, firm, and to the point in identifying reasons.
   E. Explain terms of dismissal (keys, clearing out area, final paperwork).
   F. Do not listen to the employee's opinion and emotions.
   G. If he or she insists, allow the employee to finish the work of the day.
   H. Do not engage in an in-depth discussion of performance.

3. The job description must have enough information to provide both the supervisor and the employee with a clear outline of what the job entails. Name four items that must be included in a job description.
   (1) ______________________ (3) ______________________
   (2) ______________________ (4) ______________________

4. The interview worksheet is an excellent tool to make certain that the interviews with each candidate are fair and equitable. Provide six items that should be included on any interview worksheet.
   (1) ______________________ (4) ______________________
   (2) ______________________ (5) ______________________
   (3) ______________________ (6) ______________________

CERTIFICATION REVIEW

These questions are designed to mimic the certification examinations. You can use thee questions like a small "Certification Examination Study Guide," but this is not meant to take the place of the more extensive study guides. Use this portion to determine in what areas to concentrate your efforts when studying for the certification examination.

1. A salary review is:
   a. usually conducted at the beginning of the new year
   b. virtually the same as the performance review
   c. conducted on the anniversary date of hire
   d. normally done every 3 years

2. Questions regarding drug use, arrest records, and medical history during an interview are:
   a. appropriate
   b. inappropriate
   c. illegal
   d. none of the above

3. Title VII of the Civil Rights Act addresses:
   a. overtime pay
   b. discrimination based on race, age, and sex
   c. hiring and firing practices
   d. sexual harassment

4. When a candidate accepts a position, the HR manager should write a letter outlining the specifics of the job. This letter is called:
   a. a confirmation letter
   b. a congratulatory letter
   c. a recommendation letter
   d. a reference letter

5. A person with AIDS who satisfies the necessary skills for a job and has the experience and education required will be protected from discrimination by:
   a. OSHA
   b. CLIA
   c. AAMA
   d. ADA

CASE STUDY

Since the offices of Drs. Lewis and King have expanded to cover a rapidly growing patient load, including the hiring of a co-office manager and a new clinical medical assistant, the work pace has been hectic, but challenging. At the suggestion of Dr. Lewis, the office managers decide to hold a staff meeting to talk about ways to keep the lines of communication open and process the many changes occurring at the growing medical practice. Marilyn Johnson and Shirley Brooks encourage staff to be vocal with their feedback, suggestions, and concerns.

Discuss the following:

1. What other techniques can the office managers use to prevent or solve conflicts in the workplace during this period of growth and transition?
2. Why is effective communication one of the most important goals of the HR manager?

SELF-ASSESSMENT

1. If you were put into the position of hiring a new employee, what attributes would you be looking for?
   a. Make a list of the technical skills your new employee would need.
   b. Make a list of the affective behavior skills your new employee would need, including a positive attitude, good work ethics, and so forth.

c. Determine how you could measure the technical skills you listed.

d. Determine how you could measure the softer skills of affective behavior you listed in item b above. How could you determine those qualities?

e. Which is more difficult to measure: technical or behavioral? Which is more difficult to train?

2. When you interview for a job, what technical and behavioral skills on your lists will you need to improve on?

POST-TEST

This is similar to the Pre-Test. Perform this test without looking at the book. This is just to see how well you have understood and can recall the information presented in this chapter after you have studied it and completed the workbook exercises. You will not be graded on this portion (other than the grade you give yourself), but this is an excellent preparation for your instructor's test. You may use this Post-Test to determine what areas you need to study more. Justify any "false" answers.

1. Which of the following are functions of the HR manager? (circle all the apply)
   a. creating and updating a policy manual
   b. training new personnel
   c. recruiting and hiring office personnel
   d. orienting new personnel
2. Wage and salary policies need not be in writing as long as both parties agree. (T or F)
3. A policy manual should contain general policies and practices of the office. (T or F)
4. Job descriptions are always useful and should be clearly written. (T or F)
5. Only qualified job applicants should be interviewed. (T or F)
6. It is good to ask job applicants about conflicts they have had and how they solved them. (T or F)
7. References are usually checked before the first interview. (T or F)
8. The HR manager is responsible for the exit interview, but usually not for dismissing employees. (T or F)
9. Employees do not have the right to review their personnel files unless requested by an attorney. (T or F)

CERTIFICATION CRITERIA CHECKLIST

As you go through your education and training, keep in mind the national certification examination that you will take when you graduate. Each chapter of the textbook and workbook covers a different section of the examination criteria. To keep track of your preparation for the certification examination, turn to the back of this workbook and highlight the following CMA, RMA, or CMAS certification examination criteria (if you have already highlighted them from a previous chapter, put a check mark by the criteria):

CMA

C. Psychology
  1. Basic principles

E. Communication
  6. Interviewing techniques

F. Medicolegal Guidelines & Requirements

O. Managing the Office
  1. Maintaining the physical plant

P. Office Policies and Procedures

RMA

I. General Medical Assisting Knowledge
  C. Medical Law
  D. Medical Ethics
  E. Human Relations
  F. Patient Education
    2. Patient resource materials

CMAS

1. Medical Assisting Foundation
   - Legal and ethical considerations
   - Professionalism

8. Medical Office Management
   - Human resources

COMPETENCY ASSESSMENT

Procedure 46-1 Develop and Maintain a Policy Manual

Performance Objectives: To develop and maintain a comprehensive, up-to-date policy manual of all office policies relating to employee practices, benefits, office conduct, and so forth. Perform this objective within 20 minutes (for one policy) with a minimum score of 35 points.

Supplies/Equipment: Computer, three-ring binder, paper, standard policy format

Charting/Documentation: Enter appropriate documentation/charting in the box.

Instructor's/Evaluator's Comments and Suggestions:

SKILLS CHECKLIST Procedure 46-1: Develop and Maintain a Policy Manual

Name ______________________________

Date ______________________________

No.	Skill	Check #1 20 pts ea	Check #2 10 pts ea	Check #3 5 pts ea	Notes
1	Following office format, develop precise, written office policies detailing all necessary information pertaining to the staff and their positions. Include benefits, vacation, sick leave, hours, dress codes, evaluations, rules of conduct, and grounds for dismissal.				
2	Identify procedures for reimbursing overtime, preventing discrimination and harassment, creating a safe workplace, and allowing for jury duty.				
3	Include a policy statement related to smoking and other substances.				
4	Identify steps to follow should an employee become disabled during employment.				
5	Determine what employee opportunities for continuing education will be reimbursed and include requirements for certification and licensures.				
6	Provide a copy of the policy manual for each employee.				
7	Review and update the policy manual regularly. Add or delete items as necessary, dating each revision.				
Student's Total Points					
Points Possible		140	70	35	
Final Score (Student's Total Points / Possible Points)					

	Notes
Start time:	
End time:	
Total time: (20 min goal for one policy)	

COMPETENCY ASSESSMENT

Procedure 46-2 Prepare a Job Description

Performance Objectives: To develop a precise definition of the tasks assigned to a job, to determine the expectations and level of competency required, and to specify the experience, training, and education needed to perform the job for purposes of recruiting and performance evaluation. Perform this objective within 20 minutes (for one job description) with a minimum score of 30 points.

Supplies/Equipment: Computer, three-ring binder, paper, standard job description format

Charting/Documentation: Enter appropriate documentation/charting in the box.

Instructor's/Evaluator's Comments and Suggestions:

SKILLS CHECKLIST Procedure 46-2: Prepare a Job Description

Name ______________________

Date ______________________

No.	Skill	Check #1 20 pts ea	Check #2 10 pts ea	Check #3 5 pts ea	Notes
1	Detail each task that creates the job.				
2	List special medical, technical, or clerical skills needed.				
3	Determine the level of education, training, and experience required for the position.				
4	Determine where the job fits into the overall structure of the office.				
5	Specify any unusual working conditions (hours, locations, etc.) that may apply.				
6	Describe career path opportunities.				
Student's Total Points					
Points Possible		120	60	30	
Final Score (Student's Total Points / Possible Points)					

	Notes
Start time:	
End time:	
Total time: (20 min goal)	

COMPETENCY ASSESSMENT

Procedure 46-3 Conduct Interviews

Performance Objectives: To screen applicants for training, experience, and characteristics to select the best candidate to fill the position vacancy. Perform this objective within 40 minutes with a minimum score of 85 points.

Supplies/Equipment: Interview questions; policy manual (for referencing); applicant's résumé, application, and cover letter

Charting/Documentation: Enter appropriate documentation/charting in the box.

Instructor's/Evaluator's Comments and Suggestions:

SKILLS CHECKLIST Procedure 46-3: Conduct Interviews

Name ______________________________

Date ______________________________

No.	Skill	Check #1 20 pts ea	Check #2 10 pts ea	Check #3 5 pts ea	Notes
1	Review résumés and applications received.				
2	Select candidates who most closely match the education and experience being sought.				
3	Create an interview worksheet for each candidate, listing the points to cover.				
4	Select an interview team. Include the office manager and immediate supervisor of the position being filled.				
5	Call personally to schedule the interview. This will allow you to judge the applicant's telephone voice and manners.				
6	Remind the interviewers of the various legal restrictions concerning questions that can be asked.				
7	Conduct interviews in a quiet, private setting.				
8	Put the applicant at ease by beginning with an overview about the practice and staff, briefly describing the job and answering preliminary questions.				
9	Ask questions about the applicant's work experience and educational background using the résumé and interview worksheet as a guideline.				
10	Provide the most promising applicants additional information about the benefits and a tour of the office if practical.				
11	Applicant's general salary requirements may be discussed, but avoid discussion of a specific salary until a formal offer is tendered.				
12	Inform the applicants when a decision will be made, and thank each applicant for participating in the interview.				
13	Do not make a job offer until all the candidates have been interviewed.				

No.	Skill	Check #1 20 pts ea	Check #2 10 pts ea	Check #3 5 pts ea	Notes
14	Check references of all prospective employees.				
15	Establish a second interview between the physician–employer(s) and the qualified candidate if necessary.				
16	Confirm accepted job offers in writing, specifying the details of the offer and acceptance.				
17	Notify all unsuccessful applicants by letter when the position has been filled.				
Student's Total Points					
Points Possible		340	170	85	
Final Score (Student's Total Points / Possible Points)					

	Notes
Start time:	
End time:	
Total time: (40 min goal, includes preinterview meeting of committee and postinterview meeting)	

COMPETENCY ASSESSMENT

Procedure 46-4 Orient Personnel

Performance Objectives: To acquaint new employees with office policies, staff, what the job encompasses, procedures to be performed, and job performance expectations. Perform this objective within 30 minutes with a minimum score of 45 points.

Supplies/Equipment: Policy manual

Charting/Documentation: Enter appropriate documentation/charting in the box.

Instructor's/Evaluator's Comments and Suggestions:

SKILLS CHECKLIST Procedure 46-4: Orient Personnel

Name ______________________________

Date ______________________________

No.	Skill	Check #1 20 pts ea	Check #2 10 pts ea	Check #3 5 pts ea	Notes
1	Tour the facilities and introduce the office staff.				
2	Complete employee-related documents and explain their purpose.				
3	Explain the benefits program.				
4	Present the office policy manual and discuss the key elements.				
5	Review federal and state regulatory precautions for medical facilities.				
6	Review the job description.				
7	Explain and demonstrate procedures to be performed and the use of procedures manuals supporting these procedures.				
8	Demonstrate the use of any specialized equipment (such as time clocks, key entries, etc.). Medical equipment will be demonstrated by clinical staff.				
9	Assign a mentor from the staff to help with the orientation.				
Student's Total Points					
Points Possible		180	90	45	
Final Score (Student's Total Points / Possible Points)					

	Notes
Start time:	
End time:	
Total time: (30 min goal)	

EVALUATION OF CHAPTER KNOWLEDGE

Skills	Student Self-Evaluation Good	Average	Poor
I can describe the role of the HR manager.	_____	_____	_____
I can explain the function of the office policy manual.	_____	_____	_____
I can identify methods of recruiting employees for a medical practice.	_____	_____	_____
I am familiar with the interview process.	_____	_____	_____
I can describe appropriate evaluation tools for employees.	_____	_____	_____
I can recall dismissal procedures.	_____	_____	_____
I can identify items in employee personnel files.	_____	_____	_____
I can define laws relating to personnel management.	_____	_____	_____
I understand effective strategies for conflict resolution.	_____	_____	_____

CHAPTER 47

Preparing for Medical Assisting Credentials

CHAPTER PRE-TEST

Perform this test without looking at the book. This is just to see how well you have understood and can recall the information in this chapter after you have read it, but before you have completed the workbook exercises. You will not be graded on this portion (other than the grade you give yourself). Justify any "false" answers.

1. A Registered Medical Assistant (RMA) and a Certified Medical Assistant (CMA) have the same bylaws and creed. (T or F)
2. A CMA may only work in the state in which the credentials were received. (T or F)
3. Three major areas included in the CMA examination are clinical, administrative, and general medical knowledge. (T or F)
4. Medical assistants may be trained on the job; however, physicians recognize that their offices operate much more efficiently and effectively with professionally trained and formally educated personnel. (T or F)
5. A CMA does not have to be a member of AAMA or currently employed to recertify. (T or F)
6. On meeting recertification requirements, the applicant will receive a new certificate. (T or F)
7. Once a student has become a member of AAMA, he or she may stay at the student rate for one year after graduation. (T or F)

INTRODUCTION

Certification provides established, consistent criteria for evaluating the professional competence of a medical assistant. The certification examination is offered by the American Association of Medical Assistants (AAMA). An individual who successfully passes the examination is awarded the Certified Medical Assistant (CMA) credential. In addition, the American Medical Technologists (AMT) organization conducts the examination that leads to the Registered Medical Assistant (RMA) credential. Certification is an important part of professional development and is highly valued by employers in the health care workplace. Use this workbook chapter to determine the specifics of the certification process.

PERFORMANCE OBJECTIVES

After successful completion of this chapter you will be able to explain the medical terms related to certification and recertification. You will be able to list the advantages and purposes of certification. You will be able to cite the professional organizations that sponsor the examinations and what credential is obtained by passing each examination. You will understand the requirement for recertification. *The following statements are related to your learning objectives for this chapter. Fill in the blanks in the following paragraph with the appropriate term(s).*

The CMA credential is awarded to those individuals who pass a national (1) ______________ examination offered by the Certifying Board of the (2) ______________ and administered by the (3) ______________ (abbreviated NBME). The RMA credential is offered by the (4) ______________. Only the (5) ______________ examination requires formal education. The (6) ______________ examination is available to persons with on-the-job experience. Both examinations require extensive knowledge in three basic areas: (7) ______________, (8) ______________, and (9) ______________. (10) ______________ of AAMA may take the certification examination at a reduced rate; students must enroll as members while they are still in school to take the examination at the (11) ______________ rate. Once certified, the CMA must recertify every (12) ______________ years. As of January 2005, CMAs are required to recertify by the (13) ______________ of their birth month in the (14) ______________ calendar year after certification/recertification. Recertification for the RMA credential requires an annual fee of (15) ______________. The (16) ______________ and the (17) ______________ are national professional organizations that offer many benefits to their members.

VOCABULARY BUILDER

Match each correct vocabulary term to the aspect of the certification process that best describes it.

_____ 1. Certification Examination

_____ 2. Certified Medical Assistant (CMA)

_____ 3. Continuing Education Units (CEUs)

_____ 4. National Board of Medical Examiners (NBME)

_____ 5. Recertification

_____ 6. Registered Medical Assistant (RMA)

_____ 7. Task Force for Test Construction

A. Method for earning points toward recertification

B. A standardized means of evaluating medical assistant competency

C. Maintaining current CMA status

D. Credential awarded for successfully passing the Certification Examination

E. Committee of professionals whose responsibility is to update the CMA examination annually to reflect changes in medical assistants' responsibilities and to include new developments in medical knowledge and technology

F. Credential awarded for successfully passing the AMT Examination

G. Consultants for the Certification Examination

LEARNING REVIEW

1. The AAMA Certification Examination is a comprehensive test of the knowledge actually used in today's medical office. The test is updated annually to include the latest changes in medical assistants' daily responsibilities. In addition, the updates include the latest developments in medical knowledge and technology. Name the three major areas tested in the Certification Examination and describe what each includes.

   (1) ______________________________

   (2) ______________________________

   (3) ______________________________

2. A. Health care professionals today should maintain a lifelong commitment to ______________________________.

   B. To keep their ______________ current, CMAs are required to recertify every ______________.

   C. A total of ________ points is necessary to recertify the basic CMA credential.

   D. Continuing education courses are offered by ______________ groups.

3. A. What is the address, telephone number, and web address for obtaining an application for the Certification Examination (Choose either AAMA or AMT)?

   ____

   ____

   ____

   B. What guide for the Certification Examination is available from the AAMA?

   ____

   C. What program and what bimonthly publication does the AAMA make available to members who are interested in pursuing continuing education credits?

   Program: ______________________________

   Publication: ______________________________

CERTIFICATION REVIEW

These questions are designed to mimic the certification examinations. You can use these questions like a small "Certification Examination Study Guide," but this is not meant to take the place of the more extensive study guides. Use this portion to determine in what areas to concentrate your efforts when studying for the certification examination.

1. General medical assisting knowledge on the AMT Certification Examination includes anatomy and physiology, medical terminology, and:
   a. insurance and billing
   b. medical ethics
   c. bookkeeping and filing
   d. first aid

2. The organization that develops licensure and specialty board examinations for physicians nationwide and acts as a consultant for the CMA Certification Examination is:
   a. NBME
   b. CAAHEP
   c. ABHES
   d. AMTIE

3. How many test sites are there nationwide for the CMA examination?
   a. less than 250
   b. 250
   c. 250–500
   d. more than 500

4. In what months is the CMA examination offered?
   a. June and January
   b. September and January
   c. every month
   d. June, January, and October

5. A total of how many questions are on the CMA Certification Examination?
   a. 100
   b. 300
   c. 1,000
   d. It varies year to year.

6. How often does an RMA need to recertify?
   a. every year
   b. every 6 years
   c. every 5 years
   d. beginning in 2006, every 3 years

7. A total of how many points are required to recertify the CMA credential?
   a. 45
   b. 60
   c. 100
   d. 120

8. Which of the following are grounds for denial of eligibility for the CMA credential?
   a. unauthorized possession of the examination materials
   b. copying or permitting another to copy answers
   c. falsifying information required for admission to the examination
   d. all of the above

CASE STUDY

Michele Lucas is performing an externship at Inner City Health Care under the direction of office manager Jane O'Hara. Michele has purchased a certification review study guide and has taken the sample 120-question Certification Examination available from the AAMA. From her studies, she has determined that she needs more work in the area of collections and insurance processing. Part-time administrative medical assistant Karen Ritter is responsible for these duties at Inner City Health Care, under Jane's supervision.

Discuss the following:

1. How can Michele use her externship experience to help her concentrate on improving her skills in the area of collections and insurance processing?
2. What are your own personal strengths and weaknesses in preparing for the CMA Certification Examination? What can you do to improve your areas of weakness?

SELF-ASSESSMENT

1. Think of two different places where you could get continuing education credits.
   a. Investigate each one.
   b. Write up a paragraph of the benefits and disadvantages of each method for you in your lifestyle.

2. Find out when and where your local chapter meetings are held.
   a. Attend a meeting with a classmate.
   b. Discuss what you learned from the meeting.

3. What can you do to prepare for the National Certification Examination?
   a. Write a plan in which you determine how much time you have to prepare and what you will accomplish each week/month in preparation.
   b. Make a calendar showing the steps toward your examination date.
   c. Try to stick with the plan as you progress closer to the examination date.

POST-TEST

This is similar to the Pre-Test. Perform this test without looking at the book. This is just to see how well you have understood and can recall the information presented in this chapter after you have studied it and completed the workbook exercises. You will not be graded on this portion (other than the grade you give yourself), but this is an excellent preparation for your instructor's test. You may use this Post-Test to determine what areas you need to study more. Justify any "false" answers.

1. An RMA and a CMA have different bylaws and creeds. (T or F)
2. A CMA is a national credential, so he or she may work in any state. (T or F)
3. Three major areas included in the CMA examination are clinical, administrative, and trans-disciplinary (general medical knowledge). (T or F)
4. Physicians recognize that their offices operate much more efficiently and effectively with professionally trained and formally educated personnel such as medical assistants. (T or F)
5. A CMA has to be a member of AAMA or currently employed to recertify. (T or F)
6. On meeting recertification requirements, the applicant will receive a dated seal to apply to their original certificate. (T or F)
7. Once a student has become a member of AAMA, he or she may stay at the student rate for two years after graduation. (T or F)

CERTIFICATION CRITERIA CHECKLIST

As you go through your education and training, keep in mind the national certification examination that you will take when you graduate. Each chapter of the textbook and workbook covers a different section of the examination criteria. To keep track of your preparation for the certification examination, turn to the back of this workbook and highlight the following CMA, RMA, or CMAS certification examination criteria (if you have already highlighted them from a previous chapter, put a check mark by the criteria):

CMA

D. Professionalism
   1. Displaying professional attitude

E. Communication
   4. Professional communication and behavior

RMA

I. General Medical Assisting Knowledge
   C. Medical Law

II. Administrative Medical Assisting
   C. Medical Receptionist/Secretarial/Clerical
      4. Oral and written communication

CMAS

1. Medical Assisting Foundation
   - Legal and ethical considerations
3. Medical Office Clerical Assisting
   - Communication

EVALUATION OF CHAPTER KNOWLEDGE

Skills	Student Self-Evaluation Good	Average	Poor
I can describe approved methods of training.	_____	_____	_____
I can differentiate between being certified and being registered.	_____	_____	_____
I can identify the benefits of certification.	_____	_____	_____
I understand the qualifications to sit for the AAMA Certification Examination.	_____	_____	_____
I know when the AAMA Certification Examination is offered and the registration deadlines.	_____	_____	_____
I can describe methods for obtaining Continuing Education Units.	_____	_____	_____
I understand the recertification process and its importance.	_____	_____	_____
I understand the importance of enhancing skills through continuing education and the importance of maintaining professional growth throughout my career as a medical assistant.	_____	_____	_____

CHAPTER 48

Employment Strategies

CHAPTER PRE-TEST

Perform this test without looking at the book. This is just to see how well you have understood and can recall the information in this chapter after you have read it, but before you have completed the workbook exercises. You will not be graded on this portion (other than the grade you give yourself). Justify any "false" answers.

1. Positive thinking is one of the primary keys to success in planning your career and during your job search. (T or F)
2. Job leads from friends, relatives, and neighbors are not the most successful for potential employment opportunities. (T or F)
3. Poor appearance is a reason for employers not to hire a job seeker. (T or F)
4. Employers like it when you know it all. They appreciate it when you do not ask questions. (T or F)
5. You should never expect to receive a job from an office where you are an extern. (T or F)
6. When filling out an application, it is acceptable to leave answers blank or write "see résumé." (T or F)
7. You should always plan ahead and have all your information with you when picking up an application, just in case you are asked to fill it out right there. (T or F)

INTRODUCTION

Once medical assisting students have completed their studies, it is time for them to start a career in their chosen field. There are various employment strategies that will greatly aid in obtaining a quality position in an ambulatory care setting. It is important that the job applicant adopt a strategy for job finding that includes self-assessment, job analysis and research, and budgetary needs analysis. In addition, there are several techniques that can make a difference in the success of a job-finding mission. Résumé preparation is one of the essential ingredients of the job hunt. A well-constructed résumé summarizing your work, education, and volunteer experience will make a vital connection in the interviewer's mind between what you can do and how these skills can benefit the organization. The construction of the cover letter or completion of the application form is also an important step in the success of the job-search process. The cover letter introduces the applicant to the potential employer with the goal of obtaining an interview. Once you have obtained an interview, you can prepare for it by learning what to expect in an interview and how to increase your chances for success.

PERFORMANCE OBJECTIVES

After successful completion of this chapter you will be able to explain the medical terms related to employment strategies. You will be able to list the steps involved in analyzing and researching a job. You will be able to describe a contact tracker and its usefulness; give examples of accomplishment statements; differentiate among chronologic, functional, and targeted résumés, and decide when each is the most appropriate; and be able to describe the purpose and content of a cover letter. You will be able to demonstrate effective ways to anticipate and respond to interviewer's questions, and you will be able to describe appropriate appearance for an interview and appropriate behavior at the interview. You will be able to write a good résumé, cover letter, and follow-up letter and cite the benefits of taking the time to do all well. *The following statements are related to your learning objectives. Fill in the blanks in the following paragraph with the appropriate term(s)*

One important quality an (1) ______________________ looks for in an employee is his or her (2) ______________________. Beyond having a (3) ______________________ attitude, being successful in your search for a job (4) ____________ positive thinking on your part. Having success at finding that perfect job requires (5) ________________ many hours to job strategy tactics. To begin, you need to (6) ______________ what you want in a job. Take the time to complete a (7) ______________________ worksheet, such as the one in the textbook, to help you focus on your needs. Identify your direct (8) ____________ and your (9) ________________ skills. Job leads can come from many areas, including your (10) _____________ site. As part of the job search, contact many individuals and keep track of the details in a (11) ________________. Résumés should be (12) ______________________ and concise. Yours should be short and (13) ____________ to read and understand. Use statements that are (14) ________________ and reflect confidence and portray you as a (15) ______________________________. Use (16) ______________________ statements if you have them from your (17) ______________ or work experience. References are important, and always ask (18) ____________________ before using someone's name as a (19) ______________________. Proofread, proofread, and (20) ______________________ your résumé. There are various résumé styles, such as (21) ________________, (22) ____________________, and (23) ________________. Decide which type is best suited for your needs. Applications should be neat, complete, and accurate. Never write (24) ______________ on an application, even though that might be easier. If your (25) ____________________ and (26) ________________ have created a favorable impression, you may be granted an (27)______________________. Be sure to follow the simple rules of etiquette and display a (28) __________________ manner and image at the interview. Writing a (29) ______________________ letter after the interview is an excellent way to be remembered.

VOCABULARY BUILDER

Find the words listed below that are misspelled; circle them, and then correctly spell them in the spaces provided. Then match each correct vocabulary term to the aspect of the job-seeking process that best describes it.

______	1. accomplishment statements	______	8. functional résumé
______	2. application form	______	9. interview
______	3. application/cover letter	______	10. power verbs
______	4. bullat point	______	11. refrences
______	5. carreer objective	______	12. résumé
______	6. cronological résumé	______	13. targeted résumé
______	7. contact tracker		

____

____________________ ____________________ ____________________

A. Expresses your career goal and the position for which you are applying

B. Résumé format used to highlight specialty areas of accomplishments and strengths

C. A form devised by a prospective employer to collect information relative to qualifications, education, and experience in employment

D. Individuals who have known or worked with you long enough to make an honest assessment and recommendation regarding your background history

E. Résumé format used when focusing on a clear, specific job

F. A statement that begins with a power verb and gives a brief description of what you did and the demonstrable results that were produced

G. Asterisk or dot followed by a descriptive phrase

H. A written summary data sheet or brief account of your qualifications and progress in your chosen career

I. Action words used to describe your attributes and strengths

J. A letter used to introduce yourself and your résumé to a prospective employer with the goal of obtaining an interview

K. Résumé format used when you have employment experience

L. A meeting in which you discuss employment opportunities and strengths that you can bring to the organization

M. Form used to keep track of employment contact information, such as name of employer, name of contact person, address and telephone number, date of first contact, résumé sent, interview date, and follow-up information and dates

LEARNING REVIEW

1. A variety of references should be included on your résumé or listed on a separate sheet of paper that closely matches your résumé. Give the appropriate response to the following questions.

   A. Choose references who are well-respected and are ______________________________.

   B. List three types of professional references that would make excellent reference choices.

   (1) ________________ (2) ________________ (3) ____________________

   C. Identify someone you know or have contact with who fits each professional reference type listed above.

   (1) ________________ (2) ________________ (3) ____________________

2. There are various styles of résumés that can be used, depending on your employment strengths and abilities. Each particular style has advantages and disadvantages, and can be used singly or in combination. In some cases, a medical facility may prefer a certain résumé style.

   A. Identify situations when using a targeted résumé is advantageous by circling the number next to the statements that apply.

   (1) You are just starting your career and have little experience, but you know what you want and you are clear about your capabilities.

   (2) You want to use one résumé for several different applications.

   (3) You are not clear about your abilities and accomplishments.

   (4) You can go in several directions, and you want a different résumé for each.

   (5) You are able to keep your résumé on a computer disk.

   B. Identify the situations in which using a chronologic résumé is advantageous by circling the number next to the statements that apply.

   (1) You have been in the same job for many years.

   (2) Your job history shows real growth and development.

   (3) You are trained and employed in highly traditional fields (health care, government).

   (4) You are looking for your first job.

   (5) You are staying in the same field as prior jobs.

   C. Identify the situations in which using a functional résumé is advantageous by circling the number next to the statements that apply.

   (1) You have extensive specialized experience.

   (2) Your most recent employers have been highly prestigious.

   (3) You have had a variety of different, apparently unconnected, work experiences.

   (4) You want to emphasize a management growth pattern.

   (5) Much of your work has been volunteer, freelance, or temporary.

3. If you are sending your résumé to a potential employer, you will need to mail a cover letter with it. A well-written cover letter introduces you, tells the reader why you are writing and what you are sending, highlights your qualifications and experience, and enhances the information on your résumé. There are numerous guidelines to follow when writing a cover letter for submission to a potential employer. List four guidelines that are essential when preparing an effective cover letter.

   (1) ______________________________

   (2) ______________________________

   (3) ______________________________

   (4) ______________________________

4. When Ellen Armstrong, CMA, began her job search she encountered several employers who required her to complete an application form. Ellen could recall six points that were particularly important when filling out a job application. List four items that are important when completing a job application.

   (1) ______________________________

   (2) ______________________________

   (3) ______________________________

   (4) ______________________________

5. A. Bob Thompson has an interview at Inner City Health Care for a new clinical medical assisting position. He is confident he has prepared well for the interview. On the way to the interview, Bob reminds himself of three principles he has learned about interviewing.

   (1) ______________ before answering questions, trying to provide the information requested in a ______________ manner.

   (2) ______________ carefully so that you understand what information the interviewer is requesting.

   (3) ______________ for ______________ if you are uncertain.

   B. Bob Thompson also recalls that it is not appropriate to ask questions about certain subjects during a first interview, but instead to concentrate on the value and skills one can contribute to the organization. Name four items you should not ask questions about in a first interview.

   (1) ______________ (3) ______________

   (2) ______________ (4) ______________

CERTIFICATION REVIEW

These questions are designed to mimic the certification examinations. You can use these questions like a small "Certification Examination Study Guide," but this is not meant to take the place of the more extensive study guides. Use this portion to determine in what areas to concentrate your efforts when studying for the certification examination.

1. Telling your friends, family, personal physician, dentist, and ophthalmologist that you are looking for a position in health care is called:
   a. networking
   b. references
   c. professionalism
   d. critiquing
2. Summarizing employment is acceptable on a résumé if it is prior to how many years ago?
   a. 1 year
   b. 5 years
   c. 10 years
   d. 15 years
3. The type of résumé that should be developed by someone looking for their first job is a:
   a. targeted résumé
   b. chronologic résumé
   c. functional résumé
   d. objective résumé
4. Poise includes such things as:
   a. skill level
   b. confidence and appearance
   c. a and b
   d. none of the above
5. Providing a second opportunity to express your interest in an organization and a position may be done with a:
   a. cover letter
   b. recommendation letter
   c. follow-up letter
   d. strategic letter

CASE STUDY

You are the subject of this case study. Complete the Self-Evaluation Worksheet that follows. Use your answers to help you determine the working environment you are most interested in and that best suits you. The worksheet can become a useful tool when researching prospective employers to target for your exciting first job in the medical assisting profession.

SELF-EVALUATION WORKSHEET

Respond to the following questions honestly and sincerely. They are meant to assist you in self-assessment.

1. List your strongest attributes as related to people, data, or things.
   i.e., Interpersonal skills related to people
   Accuracy related to data
   Mechanical ability related to things
   ______________________________ related to ______________
   ______________________________ related to ______________
   ______________________________ related to ______________
2. List your three weakest attributes related to people, data, or things.
   ______________________________ related to ______________
   ______________________________ related to ______________
   ______________________________ related to ______________
3. How do you express yourself? excellent, good, fair, poor
   Orally ______________ In writing ______________
4. Do you work well as a leader of a group or team? Yes ______ No ______
5. Do you prefer to work alone and on your own? Yes ______ No ______
6. Can you work under stress/pressure? Yes ______ No ______
7. Do you enjoy new ideas and situations? Yes ______ No ______
8. Are you comfortable with routines/schedules? Yes ______ No ______
9. Which work setting do you prefer?
   Single-physician setting _____ Multiphysician setting _____
   Small clinic setting _____ Large clinic setting _____
   Single-specialty setting _____ Multispecialty setting _____
10. Are you willing to relocate? _____ Willing to travel? _____

SELF-ASSESSMENT

Pretend you are interviewing a recent graduate for a medical assisting position.

1. What questions would you want to know the answers to?
2. Would you want to know the answers to some illegal or unethical questions? Do you think there is a way to obtain that information without actually asking the questions?
3. Do you think you could determine the best person for the job by meeting him or her just once? What else might you do to get to know the person better or get to know his or her work style better?

POST-TEST

This is similar to the Pre-Test. Perform this test without looking at the book. This is just to see how well you have understood and can recall the information presented in this chapter after you have studied it and completed the workbook exercises. You will not be graded on this portion (other than the grade you give yourself), but this is an excellent preparation for your instructor's test. You may use this Post-Test to determine what areas you need to study more. Justify any "false" answers.

1. Positive thinking is a good thing, but it is not all that important to success in planning your career and during your job search. (T or F)
2. Job leads from friends, relatives, and neighbors are some of the most successful for potential employment opportunities. (T or F)
3. Professional appearance is one reason for employers to want to hire a job seeker. (T or F)
4. Employers do not expect that you will know it all. They appreciate it when you ask questions. (T or F)
5. Students often receive job offers from the office where they extern. (T or F)
6. When filling out an application, it is never acceptable to leave answers blank or write "see résumé." (T or F)
7. Plan ahead and have all your information with you when you pick up an application, just in case you are asked to fill it out right there. (T or F)

CERTIFICATION CRITERIA CHECKLIST

As you go through your education and training, keep in mind the national certification examination that you will take when you graduate. Each chapter of the textbook and workbook covers a different section of the examination criteria. To keep track of your preparation for the certification examination, turn to the back of this workbook and highlight the following CMA, RMA, or CMAS certification examination criteria (if you have already highlighted them from a previous chapter, put a check mark by the criteria):

CMA

D. Professionalism
   1. Displaying professional attitude
   2. Job readiness and seeking employment

E. Communication
   6. Interviewing techniques

RMA

I. General Medical Assisting Knowledge
   C. Medical Law
   E. Human Relations

II. Administrative Medical Assisting
   C. Medical Receptionist/Secretarial/Clerical
      4. Oral and written communication

CMAS

1. Medical Assisting Foundation
   - Legal and ethical considerations
   - Professionalism

3. Medical Office Clerical Assisting
   - Communication

EVALUATION OF CHAPTER KNOWLEDGE

Skills	Student Self-Evaluation: Good	Average	Poor
I can name the steps of job analysis and research.	____	____	____
I can describe the function and use of a contact tracker.	____	____	____
I can differentiate among chronologic, functional, and targeted résumés.	____	____	____
I can implement power words to compose accomplishment statements for résumés.	____	____	____
I know the purpose and content of a cover letter.	____	____	____
I can demonstrate effective behavior during interview sessions.	____	____	____
I understand the importance of displaying professionalism.	____	____	____
I can identify benefits of follow-up letters.	____	____	____
I use self-assessment techniques to determine optimal employment goals.	____	____	____

APPENDIX A

Case Studies

INTRODUCTION

This appendix presents six case studies designed to give you experience using medical office practice management software. Using *Medical Office Simulation Software (MOSS)*, you will enroll the patients and their family members using the information provided for each patient. To complete each case study, you will also need to create appointments, post procedure charges, bill insurance companies and individual patients, and post payments received by the office.

INSTALLING MOSS ON YOUR COMPUTER

1. Take the CD from the back of the Workbook that accompanies *Thomson Delmar Learning's Comprehensive Medical Assisting, Third Edition*, and place it into your CD-ROM drive.
2. The Medical Office Simulation Software should begin setup automatically. Follow the on-screen prompts to install MOSS, Access Runtime, and SnapShot Viewer.
3. If MOSS does not begin setup automatically, follow these instructions:
   - Double-click on My Computer.
   - Double-click the Control Panel icon.
   - Double-click Add/Remove Programs.
   - Click the Install button, and follow the on-screen prompts.

USING MEDICAL OFFICE SIMULATION SOFTWARE

When you finish installing MOSS, it will be accessible through the Start menu. Select Start → All Programs → Medical Office Simulation Software → MOSS to open the software. At the logon screen, click OK to enter MOSS. Your user name and password are already loaded for you. You may change your password after you have logged in, by going to the File Maintenance area of the software.

Menu Screen

In MOSS, the user will be oriented to the general functions of most practice management software. MOSS features a Main Menu screen consisting of buttons that provide access to specific areas. Alternatively, there is an icon bar along the top left to quickly access the areas of the software, or the user may choose to navigate the software by using the pull-down menus below the software title bar.

There are eight basic components common to most practice management software. These include:

- Patient Registration
- Appointment Scheduling
- Procedure Posting
- Insurance Billing
- Posting Payments
- Patient Billing

- Report Generation
- File Maintenance

Patient Registration

The patient registration area allows the user to input information about each patient in the practice, including demographic, Health Insurance Portability and Accountability Act (HIPAA), and medical insurance information. From the Main Menu screen, click on the Patient Registration button to search for a patient, or to add a new patient, using the command buttons along the bottom of the patient selection dialog box.

Appointment Scheduling

The appointment scheduling system enables the user to make appointments and also cancel, reschedule, and search for appointments. MOSS allows for block scheduling, as well as several print features including appointment cards and daily schedules.

Procedure Posting

In the procedure posting system, patient fees for services are applied, in addition to relevant information such as service dates and place of service information. When procedures are input into the procedure posting system, the software assigns the fee to be charged according to the fee schedule for the patient's insurance.

Insurance Billing

The insurance billing system is designed to prepare claims to be sent to insurance companies for the medical office to receive payment for services provided. MOSS allows the user to generate and print a paper claim or simulate sending the claim electronically.

Posting Payments and Patient Billing

In the posting payments system, the user may input payments received by the practice from patients or insurance companies, as well as enter adjustments to the account. Once the payment from the primary insurance company has been posted, the software can generate a claim to a secondary insurance company, if applicable, or generate a bill to be sent directly to the patient to collect the outstanding balance.

File Maintenance and User Help

The File Maintenance System is a utility area of the program that contains common information used by various systems within the software. It is also an area where the setup of the software system can be adjusted or customized.

Under the Help tab, the user can turn Feedback Mode and Balloon Help Mode on or off. Feedback mode will alert the user when essential fields have not been completed before allowing data to be saved. Balloon Help offers explanations, clarification, or reminders for certain fields.

System Requirements

- Pentium II, 500 MHz minimum; Pentium III, 1 GHz recommended
- Microsoft Windows® 98, ME, 2000, XP
- 400 MB hard disk
- 64 MB RAM required, 256 MB RAM recommended
- 800 × 600 monitor display
- MS Access® 2000 recommended (MS Access Runtime supplied on MOSS CD)

Technical Support

Technical Support at Thomson Delmar Learning is available from 8:30 AM to 5:30 PM Eastern Standard Time.

- Phone: (800) 477-3692
- Fax: (518) 881-1247
- E-mail: delmarhelp@thomson.com

CASE STUDY 1: DAVID AND LOIS FITZPATRICK

The Fitzpatrick family recently moved to Douglasville from Albany, NY. Mr. Fitzpatrick has taken a promotion with his employer, the NY State Department of Corrections, which required him to relocate to the central facility.

1. **Patient Registration.** Enroll David and Lois Fitzpatrick with the Douglasville Medicine Associates practice using MOSS.

TABLE 1 PATIENT REGISTRATION INFORMATION FOR DAVID AND LOIS FITZPATRICK

Physician	Dr. Schwartz	Dr. Schwartz
Last Name	Fitzpatrick	Fitzpatrick
First Name	David	Lois
Middle Initial	J	J
SSN (Social Security number)	999-12-4567	999-21-3457
Gender	M	F
Marital Status	Married	Married
Date of Birth	01/25/49	10/17/50
Address	625 Renaud Ave.	625 Renaud Ave.
City	Douglasville	Douglasville
State	NY	NY
ZIP	01234	01234
Home Phone	(123) 456-1318	(123) 456-1318
Employer/School	NY Department of Corrections	Randall Craig Associates, LLC
Address	452 Chain Link Fence Way	29 Commerce Way
City	Douglasville	Douglasville
State	NY	NY
ZIP	01234	01234
Work Phone	(123) 456-2100, Ext 472	(123) 676-1280, Ext 21
Referring Physician	Samantha Green, MD	Samantha Green, MD
Guarantor	Self	Spouse
Relationship to Patient	Self	Spouse
Insurance—Primary	Consumer One—HRA	Consumer One—HRA
Patient Relationship to Insured	Self	Spouse
Policy Holder Information		
Last Name	Self	Fitzpatrick
First Name		David
Date of Birth		10-25-1949
ID #	999-12-4567A	999-12-4567A
Policy Number	ABC37156564	ABC37156564
Group Number	NYDOC1000	NYDOC1000
Employer Name	NY Department of Corrections	NY Department of Corrections
PCP (primary care physician)	N/A	N/A
Insurance—Secondary	N/A	N/A
Additional Information	Your practice accepts assignment, the patient's signatures are on file, and this is an in-network/PAR.	Your practice accepts assignment, the patient's signatures are on file, and this is an in-network/PAR.

2. **Insurance Verification.** Whether new or established, it is essential to verify every patient's medical insurance. Using the Online Eligibility feature in MOSS, verify the insurance eligibility for David and Lois Fitzpatrick. View and print the report.

3. **Creating Appointments.**

   a. Today is November 4, 2004. Mr. Fitzpatrick is not accustomed to the water in this area of the country and suffers from intestinal distress. He called this morning to see the doctor as soon as possible. Schedule an appointment for him for this afternoon at 2:00 PM. He is a new patient and will need a comprehensive office visit for one hour. Be sure to check Mr. Fitzpatrick in on your appointment scheduler when he arrives for his office visit.

   b. Mrs. Fitzpatrick calls one week later and requests to see her doctor. She is not sure what is wrong with her; she just feels unusually tired. Mrs. Fitzpatrick is also a new patient and will need a comprehensive office visit for one hour. Schedule an appointment for Mrs. Fitzpatrick on November 11, 2004, at 9 AM. Be sure to check Mrs. Fitzpatrick in on your appointment scheduler when she arrives for her office visit.

4. **Posting Procedures.**

   a. Mr. Fitzpatrick was diagnosed with gastroenteritis and given a prescription. Post the charges for his comprehensive, 60-minute office visit (the reference number on his superbill is 5001). Dr. Schwartz has indicated on the superbill that Mr. Fitzpatrick is to return for a follow-up appointment in one week. Make a follow-up appointment for Mr. Fitzpatrick on November 12, 2004, at 11 AM.

   b. Mrs. Fitzpatrick's visit required her physician to perform a comprehensive history and examination. The physician ordered a blood sugar test, a routine urinalysis (UA) with Micro, a complete blood cell count (CBC) with differential, and a hematocrit. She was diagnosed with generalized weakness. Post the charges for her comprehensive, 60-minute office visit (the superbill reference number is 5043). Dr. Schwartz wants to see her again in two weeks for a follow-up appointment. Make a follow-up appointment for Mrs. Fitzpatrick on November 24, 2004, at 10:30 AM.

5. **Billing.**

   a. Neither Mr. nor Mrs. Fitzpatrick made a payment at the time of their visit.

   b. Using the Insurance Billing feature in MOSS, generate and submit electronic claims to the insurance company for Mr. and Mrs. Fitzpatrick's November 4 and 11 visits.

6. **Posting Insurance Payments.** A few weeks have gone by and you receive an explanation of benefits (EOB) with a check for both of the Fitzpatricks' claims. The insurance company has paid 100% of the billed items. Post the insurance payment on December 15, 2004, to the Fitzpatricks' accounts. The reference number for the Fitzpatricks' EOB is 99123350.

CASE STUDY 2: DIANE, ROBERT, AND HANNALEY MELLO

The Mello family was referred to your practice by Dr. Reed. The Mellos have recently switched insurance plans to receive more comprehensive medical coverage. Mr. Mello is a construction worker and his wife, Diane, is a waitress at a local family restaurant. They have a daughter, Hannaley, who is asthmatic and requires a broad spectrum of health care needs.

1. **Patient Registration.** Enroll the Mellos with the Douglasville Medicine Associates practice using MOSS.

TABLE 2 PATIENT REGISTRATION INFORMATION FOR THE MELLO FAMILY

Physician	Heath	Heath	Heath
Last Name	Mello	Mello	Mello
First Name	Robert	Diane	Hannaley
Middle Initial	J	E	
SSN	999-27-4321	999-27-8002	999-32-9730
Gender	M	F	F
Marital Status	Married	Married	Single
Date of Birth	09/23/70	04/18/71	06/17/95
Address	28 Barbara Lane	28 Barbara Lane	28 Barbara Lane
Apartment/Unit			
City	Douglasville	Douglasville	Douglasville
State	NY	NY	NY
ZIP	01234	01234	01234
Home Phone	(123) 676-0332	(123) 676-0332	(123) 676-0332
Employer/School	Triple A Contractors	Grandma's Family Restaurant	Morton Elementary School
Address	435 Rhode Island Ave.	273 President Ave.	231 Main Road
City	Douglasville	Douglasville	Douglasville
State	NY	NY	NY
ZIP	01234	01234	01234
Work Phone	(123) 676-4353	(123) 676-0223	(123) 677-3210
Referring Physician	Reed	Reed	Reed
Guarantor	Self	Robert Mello	Robert Mello
Relationship to Patient	Self	Spouse	Child
Insurance—Primary	Signal HMO	Signal HMO	Signal HMO
Patient Relationship to Insured	Self	Spouse	Child
Policy Holder Information			
Last Name	Self	Mello	Mello
First Name		Robert	Robert
Date of Birth		09/23/70	09/23/70
ID #	999-27-4321BB	999-27-4321BB	999-27-4321BB
Policy Number	DE48329J	DE48329J	DE48329J
Group Number	N/A	N/A	N/A
Employer Name	Triple A Contractors	Triple A Contractors	Triple A Contractors
PCP	N/A	N/A	N/A
Copayment	$10.00	$10.00	$10.00
Insurance—Secondary	N/A	N/A	N/A
Additional Information	Your practice accepts assignment, the patient's signatures are on file, and this is an in-network/PAR.	Your practice accepts assignment, the patient's signatures are on file, and this is an in-network/PAR.	Your practice accepts assignment, the patient's signatures are on file, and this is an in-network/PAR.

2. **Insurance Verifications.** Whether new or established, it is essential to verify every patient's medical insurance. Using the Online Eligibility feature, verify the insurance eligibility for the Mellos. View and print the report.

3. **Creating Appointments.** Today is November 4, 2005. Mr. Mello called to make a same-day appointment. He has experienced persistent loose stools and vomiting. He has a temperature of 101.2°F. His wife and daughter are experiencing similar symptoms. Create appointments for all three patients at 3:00 PM, 3:15 PM, and 3:30 PM. Be sure to check all three patients in on your appointment scheduler when they arrive for their office visits.

4. **Posting Procedures.** All of the Mellos received a problem-focused history and examination. (*Hint:* Remember that the Mellos are new patients.) All were diagnosed with gastritis. Post the charges to each member's account. The superbill reference numbers are 5011, 5012, and 5013. Because Mrs. Mello exhibited the most severe symptoms, the doctor asked that she return in two weeks for a follow-up examination. Make a follow-up appointment for Mrs. Mello on November 16, 2004, at 2 PM.

5. **Billing and Payments.**

   a. Collect the copayment of $10.00 for each patient. Mr. Mello writes check number 1088 for $30.00.

   b. Prepare insurance claim forms and send electronically to their insurance company.

CASE STUDY 3: SEAN AND MANUELLA GILBERTSON

There are occasions when your providers will see patients in outside facilities such as in the hospital or a skilled nursing facility. When this occurs for new patients, it is essential that as much information as possible is gathered by the provider and verified and supplemented by the medical office staff. In the following case study, Dr. Heath made his weekly visit to the Retirement Inn Nursing Home where he met with all his patients. Today, he also saw the Gilbertsons, who recently were entered into care at that facility.

1. **Patient Registration.** Enroll the Gilbertsons with the Douglasville Medicine Associates practice using MOSS.

TABLE 3 PATIENT REGISTRATION INFORMATION FOR SEAN AND MANUELLA GILBERTSON

Physician	Heath	Heath
Last Name	Gilbertson	Gilbertson
First Name	Sean	Manuella
Middle Initial	G	A
SSN	999-11-1114	999-99-0003
Gender	M	F
Marital Status	Married	Married
Date of Birth	03/11/39	10/17/39
Address	438 Courtship Ave.	438 Courtship Ave.
Apartment/Unit		
City	Douglasville	Douglasville
State	NY	NY
ZIP	01234	01234
Home Phone	(123) 678-6765	(123) 678-6765
Employer/School	Retired	Retired
Referring Physician	Reed	Reed
Guarantor	Self	Spouse
Relationship to Patient	Self	Spouse
Insurance—Primary	Medicare—Statewide Corp	Medicare—Statewide Corp
Patient Relationship to Insured	Self	Spouse
Policy Holder Information	Self	Spouse
Last Name		Gilbertson
First Name		Sean
Date of Birth		03/11/1939
ID #	999-11-1114	999-11-1114
Policy Number		
Group Number		
Employer Name		
PCP		
Insurance—Secondary	Medicaid	Medicaid
Patient Relationship to Insured	Self	Self
Policy Holder Information	Self	Self
Last Name		
First Name		
Date of Birth		
ID #	999-11-1114M	999-99-0003M
Policy Number		
Group Number		
Employer Name		
PCP Name (if applicable)		
Additional Information	Your practice accepts assignment, the patient's signatures are on file, and Dr. Heath is a Medicare and Medicaid participating provider.	Your practice accepts assignment, the patient's signatures are on file, and Dr. Heath is a Medicare and Medicaid participating provider.

2. **Insurance Verifications.** Whether new or established, it is essential to verify every patient's medical insurance. Using the Online Eligibility feature, verify the insurance eligibility for the Gilbertsons. View and print the report.
3. **Appointments.** Today is November 2, 2005. The Gilbertsons are residents of the Retirement Inn Nursing Home. Dr. Heath makes weekly visits to his patients in the nursing home on Tuesday mornings. Today, he saw the Gilbertsons starting at 10:30 in the morning. They recently were admitted and are now under Dr. Heath's care.
4. **Posting Procedures.** Dr. Heath provided a Level 5 new patient comprehensive examination for each patient. For Mr. Gilbertson, the examination focused on his cardiac pulmonary disease; for Mrs. Gilbertson, it focused on her insulin-dependent diabetes. (*Hint:* Dr. Heath reported the procedures on an Outside Service log, as numbers 003 and 004.)
5. **Billing.**
   a. There is no copayment due at the time of service.
   b. Using the Insurance Billing feature, generate and print a paper claim to submit to Medicare.
6. **Posting Insurance Payments.** Five weeks have gone by and you receive an EOB for both Mr. and Mrs. Gilbertson, with a check for $404.80 ($202.40 for each account) and a statement that the balance for the unpaid portion has been submitted to Medicaid. Post the insurance payment on December 8, 2004, to the Gilbertson's accounts, using 972211101 as the reference number.
7. **Billing Secondary Insurance.** Using the Insurance Billing feature, generate and transmit an electronic claim to Medicaid, the Gilbertsons' secondary insurance.

CASE STUDY 4: STEPHANIE M. ROBERTSON

Stephanie Robertson is an emancipated minor who seeks free or reduced-fee care at your clinic. She has no insurance and little money in the bank. She has applied for state aid, but has not yet received it.

1. **Patient Registration.** Enroll Stephanie Robertson with the Douglasville Medicine Associates practice using MOSS.

TABLE 4 PATIENT REGISTRATION INFORMATION FOR STEPHANIE ROBERTSON

Physician	Schwartz
Last Name	Robertson
First Name	Stephanie
Middle Initial	M
SSN	999-98-2020
Gender	F
Marital Status	Single
Date of Birth	12/11/87
Address	1318 Renaud St.
Apartment/Unit	12A
City	Douglasville
State	NY
ZIP	01234
Home Phone	(123) 677-2525
Employer/School	Sloppy Joe's Burgers
Address	38 Main Road
City	Douglasville
State	NY
ZIP	01234
Work Phone	(123) 456-2708
Referring Physician	None
Guarantor	Self-Pay
Relationship to Patient	Self
Insurance—Primary	Self-Pay
Additional Information	Self-Pay

2. **Creating Appointments.** Today is November 5, 2005. Stephanie Robertson makes a 45-minute appointment for November 12, 2004, at 10:30 AM. She says that the reason is "personal." Be sure to check Ms. Robertson in on your appointment scheduler when she arrives for her office visit.

3. **Posting Procedures.** Dr. Schwartz performs a Level 4 new patient examination. He also performs a routine pelvic examination, draws blood for a Venereal Disease Research Laboratory (VDRL) test, a mononucleosis screen, and a UA with microscopy. She was seen for abdominal pain. Post the charges to her account, using 6112 as the superbill reference number.

4. **Billing.**
   a. There is no copayment due.
   b. You collect $20.00 in cash from the patient today and make arrangements to bill her $50.00 per month until the bill is paid. Post this payment to Ms. Robertson's account.

5. **Patient Billing.** Prepare Ms. Robertson's first billing statement on December 8, 2004. Be sure to include a message on her patient statement, per your agreement, to remit December's payment of $50.00.

6. **Posting Payments.** On December 17, 2004, you receive check number 151 from Ms. Robertson for the amount of $50.00. Post this amount to her account.

CASE STUDY 5: MARY AND HENRY SMITH

Occasionally there will be accounts where the guarantor and the insured party are not one and the same. This is the case with Mr. and Mrs. Smith. Mr. Smith is the unemployed spouse of Mrs. Smith, who is a real estate broker of a very successful firm. Although Mrs. Smith is the insured party, her husband is the guarantor of the account.

1. **Patient Registration.** Enroll the Smiths with the Douglasville Medicine Associates practice using MOSS. Be sure to identify Mr. Smith as the account guarantor.

TABLE 5 PATIENT REGISTRATION INFORMATION FOR HENRY AND MARY SMITH

Physician	Heath	Heath
Last Name	Smith	Smith
First Name	Henry	Mary
Middle Initial	E	M
SSN	999-00-1110	999-10-3333
Gender	M	F
Marital Status	Married	Married
Date of Birth	02/14/69	09/18/70
Address	82 Hartwell St.	82 Hartwell St.
Apartment/Unit		
City	Douglasville	Douglasville
State	NY	NY
ZIP	01234	01234
Home Phone	(123) 678-2740	(123) 678-2740
Employer/School	Unemployed	Homestead Realty, LLC
Address		4832 Home Owner Way
City		Douglasville
State		NY
ZIP		01234
Work Phone		(123) 467-4983, Ext 21
Referring Physician	Green	Green
Guarantor	Self	Spouse
Relationship to Patient	Self	Spouse
Insurance—Primary	Flexi-Health PPO	Flexi-Health PPO
Patient Relationship to Insured	Spouse	Self
Policy Holder Information		
Last Name	Smith	Self
First Name	Mary	
Date of Birth	09/18/70	
ID #	999-10-3333	999-10-3333
Policy Number		
Group Number		
Employer	Homestead Realty, LLC	Homestead Realty, LLC
PCP		
Copayment	$20.00	$20.00
Insurance—Secondary	N/A	N/A
Additional Information	Your practice accepts assignment, the patient's signatures are on file, and Dr. Heath is a participating provider of her insurance plan.	Your practice accepts assignment, the patient's signatures are on file, and Dr. Heath is a participating provider of her insurance plan.

2. **Insurance Verifications.** Whether new or established, it is essential to verify every patient's medical insurance. Using the Online Eligibility feature, verify the insurance eligibility for the Smiths. View and print the report.

3. **Creating Appointments.**

   a. Today is November 15, 2004. The Smiths have registered with your practice and want to make appointments for a general checkup. However, Mr. Smith suspects he has an upper respiratory infection of some sort, and Mrs. Smith just simply feels overtired and run down.

   b. They request an appointment during their lunch time at about 12:30 PM. You realize that this conflicts with your appointment matrix. Try to accommodate their needs. If unable to do so, schedule them in a time slot just before or after Dr. Heath's lunch.

4. **Posting Procedures.**

   a. Dr. Heath provided a Level 5 new patient comprehensive examination for each patient.

   b. Mr. Smith was diagnosed with acute bronchitis, and Mrs. Smith was diagnosed with generalized weakness, most likely due to stress. Post the charges to their accounts using 6225 and 6226 as the reference numbers.

5. **Billing and Payments.**

   a. There is $20.00 copayment for each patient. However, Mr. Smith will be paying cash for all of his charges. Post the cash payment for Mr. Smith.

   b. Post Mrs. Smith's $20.00 copayment to her account, and use the Insurance Billing feature to bill the remainder to her insurance. Generate and submit an electronic claim to Mrs. Smith's insurance company.

6. **Posting Payments.** Five weeks have gone by and you receive and EOB with a check from Flexi-Health for the balance of Mrs. Smith's account. Post the insurance check on December 20, 2004, to Mrs. Smith's account.

CASE STUDY 6: VITO AND ERMALINDA WILLIAMS

It is always nice when things work the way in which they are designed. All too often, though, they do not. Patients will cancel appointments, change appointments, or ask if they can bring a dependent beneficiary to the appointment to be seen as well. Occasionally medical office staff may fail to enter an appointment or even make an appointment for the wrong date, time, or provider. When these occurrences happen, they must be reflected and/or corrected in the medical office practice management software.

Vito and Ermalinda Williams are an older adult couple who depend on family members for help. Of particular help is their daughter, who has been their most reliable source of support. In fact, they generally make their appointments based on their daughter's availability.

1. **Patient Registration.** Enroll the Mr. and Mrs. Williams with the Douglasville Medicine Associates practice using MOSS. Note that Mr. Williams is the account guarantor. However, each patient has their individual Medicare and Medicaid medical coverage.
2. **Insurance Verifications.** Whether new or established, it is essential to verify every patient's medical insurance. Using the Online Eligibility feature, verify the insurance eligibility for Mr. and Mrs. Williams. View and print the report.
3. **Creating Appointments.**
   a. Today is November 15, 2004. Mr. Williams calls to make an appointment for both he and his wife for tomorrow, if possible. Both have similar symptoms of slight nausea, stomach pains, and chills.
   b. Today is November 16, 2004. Mr. Williams calls to say his daughter will not be able to bring him and his wife to the office today. He also states the symptoms have not worsened, and that they would like to be seen tomorrow, November 17, 2004. NOTE: For the purposes of this scenario, assume their assigned physician, Dr. Schwartz, is not available. Make an appointment for Mr. and Mrs. Williams to see Dr. Heath.
4. **Posting Procedures.**
   a. Dr. Heath provided a Level 2 new patient examination for each patient.
   b. Mr. and Mrs. Williams were diagnosed with gastritis and mild dehydration.
5. **Billing.**
   a. There is no copayment for either patient; however, it is not known if either of them has met their annual deductible.
   b. Use the Insurance Billing feature to generate and print a paper claim for all charges to Medicare for both patients.
6. **Rebilling.** As of December 30, 2004, no checks have been received from Medicare. Rebill the insurance claims for both Vito and Ermalinda Williams.

TABLE 6 PATIENT REGISTRATION INFORMATION FOR VITO AND ERMALINDA WILLIAMS

Physician	Schwartz	Heath
Last Name	Williams	Williams
First Name	Vito	Ermalinda
Middle Initial	A	A
SSN	999-99-1110	999-99-3333
Sex	M	F
Marital Status	Married	Married
Date of Birth	10/17/41	12/25/40
Address	49 Renaud St.	49 Renaud St.
Apartment/Unit	Unit 27-A	Unit 27-A
City	Douglasville	Douglasville
State	NY	NY
ZIP	01234	01234
Home Phone	(123) 679-3636	(123) 679-3636
Employer/School	Retired	Retired
Address		
City		
State		
ZIP		
Work Phone		
Referring Physician	Brennen	Brennen
Guarantor	Self	Spouse
Relationship to Patient	Self	Spouse
Insurance—Primary	Medicare Statewide Corp	Medicare Statewide Corp
Patient Relationship to Insured	Self	Self
Policy Holder Information	Self	Self
Last Name		
First Name		
Date of Birth		
ID #	999-99-1110A	999-99-3333A
Policy Number		
Group Number		
Employer Name		
PCP		
Insurance—Secondary		
Plan Name	Medicaid	Medicaid
Patient Relationship to Insured	Self	Self
Policy Holder Information	Self	Self
Last Name		
First Name		
Date of Birth		
ID #	999-99-1110B	999-99-3333B
Policy Number		
Group Number		
Employer Name		
PCP		
Additional Information	Your practice accepts assignment, the patient's signatures are on file, and Dr. Heath is a participating provider of both Medicare and Medicaid plans.	Your practice accepts assignment, the patient's signatures are on file, and Dr. Heath is a participating provider of both Medicare and Medicaid plans.

APPENDIX B

Certification Criteria Checklists

Use these checklists to keep track of where in your studies you have learned the skills and criteria listed under the examination criteria. You may choose either the AAMA Certified Medical Assistant Certification/Recertification Examination Content Outline, the AMT Registered Medical Assistant Certification Examination Content, or the AMT Certified Medical Administrative Specialist Examination Competencies. You will find that many skills will be covered in multiple courses/chapters. This checklist will help you determine which areas you might need to cover in more detail as you prepare for your certification examination.

AAMA Certified Medical Assistant Certification/ Recertification Examination Content Outline	Workbook Checklist
I. A-F GENERAL	
A. MEDICAL TERMINOLOGY	
1. Word building and definitions	
2. Uses of terminology	
B. ANATOMY AND PHYSIOLOGY	
1. Body as a whole, including multiple systems	
2. Systems, including structure, function, related conditions and diseases	
C. PSYCHOLOGY	
1. Basic principles	
2. Developmental stages of the life cycle	
3. Hereditary, cultural and environmental influences on behavior	
4. Defense mechanisms	
D. PROFESSIONALISM	
1. Displaying professional attitude	
2. Job readiness and seeking employment	
3. Performing within ethical boundaries	
4. Maintaining confidentiality	
5. Working as a team member to achieve goals	

AAMA Certified Medical Assistant Certification/ Recertification Examination Content Outline	Workbook Checklist
E. COMMUNICATION	
1. Adapting communication to an individual's ability to understand (e.g., patients with special needs)	
2. Recognizing and responding to verbal and nonverbal communication	
3. Patient instruction	
4. Professional communication and behavior	
5. Evaluating and understanding communication	
6. Interviewing techniques	
7. Receiving, organizing, prioritizing and transmitting information	
8. Telephone techniques	
9. Fundamental writing skills	
F. MEDICOLEGAL GUIDELINES & REQUIREMENTS	
1. Licenses and accreditation	
2. Legislation	
3. Documentation/reporting	
4. Releasing medical information	
5. Physician-patient relationship	
II. G-Q ADMINISTRATIVE	
G. DATA ENTRY	
1. Keyboard fundamentals and functions	
2. Formats	
3. Proofreading	
H. EQUIPMENT	
1. Equipment operation	
2. Maintenance and repairs	
I. COMPUTER CONCEPTS	
1. Computer components	
2. Care and maintenance of computer	
3. Computer applications	
4. Internet services	
J. RECORDS MANAGEMENT	
1. Needs, purposes and terminology of filing systems	
2. Process for filing documents	
3. Organization of patient's medical record	
4. Filing guidelines	
5. Medical records	
K. SCREENING AND PROCESSING MAIL	
1. US Postal Service	
2. Private services	
3. Postal machine/meter	
4. Processing incoming mail	
5. Preparing outgoing mail	

AAMA Certified Medical Assistant Certification/ Recertification Examination Content Outline	**Workbook Checklist**
L. SCHEDULING AND MONITORING APPOINTMENTS	
1. Utilizing appointment schedules/types	
2. Appointment guidelines	
3. Appointment protocol	
M. RESOURCE INFORMATION AND COMMUNITY SERVICES	
1. Services available	
2. Appropriate referrals	
3. Follow-up	
4. Patient advocate	
N. MANAGING PHYSICIAN'S PROFESSIONAL SCHEDULE AND TRAVEL	
1. Arranging meetings (e.g., dates, facilities, accommodations)	
2. Scheduling travel	
3. Integrating meetings and travel with office schedule	
O. MANAGING THE OFFICE	
1. Maintaining the physical plant	
2. Equipment and supply inventory	
3. Maintaining liability coverage	
4. Time management	
P. OFFICE POLICIES AND PROCEDURES	
1. Patient information booklet	
2. Patient education	
3. Instructions for patients with special needs	
4. Personnel manual	
5. Policy and procedures manuals/protocols	
6. Compliance plan	
Q. MANAGING PRACTICE FINANCES	
1. Bookkeeping systems (e.g., single, double entry, pegboard, computer)	
2. Coding systems	
3. Third-party billing	
4. Accounting and banking procedures	
5. Employee payroll	
III. R-Z CLINICAL	
R. PRINCIPLES OF INFECTION CONTROL	
1. Principles of asepsis	
2. Aseptic technique	
3. Disposal of biohazardous material	
4. Practice Standard Precautions	
S. TREATMENT AREA	
1. Equipment preparation and operation	
2. Principles of operation	
3. Restocking supplies	
4. Preparing/maintaining treatment areas	
5. Safety precautions	

AAMA Certified Medical Assistant Certification/ Recertification Examination Content Outline	Workbook Checklist
T. PATIENT PREPARATION AND ASSISTING THE PHYSICIAN	
1. Performing telephone and in-person screening	
2. Vital signs	
3. Examinations	
4. Procedures	
5. Explanation and instructions	
6. Instruments, supplies and equipment	
U. PATIENT HISTORY INTERVIEW	
1. Components of patient history	
2. Documentation guidelines	
V. COLLECTING AND PROCESSING SPECIMENS; DIAGNOSTIC TESTING	
1. Methods of collection	
2. Processing specimens	
3. Quality control	
4. Performing selected tests	
5. Vision testing	
6. Hearing testing	
7. Respiratory testing	
8. Medical imaging	
W. PREPARING AND ADMINISTERING MEDICATIONS	
1. Pharmacology	
2. Preparing and administering oral and parenteral medications	
3. Prescriptions	
4. Maintain medication and immunization records	
5. Medical disposal	
6. Principles of IV therapy	
X. EMERGENCIES	
1. Preplanned action	
2. Assessment and triage	
Y. FIRST AID	
1. Establishing and maintaining an airway	
2. Identifying and responding to:	
3. Signs and symptoms	
4. Management	
Z. NUTRITION	
1. Basic principles	
2. Special needs	

AMT Registered Medical Assistant Certification Examination Content	Workbook Checklist
I. GENERAL MEDICAL ASSISTING KNOWLEDGE	
A. ANATOMY AND PHYSIOLOGY	
1. Body systems	
2. Disorders and diseases	
B. MEDICAL TERMINOLOGY	
1. Word parts	
2. Definitions	
3. Common abbreviations and symbols	
4. Spelling	
C. MEDICAL LAW	
1. Medical law	
2. Licensure, certification, and registration	
3. Terminology	
D. MEDICAL ETHICS	
1. Principles of medical ethics and ethical conduct	
E. HUMAN RELATIONS	
1. Patient relations	
2. Interpersonal relations	
F. PATIENT EDUCATION	
1. Patient instruction	
2. Patient resource materials	
3. Documentation	
4. Understand and utilize proper documentation of patient encounters/instruction	
II. ADMINISTRATIVE MEDICAL ASSISTING	
A. INSURANCE	
1. Terminology	
2. Plans	
3. Claims	
4. Coding	
5. Insurance finance applications	
B. FINANCE/BOOKKEEPING	
1. Terminology	
2. Patient billing	
3. Collections	
4. Fundamental medical office accounting procedures	
5. Banking procedures	
6. Employee payroll	
7. Financial mathematics	
C. MEDICAL RECEPTIONIST/SECRETARIAL/CLERICAL	
1. Terminology	
2. Reception	
3. Scheduling	
4. Oral and written communication	

AMT Registered Medical Assistant Certification Examination Content	Workbook Checklist
5. Records and chart management	
6. Transcription and dictation	
7. Supplies and equipment management	
8. Computer applications	
9. Office safety	
III. CLINICAL MEDICAL ASSISTING	
A. ASEPSIS	
1. Terminology	
2. Bloodborne pathogens and Universal Precautions	
3. Medical asepsis	
4. Surgical asepsis	
B. STERILIZATION	
1. Terminology	
2. Sanitation	
3. Disinfection	
4. Sterilization	
5. Recordkeeping	
C. INSTRUMENTS	
1. Identification	
2. Instrument use	
3. Care and handling	
D. VITAL SIGNS	
1. Terminology	
2. Blood pressure	
3. Pulse	
4. Respirations	
5. Temperature	
6. Mensurations	
E. PHYSICAL EXAMINATIONS	
1. Medical history	
2. Patient positions	
3. Methods of examination	
4. Specialty examinations: identify examination procedures in specialty practices	
5. Visual acuity	
6. Allergy	
7. Terminology	
F. CLINICAL PHARMACOLOGY	
1. Terminology	
2. Parenteral medications	
3. Prescriptions	
4. Drugs	
G. MINOR SURGERY	
1. Surgical supplies	
2. Surgical procedures	

AMT Registered Medical Assistant Certification Examination Content	Workbook Checklist
H. THERAPEUTIC MODALITIES	
1. Modalities	
2. Alternate therapies	
3. Patient instruction	
I. LABORATORY PROCEDURES	
1. Safety	
2. Clinical Laboratory Improvement Amendments (CLIA '88)	
3. Employ Quality Control program	
4. Laboratory equipment	
5. Laboratory testing	
6. Terminology	
J. ELECTROCARDIOGRAPHY (ECG)	
1. Standard 12-lead ECG	
2. Mounting techniques	
3. Identify other ECG procedures	
K. FIRST AID AND EMERGENCY RESPONSE	
1. First aid procedures	
2. Legal responsibilities	

AMT Certified Medical Administrative Specialist Examination Competencies	Workbook Checklist
1. MEDICAL ASSISTING FOUNDATION	
Medical terminology	
Anatomy and physiology	
Legal and ethical considerations	
Professionalism	
2. BASIC CLINICAL MEDICAL OFFICE ASSISTING	
Basic health history interview	
Basic charting	
Vital signs and measurements	
Asepsis in the medical office	
Examination preparation	
Medical office emergencies	
Basic pharmacology	
3. MEDICAL OFFICE CLERICAL ASSISTING	
Appointment management and scheduling	
Reception	
Communication	
Patient information and community resources	
4. MEDICAL RECORDS MANAGEMENT	
Systems	
Procedures	
Confidentiality	
5. HEALTH CARE INSURANCE PROCESSING, CODING AND BILLING	
Insurance processing	
Insurance coding	
Insurance billing and finances	
6. MEDICAL OFFICE FINANCIAL MANAGEMENT	
Fundamental financial management	
Patient accounts	
Banking	
Payroll	
7. MEDICAL OFFICE INFORMATION PROCESSING	
Fundamentals of computing	
Medical office computer applications	
8. MEDICAL OFFICE MANAGEMENT	
Office communications	
Business organizational management	
Human resources	
Safety	
Supplies and equipment	
Physical office plant	
Risk management and quality assurance	

Made in the USA
Monee, IL
02 April 2023

30774433R00070